RNA as a Drug Target

Methods and Principles in Medicinal Chemistry

Edited by
Raimund Mannhold, Helmut Buschmann, Jörg Holenz

Previous Volumes of the Series

Daina, A., Przewosny, M., Zoete, V. (Eds.)

Open Access Databases and Datasets for Drug Discovery

2023
ISBN: 978-3-527-34839-8
Vol. 83

Bachhav, Y. (Ed.)

Targeted Drug Delivery

2023
ISBN: 978-3-527-34781-0
Vol. 82

Alza, E. (Ed.)

Flow and Microreactor Technology in Medicinal Chemistry

2022
ISBN: 978-3-527-34689-9
Vol. 81

Rübsamen-Schaeff, H., and Buschmann, H.(Eds.)

New Drug Development for Known and Emerging Viruses

2022
ISBN: 978-3-527-34337-9
Vol. 80

Gruss, M. (Ed.)

Solid State Development and Processing of Pharmaceutical Molecules Salts, Cocrystals, and Polymorphism

2021
ISBN: 978-3-527-34635-6
Vol. 79

Plowright, A.T. (Ed.)

Target Discovery and Validation Methods and Strategies for Drug Discovery

2020
ISBN: 978-3-527-34529-8
Vol. 78

Swinney, D., Pollastri, M. (Eds.)

Neglected Tropical Diseases Drug Discovery and Development

2019
ISBN: 978-3-527-34304-1
Vol. 77

Bachhav, Y. (Ed.)

Innovative Dosage Forms Design and Development at Early Stage

2019
ISBN: 978-3-527-34396-6
Vol. 76

Gervasio, F. L., Spiwok, V. (Eds.)

Biomolecular Simulations in Structure-based Drug Discovery

2018
ISBN: 978-3-527-34265-5
Vol. 75

Sippl, W., Jung, M. (Eds.)

Epigenetic Drug Discovery

2018
ISBN: 978-3-527-34314-0
Vol. 74

RNA as a Drug Target

The Next Frontier for Medicinal Chemistry

Edited by
John Schneekloth and Martin Pettersson

Series Editors
Raimund Mannhold
Helmut Buschmann
Jörg Holenz

WILEY-VCH

Volume Editors
Dr. John Schneekloth, Jr.
National Cancer Institute
Building 538, Room 249
Frederick
MD 21702-1201, USA

Dr. Martin Pettersson
Promedigen
Daejeon
South Korea

Series Editors
Prof. Dr. Raimund Mannhold
Rosenweg 7 40489
Düsseldorf
Germany

Dr. Helmut Buschmann
Sperberweg 15 52076
Aachen
Germany

Dr. Jörg Holenz
BIAL – PORTELA & CA.,
S.A. São Mamede Coronado
Portugal

Cover Image: © Oleg Nebesnyy/
Shutterstock, Courtesy of John
Schneekloth

Library of Congress Card No.: applied for

British Library Cataloguing-in-Publication Data
A catalogue record for this book is available from the British Library.

Bibliographic information published by the Deutsche Nationalbibliothek
The Deutsche Nationalbibliothek lists this publication in the Deutsche Nationalbibliografie; detailed bibliographic data are available on the Internet at <http://dnb.d-nb.de>.

Print ISBN: 978-3-527-35100-8
ePDF ISBN: 978-3-527-84043-4
ePub ISBN: 978-3-527-84044-1
oBook ISBN: 978-3-527-84045-8

Typesetting Straive, Chennai, India
Printing and Binding CPI Group (UK) Ltd, Croydon, CR0 4YY

C9783527351008_220624

Contents

Series Editors' Preface *xiii*
Preface *xv*

1 **Introduction** *1*
John Schneekloth Jr. and Martin Pettersson
References *4*

2 **RNA Structure Probing, Dynamics, and Folding** *7*
Danny Incarnato
2.1 Introduction *7*
2.1.1 Relevance of RNA Structure in Disease *8*
2.1.2 Challenges in Studying RNA Structures *8*
2.2 Experimentally Guided RNA Structure Modeling *9*
2.2.1 Structural Interrogation of RNA Nucleotides via Chemical Probing *10*
2.2.1.1 Limits of RNA Chemical Probing *12*
2.2.2 Direct Mapping of RNA–RNA Interactions *14*
2.2.2.1 Limits of RNA–RNA Interaction Mapping *16*
2.2.3 Mapping Spatially Proximal Nucleotides in RNA molecules *17*
2.2.3.1 Limits of Methods for Spatial Proximity Mapping *17*
2.3 Dealing with RNA Structure Heterogeneity *19*
2.4 Querying RNA–Small Molecule Interactions with Chemical Probing *22*
2.5 Conclusions and Future Prospects *22*
References *23*

3 **High-Resolution Structures of RNA** *29*
Lukas Braun, Zahra Alirezaeizanjani, Roberta Tesch, and Hamed Kooshapur
3.1 Introduction *29*
3.2 X-Ray Crystallography *31*
3.3 NMR Spectroscopy *34*
3.4 Cryo-EM *37*
3.5 3D Structure Prediction and Integrative Approaches *39*
3.6 Conclusions *43*
Acknowledgments *43*
Conflicts of Interest *43*
References *43*

4 Screening and Lead Generation Techniques for RNA Binders *49*
Gary Frey, Emily Garcia Sega, and Neil Lajkiewicz
4.1 Knowledge-Based Versus Agnostic Screening *49*
4.2 Virtual Screening *50*
4.3 Screening Methods *51*
4.3.1 High-Throughput Screening (HTS) *51*
4.3.1.1 Mass Spectrometry *51*
4.3.1.2 HTS of RNA Using Direct MS Approaches *52*
4.3.1.3 HTS of RNA Using Indirect MS Approaches *54*
4.3.1.4 DNA-Encoded Libraries (DELs) *56*
4.3.1.5 Microarray Screening *57*
4.3.1.6 Fragment-Based Drug Discovery *58*
4.3.1.7 Phage Display *63*
4.3.2 Orthogonal Methods *63*
4.3.2.1 Surface Plasmon Resonance *63*
4.3.2.2 Fluorescence-Based Assays *66*
4.3.2.3 Microscale Thermophoresis (MST) *70*
4.3.2.4 Isothermal Titration Calorimetry (ITC) *70*
4.4 Binding Site Identification/Target Engagement *72*
4.4.1 Covalent Methods *72*
4.4.2 Competition with an Antisense Oligonucleotide (ASO) *74*
4.5 Defining SAR and Functional Assays *75*
4.5.1 Functional Assays *75*
4.5.2 Phenotypic Screens *76*
4.6 Identifying a Lead Series *76*
4.6.1 Hit Optimization *77*
4.6.2 Risdiplam Hit-to-Lead *78*
4.6.3 Branaplam Lead Generation *79*
4.6.4 Zotatifin Lead Generation *80*
4.7 Concluding Thoughts and Outlook *80*
Acknowledgments *81*
References *81*

5 Chemical Matter That Binds RNA *93*
Emily G. Swanson Hay, Zhengguo Cai, and Amanda E. Hargrove
5.1 Introduction *93*
5.2 Natural Ligands *94*
5.2.1 Aminoglycosides *94*
5.2.2 Tetracyclines *95*
5.2.3 Macrolides *96*
5.2.4 Native Riboswitch Ligands *96*
5.3 Commercial Ligands *97*
5.3.1 Industrial Libraries *98*
5.3.2 Academic Libraries *98*

5.4 Synthetic Ligands *99*
5.4.1 Benzimidazoles and Purines *100*
5.4.2 Naphthalenes, Quinolines, and Quinazolines *101*
5.4.3 Oxazolidinones *102*
5.4.4 Amilorides *102*
5.4.5 Diphenyl Furan *103*
5.4.6 Multivalent Ligands *103*
5.5 Computational Tools for the Exploration of Chemical Space *103*
5.5.1 Similarity Searches and Principal Component Analysis *104*
5.5.2 Additional Machine-Learning Tools *105*
5.5.3 Structure-Based Ligand Design *106*
5.6 Case Studies in Examining and Expanding RNA-Targeted Chemical Space *106*
5.6.1 Using QSAR to Probe RNA-Targeting Small-Molecule Properties *107*
5.6.2 Evaluating the Chemical Space of Natural, Synthetic, and Commercial Ligands *108*
5.7 Conclusions and Outlook *111*
Acknowledgments *111*
References *111*

6 MicroRNAs as Targets for Small-Molecule Binders *119*
Maria Duca
6.1 Introduction *119*
6.2 MicroRNAs *121*
6.3 MicroRNAs Biogenesis *122*
6.4 Targeting MicroRNAs with Small-Molecule RNA Binders *123*
6.4.1 Induction of miRNAs Expression: Tackling the Decrease of Tumor Suppressor miRNAs *124*
6.4.2 Inhibition of miRNAs Production: Pre- and Pri-miRNA Binders *125*
6.4.2.1 Discovery of miRNAs Inhibitors by Intracellular Assays *125*
6.4.2.2 Target-Based *In Vitro* Assays *127*
6.4.2.3 Design of Specific Ligands of Pre- and Pri-miRNAs *131*
6.4.2.4 Fragment-Based Drug Design *138*
6.4.2.5 DNA-Encoded Libraries (DELs) *139*
6.5 Inhibition of RNA–Protein Interactions in miRNAs Pathways *140*
6.6 Adding Cleavage Properties to miRNAs Interfering Agents *142*
6.7 Conclusions *144*
References *144*

7 Pre-mRNA Splicing Modulation *151*
Scott J. Barraza and Matthew G. Woll
7.1 Introduction *151*
7.2 Overview of Splicing Biology *152*
7.2.1 The Spliceosome *152*
7.2.2 Classes of Alternative Splicing *154*

7.3 Pharmacological Mechanisms of Splicing Modulation *155*
7.3.1 *Cis*- and *Trans*-Regulatory Elements (Splicing Factors) *155*
7.3.1.1 Stabilization of *Cis*-Regulatory Elements *156*
7.3.1.2 Destabilization of *Cis*-Regulatory Elements *158*
7.3.1.3 Inhibition of *Cis*-Regulatory RNA–Protein Interactions *158*
7.3.1.4 Inhibition of *Trans*-Regulatory Elements *160*
7.3.1.5 Degradation of *Trans*-Regulatory Elements *161*
7.3.1.6 Inhibition of *Trans*-Regulatory Element Protein–Protein Interactions (PPIs) *162*
7.3.1.7 Stabilization of *Trans*-Regulatory Element RNA–Protein Interactions (RPIs) *165*
7.3.2 Kinases and Phosphatases *165*
7.3.2.1 Challenges in Targeting Kinases *167*
7.3.2.2 Inhibition of Kinases *168*
7.3.2.3 Activation and Degradation of Kinases *168*
7.3.2.4 Inhibition and Activation of Protein Phosphatases *169*
7.3.3 Epigenetic Writers and Erasers *172*
7.3.3.1 Inhibition of Epigenetic Writers *172*
7.3.4 RNA Helicases *174*
7.3.5 Drugging the Spliceosome *175*
7.3.5.1 Inhibition of U2 snRNP Recognition of the 3′-Splice Site *176*
7.3.5.2 E7107 *176*
7.3.5.3 H3B-8800 *177*
7.3.5.4 Stabilizers of U1 snRNP Recognition of the 5′-Splice Site *180*
7.3.5.5 Introduction to Spinal Muscular Atrophy (SMA) *180*
7.3.5.6 Risdiplam (Evrysdi®) *183*
7.4 Future Outlook *186*
References *188*

8 Prospects for Riboswitches in Drug Development *203*
Michael G. Mohsen and Ronald R. Breaker
8.1 Introduction *203*
8.1.1 The Known Landscape of Riboswitches *203*
8.1.2 Riboswitches in Drug Development *203*
8.1.3 The Need for Novel Antibiotics *205*
8.2 Riboswitches as Drug Targets *207*
8.2.1 Why Target Riboswitches? *207*
8.2.2 Features of a Druggable Riboswitch *208*
8.2.3 Riboswitch-Targeted Drugs *208*
8.2.3.1 Small Molecules Targeting FMN Riboswitches *208*
8.2.3.2 Other Riboswitches Targeted in Proof-of-Principle Demonstrations *209*
8.2.4 Barriers and Future Developments *210*
8.3 Riboswitches as Tools for Antibiotic Drug Development *210*
8.3.1 Riboswitches as Biosensors *210*
8.3.2 A Riboswitch-Based Fluoride Sensor Illuminates Agonists of Fluoride Toxicity *211*

8.3.3 A Riboswitch-Based ZTP Sensor Identifies Inhibitors of Folate Biosynthesis *211*
8.3.4 A Riboswitch-Based SAH Sensor Reveals an Inhibitor of SAH Nucleosidase *212*
8.3.5 Barriers and Future Developments *213*
8.4 Application of Riboswitches in Gene Therapy *213*
8.4.1 Considerations for Designer Riboswitches *213*
8.4.2 Eukaryotic Expression Platforms *214*
8.4.3 Barriers and Future Developments *216*
8.5 Concluding Remarks *217*
Acknowledgment *218*
References *218*

9 Small Molecules That Degrade RNA *227*
Noah A. Springer, Samantha M. Meyer, Amirhossein Taghavi, Jessica L. Childs-Disney, and Matthew D. Disney
9.1 Antisense Oligonucleotide Degraders *227*
9.2 Small-Molecule Direct Degraders *228*
9.2.1 *N*-Hydroxypyridine-2(1*H*)-thione (*N*-HPT) Conjugates *229*
9.2.2 Bleomycin *229*
9.2.3 Bleomycin Conjugates *231*
9.2.3.1 Bleomycin Degraders Targeting the r(CUG) Repeat Expansion That Causes DM1 *231*
9.2.3.2 Bleomycin Degraders Targeting r(CCUG) Repeat Expansion that Causes DM2 *233*
9.2.3.3 Bleomycin Degraders Targeting Oncogenic Precursor microRNAs *233*
9.2.3.4 Conclusions and Outlook for Bleomycin-Based Direct Degraders *234*
9.3 Ribonuclease Targeting Chimeras (RiboTACs) *235*
9.3.1 RNase L is an Endogenous Endoribonuclease That Functions as Part of the Innate Immune Response *236*
9.3.2 First-Generation RiboTACs Targeting Oncogenic miRNAs *236*
9.3.3 Small-Molecule-Based RiboTACs *239*
9.3.4 Comparison of Bleomycin-Based Direct Degraders and RiboTACs *242*
9.3.5 Discovery of Additional Small-Molecule RNase L Activators *242*
9.3.6 Conclusions and Outlook for RiboTACs *243*
9.4 Summary and Outlook for Small-Molecule RNA Degraders *244*
References *246*

10 Approaches to the Identification of Molecules Altering Programmed Ribosomal Frameshifting in Viruses *253*
Elinore A. VanGraafeiland, Diego M. Arévalo, and Benjamin L. Miller
10.1 Introduction *253*
10.2 Mechanisms of Frameshifting *256*
10.3 Targeting Frameshifting in HIV *257*
10.4 Targeting Frameshifting in SARS-CoV-1 and SARS-CoV-2 *263*
10.5 Conclusions *274*
References *274*

11 RNA–Protein Interactions: A New Approach for Drugging RNA Biology *281*
Dalia M. Soueid and Amanda L. Garner
11.1 Molecular Basis of RNA–Protein Interactions *282*
11.1.1 RNA Recognition Motifs (RRMs) *282*
11.1.2 Double-Stranded RNA-Binding Domains (dsRBD) *286*
11.1.3 Zinc Finger (ZnF) Domains *287*
11.1.4 K Homology (KH) Domains *289*
11.1.5 Other RBDs *290*
11.2 Regulation and Dysregulation of RNA–Protein Interactions *290*
11.2.1 Poor Quality Control Leads to Over- and Underproduction of RBPs *292*
11.2.2 RBPs Become Out of Control, mRNA Processing Gets a Makeover (and Hates It) *294*
11.2.3 RBP Shuttling of mRNA Becomes Askew *294*
11.2.4 The RBP is Lost and Wreaks Havoc on the Cell *295*
11.2.5 RBPs Dictate Which mRNAs are Translated, Favoring their Toxic Friends *295*
11.2.6 RBPs and RNA Become Very Clique-y, Form Their Own Complex and Cause Stress to the Rest of the Cell *296*
11.3 Experimental Methods to Detect and Screen for Small Molecules that Modulate RNA–Protein Interactions *297*
11.3.1 *In vitro* Fluorescence-Based Assays *297*
11.3.2 *In vitro* Chemiluminescence-Based Assays *297*
11.3.2.1 Cell-Based RPI Detection Assays *300*
11.3.3 Cell-Based RNA–Protein Interaction Screening *301*
11.4 Closing Remarks *302*
References *303*

12 Drugging the Epitranscriptome *321*
Tanner W. Eggert and Ralph E. Kleiner
12.1 Introduction *321*
12.2 Modifications on mRNA: N^6-Methyladenosine, Pseudouridine, and Inosine *325*
12.2.1 N^6-Methyladenosine (m^6A) *325*
12.2.2 Pseudouridine (Ψ) *327*
12.2.3 Inosine (I) *328*
12.3 Modifications on tRNA and rRNA *330*
12.3.1 tRNA Modifications *330*
12.3.2 rRNA Modifications *334*
12.4 Concluding Remarks *335*
References *336*

13 **Outlook** *355*
Christopher R. Fullenkamp, Xiao Liang, Martin Pettersson, and John Schneekloth Jr.
13.1 Introduction *355*
13.2 Target Selection: Identification of the Most Promising RNA Intervention Points *357*
13.3 Development of Robust Biophysical Methods, Alternative Strategies for Target Engagement, and Accurate and Reliable Functional Models *358*
13.3.1 Biophysical Methods for Interrogating Small Molecule–RNA Interactions *358*
13.3.2 Cellular Target Engagement Methods *360*
13.3.3 Unique Challenges Faced in the Development of Functional Assays for Studying Small Molecule–RNA Interactions *364*
13.4 Acquisition of High-Resolution RNA and RNA–Ligand Structures is Needed to Enable the Development and Validation of Computational Tools for RNA–Small Molecule Therapeutic Discovery *367*
13.4.1 RNA Structure Prediction *367*
13.4.2 Computational Tools for Hit Optimization *369*
13.4.3 Implementation of Molecular Dynamics Simulations, Machine Learning, and AI Tools to Interrogate RNA–Small Molecule Interactions *371*
13.5 Deposition of Small Molecule–RNA Interaction Data with Rigorous Experimental Protocols and Controls is Needed *373*
13.6 Outlook: The Future of Small Molecule-Based RNA Therapeutics is Bright *375*
References *376*

Index *385*

Series Editors' Preface

As one of the leading book series in the field, the ambition and tradition of Methods and Principles in Medicinal Chemistry has been to cover the most innovative, cutting-edge areas within the field first, and in comprehensive, hands-on format enabling the reader not only to learn deeply the field but also to practise it successfully.

The interface between small molecules and ribonucleic acid (RNA) is one of those areas that has recently gained enormous attention and has lifted medicinal chemistry to the level being *"en par"* with gene therapy or antisense approaches while maintaining the convenience and safety of oral dosing and its associated transient and reversible pharmacodynamic effects.

Prompted by the success story of Risdiplam, a pre-mRNA splicing modulator small molecule drug and a break-through medication for spinal muscular atrophy (SMA), academic as well as pharmaceutical industry research has lifted off to thoroughly explore and understand the field and to deliver new, innovative medicines to patients in difficult to drug areas of disease.

John Schneekloth, Jr., and Martin Pettersson have diligently searched for the most distinguished experts in the field to assemble the team of authors sharing their insights, while giving practical advice as well. The book follows the natural logic of the drug discovery and development path, starting from understanding the structure of RNAs and its potential interaction sites for small molecules, explaining strategies for lead generation, the features of chemical matter with increased chances of binding to RNA, and in the second part tackles the fundamentally different strategies for small molecules to interact with RNA to elicit the desired pharmacological effects. Finally, an outlook is given to capture recent trends where the field will evolve to, as well as estimate and appreciate its future impact and potential within the modalities a medicinal chemist has to interact with disease pathology.

This book is a concise, up to date, must read for every medicinal chemist! It will also give important scientific and strategic insights to all scientists, as well as managers, working in this field!

The senior editors of Methods and Principles of Medicinal Chemistry would like to express their gratitude to Martin and Jay, as well as the entire author team, for delivering what we believe will be the new reference standard for *Small Molecules targeting RNA*.

Jörg Holenz
Christa Müller
Helmut Buschmann

Preface

Once thought of as a transient messenger that did little more than carry a sequence for proteins, RNA is now recognized as a key regulator of biological homeostasis, gene expression, metabolism, and disease. While the sequencing of the human genome heralded the modern era of genomics with the promise of a drug for every gene, in practice this has been much harder to realize than originally thought. Recognition that the majority of the genome is noncoding and the majority of the proteome is at best challenging to target with small molecules has led to the perspective that RNA and RNA regulation are important new frontiers for medicinal chemistry. A key motivation for considering RNA as a drug target is the potential to develop novel small-molecule therapeutics for diseases with no treatment. This could be realized in a variety of ways, for example, by targeting the RNA that encodes for proteins that are challenging to drug (some ~85% of the proteome), targeting noncoding RNA, or pharmacologically controlling RNA-related processes like pre-mRNA splicing or posttranscriptional modifications. Additionally, broad classes of diseases, including cancers, neurodegenerative diseases, viral infections, and bacterial infections, are thought to have potential relevance in this space.

While the potential upside of targeting RNA is considerable, there are fundamental ways in which RNA differs from other targets. A broad variety of biophysical and biochemical techniques are both widely available and routinely used for protein targets, far fewer have been successfully applied to RNA. Thus, new approaches are needed to accurately identify, develop, characterize, and understand RNA-binding small molecules, and more work is needed to develop better assays that are compatible with the stringent requirements and rigor needed for drug discovery programs. Additionally, the question of what makes a good RNA target for small molecules remains an area of open debate. Still, advances in other areas, including genomics technologies such as next-generation sequencing, have allowed progress to be made at a remarkable pace, enabling the characterization and annotation of increasingly large collections of RNA structures and sequences.

We are pleased to present this exciting collection of chapters from leading experts in the field. The perspectives included here include a range of topics relevant to RNA-targeted drug discovery and medicinal chemistry. We hope this superb collection is both informative and reflective of the state of the art and brings diverse insights as to how scientists in academia, government, and industry around the world think about this important problem. Finally, we would like to extend a heartfelt thank you to all the authors and contributors for providing their important perspectives on this book. It has been an honor to work with you all, and it is a testament to the strong state of the field to have so many talented individuals willing to work on this project. Finally, we are indebted to the exceptional team at Wiley for their patience and help in guiding us through the process of editing this book. We are extremely grateful for your efforts!

John Schneekloth, Jr. (Jay)
USA

Martin Pettersson
South Korea

1

Introduction

John Schneekloth Jr.[1] *and Martin Pettersson*[2]

[1] *National Cancer Institute, Chemical Biology Laboratory, Frederick, MD 21702-1201, USA*
[2] *Promedigen, Daejeon, 34050, Republic of Korea*

The sequencing of the human genome more than 20 years ago revealed that it encodes just ~20,000 proteins, comprising only about three percent of its ~3 billion bases [1]. However, we now know that more than 80% of the genome is transcribed into RNA at some point [2]. In addition to RNAs that encode polypeptide sequences and facilitate protein biogenesis, diverse classes of non-coding RNA such as microRNAs, long non-coding RNAs (lncRNAs), small nucleolar RNAs (snoRNAs), and others continue to be discovered and characterized [3]. Numerous genome-wide association studies and other broad genomics efforts have pointed toward non-coding RNAs as relevant to diverse diseases including neurodegenerative conditions, infectious diseases, and cancer [3]. Furthermore, recent estimates indicate that only ~15% of the human proteome has been successfully targeted with small molecules, which is partly due to the lack of suitable binding pockets for small molecules on many proteins [4]. Challenges with targeting a large part of the human proteome, coupled with widespread non-coding functions of RNA in both humans and pathogenic organisms, point toward RNA and related regulatory processes as intriguing alternative drug targets for novel therapeutics.

A key promise of developing small molecules that target RNA or regulate RNA function is that, by doing so, one could potentially pharmacologically control the function of genes or signaling pathways that are challenging to modulate at the protein level [5–9]. However, understanding RNA as a small-molecule drug target comes with a number of challenges. Many RNAs are structurally dynamic, more closely resembling intrinsically disordered proteins than the ordered protein domains that are commonly associated with "traditional" drug targets [10]. Limitations in biophysical techniques to characterize RNA–ligand complexes and structural ensembles at atomic resolution complicate efforts to rationally design new potential drug molecules. In addition, the majority of RNAs are bound to and interact with RNA-binding proteins, often in a time- or stimulus-dependent fashion [11]. The RNA biopolymer consists of just four bases in contrast to the 20 canonical amino acids found in protein sequences. In addition, the chemical

RNA as a Drug Target: The Next Frontier for Medicinal Chemistry, First Edition.
Edited by John Schneekloth and Martin Pettersson.

nature of the anionic phosphodiester backbone of RNA contrasts starkly with that of the polypeptide backbone of proteins, resulting in considerably different biophysical properties of the two polymers. Still, fundamental studies aimed at understanding the targetability of RNA indicate that it is capable of folding into complex, three-dimensional structures with hydrophobic pockets that are likely suitable for small-molecule binding [7, 12]. Moreover, naturally occurring aptamers (as seen in riboswitches) and lab-evolved aptamers provide validation that RNA can interact with and sense low-molecular-weight species ranging from metal cations or halide ions to drug-like small molecules and even complex metabolites like cobalamin (vitamin B12) with exquisite selectivity [13].

Indeed, the history of drug discovery has already demonstrated the potential and significant impact that RNA-targeting medicines can have. Ribosome-targeting antibiotics, exemplified by macrolides, aminoglycosides, and tetracyclines, have been known since at least the 1940s and represent the largest class of clinically used drugs to treat infections [14]. In general, these compounds make specific contacts with ribosomal RNA (rRNA) within the large ribonucleoprotein complex of the ribosome and modulate protein synthesis. The development of these compounds has had a remarkable impact on human health. However, despite the massive clinical success of such antibiotics, efforts to develop compounds that target specific transcripts apart from the ribosome itself have proven challenging. Nevertheless, the approval of risdiplam in 2020 for the treatment of spinal muscular atrophy demonstrates that small molecules that target RNA can indeed be developed as powerful and mechanistically novel therapeutics [15].

One important factor that represents a barrier to developing RNA-targeted small molecule therapeutics is selectivity. Antisense oligonucleotides and related sequence-based probes such as peptide nucleic acids (PNAs) and locked nucleic acids (LNAs) are now routinely used as tools and provide high sequence specificity [16]. Antisense molecules have also been approved as therapeutics; however, challenges with delivery, biodistribution, and cell permeability continue to be barriers impacting the broader application and development of such molecules as therapeutics. As a complementary modality, small molecules remain highly attractive as drugs due to their ability to passively diffuse across cell membranes, achieve high metabolically stability and oral bioavailability, as well as the potential for penetration into the central nervous system (CNS). From a patient perspective, these characteristics can translate into significant benefits such as the convenience of once-a-day oral administration. The widespread recognition that RNA can directly drive disease, coupled with the potential to modulate it with small-molecule drugs, has driven significant interest in this emerging field.

This book represents a collection of perspectives from leading experts on the state of the art in understanding RNA as a target for small molecules. The chapters included represent a broad overview, covering topics ranging from how to think about and understand RNA structure, how to identify and understand druglike small molecules that bind to RNA, various approaches for controlling RNA function with small molecules, to overviews of RNA–protein interactions and post-transcriptional modifications of RNA. Finally, we provide an outlook chapter that adds perspective to the future of RNA-targeted drug discovery, including specific challenges that need to be overcome to develop RNA-targeted therapeutics.

In Chapter 2, Incarnato provides a discussion on how to think about RNA structure at the level of individual base pairs. This chapter covers methods and applications for utilizing structure probing to characterize individual RNAs (including both well-defined structures and conformationally diverse ensembles). In Chapter 3, Braun et al. report on the history and progress in determining atomic resolution structures of RNA. This space has historically been highly challenging due to the flexible nature of the RNA biopolymer. However, advances in cryoelectron microscopy and techniques in X-Ray crystallography have resulted in exciting progress in recent years. The increasing availability of atomic resolution structures of RNA ligand complexes is bound to significantly enhance the ability to effectively design high-quality small molecules that bind RNA selectively.

Chapter 4 provides a discussion on lead generation techniques for identifying small molecules that bind to RNA. These methods, including both target-based and phenotypic screens, represent diverse approaches to discover starting points for identifying lead structures for medicinal chemistry programs. In many cases, lead generation techniques used for identifying compounds that target proteins can be adapted for RNA targets, and the authors discuss specific challenges and considerations when applying these methods to RNA. This chapter also discuss several RNA-specific approaches for establishing cellular target engagement. In Chapter 5, Hay et al. discuss the types of chemical matter that binds to RNA, how to characterize it, and how it differs from (and is similar to) protein binding small molecules. Here, it is becoming clear that diverse chemotypes can interact with RNA, both within traditional druglike chemical space and beyond.

The next series of chapters describe examples of different classes of RNA targets. In Chapter 6, Duca provides an overview of microRNAs and efforts to target them. These small RNAs are an intriguing class of non-coding RNA targets that have received considerable interest from both industrial and academic groups as they play a key role in regulating mRNA levels and as a result, control expression levels of proteins. In Chapter 7, Barraza et al. describe efforts to modulate pre-mRNA splicing with small molecules. This important process is the target of clinically validated therapies for spinal muscular atrophy and holds promise for a variety of other mechanistically novel therapies for other diseases including Huntington's diseases and various cancers. While early work has focused on rare monogenic diseases, there is considerable promise in the development of splice modulators as therapeutics for a variety of diseases. Chapter 8, by Mohsen et al. describes riboswitches, which are naturally occurring, ligand-responsive RNA aptamers. These intriguing structures have been the subject of considerable study in both structural/biochemical contexts as well as drug discovery – primarily through the lens of identifying novel antibiotics. However, they also provide promise in synthetic biology as well, particularly in the exciting area of gene therapy as a potential on/off switch for gene expression.

In Chapter 9, Meyer et al. describe examples of small molecules that degrade RNA. By a mechanism analogous to targeted protein degradation strategies such as PROTACs, these molecules recruit nucleases to target RNAs for cleavage and degradation. While some RNA targeting molecules are now FDA approved, RNA-targeting chimeras (RiboTACs) are still at an earlier stage of development. However, RiboTACs may offer specific advantages over monofunctional ligands that target RNA and present opportunities to harness induced proximity pharmacology in the RNA target space and also function in a sub-stoichiometric matter.

In Chapter 10, VanGraafeiland et al. discuss how modulation of programmed frameshifting, primarily by targeting sequences in viral genomes, is an intriguing therapeutic strategy with significant potential. With the development of several potent molecules, cellular proof of concept has now been established for this unique mechanism of controlling gene expression with small molecules. In Chapter 11, Soueid et al. broadly discuss RNA–protein interactions as targets for therapeutics. RNA-binding proteins represent nearly 10% of the human genome and regulate a wide range of cellular and disease relevant processes. Here, understanding structure and patterns of recognition is key to both unraveling biology and developing therapeutics. This chapter also describes the attributes and limitations of a several assay formats that have been developed for identifying compounds that modulate RNA–protein interactions. Chapter 12, by Eggert et al. covers epitranscriptomics. In this context, epitranscriptomics is defined as chemical modifications of RNA, and how these modifications alter biological processes. Although a wide variety of RNA modifications are known, only a few have been studied extensively. Nevertheless, this is an active area of research where small molecules have already entered clinical development.

Finally, in Chapter 13, we provide an outlook on the field and discuss some of the challenges and opportunities facing the development of RNA-targeting molecules as therapeutics. Continued efforts to develop the fundamentals of medicinal chemistry and molecular design principles within this challenging space, coupled with the importance of target validation, establishing relevant functional assays, and understanding selectivity are key topics. The latter stands to benefit tremendously as more and more atomic resolution structures of RNA–small molecules complexes become availed. While many challenges remain, the potential for RNA-targeting medicines to make a broader impact on human health stands as a compelling rationale for continued efforts. Together, we hope that these chapters provide an exciting perspective on how to think about and prosecute RNA as targets for small molecules.

References

1 Lander, E.S., Linton, L.M., Birren, B. et al. (2001). Initial sequencing and analysis of the human genome. *Nature* 409: 860–921.

2 Consortium, E.P (2012). An integrated encyclopedia of DNA elements in the human genome. *Nature* 489: 57–74.

3 Iyer, M.K., Niknafs, Y.S., Malik, R. et al. (2015). The landscape of long noncoding RNAs in the human transcriptome. *Nat. Genet.* 47: 199–208.
4 Spradlin, J.N., Zhang, E., and Nomura, D.K. (2021). Reimagining druggability using chemoproteomic platforms. *Acc. Chem. Res.* 54: 1801–1813.
5 Kovachka, S., Panosetti, M., Grimaldi, B. et al. (2024). Small molecule approaches to targeting RNA. *Nat. Rev. Chem.* 8: 120–135.
6 Childs-Disney, J.L., Yang, X., Gibaut, Q.M.R. et al. (2022). Targeting RNA structures with small molecules. *Nat. Rev. Drug Discovery* 21: 736–762.
7 Warner, K.D., Hajdin, C.E., and Weeks, K.M. (2018). Principles for targeting RNA with drug-like small molecules. *Nat. Rev. Drug Discovery* 17: 547–558.
8 Connelly, C.M., Moon, M.H., and Schneekloth, J.S. Jr., (2016). The emerging role of RNA as a therapeutic target for small molecules. *Cell Chem. Biol.* 23: 1077–1090.
9 Zafferani, M. and Hargrove, A.E. (2021). Small molecule targeting of biologically relevant RNA tertiary and quaternary structures. *Cell Chem. Biol.* 28: 594–609.
10 Ganser, L.R., Kelly, M.L., Herschlag, D., and Al-Hashimi, H.M. (2019). The roles of structural dynamics in the cellular functions of RNAs. *Nat. Rev. Mol. Cell Biol.* 20: 474–489.
11 Gebauer, F., Schwarzl, T., Valcarcel, J., and Hentze, M.W. (2021). RNA-binding proteins in human genetic disease. *Nat. Rev. Genet.* 22: 185–198.
12 Hewitt, W.M., Calabrese, D.R., and Schneekloth, J.S. Jr., (2019). Evidence for ligandable sites in structured RNA throughout the Protein Data Bank. *Bioorg. Med. Chem.* 27: 2253–2260.
13 Kavita, K. and Breaker, R.R. (2023). Discovering riboswitches: the past and the future. *Trends Biochem. Sci.* 48: 119–141.
14 Wilson, D.N. (2014). Ribosome-targeting antibiotics and mechanisms of bacterial resistance. *Nat. Rev. Microbiol.* 12: 35–48.
15 Dhillon, S. (2020). Risdiplam: first approval. *Drugs* 80: 1853–1858.
16 Crooke, S.T., Baker, B.F., Crooke, R.M., and Liang, X.H. (2021). Antisense technology: an overview and prospectus. *Nat. Rev. Drug Discovery* 20: 427–453.

2

RNA Structure Probing, Dynamics, and Folding

Danny Incarnato

Department of Molecular Genetics, Groningen Biomolecular Sciences and Biotechnology Institute (GBB), University of Groningen, Groningen, The Netherlands

2.1 Introduction

RNA is pivotal for the regulation of most biological processes in the cell. Although for most of the past century researchers have mainly regarded RNA as a carrier of genetic information, a simple intermediate between DNA and proteins, recent advances in the fields of genomics and epigenomics, aided by the development of high-throughput sequencing methods, have begun shedding new light on the polyhedric nature of RNA molecules.

Messenger RNAs (mRNAs), which encode for proteins, only represent a small piece in the highly complex puzzle that is the transcriptome of a cell. The advent of RNA sequencing (RNA-seq) technologies and the dawn of the ENCODE project [1] revealed that the vast majority of the nonrepetitive genome in mammalian cells is transcribed and that most of these transcripts lack the ability to encode for proteins. The human genome is now estimated to carry over 60,000 genes, generating approximately 250,000 transcripts, of which nearly two-thirds are noncoding RNAs (ncRNAs) [2].

While the cellular roles and mechanisms of action of most of these transcripts are still largely unknown, their ability to fold into stable secondary and tertiary structures is expected to be paramount to their functions, as reported for many cellular RNAs [3]. Indeed, being a single-stranded molecule, RNA has the unique ability to fold back on itself to generate very intricate secondary structures, mediated both by direct base pairing between complementary nucleobases within the RNA strand and by base stacking. Secondary structures can then be further compacted into tertiary structures thanks to the contribution of different factors such as divalent cations, non-Watson-Crick interactions, and macromolecular crowding, among others [4]. These structures have been proven essential to mediate many of the noncoding functions of RNA molecules, including macromolecular scaffolding, sensing of the environment, and even catalysis. The ribosome is a key example of these functions as proper folding of ribosomal RNAs is crucial to provide the docking platform for ribosomal proteins and to enable efficient translation of mRNAs [5].

RNA as a Drug Target: The Next Frontier for Medicinal Chemistry, First Edition.
Edited by John Schneekloth and Martin Pettersson.

Aside from ncRNAs, mRNAs themselves carry untranslated regions (UTRs) that are populated by a myriad of regulatory RNA structure elements such as G-quadruplexes (G4), internal ribosome entry sites (IRES), iron response elements (IRE), and many more, which mediate the post-transcriptional regulation of gene expression [6].

In light of these considerations, it will become immediately evident to the reader that a complete understanding of the transcriptome is deeply entangled with our ability to interrogate and understand RNA structures in the cellular context. This chapter discusses recent advances in methods for RNA structure determination in living cells, the challenges, and the future perspectives.

2.1.1 Relevance of RNA Structure in Disease

Besides controlling gene expression in a physiological context, the deregulation of RNA structure has been widely implicated in pathogenesis. This might either involve the disruption of physiologically relevant RNA structures or the genesis of pathogenic RNA structures that are not normally present under physiological conditions. Disease-associated mutations identified within transcribed noncoding regions from genome-wide association studies (GWAS), for example, have been shown to disrupt key regulatory RNA structure elements within UTRs [7]. Mutations in the 5′UTR of the ferritin light chain (FTL) gene, associated with hyperferritinemia cataract syndrome, lead to disruption of an IRE element, hence impairing binding by an iron response protein (IRP) and, consequently, deregulating FTL expression. The expansion of CTG repeats in the 3’UTR of the dystrophin myotonin protein kinase (DMPK) gene, which drives the pathogenesis of myotonic dystrophy (DM), leads to the generation of an extended stem-loop structure [8, 9] that is capable of sequestering muscleblind proteins (MBNL) [10, 11], ultimately deregulating splicing of multiple mRNAs [12].

Aside from pathogenic RNA structures within human transcripts, studies conducted on RNA viruses highlighted how their genomes are replete with regulatory RNA structure elements that are pivotal in regulating multiple aspects of the viral life cycle, including replication, translation, and packaging [13]. Translation of the two partially overlapping ORF1a and ORF1b in coronavirus genomes, for example, is regulated by the frameshifting element (FSE), which enables pausing and backtracking of the ribosome at the end of ORF1a, leading to the synthesis of the ORF1ab polyprotein, crucial for viral replication [14]. The stem-loop A (SLA) RNA structure located at the 5′ end of flavivirus genomes acts as a promoter for the replication of the viral genome by providing the docking site for the viral RNA polymerase NS5 [15]. The Rev Response Element (RRE) of HIV-1, which interacts with the Rev protein, can switch between two alternative structures to regulate the nuclear export of the viral genome [16].

2.1.2 Challenges in Studying RNA Structures

Owing to their extreme flexibility, RNA molecules can adopt a wide variety of different conformations. An n-nucleotides long RNA can theoretically fold into up to

1.8^n distinct secondary structures [17]. This scenario is further complicated when considering that each nucleotide in the RNA chain has eight degrees of freedom and that the biologically active structures might not be strongly favored thermodynamically over competing structures [18]. This dilemma is commonly known in the field as the *RNA folding problem* [19].

At present, for most RNAs, it is nearly impossible to accurately predict their structure solely from their primary sequence. Computational approaches based on free energy minimization have been developed to predict the minimum free energy (MFE) structure, that is the thermodynamically most stable structure, using a set of thermodynamic parameters known as nearest-neighbor model (or *Turner* rules) [20]. The accuracy of MFE structure prediction is, however, limited in practice, with only ~66% of predicted base pairs found in experimentally validated structures from crystallographic studies or phylogenetic analyses [21].

One of the issues inherent to MFE-based approaches is that the MFE structure only represents one of the many conformations a given RNA can adopt. Every RNA can populate a multitude of structural *states*, each one having a certain probability of occurring, which are collectively referred to as *ensemble*. The probability that the MFE structure might occur within the ensemble might be very low, meaning that the MFE structure might not represent the most likely conformation for a given RNA. To address this limitation, methods to determine the partition function for secondary structure formation were developed, which allow predicting the probability that each possible base pair in the RNA strand might form within the ensemble. The accuracy of this type of approach is much higher, with ~91% of the base pairs occurring with a probability $\geq$0.99 in the MFE structure found in phylogenetically determined structures [21].

More recently, a new class of predictive algorithms based on machine learning has emerged. These algorithms are trained on sets of experimentally validated RNA structures [22]. However, extensive benchmarking of these algorithms suggests that their accuracy is generally biased toward certain classes of RNAs [23] and that, typically, predicted structures tend to contain more base pairs than ground truth structures [24], a trend that grows quadratically with increasing RNA lengths.

2.2 Experimentally Guided RNA Structure Modeling

Irrespective of the chosen approach, the reliability of computational RNA structure predictions is limited, and it decreases with increasing length of the RNA strand. To address these limitations, a wide variety of complementary approaches have been developed to date to experimentally interrogate the structure of RNA molecules. Data generated by these approaches can be then incorporated as *constraints* (or *restraints*) into thermodynamics-driven structure predictions to increase their accuracy [25, 26].

This chapter will solely focus on approaches suitable for the analysis of RNA structures in living cells. Particularly, I will discuss three classes of methods: chemical probing-based methods, methods for the direct mapping of RNA–RNA interactions, and methods to map nucleotide spatial proximity.

2.2.1 Structural Interrogation of RNA Nucleotides via Chemical Probing

Among the repertoire of available methods for RNA structural interrogation, chemical probing is perhaps the most popular. Methods based on chemical probing exploit specific reagents (hereafter referred to as *chemical probes*) that can react with specific functional groups in RNA nucleotides on the basis of their structural context.

Particularly, three broad classes of chemical probes can be identified. The first class of reagents includes nucleobase-specific chemical probes to measure the base-pairing status of RNA bases (Figure 2.1). These compounds act by chemically modifying functional groups involved in base pairing. One of the most popular probes in this class is dimethyl sulfate (DMS), an alkylating reagent that methylates the N1 of adenines and the N3 of cytosines when unpaired (Figure 2.1a) [27]. DMS has been widely employed to query the structure of both viral genomes [28–30] and entire cellular transcriptomes [31–34], owing both to its ability to readily permeate biological membranes and to its high efficiency, resulting in a very high signal-to-noise ratio. More recently, it has been suggested that, under mildly alkaline conditions, DMS might partially react also with unpaired guanines and uracils, although with much lower efficiency [35]. α-Ketoaldehydes such as glyoxal and N_3-kethoxal have been recently reported to form adducts with the N1 and N2 of unpaired guanines *in vivo* (Figure 2.1b) [36, 37]. Similarly, carbodiimides such as 1-ethyl-3-(3-dimethylaminopropyl)carbodiimide (EDC) are capable of forming adducts with the N1 of guanines and the N3 of uracils, both unpaired or in G:U wobbled base pairs (Figure 2.1c) [38, 39].

The second class of reagents includes selective 2′-hydroxyl acylation analyzed by primer extension (SHAPE) probes (Figure 2.1d) [40]. SHAPE reagents are electrophilic compounds capable of forming adducts with the 2′-hydroxyl (2′-OH) of the ribose moiety at structurally flexible nucleotides. These nucleotides typically lie within loops of unpaired bases, or at helix termini. A wide variety of SHAPE probes, largely differing in their hydrolysis rates in aqueous buffers, have been reported to date. Among these, acyl imidazoles such as 2-methylnicotinic acid imidazolide (NAI) and 2-aminopyridine-3-carboxylic acid imidazolide (2A3) [41, 42] and isatoic anhydrides such as 5-nitroisatoic anhydride (5NIA) [43] are the better-characterized SHAPE probes for the interrogation of RNA structures in living cells.

The third class of reagents includes compounds capable of querying the accessibility of RNA bases to the solvent. The recently characterized nicotinoyl azide (NAz), for example, forms adducts with the C8 of solvent-accessible purines upon irradiation with long-wavelength UV light (Figure 2.1e) [44]. A popular alternative to NAz involves the use of hydroxyl radicals to induce RNA strand scission at the level of solvent-accessible C3 and C4 of the ribose moiety [45]. This approach is

Figure 2.1 Reaction of different RNA chemical probes. (a) Reaction of dimethyl sulfate (DMS) with unpaired A and C bases. (b) Reaction of α-ketoaldehydes (such as glyoxal and N_3-kethoxal) with unpaired G bases. (c) Reaction of carbodiimides (such as EDC) with unpaired U bases. (d) Reaction of SHAPE reagents (such as 5NIA, NAI, and 2A3) with the 2′-OH of structurally flexible nucleotides. (e) Reaction of nicotinoyl azide (NAz) with the C-8 of solvent exposed A and G bases.

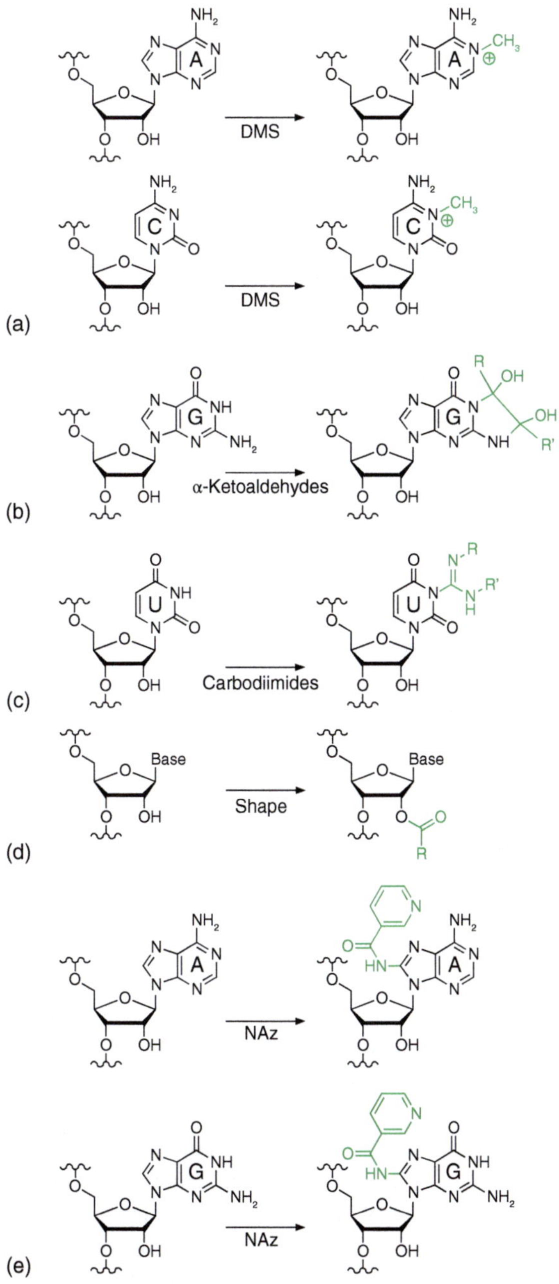

typically more challenging than NAz probing when it comes to interrogating RNA structures in living cells as it requires generating intracellular hydroxyl radicals, for example, using a high-flux synchrotron X-ray beam [46].

Irrespective of the probe choice, sites of modification on the RNA can be read out by reverse transcription experiments [47]. These experiments typically rely on the inability of the reverse transcriptase (RT) to read through probe-induced modifications, resulting in RT drop-off and premature termination of cDNA synthesis, one nucleotide downstream of the modification site. Low-throughput chemical probing experiments historically involved the interrogation of a single RNA at a time and its reverse transcription using gene-specific primers, followed by resolution of cDNAs by gel electrophoresis. Thanks to the advent of high-throughput sequencing technologies, numerous protocols have been devised to extend this procedure to the study of entire cellular transcriptomes [47]. These protocols typically involve the fragmentation of cellular RNAs, followed by reverse transcription and direct ligation of a sequencing adapter to the 3′ end of the cDNAs, allowing the high-throughput detection of RT drop-off events on a transcriptome-wide scale (Figure 2.2).

More recently, an alternative approach dubbed mutational profiling (MaP) has been introduced [32, 48, 49]. This involves adjusting the reverse transcription reaction to favor the RT read-through on the site of probe-induced modification. When reading through the modified residue, the RT incorporates a random nucleotide, typically resulting in a mutation in the synthesized cDNA. The main difference between RT drop-off and MaP methods is the ability of MaP to capture multiple sites of modification within each cDNA product. The advantages of this approach will be further discussed later on in the chapter (see Section 2.3, "Dealing with RNA structure heterogeneity").

Following the sequencing of cDNAs and mapping to the reference transcriptome, RT drop-off events (or mutations) at each position of every RNA can be counted, yielding *reactivity profiles* that can be used to constrain RNA structure prediction. Highly reactive bases are interpreted as having a high likelihood of being unpaired (or structurally flexible or accessible to the solvent). Conversely, bases with low reactivity are interpreted as having a high likelihood of being base paired (or structurally rigid or inaccessible to the solvent). Reactivity profiles can then be fed into thermodynamics-driven RNA structure prediction algorithms to adjust the thermodynamic parameters by rewarding base pairing of lowly reactive positions and penalizing base pairing of highly reactive positions [25, 26].

2.2.1.1 Limits of RNA Chemical Probing

The biggest limitation of chemical probing-based methods is the fact that lack of reactivity to the chemical probe is not necessarily correlated to the structural state of the target nucleotide. For instance, protein binding, or how deeply buried a nucleotide is within the tertiary structure of the RNA, might significantly affect the accessibility of the probe to the target nucleotide. Furthermore, systematic investigation of the structural preferences of SHAPE reagents suggests that small loops are typically more reactive to SHAPE probing as compared to longer stretches of unpaired nucleotides [50]. Interestingly, a recent study introduced a number of novel acyl imidazoles, showing that by altering the reagent scaffold, it is possible to alter the structural specificity of the SHAPE probe, for example, to reduce reactivity on loop-closing base pairs [51]. Moreover, the smallest possible scaffold, acetylimidazole, is cell permeable and capable of probing RNA structures even at the level of protein-bound regions.

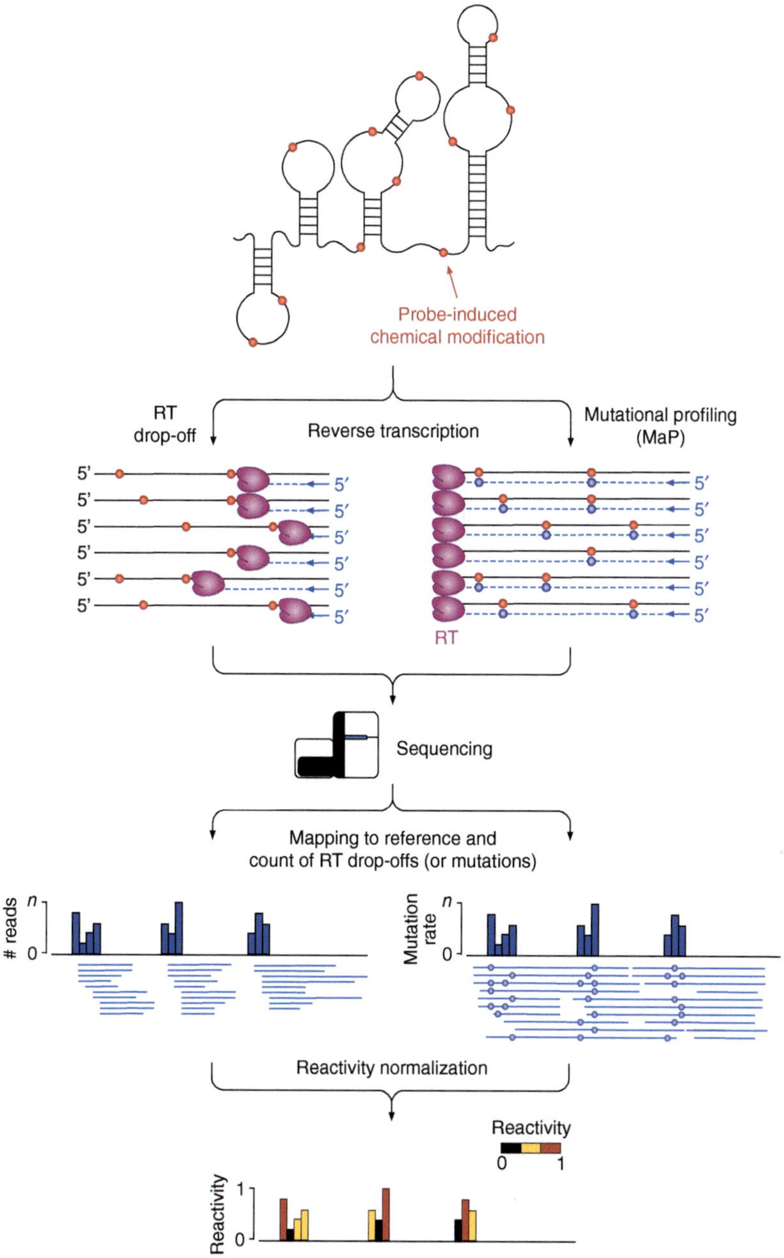

Figure 2.2 General outline of the protocol for the detection of RNA modifications following chemical probing. Modifications along the RNA are detected at reverse transcription, either because of RT drop-off on the modified nucleotide (left) or due to recording of the modification in the cDNA as mutation (right). The resulting cDNAs are then ligated to sequencing adapters and sequenced. Following mapping of the reads to the reference transcriptome, sites of RT drop-off (left, corresponding to the base 1 nucleotide upstream of the read start mapping position) or mutations (right) can be counted. Raw counts are then normalized, yielding the final reactivity profile.

These "apparent" low reactivities might be erroneously interpreted by thermodynamics-driven structure prediction algorithms as basepaired, hence resulting in inaccurate RNA structure models.

2.2.2 Direct Mapping of RNA–RNA Interactions

An alternative class of methods that allows direct mapping of RNA duplexes in living cells has been recently introduced. These methods, which include RNA proximity ligation (RPL) [52], psoralen analysis of RNA interactions and structures (PARIS) [53], sequencing of psoralen cross-linked, ligated, and selected hybrids (SPLASH) [54], ligation of interacting RNA followed by high-throughput sequencing (LIGR-seq) [55], mapping RNA interactome *in vivo* (MARIO) [56], and cross-linking of matched RNAs and deep sequencing (COMRADES) [57], to name a few, exploit psoralen, or some derivative thereof, to stabilize RNA duplexes *in vivo*. Upon long-wavelength UV light irradiation, psoralen forms covalent cross-links between adjacent pyrimidines residing on opposite strands of an RNA duplex (Figure 2.3) [58, 59], ensuring survival of cellular RNA–RNA interactions to cell lysis. RNA is then partially fragmented and/or digested with nucleases to yield short RNA duplexes, and the two strands of each duplex are joined by intramolecular ligation to generate a chimeric RNA molecule. Cross-linking can then be reversed by short-wavelength UV light irradiation, and the RNA chimeras can be ligated to adapters and sequenced. Following sequencing, chimeras will be mapped back to the reference transcriptome, providing direct evidence for the existence of certain RNA duplexes (Figure 2.4). Importantly, these approaches can be used to capture not only intramolecular but also intermolecular RNA–RNA interactions.

Aside from methods based on psoralen cross-linking, some studies have suggested that DMS chemical probing read out via MaP might also be used to obtain semi-direct evidence of base pairing between two nucleotides. RNA interaction groups measured by mutational profiling (RING-MaP) [48] and pairing ascertained from interacting RNA strands measured by mutational profiling (PAIR-MaP) [35] exploit the transient exposure of interacting bases in an RNA duplex due to equilibrium fluctuations. This "breathing" of RNA–RNA interactions results in a transient exposure of the bases that become available for modification by DMS. As modification by DMS impairs the ability of nucleobases to base pair, modification

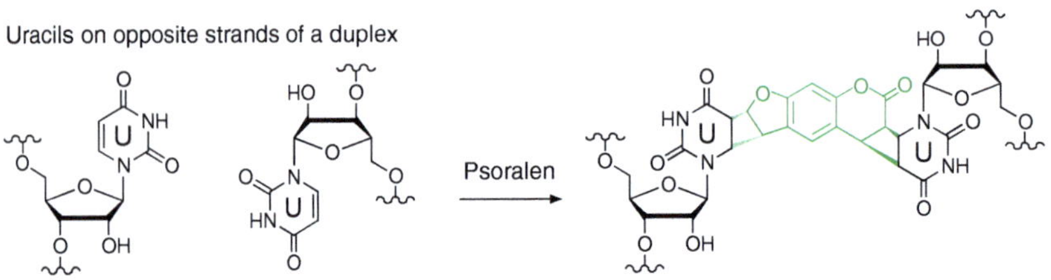

Figure 2.3 Reaction of psoralen (and its derivatives) with U bases residing on opposite strands of an RNA duplex.

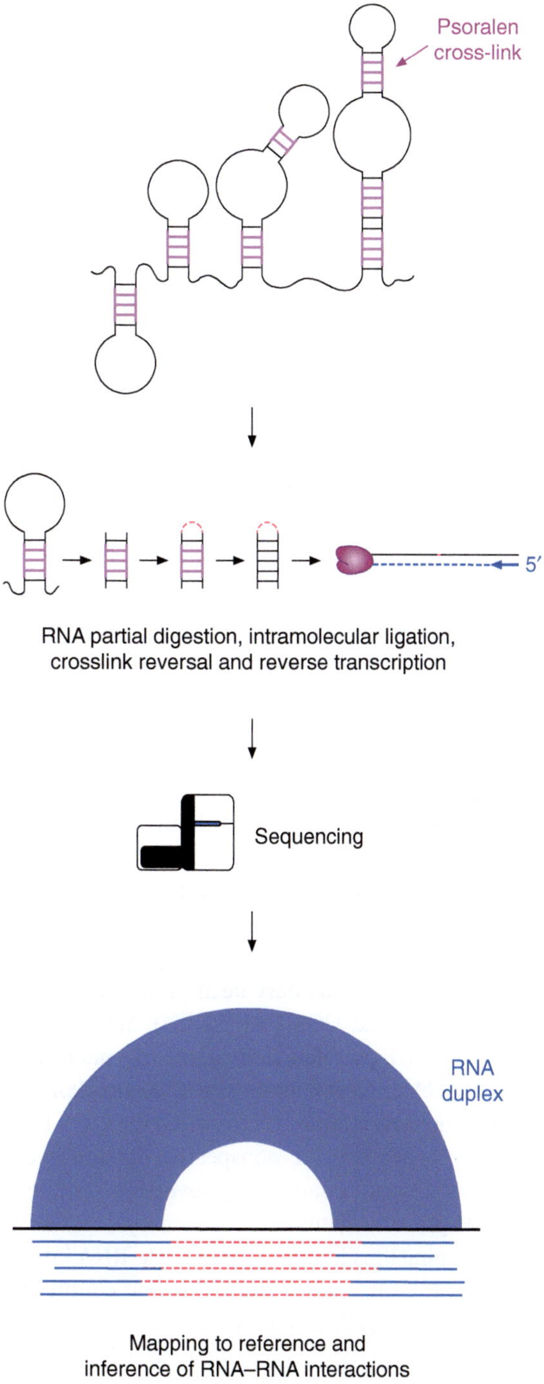

Figure 2.4 General outline of the protocol for the mapping of RNA–RNA interactions using psoralen (or its derivatives). After having stabilized RNA duplexes by psoralen cross-linking, the RNA is partially fragmented (or digested) to both remove single-stranded loops and to shorten long RNA duplexes. The resulting short RNA duplexes are joined by intramolecular ligation, generating chimeric RNA molecules. Chimeras are reverse transcribed and sequenced. Following mapping of the reads to the reference transcriptome, the two "halves" of the chimeras will map to distal regions of one (or two, in the case of intermolecular duplexes) RNA, hence enabling the direct detection of RNA duplexes.

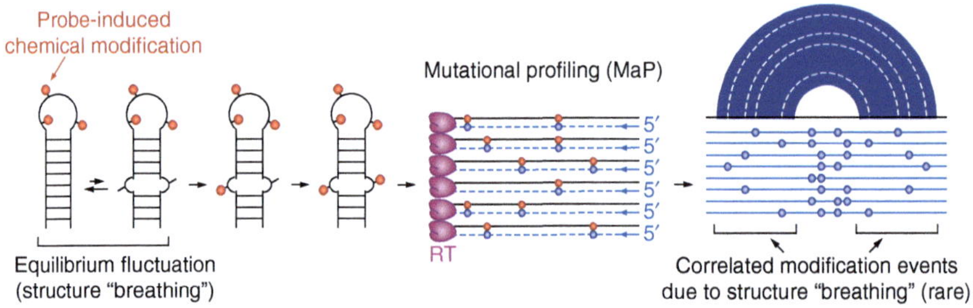

Figure 2.5 General outline of the principle exploited by RING-MaP and PAIR-MaP to indirectly infer RNA–RNA interactions from chemical probing experiments. Unpaired bases (i.e. loops) are readily modified by the chemical probe with high efficiency. In rare occasions, base-paired bases can become transiently accessible to the probe due to equilibrium fluctuations. Modification of one partner in the pair permanently destabilizes base pairing, making also the other partner available for modification. Following reverse transcription under mutational profiling (MaP) conditions, sites of modifications are recorded as mutations in the cDNA, and sites of correlated modification due to structure "breathing" can be identified and used to detect putative base-pairing interactions.

of one of the bases in a pair results in the permanent exposure of its partner, which can then be modified as well. These low-frequency correlated modification events can then be simultaneously detected as mutations within a single cDNA molecule by MaP (Figure 2.5).

2.2.2.1 Limits of RNA–RNA Interaction Mapping

Methods based on psoralen cross-linking suffer three main limitations [60]: (i) the preference of psoralen for pyrimidines, particularly uracils, can result in the preferential stabilization and capture of pyrimidine-rich duplexes, hence making these methods not quantitative; (ii) although intramolecular ligation is favored between RNA strands in a duplex, any two RNA strands in a sample can be intermolecularly ligated, resulting in a number of artifactual RNA–RNA interactions being mapped; and (iii) the vast majority of the adapter-ligated RNA fragments are non-chimeric, hence significantly increasing the required sequencing depth of these experiments. Potential workarounds have been proposed for some of these issues. For instance, SPLASH [54] and COMRADES [57], respectively, take advantage of biotin- or azido-modified psoralen derivatives to enable the streptavidin-mediated enrichment of RNA duplexes, while PARIS [53] exploits a native-denatured 2-dimensional gel electrophoresis approach to enrich the cross-linked RNA duplexes. Additionally, in order to account for nonspecific ligation events, the COMRADES approach generates a control sample by reversing psoralen cross-links and melting RNA duplexes prior to ligation.

Concerning the identification of RNA–RNA interactions via chemical probing and MaP [35, 48], the main limitation is that equilibrium fluctuations are very rare, so are correlated modification events, hence requiring extreme sequencing depths to be detected, making this type of approach only suited for the targeted analysis of individual RNAs.

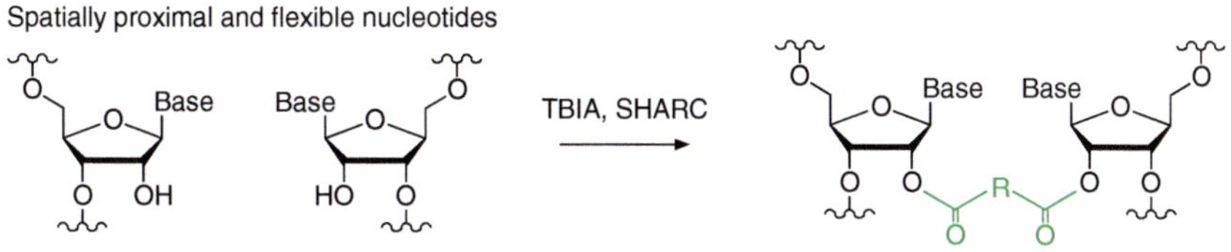

Figure 2.6 Reaction of TBIA and SHARC reagents with the ribose 2′-OH of spatially proximal and structurally flexible nucleotides.

2.2.3 Mapping Spatially Proximal Nucleotides in RNA molecules

An exciting recent evolution of SHAPE probes has led to the development of bifunctional reagents. These compounds bear two moieties capable of forming adducts with the ribose 2′-OH of two spatially proximal and structurally flexible nucleotides. These include trans-bis-isatoic anhydride (TBIA) [61] and spatial 2′-hydroxyl acylation reversible cross-linking (SHARC) reagents [62] (Figure 2.6). The length of the flexible linker between the two adduct-forming moieties of SHARC reagents can in principle be adjusted to create "molecular rulers" that can be used to measure approximate internucleotide distances.

Two readout strategies have been proposed for these experiments: selective 2′-hydroxyl acylation analyzed by primer extension and juxtaposed merged pairs (SHAPE-JuMP) and SHARC-exo (Figure 2.7). SHAPE-JuMP [61] exploits an engineered RT, RT-C8 [63], which has the ability to traverse (or *jump* across) chemical cross-links, hence recording the cross-linked sites as deletions in the cDNA. SHARC-exo [62], instead, involves partial RNA digestion with RNase III, followed by denatured-denatured 2-dimensional gel electrophoresis to enrich cross-linked RNA fragments. Fragments are then digested by RNase R to trim the 3′ ends up to ~5 nucleotides from the cross-linking site, followed by intramolecular ligation to yield chimeric RNA fragments and cross-linking reversal under mild alkaline conditions.

Data from these experiments can be used to constrain RNA 3D structure modeling, achieving significant improvements as compared to unconstrained structure models [61, 62, 64].

2.2.3.1 Limits of Methods for Spatial Proximity Mapping

The biggest limitation of these methods is, analogously to methods for RNA–RNA interaction capture, the low abundance of chimeric RNA fragments in the final library, which has been reported to be ~3–15% for SHARC-exo [62]. This is possibly the consequence of the higher frequency at which TBIA/SHARC mono-adducts, which occur when one moiety of the probe reacts with a nucleotide while the other is hydrolyzed in water [61], are formed as compared to di-adducts. This limitation significantly increases the required sequencing depths, hence posing an important challenge to the feasibility of transcriptome-wide analyses.

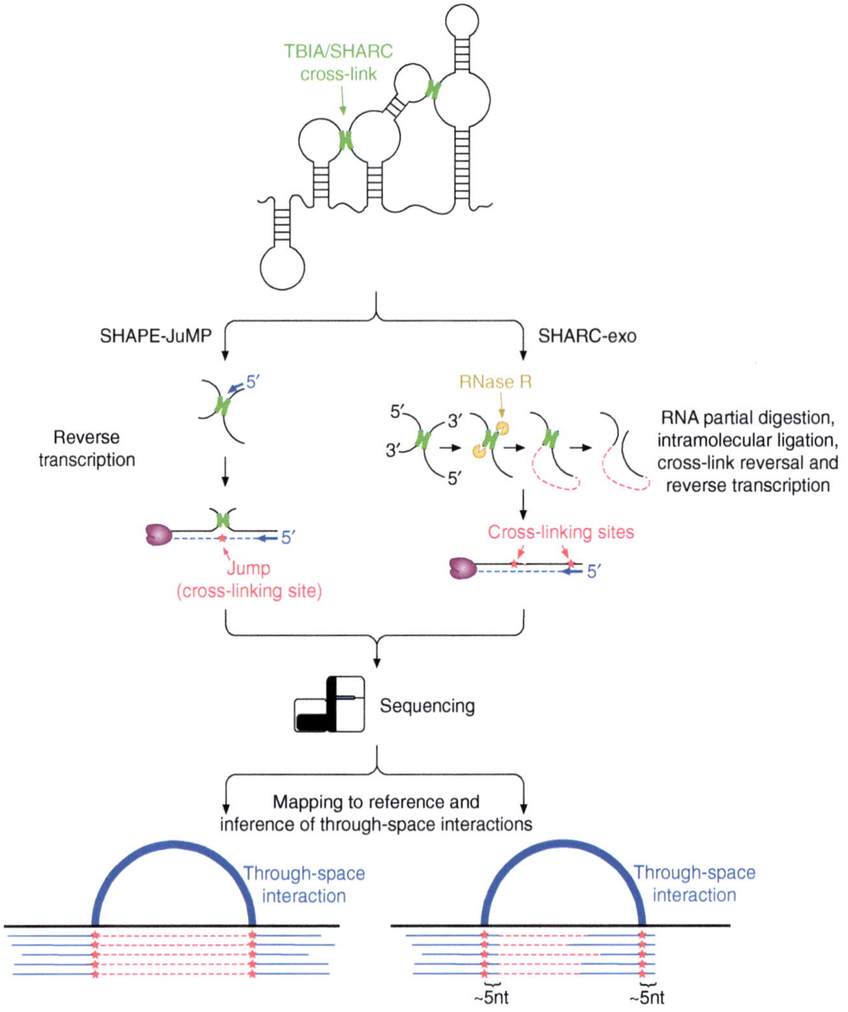

Figure 2.7 General outline of the SHAPE-JuMP and SHARC-exo protocols for the mapping of through-space interactions, following cross-linking of spatially proximal nucleotides by using either trans-bis-isatoic anhydride (TBIA) or spatial 2′-hydroxyl acylation reversible cross-linking (SHARC) reagents. The SHAPE-JuMP approach (left) uses a special RT enzyme capable of "jumping" across the reagent-induced cross-links, hence permanently recording the cross-linking site as a deletion in the cDNA. The SHARC-exo approach, instead, involves a partial digestion of the RNA, followed by enrichment of the cross-linked RNA fragments by denatured-denatured 2-dimensional gel electrophoresis. The recovered fragments are shortened down to ~5 nucleotides from the site of cross-linking at their 3′ ends by RNase R digestion and joined by intramolecular ligation. Cross-linking is then reversed, allowing reverse transcription of the chimeric RNA fragments. Following mapping of the reads to the reference transcriptome, the two "halves" of the chimeras will map to distal regions of the RNA. For SHAPE-JuMP, as the RT "jumps" across the cross-link, the coordinates of the cross-linked nucleotides can be determined from the start and end positions of the resulting deletion. For SHARC-exo, as the cross-linked RNA fragments are trimmed by RNase R digestion, the coordinates of the cross-linked nucleotides can be approximately inferred as the positions ~5 nucleotides upstream of the 3′ end of the two "halves" of the chimeras.

2.3 Dealing with RNA Structure Heterogeneity

As previously mentioned, an important feature of RNA molecules is their ability to sample a potentially very large conformational space. Many cellular RNAs are likely to populate multiple alternative structures that can coexist as part of a heterogeneous and dynamic ensemble [3, 60]. The ability to switch between alternative conformations has been reported to be crucial for several RNAs. Bacterial riboswitches [65] and RNA thermometers [66], which are capable of altering their structure in response to the presence of specific metabolites or due to temperature changes, respectively, are possibly the better characterized examples.

It is therefore paramount to point out that data generated using any of the above-described methods must not be interpreted just as a function of a single RNA structure, but rather as an aggregate of all the structures populating the ensemble for a given RNA. This point is particularly relevant for chemical probing experiments. Indeed, while RNA–RNA interaction and spatial proximity mapping methods capture individual helices or internucleotide distances, chemical probing experiments typically only provide a reactivity profile representing a weighted average of the reactivities of all the structures in the ensemble.

The recent introduction of the MaP-based readout provided an important workaround to this problem. As discussed earlier, the key advantage of MaP over the traditional RT drop-off-based readout is that multiple sites of modification within a single RNA molecule can be all recorded as mutations in a single cDNA product. Therefore, this type of approach allows preserving information about the relationship between the individual nucleotides in the RNA strand (i.e. nucleotides that were simultaneously unpaired, or structurally flexible, in a certain conformation). By analyzing the co-mutation patterns in the cDNA molecules, it is possible to learn these relationships and to determine how many alternative structures populate the ensemble for a given RNA (Figure 2.8). For instance, given a set of three nucleotides (e.g. 1, 2, and 3) on an RNA, one would expect to observe any of the three possible pairs of co-mutations (i.e. 1-2, 2-3, and 1-3) to occur with comparable probability for an RNA folding into a single structure.

Deviations from this expected behavior would suggest the presence of multiple structures. For example, if only 1-2 and 2-3 were observed to co-mutate, this would indicate that nucleotides 1 and 3 tend not to be simultaneously reactive to the chemical probe, indicating the presence of two mutually exclusive structures. After having determined the number of conformations making up the ensemble, the cDNAs can be clustered based on their co-mutation profiles, enabling the reconstruction of the reactivity profiles for the individual conformations. To date, three main computational methods exploiting this approach to reconstruct RNA structure ensembles from MaP chemical probing experiments have been developed, namely detection of RNA folding ensembles using expectation–maximization (DREEM) [67], deconvolution of RNA alternative conformations (DRACO) [68], and deconvolution and annotation of ribonucleic conformational ensembles (DANCE-MaP) [69]. A fourth method, dubbed determination of the variation of the RNA structure conformation through stochastic context-free grammar

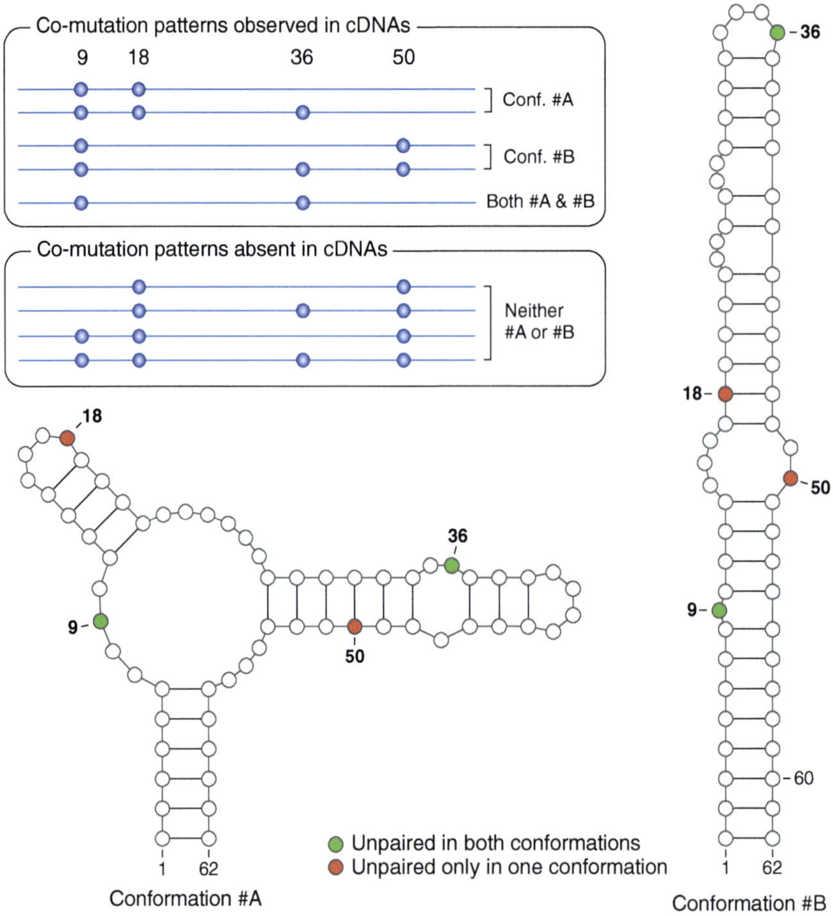

Figure 2.8 Outline of the principle exploiting chemical probing and mutational profiling (MaP) analysis for the deconvolution of coexisting alternative RNA structures. In the depicted example, the same RNA populates an ensemble of two conformations (A and B). Both conformations share a number of unpaired bases, for example, bases 9 and 36 (in green). Some bases, however, are unpaired only in one conformation and base paired in the other (in red). Among these, for example, base 18 is unpaired in conformation A and base paired in conformation B, while base 50 is base paired in conformation A and unpaired in conformation B. Chemical probing and MaP analysis of this ensemble will result in a very specific set of cDNA co-mutation patterns. For instance, co-mutations of bases 9 and 36 can be observed both for conformations A and B. Co-mutations of either (or both) bases with base 18 can only be observed for conformation A, while co-mutations with base 50 can only be observed for conformation B. However, as base pairing of bases 18 and 50 is mutually exclusive between the two conformations, reads carrying co-mutations of bases 18 and 50 will (almost) never be observed.

(DaVinci) [70], has been recently introduced. DaVinci uses a different approach, combining thermodynamics-based structure prediction and MaP data (Figure 2.9). As each sequencing read provides information on the pairing status of the nucleotides in a single RNA molecule, DaVinci predicts a structure from each

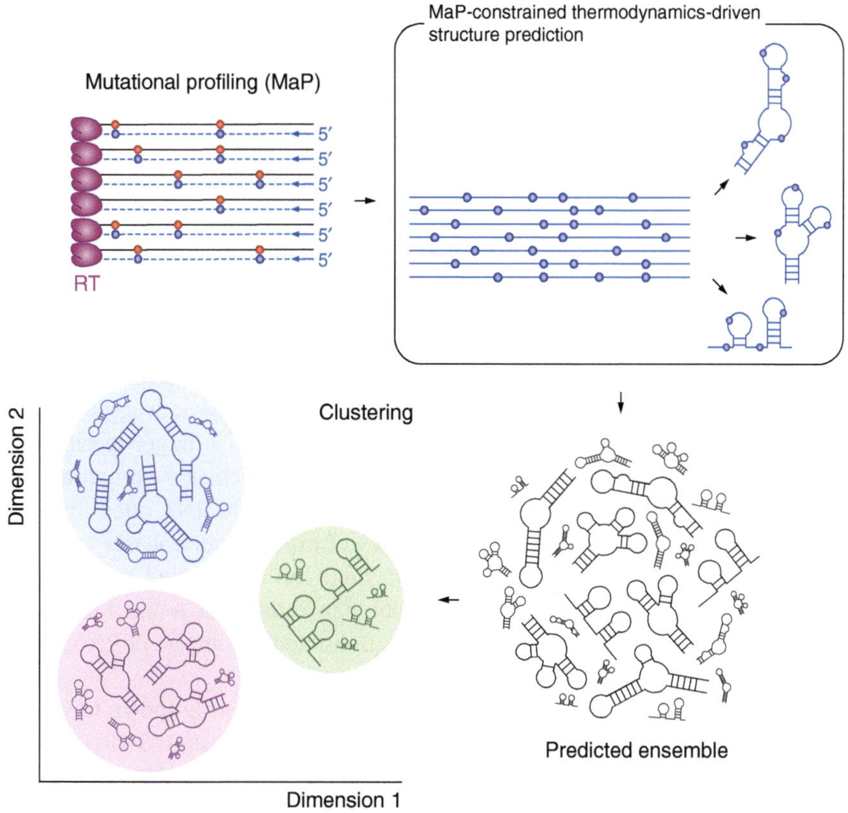

Figure 2.9 Outline of the DaVinci stochastic context-free grammar approach. Following chemical probing, mutational profiling (MaP) analysis, and sequencing, the mutational profile of each read, corresponding to the bases being simultaneously unpaired in a single original RNA molecule, is used to constrain the thermodynamics-driven structure prediction. This results in *N* predicted secondary structures, each derived from a single read (so, theoretically, from a single original RNA molecule). This predicted ensemble is then subjected to clustering. The number of clusters identified by the analysis corresponds to the number of alternative conformations making up the ensemble for the RNA in analysis.

read by constraining the mutated bases in the read to be unpaired in the predicted structure. The resulting structures are then clustered, with the number of identified clusters corresponding to the number of conformations making up the ensemble.

Although RT drop-off-based probing experiments do not preserve any information about the relationships between individual nucleotides in the RNA strand, as each cDNA molecule can only capture a single modification site, several computational methods have been devised in an attempt to mitigate this limitation [71–73]. These algorithms take advantage of a partition function-based approach to sample a large number of possible structures from the theoretical ensemble a given RNA can populate and then use the experimentally determined reactivity profile to select a parsimonious set of structures that better explains the observed experimental reactivities. All these methods have been thoroughly reviewed elsewhere [74], so they will not be discussed in detail in this chapter.

2.4 Querying RNA–Small Molecule Interactions with Chemical Probing

Determining the structure of RNA molecules in the context of living cells has recently attracted huge interest in industry [75–77]. Just like proteins, RNA structures possess ligandable pockets, amenable for targeting small molecules [78]. In this perspective, mapping which structures are functional and druggable is paramount for the development of innovative RNA-targeted therapeutic strategies, possibly opening the way to targeting proteins currently considered to be undruggable.

As learned from antibiotics such as aminoglycosides, which target specific tertiary folds in the ribosomal RNAs (rRNA) of bacteria, as well as from natural ligands of bacterial riboswitches, binding of small molecules to RNA often involves hydrogen bonding with the Watson-Crick faces of exposed nucleobases and aromatic stacking interactions [79]. These interactions can be captured and mapped by chemical probing, providing a powerful tool to investigate RNA-small molecule target engagement, as well as off-target interactions, and the impact of RNA-small molecule interactions on the structure of RNA molecules.

For example, the antibiotic spectinomycin has been previously shown to specifically interact with residues G1064 and C1192 in the *E. coli* 16S rRNA [80]. Accordingly, DMS chemical probing readout by MaP of the 16S rRNA from living bacteria treated with spectinomycin shows strong protection of C1192 from DMS due to hydrogen bonding between C1192 and spectinomycin [81]. More recently, SHAPE probing has been proposed as a rapid way to conduct high-throughput fragment-based screening of small-molecule RNA ligands [82]. In this method, a synthetic RNA molecule is designed to contain both the target RNA structure and a control structure. Nonspecific binders can be readily identified as they will result in SHAPE reactivity changes for both the target and control structures, while specific binders will only show significant reactivity changes on the target structure. An alternative SHAPE-based approach has also been proposed to map the interaction of small molecules with RNA on a transcriptome-wide scale [83]. In this approach, the small molecule of interest is functionalized with an acylimidazole-substituted linker to enable adduct formation with the ribose 2′-OH at structurally flexible nucleotides, further allowing the detection of small molecule–RNA interactions via RT drop-off or MaP-based readouts.

2.5 Conclusions and Future Prospects

Despite substantial advances, we are still far from being able to accurately map the structure of cellular transcriptomes. Of all the potential limitations and challenges of the methods discussed in this chapter, dealing with RNA structure heterogeneity in the cellular context is definitely the biggest. Although several proof-of-concept studies demonstrated the targeted deconvolution of the RNA structure ensembles of individual transcripts, to date no one has attempted exploring RNA structure heterogeneity on a transcriptome-wide scale. Achieving such resolution of the *RNA structurome* is essential in the perspective of using RNA as a drug target. Pathologically relevant RNAs might populate multiple conformations, and only one of these conformations might actually be responsible for the pathological phenotype, hence making the deconvolution of the RNA structure ensemble a crucial step in target identification. Meeting this challenge requires the cooperative development of improved experimental and computational strategies. For instance, ensemble deconvolution from MaP-based chemical probing experiments has so far been attempted mostly in conjunction with DMS probing, owing to the typically higher signal-to-noise ratio of DMS as compared to other probes, such as SHAPE reagents. This, however, poses substantial limits to our ability to efficiently identify structurally heterogeneous regions as DMS can only probe roughly half of the bases in RNA molecules. The increased signal-to-noise ratio of recently developed SHAPE probes [42], possibly combined with the development of engineered RTs with improved read-through apabilities [84], might help advance with respect to the current state of the art. Furthermore, although powerful, ensemble deconvolution from MaP-based chemical probing experiments likely only provides a coarse-grained representation of the actual ensemble, as small local structural differences might not be efficiently captured. In this regard, the ability to combine the information from orthogonal probing reagents (e.g. DMS and SHAPE), or from orthogonal experimental approaches (e.g. chemical probing and RNA duplex mapping), might help improve the resolution over each individual method, possibly providing more holistic solutions to map cellular RNA structure ensembles.

References

1 ENCODE Project Consortium, Moore, J.E., Purcaro, M.J. et al. (2020). Expanded encyclopaedias of DNA elements in the human and mouse genomes. *Nature* 583 (7818): 699–710.

2 Frankish, A., Diekhans, M., Jungreis, I. et al. (2021). GENCODE 2021. *Nucleic Acids Res.* 49 (D1): D916–D923.

3 Ganser, L.R., Kelly, M.L., Herschlag, D., and Al-Hashimi, H.M. (2019). The roles of structural dynamics in the cellular functions of RNAs. *Nat. Rev. Mol. Cell Biol.* 20 (8): 474–489.

4 Schroeder, R., Barta, A., and Semrad, K. (2004). Strategies for RNA folding and assembly. *Nat. Rev. Mol. Cell Biol.* 5 (11): 908–919.

5 Mitterer, V. and Pertschy, B. RNA folding and functions of RNA helicases in ribosome biogenesis. *RNA Biol.* 19 (1): 781–810.

6 Leppek, K., Das, R., and Barna, M. (2018). Functional 5' UTR mRNA structures in eukaryotic translation regulation and how to find them. *Nat. Rev. Mol. Cell Biol.* 19 (3): 158–174.

7 Halvorsen, M., Martin, J.S., Broadaway, S., and Laederach, A. (2010). Disease-associated mutations that alter the RNA structural ensemble. *PLos Genet.* 6 (8): e1001074.

8 Napierała, M. and Krzyzosiak, W.J. (1997). CUG repeats present in myotonin kinase RNA form metastable “slippery” hairpins. *J Biol Chem* 272 (49): 31079–31085.

9 Leppert, J., Urbinati, C.R., Häfner, S. et al. (2004). Identification of NH...N hydrogen bonds by magic angle spinning solid state NMR in a double-stranded RNA associated with myotonic dystrophy. *Nucleic Acids Res.* 32 (3): 1177–1183.

10 Timchenko, L.T., Miller, J.W., Timchenko, N.A. et al. (1996). Identification of a (CUG)n triplet repeat RNA-binding protein and its expression in myotonic dystrophy. *Nucleic Acids Res.* 24 (22): 4407–4414.

11 Roberts, R., Timchenko, N.A., Miller, J.W. et al. (1997). Altered phosphorylation and intracellular distribution of a (CUG)n triplet repeat RNA-binding protein in patients with myotonic dystrophy and in myotonin protein kinase knockout mice. *Proc. Natl. Acad. Sci. U.S.A.* 94 (24): 13221–13226.

12 Philips, A.V., Timchenko, L.T., and Cooper, T.A. (1998). Disruption of splicing regulated by a CUG-binding protein in myotonic dystrophy. *Science* 280 (5364): 737–741.

13 Boerneke, M.A., Ehrhardt, J.E., and Weeks, K.M. (2019). Physical and functional analysis of viral RNA genomes by SHAPE. *Annu. Rev. Virol.* 6 (1): 93–117.

14 Manfredonia, I. and Incarnato, D. (2020). Structure and regulation of coronavirus genomes: state-of-the-art and novel insights from SARS-CoV-2 studies. *Biochem. Soc. Trans.* 49 (1): 341–352.

15 Lee, E., Bujalowski, P.J., Teramoto, T. et al. (2021). Structures of flavivirus RNA promoters suggest two binding modes with NS5 polymerase. *Nat. Commun.* 12 (1): 2530.

16 Sherpa, C., Rausch, J.W., Le Grice, S.F.J. et al. (2015). The HIV-1 Rev response element (RRE) adopts alternative conformations that promote different rates of virus replication. *Nucleic Acids Res.* 43 (9): 4676–4686.

17 Zuker, M. and Sankoff, D. (1984). RNA secondary structures and their prediction. *Bull. Math. Biol.* 46 (4): 591–621.

18 Chen, S.-J. (2008). RNA folding: conformational statistics, folding kinetics, and ion electrostatics. *Annu. Rev. Biophys.* 37: 197–214.

19 Herschlag, D. (1995). RNA chaperones and the RNA folding problem. *J. Biol. Chem.* 270 (36): 20871–20874.

20 Xia, T., SantaLucia, J., Burkard, M.E. et al. (1998). Thermodynamic parameters for an expanded nearest-neighbor model for formation of RNA duplexes with Watson-Crick base pairs. *Biochemistry* 37 (42): 14719–14735.

21 Mathews, D.H. (2004). Using an RNA secondary structure partition function to determine confidence in base pairs predicted by free energy minimization. *RNA* 10 (8): 1178–1190.

22 Zhang, J., Fei, Y., Sun, L., and Zhang, Q.C. (2022). Advances and opportunities in RNA structure experimental determination and computational modeling. *Nat. Methods* 19 (10): 1193–1207.

23 Szikszai, M., Wise, M., Datta, A. et al. (2022). Deep learning models for RNA secondary structure prediction (probably) do not generalize across families. *Bioinformatics* 38 (16): 3892–3899.

24 Flamm, C., Wielach, J., Wolfinger, M.T. et al. (2022). Caveats to deep learning approaches to RNA secondary structure prediction. *Front. Bioinf.* 2: 835422.

25 Mathews, D.H., Disney, M.D., Childs, J.L. et al. (2004). Incorporating chemical modification constraints into a dynamic programming algorithm for prediction of RNA secondary structure. *Proc. Natl. Acad. Sci. U.S.A.* 101 (19): 7287–7292.

26 Deigan, K.E., Li, T.W., Mathews, D.H., and Weeks, K.M. (2009). Accurate SHAPE-directed RNA structure determination. *Proc. Natl. Acad. Sci. U.S.A.* 106 (1): 97–102.

27 Wells, S.E., Hughes, J.M., Igel, A.H., and Ares, M. (2000). Use of dimethyl sulfate to probe RNA structure in vivo. *Methods Enzymol.* 318: 479–493.

28 Simon, L.M., Morandi, E., Luganini, A. et al. (2019). In vivo analysis of influenza A mRNA secondary structures identifies critical regulatory motifs. *Nucleic Acids Res.* 47 (13): 7003–7017.

29 Manfredonia, I., Nithin, C., Ponce-Salvatierra, A. et al. (2020). Genome-wide mapping of SARS-CoV-2 RNA structures identifies therapeutically-relevant elements. *Nucleic Acids Res.* 48 (22): 12436–12452.

30 Lan, T.C.T., Allan, M.F., Malsick, L.E. et al. (2022). Secondary structural ensembles of the SARS-CoV-2 RNA genome in infected cells. *Nat. Commun.* 13 (1): 1128.

31 Rouskin, S., Zubradt, M., Washietl, S. et al. (2014). Genome-wide probing of RNA structure reveals active unfolding of mRNA structures in vivo. *Nature* 505 (7485): 701–705.

32 Zubradt, M., Gupta, P., Persad, S. et al. (2017). DMS-MaPseq for genome-wide or targeted RNA structure probing in vivo. *Nat. Methods* 14 (1): 75–82.

33 Beaudoin, J.-D., Novoa, E.M., Vejnar, C.E. et al. (2018). Analyses of mRNA structure dynamics identify embryonic gene regulatory programs. *Nat. Struct. Mol. Biol.* 25 (8): 677–686.

34 Incarnato, D., Morandi, E., Simon, L.M., and Oliviero, S. (2018). RNA Framework: an all-in-one toolkit for the analysis of RNA structures and post-transcriptional modifications. *Nucleic Acids Res.* 46 (16): e97.

35 Mustoe, A.M., Lama, N.N., Irving, P.S. et al. (2019). RNA base-pairing complexity in living cells visualized by correlated chemical probing. *Proc. Natl. Acad. Sci. U.S.A.* 116 (49): 24574–24582.

36 Mitchell, D., Ritchey, L.E., Park, H. et al. (2018). Glyoxals as in vivo RNA structural probes of guanine base-pairing. *RNA* 24 (1): 114–124.

37 Weng, X., Gong, J., Chen, Y. et al. (2020). Keth-seq for transcriptome-wide RNA structure mapping. *Nat. Chem. Biol.* 16 (5): 489–492.

38 Mitchell, D., Renda, A.J., Douds, C.A. et al. (2019). In vivo RNA structural probing of uracil and guanine base-pairing by 1-ethyl-3-(3-dimethylaminopropyl) carbodiimide (EDC). *RNA* 25 (1): 147–157.

39 Wang, P.Y., Sexton, A.N., Culligan, W.J., and Simon, M.D. (2019). Carbodiimide reagents for the chemical probing of RNA structure in cells. *RNA* 25 (1): 135–146.

40 Merino, E.J., Wilkinson, K.A., Coughlan, J.L., and Weeks, K.M. (2005). RNA structure analysis at single nucleotide resolution by selective 2′-hydroxyl acylation and primer extension (SHAPE). *J. Am. Chem. Soc.* 127 (12): 4223–4231.

41 Spitale, R.C., Crisalli, P., Flynn, R.A. et al. (2013). RNA SHAPE analysis in living cells. *Nat. Chem. Biol.* 9 (1): 18–20.

42 Marinus, T., Fessler, A.B., Ogle, C.A., and Incarnato, D. (2021). A novel SHAPE reagent enables the analysis of RNA structure in living cells with unprecedented accuracy. *Nucleic Acids Res.* 49 (6): e34.

43 Busan, S., Weidmann, C.A., Sengupta, A., and Weeks, K.M. (2019). Guidelines for SHAPE reagent choice and detection strategy for RNA structure probing studies. *Biochemistry* 58 (23): 2655–2664.

44 Feng, C., Chan, D., Joseph, J. et al. (2018). Light-activated chemical probing of nucleobase solvent accessibility inside cells. *Nat. Chem. Biol.* 14 (3): 276–283.

45 Costa, M. and Monachello, D. (2014). Probing RNA folding by hydroxyl radical footprinting. *Methods Mol. Biol.* 1086: 119–142.

46 Adilakshmi, T., Lease, R.A., and Woodson, S.A. (2006). Hydroxyl radical footprinting in vivo: mapping macromolecular structures with synchrotron radiation. *Nucleic Acids Res.* 34 (8): e64.

47 Strobel, E.J., Yu, A.M., and Lucks, J.B. (2018). High-throughput determination of RNA structures. *Nat. Rev. Genet.* 19 (10): 615–634.

48 Homan, P.J., Favorov, O.V., Lavender, C.A. et al. (2014). Single-molecule correlated chemical probing of RNA. *Proc. Natl. Acad. Sci. U.S.A.* 111 (38): 13858–13863.

49 Siegfried, N.A., Busan, S., Rice, G.M. et al. (2014). RNA motif discovery by SHAPE and mutational profiling (SHAPE-MaP). *Nat. Methods* 11 (9): 959–965.

50 Xiao, L., Fang, L., and Kool, E.T. (2022). Acylation probing of "generic" RNA libraries reveals critical influence of loop constraints on reactivity. *Cell Chem. Biol.* 29 (8): 1341–1352.

51 Xiao, L., Fang, L., Chatterjee, S., and Kool, E.T. (2022). Diverse reagent scaffolds provide differential selectivity of 2′-OH Acylation in RNA. *J. Am. Chem. Soc.* https://doi.org/10.1021/jacs.2c09040.

52 Ramani, V., Qiu, R., and Shendure, J. (2015). High-throughput determination of RNA structure by proximity ligation. *Nat. Biotechnol.* 33 (9): 980–984.

53 Lu, Z., Zhang, Q.C., Lee, B. et al. (2016). RNA duplex map in living cells reveals higher order transcriptome structure. *Cell* 165 (5): 1267–1279.

54 Aw, J.G.A., Shen, Y., Wilm, A. et al. (2016). In vivo mapping of eukaryotic RNA interactomes reveals principles of higher-order organization and regulation. *Mol. Cell* 62 (4): 603–617.

55 Sharma, E., Sterne-Weiler, T., O'Hanlon, D., and Blencowe, B.J. (2016). Global mapping of human RNA-RNA interactions. *Mol. Cell* 62 (4): 618–626.

56 Nguyen, T.C., Cao, X., Yu, P. et al. (2016). Mapping RNA–RNA interactome and RNA structure in vivo by MARIO. *Nat. Commun.* 7 (1): 12023.

57 Ziv, O., Gabryelska, M.M., Lun, A.T.L. et al. (2018). COMRADES determines in vivo RNA structures and interactions. *Nat. Methods* 15 (10): 785–788.

58 Cimino, G.D., Gamper, H.B., Isaacs, S.T., and Hearst, J.E. (1985). Psoralens as photoactive probes of nucleic acid structure and function: organic chemistry, photochemistry, and biochemistry. *Annu. Rev. Biochem.* 54: 1151–1193.

59 Nilsen, T.W. (2014). Detecting RNA-RNA interactions using psoralen derivatives. *Cold Spring Harb. Protoc.* 9: 996–1000.

60 Spitale, R.C. and Incarnato, D. (2022). Probing the dynamic RNA structurome and its functions. *Nat. Rev. Genet.* 1–19.

61 Christy, T.W., Giannetti, C.A., Houlihan, G. et al. (2021). Direct mapping of higher-order RNA interactions by SHAPE-JuMP. *Biochemistry* 60 (25): 1971–1982.

62 Van Damme, R., Li, K., Zhang, M. et al. (2022). Chemical reversible crosslinking enables measurement of RNA 3D distances and alternative conformations in cells. *Nat. Commun.* 13 (1): 911.

63 Houlihan, G., Arangundy-Franklin, S., Porebski, B.T. et al. (2020). Discovery and evolution of RNA and XNA reverse transcriptase function and fidelity. *Nat. Chem.* 12 (8): 683–690.

64 Christy, T.W., Giannetti, C.A., Laederach, A., and Weeks, K.M. (2021). Identifying proximal RNA interactions from cDNA-encoded crosslinks with Shape-Jumper. *PLoS Comput. Biol.* 17 (12): e1009632.

65 Serganov, A. and Nudler, E. (2013). A decade of riboswitches. *Cell* 152 (1): 17–24.

66 Kortmann, J. and Narberhaus, F. (2012). Bacterial RNA thermometers: molecular zippers and switches. *Nat. Rev. Microbiol.* 10 (4): 255–265.

67 Tomezsko, P.J., Corbin, V.D.A., Gupta, P. et al. (2020). Determination of RNA structural diversity and its role in HIV-1 RNA splicing. *Nature* 582 (7812): 438–442.

68 Morandi, E., Manfredonia, I., Simon, L.M. et al. (2021). Genome-scale deconvolution of RNA structure ensembles. *Nat. Methods* 18 (3): 249–252.

69 Olson, S.W., Turner, A.-M.W., Arney, J.W. et al. (2022). Discovery of a large-scale, cell-state-responsive allosteric switch in the 7SK RNA using DANCE-MaP. *Mol. Cell* 82 (9): 1708–1723.e10.

70 Yang, M., Zhu, P., Cheema, J. et al. (2022). In vivo single-molecule analysis reveals COOLAIR RNA structural diversity. *Nature* .

71 Spasic, A., Assmann, S.M., Bevilacqua, P.C., and Mathews, D.H. (2018). Modeling RNA secondary structure folding ensembles using SHAPE mapping data. *Nucleic Acids Res.* 46 (1): 314–323.

72 Li, H. and Aviran, S. (2018). Statistical modeling of RNA structure profiling experiments enables parsimonious reconstruction of structure landscapes. *Nat. Commun.* 9 (1): 606.

73 Yu, A.M., Gasper, P.M., Cheng, L. et al. (2021). Computationally reconstructing cotranscriptional RNA folding from experimental data reveals rearrangement of non-native folding intermediates. *Mol. Cell* 81 (4): 870–883.e10.

74 Aviran, S. and Incarnato, D. (2022). Computational approaches for RNA structure ensemble deconvolution from structure probing data. *J. Mol. Biol.* 167635.

75 Mullard, A. (2017). Small molecules against RNA targets attract big backers. *Nat. Rev. Drug Discovery* 16 (12): 813–815.

76 Warner, K.D., Hajdin, C.E., and Weeks, K.M. (2018). Principles for targeting RNA with drug-like small molecules. *Nat. Rev. Drug Discovery* 17 (8): 547–558.

77 Childs-Disney, J.L., Yang, X., Gibaut, Q.M.R. et al. (2022). Targeting RNA structures with small molecules. *Nat. Rev. Drug Discovery* 21 (10): 736–762.

78 Hewitt, W.M., Calabrese, D.R., and Schneekloth, J.S. (2019). Evidence for ligandable sites in structured RNA throughout the Protein Data Bank. *Bioorg. Med. Chem.* 27 (11): 2253–2260.

79 Padroni, G., Patwardhan, N.N., Schapira, M., and Hargrove, A.E. Systematic analysis of the interactions driving small molecule–RNA recognition. *RSC Med. Chem.* 11 (7): 802–813.

80 Brink, M.F., Brink, G., Verbeet, M.P., and de Boer, H.A. (1994). Spectinomycin interacts specifically with the residues G1064 and C1192 in 16S rRNA, thereby potentially freezing this molecule into an inactive conformation. *Nucleic Acids Res.* 22 (3): 325–331.

81 Sengupta, A., Rice, G.M., and Weeks, K.M. (2019). Single-molecule correlated chemical probing reveals large-scale structural communication in the ribosome and the mechanism of the antibiotic spectinomycin in living cells. *PLoS Biol.* 17 (9): e3000393.

82 Zeller, M.J., Favorov, O., Li, K. et al. (2022). SHAPE-enabled fragment-based ligand discovery for RNA. *Proc. Natl. Acad. Sci. U.S.A.* 119 (20): e2122660119.

83 Fang, L., Velema, W.A., Lee, Y., Lu, X., Mohsen, M.G., Kietrys, A.M., and Kool, E.T. (2022) Pervasive transcriptome interactions of protein-targeted drugs. https://doi.org/10.1101/2022.07.18.500496 .

84 Guo, L.-T., Adams, R.L., Wan, H. et al. (2020). Sequencing and structure probing of long RNAs using MarathonRT: a next-generation reverse transcriptase. *J. Mol. Biol.* 432 (10): 3338–3352.

3

High-Resolution Structures of RNA

Lukas Braun[1], Zahra Alirezaeizanjani[2], Roberta Tesch[2], and Hamed Kooshapur[2]

[1] *Bayer AG Pharmaceuticals, Research and Development, 13353 Berlin, Germany*
[2] *Bayer AG Pharmaceuticals, Research and Development, 42113 Wuppertal, Germany*

3.1 Introduction

Structural biology has become one of the cornerstones of modern drug discovery. Knowing the binding pose of a small molecule with atomistic detail not only helps to understand its mode of action but also makes rational improvements of the compound more straightforward (structure-based drug design [SBDD]). Even in the absence of ligands, structural insights provide a deeper understanding of a drug target and facilitate the generation of new hypotheses. While this holds true for all macromolecules, much of the past work has focused on determining protein structures. This is clearly reflected in the number of deposited structures in the Protein Data Bank (PDB) [1]: the number of RNA structures in the database is orders of magnitude smaller than for proteins. This disparity can be partially attributed to the longstanding belief that most RNAs are largely unstructured or at least too flexible for structure determination. In the 1970s, the crystal structure of phenylalanine transfer RNA (tRNA) was the first direct proof that RNAs can indeed adopt a stable, complex three-dimensional (3D) fold [2–4]. Since then, an ever-growing number of structures have been solved. These contributions have helped to understand how ribozymes achieve their catalytic function, how small molecules regulate riboswitches, and how single-point mutations alter the biological function of noncoding RNAs, to name a few (Figure 3.1) [5–7]. This progress was only possible by applying a broad arsenal of methods, often integrating data from multiple experimental and computational approaches. Recent technological breakthroughs have further helped to accelerate the advances in the field. These improvements come at a time when the first-in-class, small-molecule splicing modifier Risdiplam was successfully brought to the market [8]. While the compound was discovered through a target-agnostic phenotypic screen followed by ligand-based optimization, retrospective structural studies have shown that it binds directly to RNA and modulates its structure [9]. This proof-of-concept has sparked the interest of many academic and industrial research groups in this modality and with it into RNA.

RNA as a Drug Target: The Next Frontier for Medicinal Chemistry, First Edition.
Edited by John Schneekloth and Martin Pettersson.

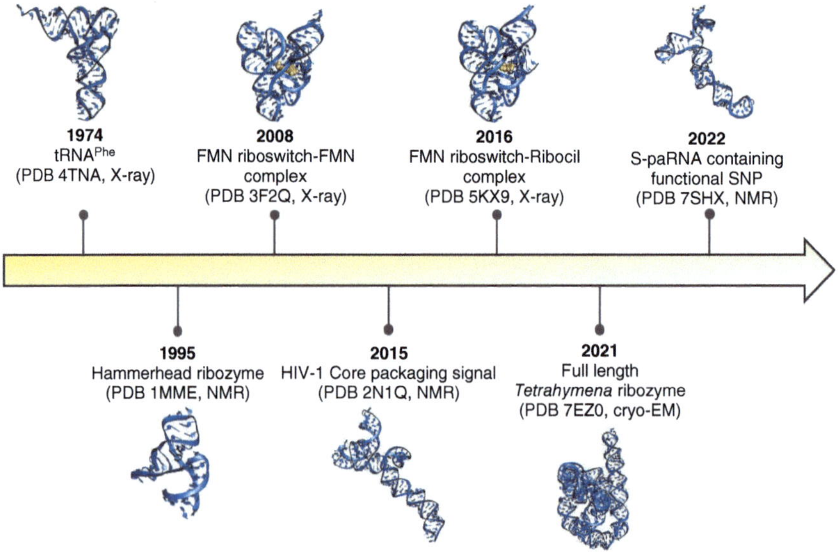

Figure 3.1 A selection of important RNA structures elucidated over the years using different structural biology methods.

The COVID-19 pandemic has brought another boost for RNA structure. After the outbreak, it was quickly realized that the genomic RNA of SARS-CoV-2 contains highly conserved, functional structures that constitute potential drug targets. In record time, a multitude of structures/models of different RNA segments was determined using X-ray crystallography, nuclear magnetic resonance (NMR), cryogenic electron microscopy (cryo-EM), and computational structure prediction [10–12]. Due to this increased focus from a wider community, we will certainly see an uptick in the number of RNA-containing structures over the next years. This not only holds the promise of finding novel ways to treat a wide range of diseases but also new insights into the molecular details of RNA biology.

Considering that RNA is made from only four building blocks, the multitude of complex, intricate folds that it can adopt are truly astonishing. The aromatic bases with their decorations of hydrogen bond donors and acceptors as well as the charged phosphate groups and polar sugar moieties in the backbone give rise to many possible interactions. The best known are certainly Watson-Crick (W-C) base pairs in which the edges of complementary bases interact via matching hydrogen bonds. The base-paring pattern is also referred to as the secondary or 2D structure. Although W-C pairs are ubiquitous in structured RNAs, it is important to note that they are not the main drivers of folding [13]. This role is attributed to stacking interactions between the bases [13, 14]. The faces of these aromatic ring systems are highly hydrophobic. Placing them on top of each other shields them from the solvent and allows for favorable interactions with their π-orbitals [15]. Due to this driving force, the ends of adjacent helices tend to stack on top of each other (co-axial stacking). Likewise, it is often more favorable for unpaired bases in junctions or (internal) loops to be buried into the structure. This can lead to kinks and distortions in the fold or bring sequentially distant regions of the molecule in close spatial proximity [13, 14]. This tertiary structure is then further stabilized by a multitude of polar and charged interactions. These include non-W-C base pairs, base triples or even quadruples, extensive hydrogen bonding between the backbone sugars, or charge-assisted hydrogen bonds with the phosphate groups.

In solution, biomolecules are best described as a dynamic ensemble of interconverting conformations. The relative population of each conformation is dictated by the underlying free energy landscape [16]. Even lowly populated states with short lifetimes can be functionally important. Some RNA sequences encode a free energy landscape with few deep valleys leading to stable folds with slow transitions between different states. Others have a flatter landscape with rapid interconversion of conformations. In general, RNAs are more flexible than globular proteins [17]. The relative abundance of conformations in an RNA ensemble can be strongly modulated by cellular conditions (e.g. pH), binding partners, and posttranscriptional modifications. For RNA folding, the presence of mono- and divalent cations that help to shield the strong electrostatic repulsion of the negatively charged backbone is often required to stabilize the final fold [18]. Within cells, most RNAs associate with proteins and function as ribonucleoprotein complexes (RNPs). Protein binding can also shift the population of a given state, as was shown for the HIV-1 RNA (see Section 3.3). The ensemble view on RNA is important for a mechanistic understanding of how it folds, functions, and binds to small molecules [19]. Since most RNAs do not have catalytic activity, blocking of an active site is typically not a path forward for drug design. Instead, a ligand could stabilize a conformation of the ensemble that leads to the desired biological outcome.

Nowadays, structural biologists have a large toolbox for elucidating RNA structures and dynamics, each with their own strengths and limitations. In this chapter, we provide an overview of the main experimental and computational methods for determining RNA structures at (near) atomistic level and highlight key achievements in the field. Despite the essential role of RNA–protein interactions in many biological processes, discussing RNPs would go beyond the scope of this chapter. Therefore, we will focus on systems containing only RNA.

3.2 X-Ray Crystallography

X-ray crystallography, the oldest method in structural biology, delivered the first breakthrough in RNA structure determination: the structure of the yeast phenylalanine tRNA ($tRNA^{Phe}$). In the 1970s, for the first time, scientists were able to see that the cloverleaf secondary structure adopts an L-shaped conformation in 3D [2–4]. However, due to the dynamic nature of many RNAs, the formation of well-diffracting crystals remains generally challenging. Crystallization is further impaired by the uniformity of the charged phosphate backbone, which can impede the formation of crystal contacts. To overcome these challenges, different engineering techniques have been developed over the years. For a recent review see [20].

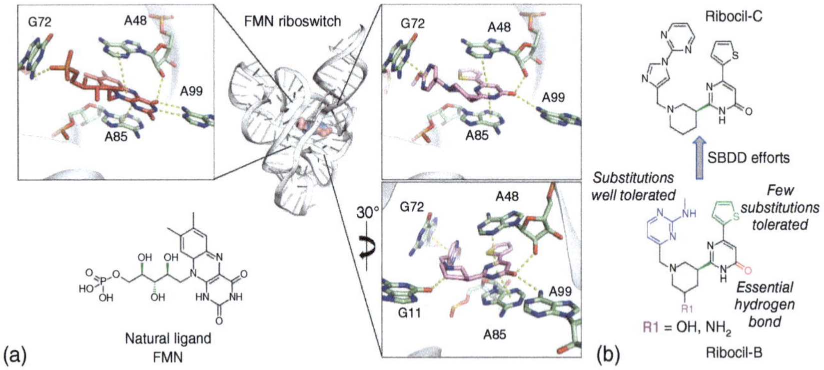

Figure 3.2 (a) X-ray structure of FMN riboswitch bound to the natural ligand FMN (left, PDB: 3F2Q) and ribocil (right, PDB: 5C45). Interactions are highlighted as yellow dashes. Distance between the piperidinyl ring of ribocil (light pink) and G11 (light green) guides the addition of hydroxyl group in that region. (b) SAR profile of ribocil-B analogs leading to the higher potent compound ribocil-C.

X-ray crystallography has been most successful for the structure determination of riboswitches. Riboswitches are regions of mRNA that contain a ligand-binding aptamer domain that senses small molecules (such as metabolites) and an expression platform that responds by undergoing a conformational change, thereby modulating gene expression [21, 22]. The elucidation of diverse riboswitch structures has provided important molecular insights into RNA ligand recognition that could be leveraged for the design of RNA-targeting drugs [23].

The presence of a ligand-binding site in riboswitches provides an opportunity for developing small molecules that bind to these pockets and inhibit the biological function of these regulatory elements. Ribocil is a member of a new class of antibiotics that modulates the bacterial flavin mononucleotide (FMN) riboswitch [24]. In the crystal structure, ribocil adopts a constrained U-shaped conformation with a key interaction between the pyrimidonyl oxygen and A48 and A99. When comparing the FMN and ribocil-bound structures, FMN and ribocil overlap in terms of interaction with the RNA-binding pocket, but ribocil has additional stacking interactions with other bases [6, 25] (Figure 3.2).

Moreover, the racemic mixture of ribocil was used during the crystallization experiments but only one of the isomers ((S)-isomer, ribocil-B) was bound to RNA based on the electron density map. This was further confirmed with the microbiological activity of the separated enantiomers. Following this, SBDD was applied with the crystal structure of analogs to improve the inhibitory activity of ribocil-B. Modifications of the amino-pyrimidine moiety were more tolerated than those on the thiophene ring, and a hydroxyl group attached to the piperidine ring allowed additional interactions with G11. The medicinal chemistry efforts together with the established structure–activity relationship (SAR) led to ribocil-C with eightfold higher potency than the lead compound [25] (Figure 3.2).

X-ray crystallography has revealed another structural element that could have an impact on RNA-targeted drug discovery: the triple helix [26, 27]. Specifically,

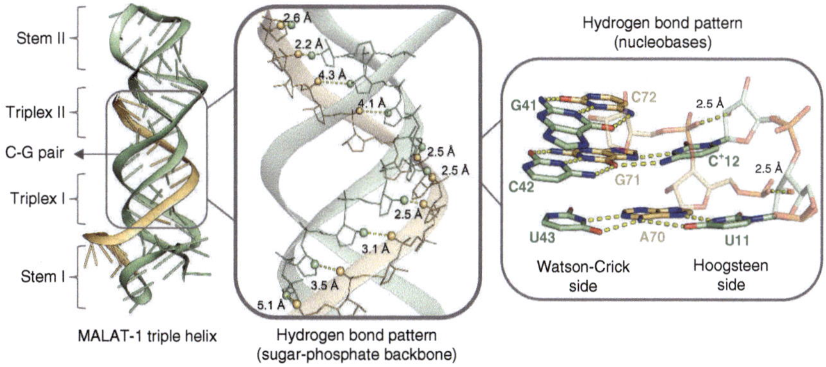

Figure 3.3 X-ray structure of MALAT-1 ENE core (PDB: 4PLX). The A-rich tail is colored in light yellow. Distances between the 2′-hydroxyl (light green spheres) of the double helix and the backbone phosphate (light yellow spheres) of the A-rich strand are indicated. The hydrogen bond network of U-A-U, C⁺-G-C, and C-G pairs is shown.

MALAT-1 (metastasis associated lung adenocarcinoma transcript 1) is one of the most studied long noncoding RNAs (lncRNAs) and has been described as a potential predictive biomarker for metastasis development in numerous cancers [28]. The 3′-end of MALAT-1 contains a motif known as the expression and nuclear retention element (ENE). The ENE stabilizes the RNA by inhibiting its degradation through the formation of a triple helix with an A-rich tail.

The crystal structure of MALAT-1 ENE revealed different structural elements, specifically a bipartite triple helix that is interrupted by a C-G pair leading to the formation of independent triple helices (triplex I and II) [29]. These helices are comprised of U-A-U triples that have a combination of W-C and Hoogsteen base pairs. Triplex I has an additional triple interaction formed by C^+-G-C and is stabilized by a C-G pair (C72-G41). Moreover, mutations in C-G and C^+-G-C lead to an increase in the RNA decay, indicating an important functional and structural role for these base pairs. The disruption of the U-A-U triple also changes the distance profile between the backbone phosphate of the A-rich tail and the 2′ hydroxyl of the double helix (represented as spheres in Figure 3.3). This distance profile is important for minimizing the electrostatic clashes in the sugar-phosphate backbone [29].

Since MALAT-1 has been implicated in different malignancies, the triple helix structure is a potential drug target. The available crystal structure presented an opportunity for identifying MALAT-1 ligands through virtual screening methods and studying the potential binding mode of new drug molecules One example is the work of Le Grice and collaborators that combined small-molecule microarray (SMM) screening, biophysical, and computational methods to identify chemotypes that affect the stabilization of the MALAT-1 ENE triplex [30]. The most promising compounds that were identified bind MALAT-1 ENE triplex but do not affect NEAT1, a lncRNA with a similar triple helix structure. Docking of these compounds on the RNA showed preference for distinct regions. In addition, saturation transfer difference (STD) NMR confirmed the binding of one of the hit compounds to MALAT-1 ENE triplex but not to other known triple helices. The compounds identified in this work not only affect the levels of MALAT-1 in a cellular context but also modulate previously identified downstream targets. However, the main challenge is understanding the biological mechanisms of poly(A) protection by the formation of the triplex structure. Nevertheless, the increasing knowledge of ENE structures and its presence in equivalent motifs from other RNAs [31] together with the discovery of new chemical tools could lead to new drug discovery programs.

3.3 NMR Spectroscopy

NMR spectroscopy is a highly versatile technique that provides atomic-resolution insight into structure, dynamics, and interactions of biomolecules and has played a pivotal role in RNA structural biology. Since the first solution structure of an RNA molecule (a 12 nt hairpin) reported in 1990 [32], several hundred NMR structures of RNA in the free form and in complex with various binding partners have been reported. Currently, around one-third of RNA-only structures deposited in the PDB are obtained by NMR spectroscopy. Further, NMR can readily report on base pairing and determine the secondary structures of RNA.

Despite the great success, structure determination of RNA by NMR remains challenging [33]. Compared to proteins that are made of 20 amino acids, RNA is composed of only four nucleotides with similar chemical structures; this leads to lower chemical shift dispersion and overlap of NMR signals. In addition, there is a lower density of protons in RNA and they typically form extended structures; thus, the number of intramolecular contacts that can be obtained is limited. These challenges are exacerbated in large RNAs (>50 nt) where the NMR signals are broadened owing to slower tumbling of larger molecules in solution. As of now, the average size of NMR-derived RNA structures is 29 nt, the largest RNA structure determined by NMR is 155 nt, and fewer than ten structures above 100 nt have been deposited in the PDB.

Several approaches have been developed for reducing signal overlap and simplifying NMR spectroscopy of large RNAs. One strategy is "divide-and-conquer" in which the RNA is divided into domains that are studied separately. This is only applicable when the conformation of the domains is maintained in the context of the intact RNA. As an example, for determining the structure of the 77 nt (~25 kDa) domain II of the hepatitis C virus (HCV) internal ribosome entry site (IRES), the RNA was divided into two subdomains that were analyzed individually for assigning the chemical shifts (CS) and obtaining short-range distance information based on nuclear Overhauser effect (NOE) and other local restraints. These were then combined with long-range residual dipolar coupling (RDC) restraints obtained from the full-length RNA [34]. For cases where divide-and-conquer is not applicable, segmental labeling is the method of choice. Here isotopically labeled and unlabeled regions of an RNA are ligated to form the full-length RNA that is only partially labeled and hence visible in the NMR spectra [35]. Although sample preparation can be laborious, such labeling strategies can drastically improve the quality of NMR spectra by reducing the number of signals. Another selective isotope-labeling approach that has made a huge impact on the application of NMR to larger RNAs is selective deuteration of nucleotides that reduces signal overlap and narrows the linewidth of NMR signals [36]. This deuterium-edited NMR approach enabled the structure determination of the HIV-1 core packaging signal, the largest RNA structure solved by NMR [37], and has been applied to RNAs as large as 232 kDa [38]. Combined with selective isotope-labeling methods, advances in NMR methodology, computation, and integrative structural biology have allowed NMR structural studies of RNAs with increasing size.

An advantage of NMR over other structural biology methods discussed here is that it provides atomic-resolution insights of RNAs under native-like conditions in solution. In one study, NMR analysis of a class II GTP riboswitch revealed that a protonated adenine (A+) with a pK_a value that is shifted by more than five pH units (relative to the nucleotide in single-stranded RNA) stabilizes the tertiary structure [39]. This exceptionally large shift in pK_a is comparable to the largest shifts observed for amino acid sidechains. Consistent with the NMR data, the affinity of the RNA for GTP was found to be highly pH-dependent. The NMR structure of this aptamer in complex with GTP showed that the A+ is stabilized by the structure of a unique base quartet (G:A+:C:G) where the N1 atom of adenine is protonated. Other structural features of this aptamer are two base triplets, one of which includes the GTP-binding site and a *trans* A:A base pair (Figure 3.4). This work highlights the importance of protonated nucleotides as building blocks in RNA tertiary structure and illustrates how the RNA fold can dramatically shift the protonation state of nucleotides with functional implications.

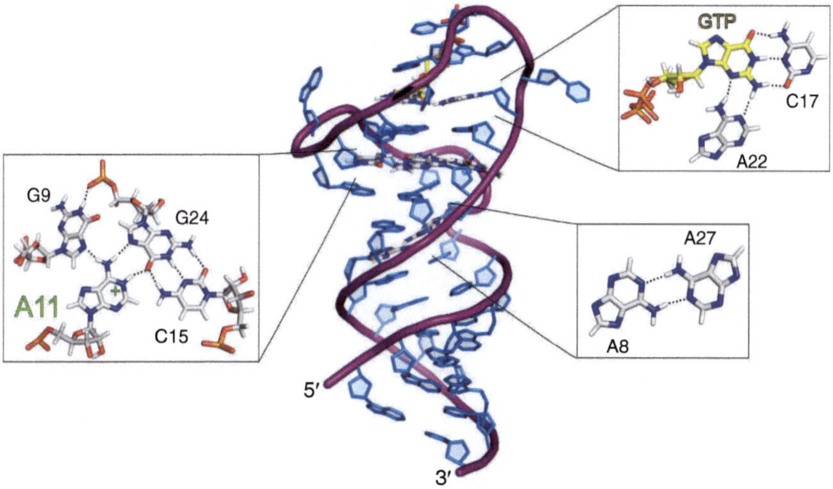

Figure 3.4 NMR structure of the class II GTP aptamer in complex with GTP (PDB: 5LWJ). Hydrogen bonds in unique structural features are highlighted. These include a unique base quartet formed by a protonated adenine (A11+), a base triplet formed by GTP and a *trans* A:A base pair.

NMR spectroscopy has been instrumental in probing RNA–small molecule interactions [40]. Because it can detect weak interactions, NMR-based screening is a popular method in early drug discovery campaigns, as exemplified by the work on targeting the SARS-CoV-2 RNA [41]. A recent study based on NMR chemical shift mapping and structure-based survey revealed that drug-like small molecules form hydrogen bonds with functional groups that are exposed in stem-loop RNAs [42].

Several NMR structures of RNA bound to aminoglycoside antibiotics have been reported [43–45], but perhaps the most important structure of an RNA-drug complex solved by NMR spectroscopy is that of the RNA duplex formed by the U1 snRNA 5′-end and the 5′ splice site of *SMN2* pre-mRNA exon 7 (E7) in complex with a splicing modifier [9]. The solution structures of the RNA duplex free and bound to SMN-C5 (an analog of Risdiplam) revealed that the drug stabilizes an unpaired (bulged) adenine at position -1 at the exon-intron junction in the major groove of the RNA helix. The structural studies suggest that SMN-C5 strengthens the interaction between U1 snRNP and the 5′ splice site of *SMN2* E7, thereby promoting E7 inclusion in a mechanism referred to as "5′ splice site bulge repair" (Figure 3.5). However, it is important to note that these NMR experiments have been conducted in a system containing only RNA and the compound. In a cellular context, interactions with protein components of U1 snRNP and splicing modulators are likely to play a significant role. A deeper understanding of these interactions is needed to fully understand the mechanism of action of Risdiplam and its analogs. Nevertheless, this work is an important step in this direction and highlights the strength of NMR spectroscopy in providing atomic-resolution insight into RNA–drug interactions.

NMR spectroscopy is unique as it can provide atomic-resolution insight into the dynamics of RNAs over a wide range of timescales enabling a quantitative description of the RNA conformational landscape [47–49]. The highly conserved HIV-1 trans-activation response (TAR) element RNA is an important target for development of antiviral drugs and has served as a model system for NMR studies on RNA conformational dynamics. TAR undergoes large interhelical motions in solution and

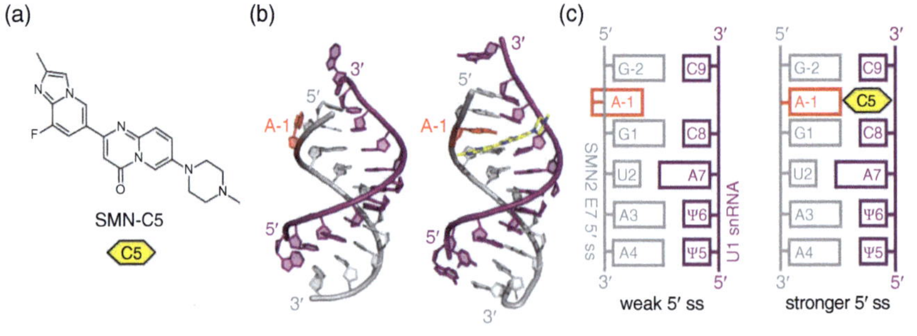

Figure 3.5 (a) Chemical structure of SMN-C5. (b) NMR structure of the duplex involving U1 snRNA 5′-end (purple) and 5′ splice site of *SMN2* E7 (gray) in the free form (left, PDB: 6HMI) and bound to SMN-C5 (right, PDB: 6HMO). (c) The 5′ splice site bulge-repair mechanism proposes that splicing modifiers, such as SMN-C5, bind to a bulged nucleotide and strengthen the interaction of U1 snRNP and the 5′ splice site (ss), thereby converting a weak splice site to a stronger one. Source: Adapted from [46].

binds to diverse ligands such as arginine derivatives and peptides derived from its cognate partner Tat [50–52]. NMR studies have shown that these molecules capture "pre-existing" conformations in TAR and shift the conformational equilibrium [53].

There is growing evidence that RNA conformations with exceptionally low populations (even below 1%) and short lifetimes (as low as a few microseconds), known as excited states (ES), play an important regulatory role [54]. Such states are not detectable by conventional structural biology approaches. However, advanced NMR methods based on relaxation dispersion (RD) allow the characterization of the ES conformation, population, and lifetime providing a quantitative description of exchange processes such as ligand binding [47].

A mechanistic understanding of ES would provide new opportunities for RNA-targeted therapeutics. In one study, the affinity of argininamide (ARG) to a TAR ES in the dynamic ensemble was estimated to be significantly higher than the apparent overall weak affinity of ARG for this RNA [55]. In another study, Al-Hashimi and coworkers showed that small molecules, such as ARG, can preferentially bind and stabilize the ES over the ground state (GS) conformation of a TAR mutant [56]. These studies demonstrate that, in principle, RNA ES can be targeted by small molecules and suggest that preferential binding to the ES may be a general mechanism by which ligands achieve selectivity for their target RNAs.

Another example that highlights the functional importance of ES is the *Bacillus cereus* fluoride riboswitch aptamer domain. This RNA adopts identical structures in the ligand-free (*apo*) and ligand-bound (*holo*) forms, but with distinct functional outcomes. NMR chemical exchange saturation transfer (CEST) experiments revealed that the *apo* form transiently samples an ES that had not been detected by conventional biophysical methods. The *apo* ES unlocks a highly conserved "linchpin" base pair, thereby providing a kinetically favorable path that leads to transcription termination. Upon fluoride binding, conformational transition to the ES is suppressed, and transcription is activated [57]. This study not only uncovers a new mode of RNA regulation that is based on ligand-induced suppression of an ES but also highlights the power of NMR spectroscopy in providing atomic-resolution insights into conformational states that are invisible to other structural biology techniques.

3.4 Cryo-EM

Recent hardware and software breakthroughs in single-particle cryo-EM have led to a dramatic increase in the number of high-resolution structures of proteins and complex macromolecular assemblies. However, the number of RNA-only structures has grown at a much slower pace; currently, only a handful of structures below 3.5 Å resolution are available in the PDB [1] and the Electron Microscopy Data Bank (EMDB) [58].

Despite the challenges, recent studies have shown the great potential of cryo-EM for obtaining atomic insights into RNA structures. An important achievement was determining the structure of the complete *Tetrahymena* group I self-splicing intron, the first discovered ribozyme [59], that had remained unknown for forty years. The cryo-EM map at 3.1 Å resolution revealed previously unseen tertiary interactions and enabled the localization of metal ions that are important for the stability and catalytic activity of this ribozyme [60]. This study illustrates the power of modern single-particle cryo-EM in determining atomic-resolution structures of RNAs that had previously been intractable.

An important parameter in cryo-EM structure determination is the size of the particle. Most macromolecular structures solved by cryo-EM are larger than ~200 kDa, although the size limit has been continuously reduced over the years [61]. The size, shape and flexibility of many biological RNAs pose challenges for cryo-EM. To overcome these a method called "RNA oligomerization-enabled cryo-EM via installing kissing-loops" (ROCK) was proposed. It is based on insertion of kissing-loop sequences in peripheral helices of the RNA to mediate self-assembly into a homo-oligomeric ring [62]. This strategy increases the molecular weight of the RNA while reducing the flexibility of each monomer in the assembly. Further, the assembled RNAs have a characteristic symmetric shape that can facilitate cryo-EM data processing. The key step in the ROCK approach is RNA construct engineering that relies on computational modeling or prior structural information. At least two helices are needed for installing the kissing-loop sequences and the length of these must be optimized to ensure ring formation. Using ROCK, Liu et al. obtained a high-quality sub-3 Å resolution map of the *Tetrahymena* ribozyme that allowed de novo model building of the whole RNA. However, given the challenges associated with construct engineering and potential changes to the native RNA structure, the general applicability of this approach remains to be seen.

Because cryo-EM samples are rapidly cooled, the different conformers that are present in the ensemble are preserved and can, in theory, be visualized. Recently the Kieft group reported on the structure and dynamics of the brome mosaic virus tRNA-like structure (BMV TLS) that is aminoacylated by the host's tyrosyl-tRNA synthetase (TyrRS) [17, 63]. Surprisingly, the cryo-EM structure of the BMV TLS RNA revealed that it lacks a typical L-shaped tRNA fold. Further analysis of the data tailored towards detecting the conformational variability showed that one stem of the TLS RNA is highly dynamic, perhaps explaining why it had escaped crystallization. In addition, structures of the TLS-TyRS complex demonstrated that the RNA undergoes a large rearrangement upon binding to the enzyme and that the complex also samples multiple conformations [17]. This work highlights the utility of cryo-EM for characterizing conformational dynamics of RNAs and RNPs. A recent study has shown that cryo-EM can also visualize RNA folding intermediates [64]. Whether cryo-EM sample freezing and radiation biases the conformational ensemble of RNA requires further investigation.

Cryo-EM maps of small RNA-only systems are generally of low resolution, thus prohibiting accurate de novo model building. Therefore, a hybrid approach is often necessary for obtaining atomic-resolution information. In one study a hybrid NMR/cryo-EM approach was used to determine the structure of the 30 kDa HIV-1 RNA dimerization signal [65]. In this work, the cryo-EM map at 9 Å resolution, which reports on the global RNA topology, was used as a restraint and combined with NMR-derived local distance restraints to generate a structure with atomic level information. The structure revealed features such as a previously unobserved bulged nucleotide. Further applications of cryo-EM in integrative structural biology are discussed in the next section.

3.5 3D Structure Prediction and Integrative Approaches

Advances in RNA sequencing have led to a rapid growth in the number of newly described RNA families [66]. For most of these families not a single structure has been solved yet, hampering our understanding of their molecular function. Since experimental structure determination is laborious and time-consuming, this gap will only expand in the future. Recent breakthroughs in artificial intelligence (AI) based protein structure prediction have shown that computational tools have the potential to generate models with often astonishing quality at an extremely high throughput. Although RNA 3D structure prediction methods have not reached the level of their protein counterparts yet, significant progress has been made over the last couple of years.

The most straightforward approach to predict the fold of a new RNA (target) is to rely on the already solved structure of a close homologue (template). Just like for protein homology modelling, the underlying assumption is that similar sequences result in similar structures. For this purpose, the target sequence is threaded onto the template structure [67]. This method allows, for example, the exchange of a GC for an AT pair in a helical region of the template structure, while maintaining its local geometry. Changes in non-W-C base pairs or differences in loop regions usually need to be modelled with different approaches. This means that except for very closely related RNAs, homology modeling will not suffice. Its applicability is further reduced by the small number of available templates. However, the modular nature of RNA folds sometimes allows the identification of small, conserved motifs in otherwise unrelated molecules. An example is the tetraloop-receptor interaction, a tertiary motif occurring in a wide range of RNAs [68]. Finding these motifs requires expert knowledge but can dramatically improve the success of downstream modelling efforts.

Existing structural information can also be used to produce models of completely unrelated RNAs by focusing on local sequence similarities. To this end, structures of nonhomologous RNAs are broken down into small motifs. These fragment libraries are then matched against the target sequence and recombined to assemble a model of the target molecule that is subsequently refined against a semi-empirical (knowledge-based) scoring function. A popular implementation of this method is the Rosetta-based FARFAR2 (Fragment Assembly of RNA with Full Atom Refinement) algorithm [69]. Other nonfragment-based methods generate models by sampling conformations, e.g. through discrete molecular dynamics (MD) simulations [70].

Independent of the methodological details, the goal of computational modeling is to minimize a physics-based potential or a knowledge-based scoring function.

The first challenge is that these high-dimensional functions cannot be solved analytically and need to be explored by (stochastic) sampling. Unfortunately, the conformational space of a longer RNA becomes extremely large. The reliance on fragment libraries and providing the algorithm with a 2D structure reduce the degrees of freedom. However, the intricate folds of complex RNAs are often mediated by long-range tertiary contacts that are difficult to predict. Thus, many models need to be generated to ensure sufficient sampling. This makes the approach computationally expensive and inaccessible for many larger RNAs. The second challenge is the quality of the potential/scoring function itself. Benchmark studies show that their accuracy is often still inadequate [71]. This means that the algorithm sometimes generates near-native structures but is not able to recognize them as such. Recent advances in deep learning-based RNA model scoring improve the situation, but these learned scoring functions are still far from ideal [71].

The performance of computational structure prediction methods can be significantly enhanced by integrating experimental data from biophysical and biochemical methods. These data can help to generate better models by restricting sampling closer to the native state (Figure 3.6 (a)) or to improve the underlying scoring function (Figure 3.6 (b)). The chance to generate a high-quality model is increased if more of the computing power is spent to explore the conformational space close to the native state by enforcing experimental constraints. Often, just a few constraints are sufficient to improve model quality dramatically, especially if they allow to identify tertiary and non-W-C contacts. The types of constraints can be roughly grouped into two sets. The first type is based on interbase/interatomic distances, while the second type is based on the 3D shape and topology of the whole RNA molecule.

Distance constraints can be derived from a multitude of biophysical/chemical experiments and integrated as pseudo-energy terms to drive the conformational sampling toward the right direction. One of the chemical labeling methods developed to detect tertiary contacts is multiplexed hydroxyl radical (˙OH) cleavage analysis with paired-end sequencing (MOHCA-seq) [72, 73]. Here, an iron (Fe(III)) chelate is randomly attached to different positions of the RNA backbone. Subsequent reduction of the Fe(III) to Fe(II) locally produces hydroxyl radicals that cleave proximal regions of the RNA. It is then possible to deconvolute the position of the cleavage sites and the radical sources and turn them into distance constraints. This method has allowed to structurally characterize a partially folded state of the *Tetrahymena* ribozyme for the first time and to recover complex RNA folds at subnanometer resolution. The advantage of this approach is that it relies just on spatial proximity and not on base-pairing interactions. However, this comes at the price of reduced resolution and noisier data.

Shape constraints can, for example, be derived from mid-resolution cryo-EM maps that do not allow a direct atomistic model building. In this case, an additional pseudo-energy term that enforces a fit to the density map can be employed to guide model building. The Das group developed the Rosetta-based auto-DRRAFTER application that is based on this principle and uses an iterative algorithm to build models directly into the map [74]. Using the published 9 Å resolution map of the

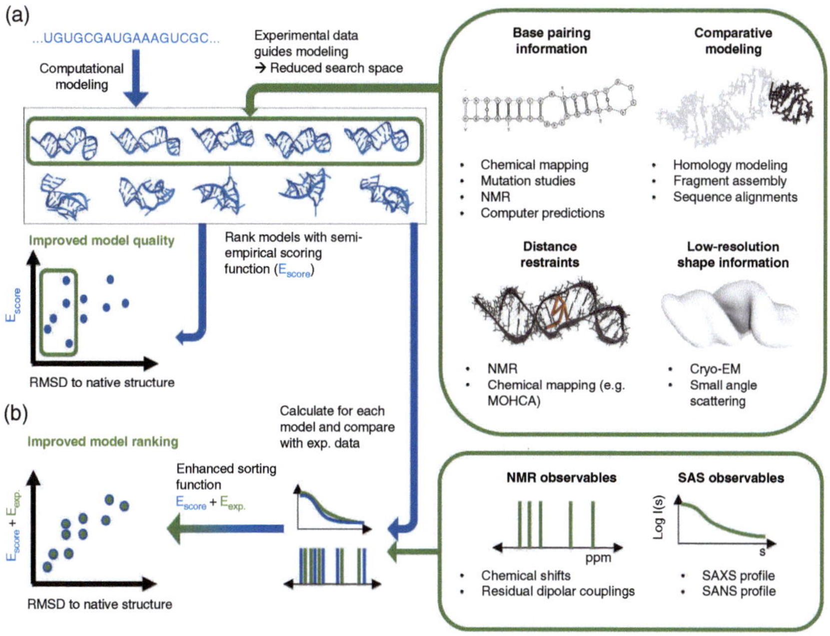

Figure 3.6 Schematic workflow for integrative modeling approaches, combining computational structure prediction with experimental data. (a) In principle, the only required input for computational modeling tools is the primary sequence of the RNA. The algorithm then produces models by sampling the conformational space guided by a scoring function (black box). In the absence of additional constraints, many of the models will deviate significantly from the native structure. The integration of experimental data improves model quality by restricting sampling to regions of the conformational space that agree with these data (left green box). The green box on the right shows examples for different types of experimental restraints. Once a model has been generated, its quality is assessed by the scoring function. Inaccuracies in these functions can prevent the identification of the best model. (b) This issue can be remedied by enhancing the scoring function by a term that rewards closer agreement with experimental data (examples in green box on the right). To this end, the relevant parameters are back-calculated for each model and then compared with the measured values. This rescoring often produces a more accurate model ranking.

HIV-1 RNA dimerization signal (see Section 3.4), they found that the DRRAFTER model agreed well with the NMR-based structure. Based on this, they developed a pipeline named Ribosolve that integrates cryo-EM with chemical mapping information obtained from mutate-and-map by next-generation sequencing (M2-seq) and DRRAFTER [74]. The Ribosolve pipeline can accelerate cryo-EM structure determination of RNA-only systems. Using this pipeline, the authors solved eleven previously unknown RNA structures at 4.7–11 Å resolution. Although the maps are of low resolution, they enable determination of the overall fold and global architecture of RNAs. Recently, the structure of the 28 kDa (88 nt) frameshift stimulation element (FSE) from the SARS-CoV-2 RNA genome was determined using Ribosolve [10]. The 6.9 Å cryo-EM map of this RNA showed helical grooves and guided the design of antisense oligonucleotides (ASOs) that inhibit SARS-CoV-2 replication.

This work exemplifies how structural information of RNA, even at low resolution, can inform strategies for RNA-based therapeutics.

For some types of experimental data, it is more convenient to first generate a set of unbiased models and then use additional information to judge their quality post hoc. Different NMR observables are popular data sources for this method. In the CS-Rosetta-RNA method, CS for nonexchangeable protons are calculated for each model. The scoring function is then extended by a term that compares the calculated CS to the experimental data [75]. This approach has allowed to recover near native models of a diverse set of RNAs that were not recognized by the original scoring function. Shi et al. have demonstrated that a similar approach using NMR RDCs can be used to identify an ensemble of structures from a pool of unbiased models that best describe the experimental data [48]. This FARFAR-NMR approach was used to generate an ensemble structure of the HIV-1 TAR at atomic resolution (PDB: 7JU1), and its general applicability was demonstrated for few RNAs with complex 3D structures.

Complementary data from orthogonal experimental techniques can also generate new insights into RNA structure. Small-angle X-ray/neutron scattering (SAXS/SANS), here referred to as SAS, provides information about the overall shape and dimensions of molecules in solution [76]. Although the structural information provided by SAS is relatively of low resolution, it can be combined with high-resolution data obtained from other biophysical techniques. SAS is highly complementary to solution NMR spectroscopy as it is also performed on samples in solution with the advantage that there are no size limitations [77]. Combining NMR and SAS is a powerful approach for studying the structure and dynamics of RNA and protein-RNA complexes in solution. For example, the structure of the 111 nt U2/U6 snRNA complex was determined by combining NMR, SAXS, and computational modeling [78]. Here, a large number of RNA models were generated using the MC-Fold/MC-Sym pipeline [79], these models were then filtered based on agreement with NMR and SAXS data and further refined. A similar approach was applied to model the structure of the primary miRNA 18a [80].

Describing an RNA ensemble is challenging and requires significant efforts to deconvolute the relative contribution of each conformational state. As mentioned earlier, one way to approach this is by producing a set of computational models and then picking a weighted subset that best describes the experimental data (for a recent review see [81]). Besides methods like FARFAR2, MD simulations are another popular method to produce structural ensembles that can then be reweighted by experimental data. However, simple MD simulations often do not achieve sufficient sampling so that important states of the ensemble can be missed. To overcome this challenge, different enhanced sampling methods can be used to drive the system into new conformational states. Unfortunately, MD forcefields for nucleic acids are not as mature as those for proteins, which can lead to structural artifacts. To avoid this issue, simulations can be constrained by experimental data on-the-fly [82]. This maintains the structure in a conformation that agrees with the experimental data, while the system can still explore other degrees of freedom. The growing interest in RNA structure and dynamics will hopefully lead to advances in the development of RNA-specific forcefields and simulation protocols.

3.6 Conclusions

Soon, half a century will have passed since the determination of the first high-resolution RNA structure. In the five decades since then, structural biology has had a tremendous impact on our understanding of the role of RNA in molecular biology. As the field advances to larger and more complex structures, it will be increasingly difficult to solve them using a single technique. Thus, integrating different experimental and computational approaches is likely to become the key for success. RNA structure determination is and will be a highly interdisciplinary endeavor, bringing together scientists with different experimental and computational expertise. We argue that another important consequence of more available structures is that they will help change the perception of RNA as a “floppy” unstructured molecule. “Seeing is believing” and being exposed to more RNA structures will help us update our mental models. This is especially crucial to garner broad interest in RNA as a drug target. Only if people are convinced that RNA forms functional structures that can potentially be manipulated by a small molecule, will there be broad buy-in into the field of RNA-targeted drug discovery. The recent approval of Risdiplam provides an important proof-of-concept that will drive further investments into this modality. RNA structural biology will certainly play an integral role in finding novel entry points to treat currently untreatable diseases.

Acknowledgments

We are grateful to John O’Donnell for helpful comments. We thank Razvan Nutiu and the entire RNA community at Bayer AG for support.

Conflicts of Interest

All authors of this chapter are employees of Bayer AG.

References

1 Berman, H.M., Westbrook, J., Feng, Z. et al. (2000). The protein data bank. *Nucleic Acids Res.* 28 (1): 235–242.

2 Kim, S.H., Quigley, G.J., Suddath, F.L. et al. (1973). Three-dimensional structure of yeast phenylalanine transfer RNA: folding of the polynucleotide chain. *Science.* 179 (4070): 285–288.

3 Kim, S.H., Suddath, F.L., Quigley, G.J. et al. (1974). Three-dimensional tertiary structure of yeast phenylalanine transfer RNA. *Science.* 185 (4149): 435–440.

4 Robertus, J.D., Ladner, J.E., Finch, J.T. et al. (1974). Structure of yeast phenylalanine tRNA at 3 A resolution. *Nature* 250 (467): 546–551.
5 Golden, B.L., Gooding, A.R., Podell, E.R., and Cech, T.R. (1998). A preorganized active site in the crystal structure of the Tetrahymena ribozyme. *Science.* 282 (5387): 259–264.
6 Serganov, A., Huang, L., and Patel, D.J. (2009). Coenzyme recognition and gene regulation by a flavin mononucleotide riboswitch. *Nature* 458 (7235): 233–237.
7 Sharma, S., Pisignano, G., Merulla, J. et al. (2022). A functional SNP regulates E-cadherin expression by dynamically remodeling the 3D structure of a promoter-associated non-coding RNA transcript. *Nucleic Acids Res.* 50 (19): 11331–11343.
8 Dhillon, S. (2020). Risdiplam: first approval. *Drugs* 80 (17): 1853–1858.
9 Campagne, S., Boigner, S., Rudisser, S. et al. (2019). Structural basis of a small molecule targeting RNA for a specific splicing correction. *Nat. Chem. Biol.* 15 (12): 1191–1198.
10 Zhang, K., Zheludev, I.N., Hagey, R.J. et al. (2021). Cryo-EM and antisense targeting of the 28-kDa frameshift stimulation element from the SARS-CoV-2 RNA genome. *Nat. Struct. Mol. Biol.* 28 (9): 747–754.
11 Wacker, A., Weigand, J.E., Akabayov, S.R. et al. (2020). Secondary structure determination of conserved SARS-CoV-2 RNA elements by NMR spectroscopy. *Nucleic Acids Res.* 48 (22): 12415–12435.
12 Bottaro, S., Bussi, G., and Lindorff-Larsen, K. (2021). Conformational ensembles of noncoding elements in the SARS-CoV-2 genome from molecular dynamics simulations. *JACS* 143 (22): 8333–8343.
13 Vicens, Q. and Kieft, J.S. (2022). Thoughts on how to think (and talk) about RNA structure. *PNAS* 119 (17): e2112677119.
14 Westhof, E. and Fritsch, V. (2000). RNA folding: beyond Watson-Crick pairs. *Structure* 8 (3): R55–R65.
15 Schweizer, M.P., Chan, S.I., and Ts'o, P.O. (1965). Interaction and association of bases and nucleosides in aqueous solutions. IV. Proton magnetic resonance studies of the association of pyrimidine nucleosides and their interactions with purine. *JACS* 87 (22): 5241–5247.
16 Frauenfelder, H., Sligar, S.G., and Wolynes, P.G. (1991). The energy landscapes and motions of proteins. *Science* 254 (5038): 1598–1603.
17 Bonilla, S.L. and Kieft, J.S. (2022). The promise of cryo-EM to explore RNA structural dynamics. *J. Mol. Biol.* 434 (18): 167802.
18 Draper, D.E. (2008). RNA folding: thermodynamic and molecular descriptions of the roles of ions. *Biophys. J.* 95 (12): 5489–5495.
19 Ganser, L.R., Kelly, M.L., Herschlag, D., and Al-Hashimi, H.M. (2019). The roles of structural dynamics in the cellular functions of RNAs. *Nat. Rev. Mol. Cell Biol.* 20 (8): 474–489.
20 Pujari, N., Saundh, S.L., Acquah, F.A. et al. (2021). Engineering crystal packing in RNA Structures I: past and future strategies for engineering RNA packing in crystals. *Crystals (Basel)* 11 (8).

21 Garst AD, Edwards AL, Batey RT. *Riboswitches: Structures and Mechanisms.* Cold Spring Harb Perspect Biol. 2011;3(6).

22 Kavita, K. and Breaker, R.R. (2022). Discovering riboswitches: the past and the future. *Trends Biochem. Sci.*

23 Serganov, A. and Nudler, E. (2013). A decade of riboswitches. *Cell* 152 (1–2): 17–24.

24 Howe, J.A., Wang, H., Fischmann TO et al. (2015). Selective small-molecule inhibition of an RNA structural element. *Nature* 526 (7575): 672–677.

25 Howe, J.A., Xiao, L., Fischmann TO et al. (2016). Atomic resolution mechanistic studies of ribocil: a highly selective unnatural ligand mimic of the E. coli FMN riboswitch. *RNA Biol.* 13 (10): 946–954.

26 Brown, J.A. (2020). Unraveling the structure and biological functions of RNA triple helices. *Wiley Interdiscip. Rev.: RNA* 11 (6): e1598.

27 Conrad, N.K. (2014). The emerging role of triple helices in RNA biology. *Wiley Interdiscip. Rev.: RNA* 5 (1): 15–29.

28 Arun, G., Aggarwal, D., and Spector, D.L. (2020). MALAT1 long non-coding RNA: functional implications. *Noncoding RNA* 6 (2).

29 Brown, J.A., Bulkley, D., Wang, J. et al. (2014). Structural insights into the stabilization of MALAT1 noncoding RNA by a bipartite triple helix. *Nat. Struct. Mol. Biol.* 21 (7): 633–640.

30 Abulwerdi, F.A., Xu, W., Ageeli, A.A. et al. (2019). Selective small-molecule targeting of a triple helix encoded by the long noncoding RNA, MALAT1. *ACS Chem. Biol.* 14 (2): 223–235.

31 Tycowski, K.T., Shu, M.D., Borah, S. et al. (2012). Conservation of a triple-helix-forming RNA stability element in noncoding and genomic RNAs of diverse viruses. *Cell Rep.* 2 (1): 26–32.

32 Cheong, C., Varani, G., and Tinoco, I. Jr. (1990). Solution structure of an unusually stable RNA hairpin, 5'GGAC(UUCG)GUCC. *Nature* 346 (6285): 680–682.

33 Lukavsky, P.J. and Puglisi, J.D. (2005). Structure determination of large biological RNAs. *Methods Enzymol.* 394: 399–416.

34 Lukavsky, P.J., Kim, I., Otto, G.A., and Puglisi, J.D. (2003). Structure of HCV IRES domain II determined by NMR. *Nat. Struct. Biol.* 10 (12): 1033–1038.

35 Xu, J., Lapham, J., and Crothers, D.M. (1996). Determining RNA solution structure by segmental isotopic labeling and NMR: application to *Caenorhabditis elegans* spliced leader RNA 1. *PNAS* 93 (1): 44–48.

36 Lu, K., Heng, X., Garyu, L. et al. (2011). NMR detection of structures in the HIV-1 5'-leader RNA that regulate genome packaging. *Science.* 334 (6053): 242–245.

37 Keane, S.C., Heng, X., Lu, K. et al. (2015). RNA structure. Structure of the HIV-1 RNA packaging signal. *Science.* 348 (6237): 917–921.

38 Brown, J.D., Kharytonchyk, S., Chaudry, I. et al. (2020). Structural basis for transcriptional start site control of HIV-1 RNA fate. *Science.* 368 (6489): 413–417.

39 Wolter, A.C., Weickhmann, A.K., Nasiri, A.H. et al. (2017). A stably protonated adenine nucleotide with a highly shifted pKa value stabilizes the tertiary structure of a GTP-binding RNA aptamer. *Angew. Chem. Int. Ed. Engl.* 56 (1): 401–404.

40 Thompson, R.D., Baisden, J.T., and Zhang, Q. (2019). NMR characterization of RNA small molecule interactions. *Methods* 167: 66–77.

41 Sreeramulu, S., Richter, C., Berg, H. et al. (2021). Exploring the druggability of conserved RNA regulatory elements in the SARS-CoV-2 genome. *Angew. Chem. Int. Ed. Engl.* 60 (35): 19191–19200.

42 Kelly, M.L., Chu, C.C., Shi, H. et al. (2021). Understanding the characteristics of nonspecific binding of drug-like compounds to canonical stem-loop RNAs and their implications for functional cellular assays. *RNA* 27 (1): 12–26.

43 Fourmy, D., Recht, M.I., Blanchard, S.C., and Puglisi, J.D. (1996). Structure of the A site of *Escherichia coli* 16S ribosomal RNA complexed with an aminoglycoside antibiotic. *Science.* 274 (5291): 1367–1371.

44 Yoshizawa, S., Fourmy, D., and Puglisi, J.D. (1998). Structural origins of gentamicin antibiotic action. *EMBO J.* 17 (22): 6437–6448.

45 Varani, L., Spillantini, M.G., Goedert, M., and Varani, G. (2000). Structural basis for recognition of the RNA major groove in the tau exon 10 splicing regulatory element by aminoglycoside antibiotics. *Nucleic Acids Res.* 28 (3): 710–719.

46 Malard, F., Mackereth, C.D., and Campagne, S. (2022). Principles and correction of 5'-splice site selection. *RNA Biol.* 19 (1): 943–960.

47 Liu, B., Shi, H., and Al-Hashimi, H.M. (2021). Developments in solution-state NMR yield broader and deeper views of the dynamic ensembles of nucleic acids. *Curr. Opin. Struct. Biol.* 70: 16–25.

48 Shi, H., Rangadurai, A., Abou Assi, H. et al. (2020). Rapid and accurate determination of atomistic RNA dynamic ensemble models using NMR and structure prediction. *Nat. Commun.* 11 (1): 5531.

49 Dethoff, E.A., Chugh, J., Mustoe, A.M., and Al-Hashimi, H.M. (2012). Functional complexity and regulation through RNA dynamics. *Nature* 482 (7385): 322–330.

50 Aboul-ela, F., Karn, J., and Varani, G. (1995). The structure of the human immunodeficiency virus type-1 TAR RNA reveals principles of RNA recognition by Tat protein. *J. Mol. Biol.* 253 (2): 313–332.

51 Pitt, S.W., Majumdar, A., Serganov, A. et al. (2004). Argininamide binding arrests global motions in HIV-1 TAR RNA: comparison with Mg2+-induced conformational stabilization. *J. Mol. Biol.* 338 (1): 7–16.

52 Bardaro, M.F. Jr., Shajani, Z., Patora-Komisarska, K. et al. (2009). How binding of small molecule and peptide ligands to HIV-1 TAR alters the RNA motional landscape. *Nucleic Acids Res.* 37 (5): 1529–1540.

53 Al-Hashimi, H.M., Gosser, Y., Gorin, A. et al. (2002). Concerted motions in HIV-1 TAR RNA may allow access to bound state conformations: RNA dynamics from NMR residual dipolar couplings. *J. Mol. Biol.* 315 (2): 95–102.

54 Dethoff, E.A., Petzold, K., Chugh, J. et al. (2012). Visualizing transient low-populated structures of RNA. *Nature* 491 (7426): 724–728.

55 Orlovsky, N.I., Al-Hashimi, H.M., and Oas, T.G. (2020). Exposing hidden high-affinity RNA conformational states. *JACS* 142 (2): 907–921.

56 Ganser, L.R., Kelly, M.L., Patwardhan, N.N. et al. (2020). Demonstration that small molecules can bind and stabilize low-abundance short-lived RNA excited conformational states. *J. Mol. Biol.* 432 (4): 1297–1304.

57 Zhao, B., Guffy, S.L., Williams, B., and Zhang, Q. (2017). An excited state underlies gene regulation of a transcriptional riboswitch. *Nat. Chem. Biol.* 13 (9): 968–974.

58 Lawson, C.L., Patwardhan, A., Baker, M.L. et al. (2016). EMDataBank unified data resource for 3DEM. *Nucleic Acids Res.* 44 (D1): D396–D403.

59 Kruger, K., Grabowski, P.J., Zaug, A.J. et al. (1982). Self-splicing RNA: autoexcision and autocyclization of the ribosomal RNA intervening sequence of Tetrahymena. *Cell* 31 (1): 147–157.

60 Su, Z., Zhang, K., Kappel, K. et al. (2021). Cryo-EM structures of full-length *Tetrahymena ribozyme* at 3.1 A resolution. *Nature* 596 (7873): 603–607.

61 Wu, M. and Lander, G.C. (2020). How low can we go? Structure determination of small biological complexes using single-particle cryo-EM. *Curr. Opin. Struct. Biol.* 64: 9–16.

62 Liu, D., Thelot, F.A., Piccirilli, J.A. et al. (2022). Sub-3-A cryo-EM structure of RNA enabled by engineered homomeric self-assembly. *Nat. Methods* 19 (5): 576–585.

63 Bonilla, S.L., Sherlock, M.E., MacFadden, A., and Kieft, J.S. (2021). A viral RNA hijacks host machinery using dynamic conformational changes of a tRNA-like structure. *Science.* 374 (6570): 955–960.

64 Bonilla, S.L., Vicens, Q., and Kieft, J.S. (2022). Cryo-EM reveals an entangled kinetic trap in the folding of a catalytic RNA. *Sci. Adv.* 8 (34): eabq4144.

65 Zhang, K., Keane, S.C., Su, Z. et al. (2018). Structure of the 30 kDa HIV-1 RNA dimerization signal by a hybrid cryo-EM, NMR, and molecular dynamics approach. *Structure* 26 (3): 490–8 e3.

66 Kalvari, I., Argasinska, J., Quinones-Olvera, N. et al. (2018). Rfam 13.0: shifting to a genome-centric resource for non-coding RNA families. *Nucleic Acids Res.* 46 (D1): D335–D342.

67 Watkins, A.M., Rangan, R., and Das, R. (2019). Using Rosetta for RNA homology modeling. *Methods Enzymol.* 623: 177–207.

68 Fiore, J.L. and Nesbitt, D.J. (2013). An RNA folding motif: GNRA tetraloop-receptor interactions. *Q. Rev. Biophys.* 46 (3): 223–264.

69 Watkins, A.M., Rangan, R., and Das, R. (2020). FARFAR2: improved de novo Rosetta prediction of complex global RNA folds. *Structure* 28 (8): 963–76 e6.

70 Krokhotin, A., Houlihan, K., and Dokholyan, N.V. (2015). iFoldRNA v2: folding RNA with constraints. *Bioinformatics* 31 (17): 2891–2893.

71 Townshend, R.J.L., Eismann, S., Watkins, A.M. et al. (2021). Geometric deep learning of RNA structure. *Science.* 373 (6558): 1047–1051.

72 Das, R., Kudaravalli, M., Jonikas, M. et al. (2008). Structural inference of native and partially folded RNA by high-throughput contact mapping. *PNAS* 105 (11): 4144–4149.

73 Cheng, C.Y., Chou, F.C., Kladwang, W. et al. (2015). Consistent global structures of complex RNA states through multidimensional chemical mapping. *Elife* 4: e07600.

74 Kappel, K., Zhang, K., Su, Z. et al. (2020). Accelerated cryo-EM-guided determination of three-dimensional RNA-only structures. *Nat. Methods* 17 (7): 699–707.

75 Sripakdeevong, P., Cevec, M., Chang, A.T. et al. (2014). Structure determination of noncanonical RNA motifs guided by (1)H NMR chemical shifts. *Nat. Methods* 11 (4): 413–416.

76 Putnam, C.D., Hammel, M., Hura, G.L., and Tainer, J.A. (2007). X-ray solution scattering (SAXS) combined with crystallography and computation: defining accurate macromolecular structures, conformations and assemblies in solution. *Q. Rev. Biophys.* 40 (3): 191–285.

77 Mertens, H.D.T. and Svergun, D.I. (2017). Combining NMR and small angle X-ray scattering for the study of biomolecular structure and dynamics. *Arch. Biochem. Biophys.* 628: 33–41.

78 Burke, J.E., Sashital, D.G., Zuo, X. et al. (2012). Structure of the yeast U2/U6 snRNA complex. *RNA* 18 (4): 673–683.

79 Parisien, M. and Major, F. (2008). The MC-Fold and MC-Sym pipeline infers RNA structure from sequence data. *Nature* 452 (7183): 51–55.

80 Kooshapur, H., Choudhury, N.R., Simon, B. et al. (2018). Structural basis for terminal loop recognition and stimulation of pri-miRNA-18a processing by hnRNP A1. *Nat. Commun.* 9 (1): 2479.

81 Gama Lima Costa, R. and Fushman, D. (2022). Reweighting methods for elucidation of conformation ensembles of proteins. *Curr. Opin. Struct. Biol.* 77: 102470.

82 Bernetti, M. and Bussi, G. (2022). Integrating experimental data with molecular simulations to investigate RNA structural dynamics. *Curr. Opin. Struct. Biol.* 78: 102503.

4

Screening and Lead Generation Techniques for RNA Binders

Gary Frey, Emily Garcia Sega, and Neil Lajkiewicz

Arrakis Therapeutics, 828 Winter Street, Waltham, MA 02451, United States

Analogous to the "protein world" of drug discovery, academic and industrial research groups employ screening and lead generation techniques to discover molecules that bind RNA. This chapter describes methods and strategies researchers that are used to discover lead molecules that bind structured regions of RNA. A general screening funnel is outlined in Figure 4.1.

This chapter will focus on knowledge-based screening approaches (e.g. virtual screens) and agnostic screening approaches (e.g. high-throughput screens), which can be done separately or in parallel to identify RNA binders. Next, we will describe methods to confirm the binding of a ligand to an RNA target, summarized in Table 4.1. Moreover, methods for target engagement along with binding site identification/target engagement will be discussed. This chapter will also explore functional assays used to determine if an RNA binder induces a desired pharmacological effect. Finally, the identification of a lead series will be explored along with examples of hit optimization from literature. Primarily, we will focus on tools specific to identifying small molecules that bind to RNA.

4.1 Knowledge-Based Versus Agnostic Screening

The decision to use agnostic or knowledge-based screening approaches depends on the depth of information already known for a given RNA target. For example, if screening against an RNA with a known high-resolution structure that includes a desired binding site, initiation of a virtual screen may be appropriate. Conversely, if little information is known regarding the desired RNA target, high-throughput screens would likely be more appropriate. Some commonly used high-throughput screening techniques include affinity mass spectrometry (ASMS), fluorescence-based biochemical methods, phenotypic screens, small-molecule microarrays (SMMs), and fragment screening.

RNA as a Drug Target: The Next Frontier for Medicinal Chemistry, First Edition.
Edited by John Schneekloth and Martin Pettersson.

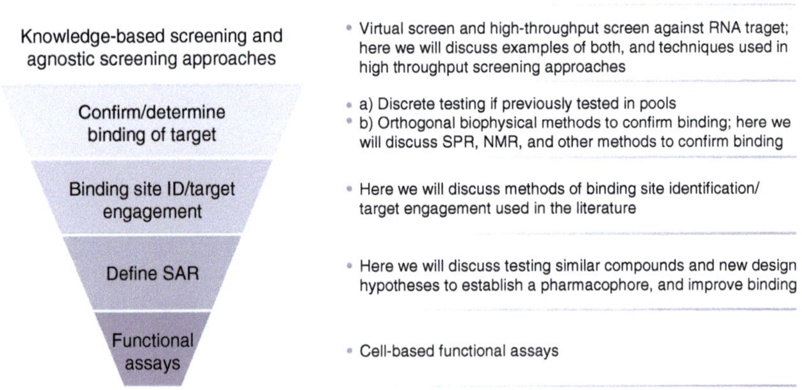
Knowledge-based screening and agnostic screening approaches
Confirm/determine binding of target
Binding site ID/target engagement
Define SAR
Functional assays
Virtual screen and high-throughput screen against RNA traget; here we will discuss examples of both, and techniques used in high throughput screening approaches
a) Discrete testing if previously tested in pools
b) Orthogonal biophysical methods to confirm binding; here we will discuss SPR, NMR, and other methods to confirm binding
Here we will discuss methods of binding site identification/ target engagement used in the literature
Here we will discuss testing similar compounds and new design hypotheses to establish a pharmacophore, and improve binding
Cell-based functional assays

Figure 4.1 A general screening funnel for screening and lead generation techniques for RNA binders.

Table 4.1 Summary of assays used to find RNA binders.

Screening Method	Amount of RNA[a)b)]	Preferred RNA Size	Through-put	RNA sample prep
ASMS	10 pmoles	—	High	—
MST	10–20 pmoles	—	Med–High	Fluorophore Labeling of RNA
SPR	200 pmoles	<150 nts	Med	Biotinylation of RNA
SMM	2.5 nmoles	—	High	Labeling of RNA
NMR	2.5 nmoles	<50 nts[c)]	Low–Med	—
ITC	5 nmoles	>10 nts	Low	—
SAXS	2–5 nmoles	<300 nts	Low	—
X-ray Crystallography	20 nmoles	—	Low	Novel construct design or RNA-protein complex may be needed
DEL	50 nmoles per screen	—	High	Labeling of RNA (e.g. biotin, fluorophore)

a) Amount per sample per assay.
b) Estimated amount per sample per assay.
c) RNA-observed NMR spectroscopy.

4.2 Virtual Screening

Molecular docking is a computational technique that can be used to identify potential binders and predict ligand binding modes among very large virtual libraries of molecules, often in the millions. While virtual screening is widely used in protein-based drug discovery, its use has been more limited for RNA targets. While the number of available RNA structures is increasing, there are many more structural examples of proteins. Without a high-resolution structure of the binding pocket, ideally with a bound ligand, the current scope of virtual screens for RNA targets is limited, especially for those targets with unknown or structurally complex binding pockets. Molecular docking against an RNA target has been used successfully by Peter Daldrop and co-authors [1]. The authors utilized a protein-ligand docking program with minor changes, and notably the problems encountered in this study were well-known problems also encountered in protein-ligand docking, e.g. the role of water molecules and protonation state variation [1]. In their study, the authors identified four ligands targeting the xpt-pbuX guanine riboswitch, some of which were structurally distinct from known ligands. They were then experimentally shown to bind to the *Bacillus subtilis xpt-pbuX* guanine riboswitch carrying a C74U mutation (GRA) [2].

4.3 Screening Methods

4.3.1 High-Throughput Screening (HTS)

Since the mid-1980s, high-throughput screening has been an effective method for identifying small molecules that serve as starting points for drug development [3]. Many of the standard methods developed for the high-throughput screening of protein targets have been applied to RNA. Since many of the RNAs being targeted lack an inherent function in isolation, such as the enzymatic activity or receptor binding functions of their protein counterparts, many of the assays rely on direct binding methods. In this section, we outline the methods used for assaying RNA.

4.3.1.1 Mass Spectrometry

RNA targets used for high-throughput screening often consist of a fragment of a larger RNA target with the potential to form a small-molecule-binding pocket. These RNA fragments often lack an intrinsic function. Therefore, it is necessary to use direct binding methods to identify ligands. Mass spectrometry is an attractive option as it can detect binders to all potential surfaces of the RNA and is amenable to high-throughput screening. It is highly sensitive, thereby minimizing the amount of RNA consumed in the screen. There are no requirements for labeling the target or ligand, eliminating the concern about RNA modifications affecting proper folding. Molecules are detected by their intrinsic mass, so pools of compounds can be screened simultaneously, as any binders can be uniquely identified.

Electrospray ionization mass spectrometry (ESI-MS) is a soft ionization technique that has shown broad applicability in the analysis of macromolecules. Ever since its development [4], the applications for mass spectrometry in the analysis of biomolecules have been growing [5]. In ESI-MS, samples are ionized in an electric field followed by dispersion into a fine spray. The ionized droplets are subsequently reduced in size, eventually transferring the ions from solution to gas phase via a combination of temperature, reduced pressure, coulombic repulsion, and/or dry nitrogen gas, before being accelerated toward a mass analyzer. The analysis will provide information on both the molecular mass and the ion intensity of the sample.

Integration of mass peaks can provide quantitative information that can be particularly important in the analysis of binding interactions. The establishment of ESI-MS as a method that can detect the noncovalent association of macromolecule–ligand complexes has enabled its use in high-throughput screening in drug discovery [6]. Initially used in the detection of enzyme–ligand complexes [7], ESI-MS has subsequently been used in drug discovery to target RNA.

Brief Background on RNA HTS Screening by Mass Spectrometry HTS mass spectrometry techniques that have been applied to RNA can be divided into two categories: those that measure the mass of the intact RNA:ligand complex (direct) and those that first separate the ligand from the complex and then subject the ligand to mass analysis (indirect) (see Figure 4.2). With direct methods, both the bound complex and unbound fraction of the RNA are measured. This allows one to calculate a single point K_D of the interaction, providing an estimate of the true K_D and a convenient way to rank order compounds in a high throughput screen. Also, since the mass of the intact complex is detected, binding stoichiometry as well as whether compounds are binding to independent sites on the target can be determined. Multiple targets can be screened within a single sample as long as there are sufficient mass differences between the targets. This allows for controls to be run along with the target in a single sample well which can greatly increase throughput. The major drawback with this approach is that samples are directly injected for mass spectrometric analysis, requiring that all components of the sample be fully compatible with mass spectrometry instrumentation. Components such as metal ions, nonvolatile buffer components, and other co-factors which cause issues must therefore be avoided. Often such components play an important role in the proper folding of the RNA [8]. Direct approaches are also limited to smaller targets (<100 nucleotides) due to difficulties in ionization and detection of larger targets.

By contrast, indirect methods measure the mass of the bound ligand by separating it from the complex through a series of chromatographic steps. In a typical experiment, the RNA along with any bound compounds are separated from unbound compounds using size exclusion chromatography (SEC). Any compounds associated with the RNA are then separated through denaturation of the complex followed by an HPLC purification step. Peaks from the HPLC column are subsequently injected for mass spectrometry analysis. Components that are not compatible with mass spectrometry can be included in the original sample as they are removed during the ligand separation process. However, important information is lost by separating the ligand from the RNA such as the identity of the target and binding stoichiometry. This limits the technique to either single-target screening or multitarget screening that require follow-up experiments to identify the target. Both approaches have been adapted to RNA drug discovery and are discussed later.

4.3.1.2 HTS of RNA Using Direct MS Approaches

Hofstadler et al. developed a direct mass spectrometry approach they termed multitarget affinity/specificity screening (MASS) [9]. The method takes advantage of the extremely high mass accuracy of electrospray ionization Fourier transform

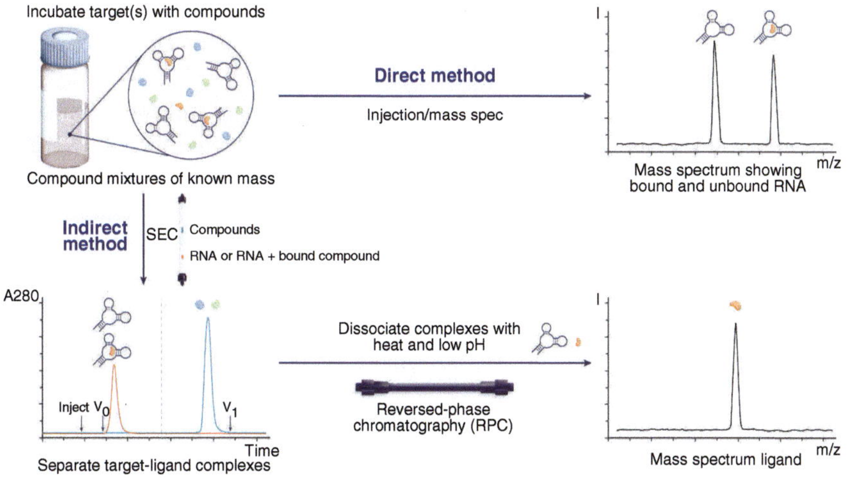

Figure 4.2 Comparison of direct and indirect methods for HTS by mass spectrometry. Both methods start with the equilibration of RNA and small molecules. Using direct methods, the equilibrated sample is injected directly for mass spectrometry analysis. The resulting spectrum will contain information on any bound complex in addition to free RNA. Using indirect methods, the equilibrated sample is first separated using SEC. The conditions are chosen so that the RNA fraction will elute in the void volume (V_0) of the column. This fraction is then subjected to denaturing conditions and directed to a reversed-phase HPLC column where any bound small molecules will be resolved according to hydrophobicity and then directed for mass spectrometry analysis. The resulting mass spectrum will contain information on the mass of the small molecule and the amount present.

ion cyclotron resonance mass spectrometry (ESI-FTICR-MS) [10]. The method allows for the determination of the masses of the intact RNA:ligand complexes, and they are able to measure the binding of mixtures of compounds against multiple RNA targets simultaneously [9]. In brief, RNA and compounds are equilibrated in ammonium acetate buffer. Prior to injection, isopropanol is added to aid in desolvation. In a typical experiment, RNA concentration at a concentration of 2.5 μM was mixed with a 10-fold excess of the compound. By optimizing the ESI conditions, very weak binding interactions could be detected. Griffey et al. were able to measure RNA:ligand complexes with affinities as weak as 15 mM using this method [11]. Overall, their technique captured K_D ranges from very weak (mM) to low nM [12]. The resulting mass spectrum obtained using MASS contains peaks corresponding to both bound RNA:ligand complexes and unbound RNA. Integration of the peaks allows for compound identification and single-point K_D estimates, which can be used to rank order compounds in the screen. Follow-up studies on hit compounds by titration experiments can be performed to obtain more accurate K_D calculations.

Using MASS, Hofstadler et al. measured the binding of a series of aminoglycosides to a 27-nucleotide RNA fragment corresponding to a structured hairpin on the procaryotic 16S rRNA [13]. They were able to show the preferential binding of the aminoglycosides to the 16S RNA fragment over the eukaryotic 18S RNA fragment by including both targets in the reaction mixture. Similarities in the molecular weights of the two targets when bound to a mixture of compounds complicated analysis due to the overlap of mass peaks. To overcome this, a "neutral mass tag" consisting of a PEG moiety was attached to the 5′ terminus of one of the target RNAs. This provided sufficient mass separation to facilitate analysis.

MASS has also been used for the high-throughput screening and development of small molecules targeting the Hepatitis C virus internal ribosome entry site (IRES) [14]. Seth et al. specifically targeted a 29-nucleotide structured region corresponding to the IRES IIa subdomain. A multitarget approach was employed in the screen, which contained both the structured IIa 29-mer RNA target and a 33-mer structured control RNA. Both a single-point K_D and a selectivity score (the ratio of ligand K_D for the 33-mer RNA versus 29-mer RNA) were employed in the identification of hits. HTS of an 18,000 compound library led to the identification of a relatively weak binding benzimidazole compound with a K_D of approximately 100 μM. With SAR driven by quantitative binding measurements using MASS, they were able to identify several analogs with K_Ds below 1 μM activity in an HCV replicon assay and low toxicity.

In addition to its application to high-throughput screening, MASS has also been used in follow-up work using multipoint K_D determination [15]. Sannes-Lowery et al. determined the K_D values for two aminoglycosides, tobramycin, and paromomycin to the 16S rRNA fragment using MASS. They also showed that tobramycin contained two nonequivalent sites and were able to determine K_Ds for both sites.

4.3.1.3 HTS of RNA Using Indirect MS Approaches

Annis et al. developed a HTS approach using indirect mass spectrometry termed ALIS (automated ligand identification system) [16]. Originally used for the discovery of small-molecules targeting the *E. coli* enzyme dihydrofolate reductase, it has since been adapted to the high-throughput discovery of novel compounds targeting noncoding RNA [17]. Being an indirect MS approach, ALIS employs two chromatographic steps prior to sample injection for mass spectrometry analysis. In a typical experiment, RNA and small molecule are combined and equilibrated. This step can incorporate any buffers and cofactors necessary for proper RNA folding, as the buffers and cofactors will be separated away in the subsequent steps prior to mass spectrometry analysis. Following equilibration, the RNA fraction is separated from any unbound ligands using SEC. This column is typically run in ammonium acetate, a mass spectrometry-compatible buffer, and it is in this step where the noncompatible components in the sample buffer are removed. The RNA fraction, which contains any potential complexed ligands, is loaded onto a second chromatographic step, a reversed-phase (RP) liquid chromatography column, typically C18. The separation can be performed at high temperature (>60 °C) and at low pH, which will lead to denaturation of the RNA over the C18 column. During the loading of the RP column in aqueous conditions, the small-molecule ligand will be captured on the C18 column, and the RNA will be rejected to waste. Small molecule peaks from the C18 column are then subjected to mass spectrometry analysis. During analysis, data files are scanned for selected ion traces that match the compounds in the sample mixture. The entire system can be automated, with screening rates of >250,000 compounds per day reported [16]. Since the method measures the mass of the dissociated ligand, ligands that work by a covalent mechanism will not be detected as they will be retained on the RNA.

One of the advantages of ALIS is the overall low hit rate combined with a low false-positive rate. One reason for this is the unambiguous determination of binders based on their intrinsic mass. More importantly, however, bound ligands must survive separation by SEC. During the separation process, compounds continue to dissociate from the target with a half-life that is determined by the off-rate for the interaction (Eq. (4.1)):

$$t_{1/2} = \frac{0.693}{k_{\text{off}}} \tag{4.1}$$

$$[\text{RNA}] + [\text{ligand}] \underset{k_{\text{off}}}{\overset{k_{\text{on}}}{\rightleftharpoons}} [\text{RNA} : \text{ligand}]$$

Only complexes with sufficiently slow off-rates will still contain enough compound after SEC to be detected by mass spectrometry. The SEC conditions must be carefully chosen to ensure the success of ALIS. The separation of RNA from unbound molecules must have sufficient resolution so that the unbound fraction does not bleed into the bound fraction, resulting in false positives. The speed of the separation is also critical. As an example, for a k_{off} rate of 0.1 s^{-1}, only 50% of the complex remains after ~7 seconds (Figure 4.3). The issue of ligand dissociation on the column can be dealt with in several ways. First, a higher starting concentration of RNA, typically 1–5 μM, will mean a higher concentration remaining after decay. Second, employing rapid SEC separations to decrease column residence time will help to minimize the amount of decay. Below-ambient temperature of the SEC column can be used to slow the rate of ligand-receptor dissociation, assisting detection. Modern HPLC sizing columns allow for small column volumes and high flow rates which enable rapid separation of complexes. Column resins are selected so that the RNA runs in the void volume, the earliest fraction on a sizing column. RNA presence in the void volume can be verified via placement of a UV spectrophotometer post-SEC in the chromatographic system; detection of RNA via UV absorption is also useful as a quality control metric during routine analysis.

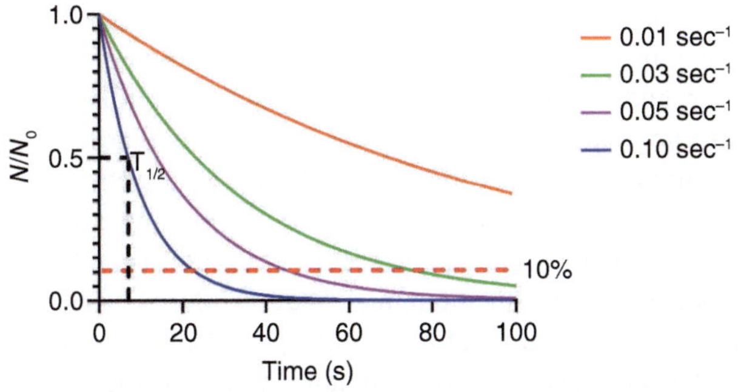

Figure 4.3 Simulated decay curves for complexes with varying dissociation rates. The half-life for a complex with a k_{off} rate constant of 1×10^{-1} s^{-1} (approximately 7 second half life) is illustrated. The red line shows the point at which only 10% of the complex remains.

O'Connel et al. estimated that with a 5-second column separation and the ability to observe binders for approximately 5 half-lives they were able to capture compounds with off-rates of $0.7\,s^{-1}$ or slower [18].

Two other considerations in ALIS, both of which can result in false positives, are compound breakthrough and compound carryover. Compound breakthrough refers to small molecules that elute in the void volume in the absence of RNA. This can be caused by nonideal behavior of the small molecule by mechanisms such as aggregation. Another nonideal behavior is carryover, where the compound shows adherent behavior within the system and becomes detectable in immediately subsequent experimental runs. Both issues can be addressed with the appropriate placement of controls and blank injections.

In addition to high-throughput screening, ALIS can be used to obtain quantitative binding measurements. Several approaches can be used. The first is the calculation of a direct K_D measurement using multipoint titrations. Alternatively, if the target of interest contains a ligand with a known affinity, a competition-based method for affinity ranking can be used [19]. In these experiments, a constant concentration of the ligand of interest is titrated with increasing concentrations of competitor ligand. The resulting titration curve yields an ACE_{50}, defined as the affinity competition 50% inhibitory concentration. In this case, a higher ACE_{50} concentration indicates a higher affinity for the ligand of interest. Rizvi et al. used competition titration experiments to rank order a series of small molecules binding to the FMN riboswitch [17]. Finally, if the goal is to rank order compounds without the need for a quantitative binding constant, then relative affinity ranking can be performed by titrating the target molecule against fixed concentrations of compounds. As the target concentration decreases, competition among compounds increases with weaker compounds disappearing first. The advantage of this method is its quickness and the ability to screen high numbers of compounds in a single experiment.

4.3.1.4 DNA-Encoded Libraries (DELs)

Recently, researchers have used DNA-encoded libraries (DELs) to discover RNA binders. A DEL is a mixture of small molecules conjugated to unique DNA tags, wherein the structure information is encoded within DNA sequences. This allows the screening of billions of compounds simultaneously in a single vessel [20]. Researchers have not typically used DEL screening to discover RNA binders [21], but Mukherjee, Blain, Petter, and co-workers utilized the Vipergen yoctoReactor DNA-encoded library (DEL) approach [22] to screen for compounds that bound Aptamer 21 [23]. Among the primary hits identified from this DEL screen, one compound was selected for photoprobe development based on its binding affinity in confirmatory SPR assays (K_D = 130 nM). More recently, Dou and co-authors used DEL technology on the *E. coli* flavin mononucleotide (FMN) Riboswitch to find compounds with mid-nanomolar binding affinity [24]. Originally, Dou and co-authors screened a DEL consisting of 10.38 billion ligands against HIV1 trans-acting responsive region (TAR) RNA and found significant false-positive signals due to DNA–RNA base-pairing interactions. To solve this issue, Dou and co-authors developed an algorithm to differentiate DNA–RNA-binding signals from small molecule–RNA binding and they realized certain compounds were enriched because their DNA tags (rather than the small molecules) were interacting with the TAR RNA from base 21 to 29 through the "GGCAGAGAG" motif. In view of this, Dou and co-authors were able to reduce false positive signals by preincubating the DELs with RNA fragments from the RNA target and using competitive elution with 50 μM Pra-tat. Using this protocol, they did not find any active compounds from screening the DEL against TAR but found compounds with mid-nanomolar binding affinity against FMN riboswitch after applying what they learned from screening HIV1 TAR.

Paegel, Disney, and co-authors have recently reported success in screening a DEL of 73,728 ligands against a library of RNA structures (4096 targets) [25]. They pooled, amplified, sequenced, and decoded the DEL hits to identify hit structures for synthesis and subsequent validation. One of the hits bound a 5′G$\underline{A}$G/3′C$\underline{C}$C internal loop that is present in primary microRNA-27a (pri-miR-27a), the oncogenic precursor of microRNA-27a with a K_D of 40 ± 30 nM as measured by a competitive binding assay with a constant concentration of compound, a cyanine5 (Cy5)-labeled model of pri-miR-27a's Drosha site, and varying concentrations of unlabeled miR-27a precursor. This compound was cell active, inhibiting pri-miR-27a processing in MCF-10a cells transfected with a plasmid encoding wild-type pri-miR-27a. Further, the compound inhibited pri-miR-27a biogenesis in MDA-Mb-231 TNBC cells with a measured IC_{50} of ~1 μM. Most recently, Paegel, Disney, and co-authors used a solid phase DEL [26] to find binders of the RNA repeat expansion r(CUG)^{exp}, widely considered the cause of the most common form of adult-onset muscular dystrophy, myotonic dystrophy type 1 (DM1) [27].

4.3.1.5 Microarray Screening

SMM is a high-throughput method that can be used to identify ligands for a given RNA target. SMMs work through the immobilization of a library of compounds in an array onto a glass surface [28]. Labeled RNA is then exposed to the immobilized library. Through the detection of the labeled RNA, compounds that bind are identified.

A clear advantage to the use of SMM is the minute amount of material required for each assay, as well as the large number of samples that can be evaluated at a time via high throughput screens. However, SMMs also present a few challenges. First, careful consideration of label type and location along with proper quality control of RNA structure should be employed to alleviate concerns about labeled RNA not replicating native RNA folds. Second, a compound needs to contain an appropriate functional group to adhere to the microarray surface. This functional group cannot be essential to the interaction with the RNA target, as association with the surface may inhibit the interaction with the RNA. Further concerns exist around the binding capacity of the immobilized ligands, as this environment varies from a small molecule binding to RNA completely in solution. Recently, a technique called AbsorbArray was described illustrating the potential for unmodified compounds to be screened in a microarray-based approach [29]. Using AbsorbArray, compounds are noncovalently adhered onto hydrated agarose-coated microarray surfaces and subsequently dried. In this study, FDA-approved drugs were screened against various RNA motifs, and approved anticancer drugs were identified that target the oncogenic noncoding RNA microRNA-21.

Despite these concerns, SMMs have been used successfully for numerous RNA targets. Though SMMs have long been used to identify ligands for protein targets, they were first used with RNA by Disney and co-authors to look at the interactions between aminoglycosides and bacterial rRNA [30]. Since then, microarrays for RNA targets have evolved to assess binding with drug-like compounds. To our knowledge, the first use of an SMM for RNA targeting specifically with drug-like compounds was completed by Schneekloth and co-authors [31]. This work focused on targeting an HIV TAR hairpin structure and identified two hits from a library of 20,000 compounds. Most notably, one of the hits was found to be structurally distinct from any ligands previously known to bind the HIV TAR hairpin. Additional SMM screens completed by Schneekloth and co-authors identified ligands for microRNA-21 [32], pre-Q1 riboswitches [33], MALAT-1 [34], and the ZTP riboswitch [35]. Additionally, Disney and co-authors more recently used SMM to screen a newly designed RNA fragment library against a variety of RNA structures displaying randomized regions of 3×3 or 3×2 internal loops. This study illustrated that even compounds with low molecular weight have the potential to selectively affect RNA-mediated pathways [36].

4.3.1.6 Fragment-Based Drug Discovery

Fragment-based drug discovery (FBDD) is a high-throughput method that uses fragments to screen potential drug targets. In FBDD, a library of fragments is screened, often in pools. Once a fragment is identified as a hit, if screened in pools, binding is subsequently verified in singleton form, and then via an orthogonal binding assay. Binding elucidation may then be used to help guide fragment optimization to enhance binding affinity as part of the fragment-to-lead stage of FBDD. Overall, FBDD requires careful consideration of a fragment library, screening and validation of fragment binders by two separate methods, elucidation of a fragment's mode of binding, and optimization of fragment(s) to drug-like candidates. FBDD can lead to the identification of fragments with high ligand efficiency to their target, therefore helping to identify compounds that bind in a more specific fashion.

FBDD as a method has become a crucial part of early-stage drug discovery. One clear advantage of fragment libraries is that they can cover a greater percentage of chemical space per molecule when compared to HTS of drug-like molecules. It has been estimated that there are between 10^{60} and 10^{200} possible drug-like compounds like those used in HTS (between 300 and 500 Da), but only 10^7 possible molecules that meet the "Rule of 3" parameters used for fragment libraries [37–39]. Therefore, a fragment screen using a carefully selected couple of thousands of compounds can be more effective at exploring the available chemical space when compared to a library of hundreds of thousands of HTS compounds.

The number of examples of successful FBDD screening against drug targets, both protein and RNA-based, is rapidly increasing, as is the number of examples of successful progression from fragment to lead. This indicates that FBDD may be a very useful tool in helping to assess the ligandability of RNA structures as well as helping to identify and develop lead compounds for these targets. FBDD has been used in numerous instances to illustrate small molecule binding specifically to RNA targets. A few examples where FBDD has been used for RNA targets include the identification of novel ligands to the TPP riboswitch, TERRA, HIV TAR, and the Influenza A virus [40–44].

Fragment Library Design Fragment libraries consist of a set of compounds which all fall under the parameters found within the "Rule of 3" (Ro3). The "Rule of 3" indicates that a fragment is less than or equal to 300 Da, has a cLogP less than or equal to 3, and contains no more than 3 H-bond donors and acceptors. Fragment library design should consider the Ro3 guidelines [45], three-dimensional space, and the ease of chemical elaboration [46]. Since hits coming from fragment-based screening are small, they often need to be grown, linked, or merged. Therefore, molecules containing favorable functionality to serve as growth vectors are preferred. However, care must also be taken to avoid reactive or unstable scaffolds.

The largest RNA-specific fragment library we are aware of was recently developed by the Disney lab [36]. In addition to this fragment library, there are numerous studies of small molecule libraries used for RNA that can help design the generation of a fragment library specifically focused around targeting RNA [29, 47, 48]. Additionally, RNA-binding sites can be similar in size and hydrophobicity to druggable protein-binding sites. For this reason, general purpose fragment libraries should deliver sufficient hits. However, there are some known privileged scaffolds for RNA ligands that could lead to higher hit rates [49]. For example, Giacomo Padroni and co-authors claim that the H-bonding and hydrophobic effects of sulfur-mediated interactions are underexplored for RNA-targeted drug discovery [50]. Additionally, Hamid Nasiri and co-authors ran a study on cMYC illustrating a higher propensity for binding the target with fragments containing either 5- and 6-membered heterocyclic rings, two fused 6-membered heterocyclic rings, or four substituted aniline derivatives [51].

Fragment Screening Methods Fragment screening is different from traditional high-throughput screening in various ways. First, fragments tend to bind targets with low affinity. To identify these low-affinity compounds, it is necessary to screen them at high concentrations, typically up to 1 or 2 mM [52]. Unfortunately, these circumstances create unsuitable conditions for some traditional biophysical or biochemical assays such as fluorescent-based competition assays or cell-based assays. Additionally, adverse effects of using such high concentrations include an increased rate of false positives due to aggregation and the identification of nonspecific binders. For this reason, it is essential to verify the binding results of the primary screen utilizing at least one orthogonal screening method. Compounds identified by at least two screening methods can more confidently be confirmed as hits and optimized via medicinal chemistry. There are many screening methods used for fragment screening but NMR, SPR, and virtual screens are the most utilized methods. We will focus on these methods later.

NMR for Fragment Screening NMR is a commonly used screening method for FBDD due to its sensitivity and capability to characterize fragments with a broad range of RNA and fragment binding affinities, from μM to mM. Additionally, NMR screening data can provide structural information on the binding interface and modes. There are two main NMR techniques used for FBDD: RNA-observed NMR spectroscopy and ligand-observed NMR spectroscopy.

^{1}H NMR-binding assays are widely used as RNA imino protons that arise from the formation of base pairs are resolved from typical proton peaks from the fragments. For this reason, the chemical shifts of the imino protons are sensitive, often with clear shifts upon binding to fragments. RNA target size can vary for RNA-observed NMR screens, though they typically favor small, well-folded RNA less than 50 nucleotides long as peak overlap issues may arise for longer RNA [53]. For this screening method, a pooled set of fragments (typically 5–10) can be screened simultaneously as long as there is minimal signal overlap among the ^{1}H resonances of each fragment in the pool. Binding is observed through shifts in imino ^{1}H resonances based on interaction with the RNA target. If the initial screen was carried out in pools, once a binding event is observed, screening of individual fragments must be carried out from the positive pools to confirm binding. Since each imino proton corresponds to a base pair, the binding site on the RNA target can be immediately mapped based on the assignment. Unfortunately, this method is less sensitive if the fragment only binds with a loop or a bulge residue due to lack of imino proton signals from these regions [54].

Another NMR screening method is ligand-observed NMR spectroscopy. This method has the advantage that the target structure is not required, there is no RNA size limit, less RNA sample is required, and no isotopic labeling is required. There are several widely used ligand-observed NMR methods, including line broadening, saturation transfer difference (STD), water-ligand observed via gradient spectroscopy (WaterLOGSY), and Carr–Purcell–Meiboom–Gill (CPMG). These NMR methods can not only provide information regarding if the fragment binds with RNA (Figure 4.4) but can also generate binding information on the fragment molecules. Due to the high sensitivity of detecting weak binding affinity in the mM range, a combination of multiple methods is recommended during screening to

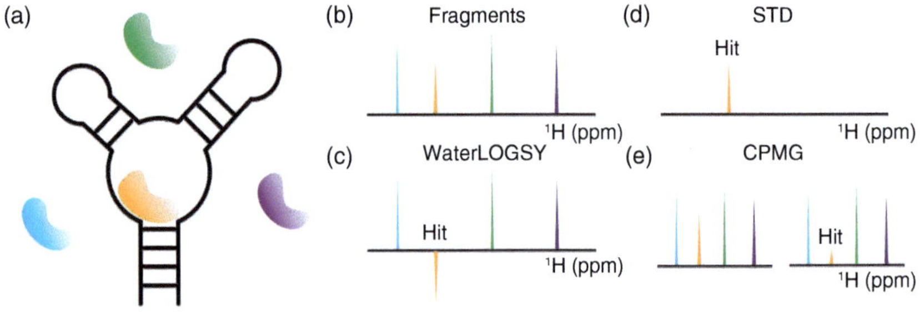

Figure 4.4 ^{1}H NMR methods used to identify fragments that bind to a given RNA structure.

lower the rate of false positive hits. It is worth mentioning that 19F NMR has also been widely used for ligand-observed screening due to its higher sensitivity and throughputs (up to 20 fragments per pool).

Surface Plasmon Resonance (SPR) for Fragment Screening SPR is often utilized for screening fragments and is especially beneficial because it is a sensitive method that does not require large amounts of RNA. However, SPR is relatively low throughput and when screening large fragment libraries, higher throughput methods of screening are often more efficient. For this reason, SPR may more commonly be utilized as a follow-up screen for binding verification. Another utilization of SPR within fragment screening is for competition experiments [55]. In these competition experiments, a known ligand is tethered to the chip surface. The RNA is then added and allowed to form a complex. Addition of a competing fragment will result in decomplexation and a large signal change can be observed. This can provide additional information regarding fragment binding and overlap (cf. Section 4.3.2.1).

Fragment Hit Validation/Elucidation of Binding

X-ray Crystallography and SAXS of Fragments X-ray crystallography provides a unique atomic level structure elucidation that is often crucial for not only validating a hit but also evolving the hit to a lead compound. Relative to proteins there are fewer X-ray crystal structures of RNA. This limits the use of X-ray crystallography as a method of validation. However, once a crystallization condition is established for a given RNA, obtaining high-resolution structures with different fragments becomes much more feasible. This is illustrated in the successful use of X-ray crystallography for fragment hit validation achieved in 2014 against the thiM riboswitch [41]. In addition to X-ray crystallography, the authors used small-angle X-ray scattering (SAXS) [56]. SAXS provides lower resolution structural determination and can be especially useful when determining RNA 3D topological structure due to the stronger X-ray scattering observed in the sugar-phosphate backbone of RNA [57, 58]. Utilizing SAXS, the authors were able to observe the induction of a conformational change resulting in a structure intermediate between that of the free and that of the native ligand-bound riboswitch. Recently, Menichelli and coauthors successfully co-crystallized the theophylline aptamer with theophylline and four unique binders that have up to 340-fold greater affinity compared to theophylline [59]. These results show that the same approaches to drug discovery that are used for proteins may also be applied to RNA.

Virtual Screening of Fragments In FBDD of proteins, virtual screening can be a great tool to identify and elaborate fragments as well as to predict binding modes of ligands from large libraries. Due to many complexities of structure modeling, including water displacement, protonation states, and accounting for multiple possible binding modes, virtual screening is more useful for later stages in screening such as the elaboration of fragments rather than initial fragment screening. For RNA-specific targets, there are only limited examples of virtual screens.

Target Engagement of Fragments Target engagement is discussed in more detail in another section of this chapter (cf. Section 4.4). However, in the context of RNA-focused fragment screening, Suresh et. al published a technique termed Chem-CLIP-Frag-Map [60]. This technique utilizes a fragment library where each fragment contains a photoaffinity group, which enables covalent attachment of the fragments to the target. In this technique, each fragment also contains an azide to bind to streptavidin-coated magnetic beads, allowing for isolation and further evaluation of the covalently bound fragment and target [60]. While this technique can be useful to efficiently identify fragments that bind to a target, the library is limited by the requirements to have multiple functionalities for target attachment and isolation.

Fragment Hit Optimization While fragment screens are widely reported for identifying binders to a variety of RNA targets, little has been reported regarding optimization of these fragments. However, the strategies discussed below are commonly applied to protein-binding fragments, and the same techniques are anticipated to also be useful for RNA-binding fragments. Once a set of binding fragments is confirmed via two orthogonal assays, analysis of the binders can help prioritize which fragments to explore. Analysis of binders includes assessing solubility and ligand efficiency. Many fragments are prioritized because of their good aqueous solubility. This should lead to a lower rate of false positives from aggregation, which is a common problem in HTS programs [55]. FBDD helps to identify small compounds with high ligand efficiency. However, most fragments due to their small size bind with low affinity. In order to optimize fragment–target interactions, the fragment(s) often go through an optimization where the fragment is merged, linked, or grown.

Merging starts with compounds with overlapping features; for example, common binding interactions of functional groups. The compounds can be merged where they overlap to create a compound with increased binding interactions and higher affinity. Merging has also been shown to be helpful for improving selectivity of protein ligands [61].

Linking of fragments involves the joining of two fragments that do not bind at overlapping sites. Finding an ideal linker can be very demanding and requires exploring multiple parameters. First, a linker may not alter the orientation of each fragment to the binding site. Doing so could reduce important binding interactions and favorable geometry thereby reducing binding affinity. Second, flexibility must be carefully considered. A rigid linker that reduces the degrees of freedom can serve to reduce the entropic cost paid upon binding. Alternatively, a flexible linker could cause hydrophobic surfaces to become buried intramolecularly. In this case, the resulting conformation would create an energetic barrier for binding. An ideal linker would maintain a careful balance of rigidity and flexibility while also incorporating additional opportunities for favorable interactions with the RNA target.

Growing fragments employs synthesis to capture additional interactions with the RNA target. Before growing a fragment, close analogs of the fragment hit should be tested to find the highest affinity starting point. These investigations may lead to the identification of novel growth vectors, which can include the addition of functional groups or moieties that provide increased opportunities for binding-site interactions. In order to grow the fragment, one should consider ligand efficiency, synthetic tractability, and drug-like properties. It is important to have structural information on the macromolecular target and the fragment binding mode. Without this information optimization becomes very difficult. Often NMR, X-ray crystallography, and target engagement assays are used to help guide fragment optimization.

As with other binding first approaches, FBDD does not account for any potential biological impacts the binding may have. Given the complexity and flexibility of RNA structures, binding does not necessarily indicate function. Care must be taken to consider biological targets and verify functional activity upon binding confirmation. Despite this distinction, FBDD can still be extremely useful in the design and development of RNA-binding small molecules, and it has become an accepted part of early-stage drug discovery.

4.3.1.7 Phage Display

Phage display uses bacteriophages to link proteins with the genetic information that encodes them [62]. It has been used to discover protein and peptide binders to proteins, DNA, and RNA. In this technique, a gene encoding a protein is inserted into a phage coat protein gene, causing the phage to "display" the protein on its surface while containing the gene that codes the protein genome, thus linking genotype and phenotype. These displaying phages can be screened against an immobilized RNA sequence to enrich for those displaying protein sequences that bind the RNA. Phage display can be performed iteratively by using the enriched phage from one round as input for the next. After screening, the coat protein gene from the enriched phage is sequenced to determine the protein or peptide sequences of the binders.

Previously, Chow and co-authors have used a heptapeptide M13 phage-display library to find ligands for the tRNA-binding site of bacterial 16S ribosomal RNA [63, 64]. Galleni, Vandevenne, and co-authors used a phage display selection of a synthetic nanobody gene library (dedicated for nucleic acid binding) to find one nanobody (a camelid heavy-chain antibody named $cAb_{BC1rib}3$) that binds structured RNA φBC1 with nM affinity as measured by biolayer interferometry (BLI) [65].

4.3.2 Orthogonal Methods

4.3.2.1 Surface Plasmon Resonance

Following the identification of small-molecule binders, the next step in drug discovery is to characterize the affinity, stoichiometry, and specificity of the binding interaction. Unlike many protein targets, which may have an intrinsic function like enzymatic activity or receptor binding, many of the RNAs being targeted lack an inherent function in isolation. This limits the options to assays with the ability to measure direct binding. One method that can address all these factors is surface plasmon resonance (SPR). The technique measures the interaction of molecules to a target in real time and can determine both equilibrium binding and kinetic constants. The signals observed in an SPR experiment are proportional to the molecular weights of the binding partners, which can be used to determine the stoichiometry of

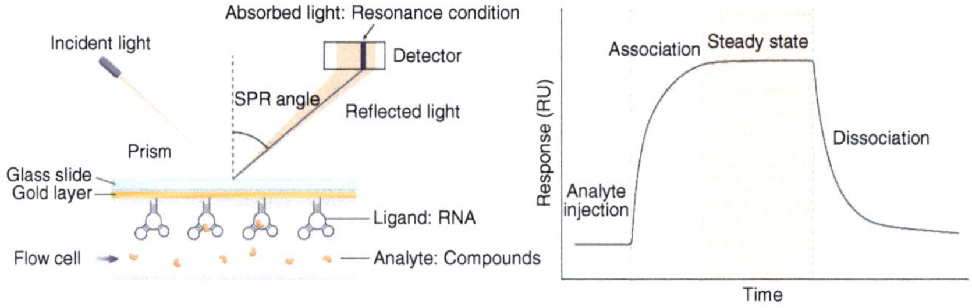

Figure 4.5 (a) SPR configuration. Polarized light is focused onto a biosensor surface through a glass prism, resulting in the creation of surface plasmons. Absorption of light occurs at the resonance condition. The location of the absorbed light can be defined in terms of an SPR angle with the location being in part determined by the refractive index close to the biosensor surface. Binding interactions occurring near the biosensor surface will change the refractive index, which results in a shift of the absorbed light, thus changing the SPR angle. (b) SPR sensorgram. The SPR angle is monitored in real time and represented on the *y*-axis as response units (RU). Following injection of analyte, the sensorgram can be divided into three phases: association, steady state, and dissociation.

the interaction based on the observed signal. In addition, inspection of sensorgrams can be informative, often detecting the presence of nonspecific binding interactions.

A Brief Overview of SPR Theory SPR is a microfluidic system in which an analyte (A) is flowed over a ligand (L) that is immobilized to the surface of a bio-sensor chip (Figure 4.5a). The biosensor detects molecular interactions through the generation of a SPR, which is highly sensitive to changes in the refractive index close to the surface of the biosensor chip [66]. Analyte molecules that interact with the immobilized ligand alter the refractive index at the chip surface, resulting in a change in the SPR angle, which is measured in real time and represented in the form of a sensorgram (Figure 4.5b). Analysis of the sensorgram steady-state phase will provide information on equilibrium binding, and analysis of the association and dissociation phases can provide kinetic parameters. The determination of kinetic constants requires sufficient curvature in the association and dissociation phases of the sensorgram (cf. Figure 4.5b).

The ability to match the K_Ds determined from both kinetic and equilibrium fitting can increase confidence in the values being measured. Early-stage compounds typically exhibit fast kinetics with very steep association and dissociation phases which precludes the robust measurement of kinetic parameters.

In addition to measuring equilibrium binding and rate constants, sensorgrams can also provide information about the stoichiometry of the interaction. The signals in an SPR binding experiment are related to the molecular weights of the ligand and analyte according to Eq. (4.2):

$$R_{max}\,\text{analyte} = \frac{\text{Mr}_{\text{analyte}} R_{\text{ligand}} \text{Valency}_{\text{ligand}}}{\text{Mr}_{\text{ligand}}} \tag{4.2}$$

R_{ligand} refers to the immobilization level for the ligand in response units, valency is the number of binding sites, and $\text{Mr}_{\text{analyte}}$ and $\text{Mr}_{\text{ligand}}$ refer to the molecular weights of the analyte and ligand, respectively. The equation will calculate R_{max}analyte, which is the theoretical maximum signal one would expect if all the ligand binding sites were occupied by the analyte. This relationship allows one to infer whether they are observing the expected stoichiometry. It should be noted that the above equation assumes that the refractive index increment (RII) between the ligand and the analyte is equal. Studies have shown that for small molecules in particular, this assumption may not always hold and could be off by a factor as great as two [67]. In addition, the percentage of properly folded RNA on the chip surface is not known definitively and may not be expected to be 100%.

Additional Considerations for Using SPR to Measure Small Molecule–RNA Interactions For the screening of small molecules against an RNA target, typically the RNA is immobilized to the chip surface (ligand). A variety of coupling chemistries are available for the immobilization of nucleic acids to biosensor chips. RNA modified with biotin can be immobilized to chips precoated with streptavidin. Amine-modified RNA molecules can be coupled to CM5 chips with the use of EDC/NHS chemistry [68]. As the signal observed in an SPR experiment is related to the molecular weights of the ligand and analyte according to Eq. (4.2), high levels of RNA must be immobilized on the sensor chip to obtain a signal sufficient for measuring small molecule binding. Both coupling methods can provide the high levels of immobilization required for the measurement of RNA–small molecule interactions.

The effects of DMSO must be considered when running an SPR experiment. Small molecules are typically stored as stock concentrations dissolved in DMSO and the inclusion of DMSO in the running buffer can aid with solubility of the small molecule. The signals produced from low-molecular-weight molecules are small in accordance with Eq. (4.2), and the signal change due to the bulk refractive index of DMSO is very large by comparison [69]. Careful matching of the DMSO concentration in the running buffer and the sample is critical. Running DMSO blank injections and subtracting the blank data from the experimental data, referred to as double referencing [70], are used to help deal with the issue. Lastly, due to the small but significant volume differences in the experimental and reference channels as the result of ligand immobilization, differences in DMSO bulk solvent contributions between the two channels must be accounted for. This is accomplished by performing a solvent correction, which is then applied to the experimental data.

Dealing with Nonspecific Interactions by SPR SPR can measure not only specific binding interactions but also nonspecific binding interactions. Small molecules can bind to RNA nonspecifically due to a variety of mechanisms, including electrostatic interactions, stacking interactions, and intercalation. By definition, the stoichiometry of nonspecific binding exceeds 1 : 1. This can be particularly problematic for weaker binding compounds that also display high levels of nonspecific binding, where the signal from the nonspecific binding component can match or exceed that of the specific component (Figure 4.6). Arney and Weeks showed that by including a carefully designed control RNA in the reference channel, much of the effects of

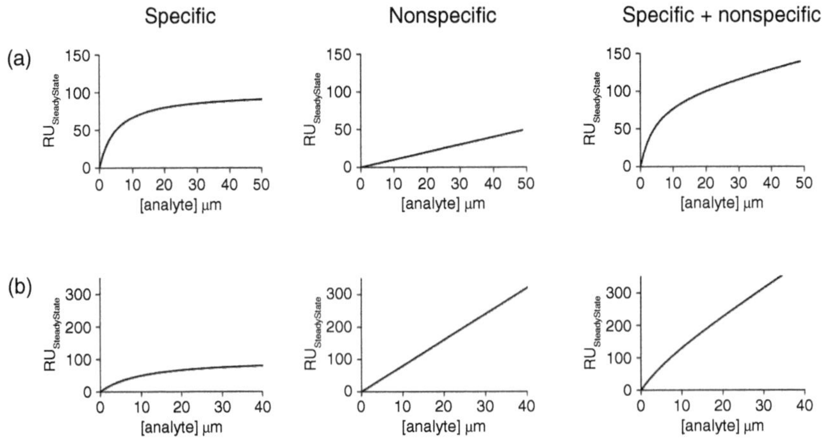

Figure 4.6 Simulated binding curves illustrating the contributions of specific and nonspecific components to a binding curve. High levels of nonspecific binding can mask the specific binding interaction, preventing its measurement in an SPR experiment. (a) Higher affinity-specific interaction with moderate levels of nonspecific binding. In the resultant curve, the specific component is not completely masked and can be fit to equations including the nonspecific component. (b) A weaker affinity-specific interaction with high levels of nonspecific binding. In the resultant curve, the specific interaction is almost completely masked and is not measurable.

nonspecific binding observed in the SPR experiment could be mitigated [71]. Using the SAM-1 and TPP riboswitches as model systems, they showed that by including the appropriate binding site mutant in the reference channel, they were able to significantly reduce the effects of nonspecific binding and were able to extract K_D measurements that were in better agreement with other biophysical methods. Design of an appropriate reference RNA construct requires knowledge of the precise binding site on the RNA. The authors explored the use of noncognate RNAs in the reference channel to address this. While the inclusion of the SAM-III riboswitch in the reference channel gave results comparable to the binding site mutant for the TPP riboswitch, the use of a generic structured RNA in the reference channel had a more modest effect. Thus, it appears that the design of the reference channel RNA is critical, and method development is required for achieving a correct reference channel match for a given RNA target.

4.3.2.2 Fluorescence-Based Assays

Fluorescence-based assays are widely used to provide insight into the binding and specificity of RNA-binding small molecules. Understanding the interactions between an RNA and small molecule ligands is important to the development of new small molecules aimed at targeting RNA. In a complex cellular environment observation of a single interaction event can be very difficult to observe. For this reason, many in vitro studies utilizing fluorescence have been developed. Some of these assays require RNA modification, such as Förster resonance energy transfer (FRET) and site-specific labeling assays such as the 2-aminopurine (2-AP) assay. In these assays, care must be taken to thoroughly evaluate any fluorescently labeled

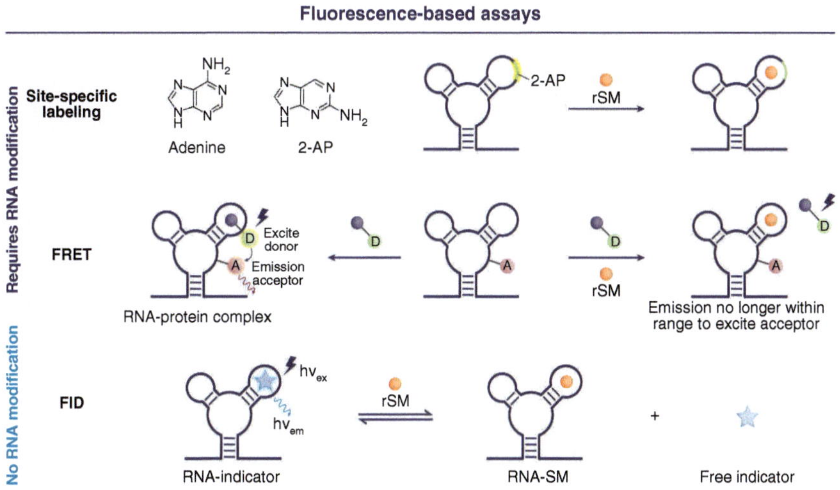

Figure 4.7 Fluorescence-based assays include site-specific labeling assays such as the 2-AP assay and Förster resonance energy transfer (FRET) assays, as well as fluorescence indicator displacement assays.

component to ensure proper structure and similar binding affinity, as labeled RNA may not fold or interact exactly as the native RNA. Other fluorescence-based techniques do not require any modification of the RNA, such as many fluorescent indicator displacement (FID) techniques (Figure 4.7). The use of these assays has aided in the advancement of our understanding of RNA-binding ligand properties as well as in the identification of small molecules structurally distinct from a cognate ligand. Each of the assays mentioned above has distinct advantages and disadvantages, as well as examples of RNA-specific applications.

FRET Assay FRET [72] is a quantum-mechanical phenomenon that occurs when two chromophores are in molecular proximity. FRET uses a distance-dependent transfer of energy from a donor fluorophore to an acceptor molecule. Based on this transfer it is possible to collect information regarding the molecular interactions for a given system. For this reason, its applications within bioscience are widespread and frequently used to study various cellular functions [73]. In FRET, the transfer of energy is radiation-less and occurs when an excited-state donor chromophore transfers some fluorescence energy to an acceptor. For this transfer to occur, the FRET donor/acceptor pair must be in close proximity and the excitation spectrum of the acceptor must overlap with the fluorescence emission spectrum of the donor (Figure 4.8). This transfer results in an increase in the acceptor's emission intensity. By placing the donor and acceptor chromophores on different components and monitoring the changes in fluorescence intensity, one can observe changes in interactions within a given system. Some examples of the interactions previously monitored by FRET for RNA include RNA conformational changes associated with binding events such as those with domain II of the HCV IRES [74, 75], RNA-ligand binding such as the use of FRET-based quenching for binding of small

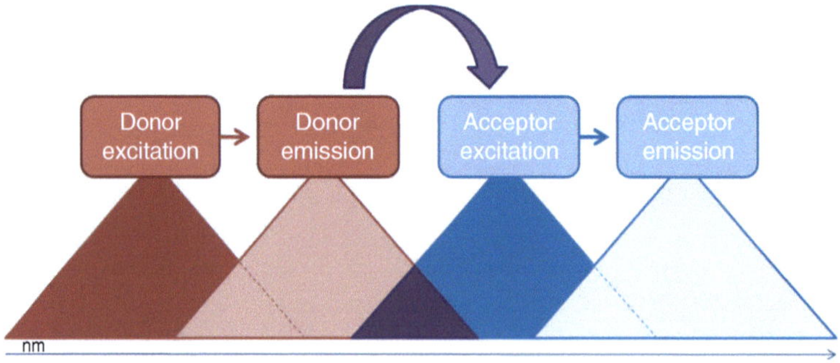

Figure 4.8 Spectral overlap necessary for a successful FRET pair.

molecules to exon 10-intron 10 hairpin [76], and RNA-protein interactions between muscleblind-like1 (MBNL1) and an expanded CUG repeat RNA as a target for myotonic dystrophy type I (DM1) [77].

Site-specific Labeling Assays (2-AP) 2-Aminopurine (2-AP) is a fluorophore with high structural similarity to the natural nucleobase adenine, differing from adenine (6-aminopurine) by the position of the exocyclic amine group. Though they are structurally similar, 2-AP has an emission 1000 times the fluorescence intensity of adenine [78]. For this reason 2-AP can be incorporated into RNA strands with minimal structural disturbance and be used as a very sensitive fluorescent probe to provide information regarding the local microenvironment experienced by the probe. 2-AP has been used extensively in both DNA and RNA structures to help gain information regarding both secondary and tertiary structure, including helping to track changes in configuration upon ligand binding. One example includes the use of the 2-AP assay in subdomain IIa of the HCV IRES to provide insight into the folding state of the internal loop of the structure [79]. Another example used 2-AP within the A-bulge of tau as a target for neurodegenerative diseases [76]. While 2-AP is well-studied and remains the most used nucleobase probe, efforts have been made to develop additional fluorescent base analogs [80–82]. Additionally, work has recently been carried out to enhance the effectiveness of 2-AP, with a strong focus on the ideal positions of the probe [83, 84].

Fluorescence Indicator Displacement (FID) Assay Fluorescence indicator displacement (FID) is a widely used method that relies on a change in fluorescence of an indicator upon binding with a given receptor, in this case RNA. It is a sensitive, quantitative, and high-throughput assay. Since FID does not have to be immobilized, the RNA is not limited to binding or conformational restraints. There are a wide variety of RNA-binding indicators with various levels of fluorescence. This large variety of tool ligands provides a great opportunity for fine-tuning for individual assay/RNA needs. Some key classes of fluorescent compounds used in FID include cyanine dyes, xanthone derivatives, metabolites, intercalators, and dye-labeled aminoglycosides [85]. FID can also use dye-labeled peptides. Here we will highlight some examples of cyanine dyes and xanthone derivatives used for FID assays with RNA.

Cyanine dyes are compounds containing two nitrogen-containing heterocyclic rings linked by a polymethine bridge [86]. When in aqueous environments, free cyanine dyes illustrate very little to no fluorescence. However, upon binding nucleic acids, the structure is restricted ultimately leading to a 100- to 1000-fold enhancement in fluorescence [87]. The broad spectroscopic range of cyanine dyes provides the opportunity to detect these at a large range of wavelengths. Additionally, these dyes can be further tuned through synthetic modifications including variation of chain length, changing the identity of cyclic heteroatoms, and adding substituents to one or both heterocycles. These features provide the opportunity to easily access commercial sources as well as modify synthetically to modulate these dyes for specific use [87]. There are many examples of different cyanine dyes used in FID experiments for RNA-binding small molecules.

An early example of cyanine dyes used in FID for RNA targets includes the work of the Stojanovic and Datta laboratories demonstrating the detection of selective ligands with RNA aptamers [88, 89]. Additional work carried out by Asare-Okai and Chow evaluated bacterial RNA targets including the ribosomal A-site, helix 31 of the 16S, and helix 69 of the 23S ribosomal RNA in addition to the HIV-1TAR element. Utilizing known RNA–ligand pairs the authors demonstrated that FID utilizing the cyanine dye TO-PRO-1 is an effective, sensitive, high-throughput method for capturing relative binding affinities of various ligands to RNA targets [90–92].

Xanthones are a class of compounds with a fused tricyclic scaffold containing oxygenated heterocycles. A wide variety of xanthone derivatives have been highlighted as not only pharmacological tools but also as therapeutic agents [93]. Initial studies on xanthones with DNA illustrated that the addition of electron-donating amino groups generated the potential for use as biological indicators [94]. These have been extensively studied in the Nakatani laboratory [95–99]. In one study, Nakatani and co-workers demonstrated the use of a xanthone derivative 2,7-disubstituted 9H-xanthen-9-one (X2S) as a fluorescent indicator to identify a unique set of hits for two distinct RNA targets. Importantly, the X2S FID assay is suitable for high-throughput screenings and has illustrated its potential to generate qualitative results consistent with those of ITC analysis [95]. This indicator was illustrated to bind more efficiently to unpaired regions of RNA compared to double-stranded regions. Upon binding to RNA, fluorescence decreases, providing a qualitative evaluation of ligand–RNA interactions which the authors illustrate are consistent with ITC analysis, and provide the advantage that FID is suitable for high- throughput analysis.

One key limitation of FID is that it provides only binding affinity information. While this is incredibly valuable information, other assays such as ITC, SPR, or NMR can provide additional details such as stoichiometry, thermodynamic, or kinetic binding parameters. Additionally, FID requires controls to ensure that there are no interactions between the indicator and small molecule, as well as verification that the small molecule does not fluoresce. Overall, FID for RNA targets has been widely explored. This exploration has provided the opportunity to easily adapt FID to new RNA targets and therefore continue to gain a deeper understanding of small molecule binding with RNA.

4.3.2.3 Microscale Thermophoresis (MST)

Microscale thermophoresis (MST) is a highly sensitive biophysical method that can measure K_D values down to 1 picomolar [100]. MST is based on the detection of a temperature-induced change (induced by an infrared laser) in the fluorescence of a target (either intrinsically fluorescent or containing a conjugated fluorophore) as a function of the concentration of a nonfluorescent ligand. The term "thermophoresis" describes a directed movement of particles along a temperature gradient [101]. A temperature difference ΔT in space leads to a depletion of solvated biomolecules in the region of elevated temperature, quantified by the Soret coefficient S_T, wherein $c_{hot}/c_{cold} = \exp(-S_T\Delta T)$. The values c_{hot} and c_{cold} represent the concentrations in the heated and nonheated regions, respectively. This depletion of solvated biomolecules depends on the interface between molecule and solvent. Under constant buffer conditions, thermophoresis probes the size, charge, and solvation entropy of the molecules. The thermophoresis of a target molecule (e.g. an RNA with a fluorescence tag) can differ significantly from the thermophoresis of a target molecule–ligand complex due to binding-induced changes in size, charge, and solvation energy. For proteins, even if binding does not significantly change the size or charge of a target molecule, MST can still detect binding due to binding-induced changes in the target molecule's solvation entropy. Some advantages to MST include compatibility with complex bioliquids (e.g. cell lysates), low sample consumption, and no need to prepare immobilized RNA targets.

For RNA binders, researchers have used MST to confirm binding and determine K_D values. Schneekloth and co-workers measured K_D values of peptide–RNA interactions (e.g. HIV type 1 Rev response element (RRE) RNA with fluorescein-labeled Rev peptide), RNA–small molecule interactions (e.g. Cy5 labeled *Bs* preQ_1 riboswitch with preQ_1; Cy5 labeled *Tt* preQ_1 riboswitch with preQ_1; and others), and displacement of an RNA-bound peptide by a small molecule (e.g. ,displacement of Fl labeled Rev from RRE with neomycin) [102]. Disney and co-workers have recently used MST to determine the K_Ds of various ligands to their target RNAs [25, 27, 103]. Some drawbacks to MST are the preparation of fluorescently labeled RNA or ligand and the relatively unstudied effect of solvation of an RNA–ligand complex for uncharged ligands that do not possess net charge upon solvation in aqueous media. Thus, MST can serve as an assay to confirm binding and to help optimize binding within a series of molecules.

4.3.2.4 Isothermal Titration Calorimetry (ITC)

Isothermal calorimetry (ITC) is a highly versatile, label-free method often viewed as the gold standard for characterizing the stoichiometry, affinity, and full thermodynamic profile of a ligand binding event. The thermodynamic information obtained in an ITC experiment provides valuable insight into both the enthalpic and entropic contributions to small molecule–macromolecule and macromolecule–macromolecule interactions, including RNA–RNA, RNA–small molecule, and RNA–protein interactions. A close look at these contributions may lead to a better understanding of the binding mode of a ligand as well as its effects on the conformation and folded state of an RNA target [104]. Ultimately, this information can provide valuable feedback regarding compound design to improve binding selectivity, minimize the entropic cost of binding, and maximize enthalpic favorability.

ITC works through the use of two cells: the first is a reference cell with water and the second is a sample cell containing macromolecule (RNA) and can have a ligand (compound) injected in. Each cell is connected to a power source that seeks to maintain a constant temperature for both cells [105]. The enthalpy (heat, ΔH) of the interaction is directly measured through this method by the integration of differential power with respect to time for each injection, and stoichiometry, ΔS and $\Delta G/K_D$ are later calculated by the careful fitting of the titration series from start to saturation. If the titration is run at multiple temperatures, the heat capacity change upon binding (ΔC_p) may be derived from the slope of $\Delta\Delta H$ with respect to sample temperature [106]. This parameter can be useful for understanding how the degrees of freedom, or flexibility, of the biomolecule changes upon binding.

The major advantage of ITC over other label-free methods is that it can derive a full set of thermodynamic parameters using just the interaction heat as the reporter. However, ITC's high sensitivity to changes in heat is also one of its drawbacks. For example, even the heat of dilution of a 1% mismatched buffer in the syringe injected into the cell can completely mask the binding signal [104]. Another potential limitation is in the case of thermoneutral events such as running a titration at the isoenthalpic temperature, where there is no detectable net heat of binding even though binding is still occurring. Additionally, a relatively large sample quantity is required for an effective experiment. While the amount of RNA required for ITC is dependent on the instrument used, it is typically less than required for NMR and X-ray, but more than needed for other experiments including gel shifts, SPR, UV-melts, and fluorescence-based assays. Best results are typically obtained when using ligand concentrations that are 15–20 times the concentration of RNA. Additionally, the amount of RNA used in the experiment should be at least three times of the expected KD value [107, 108]. However, due to the relatively large quantity of RNA required for each experiment, ITC is best used following a preliminary binding study such as SPR or UV melts, with the aim of further understanding the thermodynamics and stoichiometry of the ligand–RNA interaction.

Since the ΔH measured will be the sum of all enthalpic events during the titration, including solvent effects, molecular reorganization, conformational changes, heat of dilution and mechanical artifacts, sample quality, and purity are essential [105]. The RNA sample should have undergone adequate quality control to ensure sample homogeneity and that no alternative long-lived conformations exist. Gel shifts often provide a good assessment of these factors [105]. Without these quality control steps, there is lower confidence that thermal changes observed via ITC are reflective of a binding event to the species and structure of interest and not alternative oligomers or a mixture of nonexchanging, discrete conformational states. To avoid observing excess heat of dilution due to buffer mismatch during a titration, it is also very important that the RNA samples are dialyzed into the assay buffer and that the remaining dialysis buffer is used to dissolve the ligand. Bubbles can add noise to the experimental baseline so they should be removed by degassing the syringe and cell species prior to the assay.

In the case of a binding event that may involve protonation or deprotonation, pH and buffer should be carefully considered to ensure that the measured enthalpy is not due to the buffer-dependent and solvent dilution events instead of the binding event. To consider this experimentally, the experiment should be run at various buffer conditions and pHs. Cacodylate, phosphate, and HEPES buffers are often preferred for their low heat of ionization. Comparison of the binding event at various pH conditions can provide insight regarding the enthalpy of the binding event compared to the background noise. Similar factors must be considered when metal ions are needed for proper RNA folding, where ionic interactions may or may not contribute to the binding thermodynamics.

ITC has been used to characterize RNA interactions with various binding partners including small molecules or ions, proteins, and other RNAs [106]. Small molecule–RNA interactions studied using ITC include the evaluation of various $preQ_1$ riboswitch classes for the pyrrolopyrimidine effector $preQ_1$ [109] and the evaluation of aminoglycoside-RNA-binding interactions among others [110–112]. These studies illustrate the important thermodynamic interactions that ITC can help characterize in order to optimize RNA–small molecule interactions.

4.4 Binding Site Identification/Target Engagement

Binding site identification and target engagement involve finding sites where a ligand binds a target RNA and is critical to elucidate a compound's mechanism of action. Herein, we will focus on several covalent methods to assess target engagement: Δ selective 2′-hydroxyl acylation and primer extension (ΔSHAPE) [31]/ΔDMS, photoaffinity evaluation of RNA ligation-sequencing (PEARL-seq) [23], and chemical cross-linking and isolation by pulldown (Chem-CLIP) [113]. Lastly, competition with gapmer anti-sense oligonucleotides (ASOs) may also be used to assess target engagement. These methods can be done in-cells, in cell lysates, and in vitro. Ideally, a lead molecule should demonstrate in-cell target engagement to validate its mechanism of action.

4.4.1 Covalent Methods

Target engagement may be assessed using covalent methods such as ΔSHAPE or ΔDMS (see Figure 4.9). For decades, researchers have used chemical probing reagents like dimethyl sulfate (DMS) and selective 2′-hydroxyl acylation and primer extension (SHAPE) reagents for mapping the structural features of nucleic acids (cf. Chapter 2). Treating target RNA with both a probing reagent and an RNA binder may reveal binding sites when the RNA binder evokes a protective effect (i.e. a reduction in chemical probe reacting with RNA at or near the binding

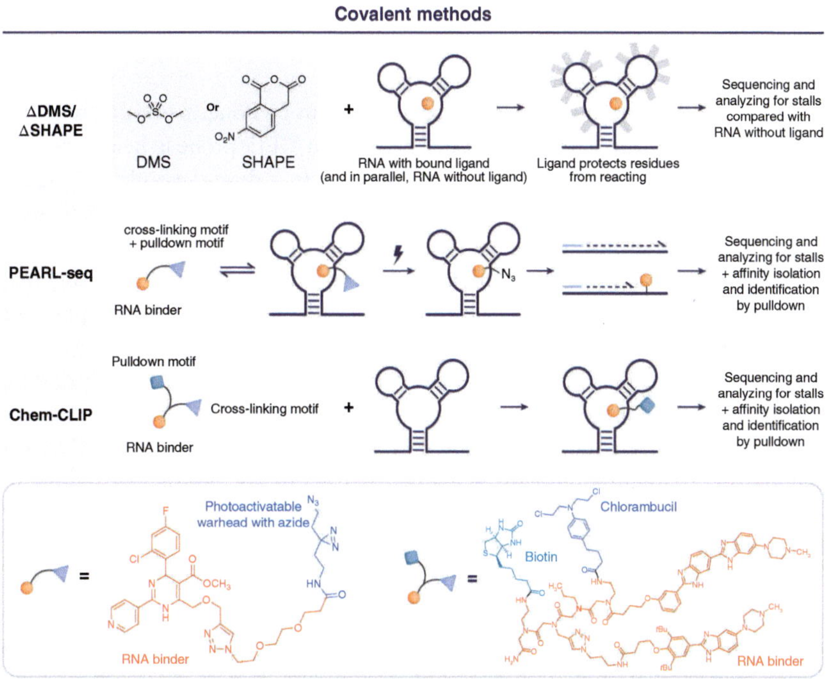

Figure 4.9 Covalent methods used to ascertain target engagement. ΔDMS/ΔSHAPE are probing methods that use DMS or SHAPE reagents to identify the binding site of a ligand. PEARL-seq and Chem-CLIP require the synthesis of probes featuring a cross-linking motif, a pulldown motif, and an RNA binder to identify the site of binding and assess the selectivity of a ligand.

site as measured by reverse transcription) or a deprotective effect representing a conformational change. For example, Sztuba-Solinska and co-workers identified biologically active RNA binders targeting the HIV transactivation response (TAR) RNA using ΔSHAPE [31].

Covalent methods like in-cell click selective cross-linking with RNA sequence profiling (icCL-seq) [114], PEARL-seq and Chem-CLIP may also be used to assess target engagement. These methods use an RNA binder conjugated with: (i) a cross-linking motif (for example, diazirine or chlorambucil) and (ii) a pulldown substituent (e.g. an alkyne, an azide, or biotin). IcCL-seq and PEARL-seq use a diazirine moiety with a pendant aliphatic azide moiety (that survives irradiation), while Chem-CLIP typically uses chlorambucil and biotin as the cross-linking motif and pulldown substituent, respectively. The RNA binder interacts with the target RNA and brings the cross-linking motif into proximity with the RNA such that they react either directly (e.g. in the case of chlorambucil) or upon irradiation (e.g. in the case of diazirine). A reverse-transcription (RT) pausing assay can then be used to determine the sites of covalent modification. The pulldown substituent enables downstream labeling of the RNA adducts, allowing for subsequent affinity isolation and identification of RNA-binding partners from complex mixtures. Effectively, PEARL-seq and Chem-CLIP elucidate both binding site and ligand selectivity in a single sequencing experiment.

For further validation, competitive experiments can be done in parallel wherein the RNA binder is titrated and the PEARL-seq/Chem-CLIP probe is held constant. If the two molecules compete for the same binding site, a dose-dependent decrease in target enrichment will be observed as the RNA-binder concentration increases. These methods can also be used in cells and with cell lysate.

In their mechanistic studies of small-molecule modulation of SMN2 splicing, Schultz, Johnson, and Wang used a biotinyl (pulldown substituent) and pendant diazirine (cross-linking motif) probe derived from SMN-C2 (an analog of an FDA-approved drug for treatment of spinal muscular atrophy (SMA)), risdiplam (cf. Section 4.6.2 and Chapter 7). Using the competitively treated cells as a reference control (2 μM SMN-C2 probe + 100 μM SMN-C3, a related analog of SMN-C2 (cf. Figure 4.11)), alignment of the sequencing reads of the probe-only sample to the human genome did not reveal an enrichment of exon 7. However, Schultz and co-workers identified AGGAAG as a binding motif for SMN-C2 probe in a genome-wide analysis of the captured pre-mRNA [115]. Further, ΔSHAPE analysis revealed a conformational change in two to three unpaired nucleotides at the junction of intron 6 and exon 7 in both in vitro and in-cell models. Other examples of target engagement include Myers and co-workers' use of icCL-seq to map binding sites for tetracycline derivatives on key human rRNA substructures [114]. Disney and co-authors used Chem-CLIP to identify binding sites of oncogenic microRNA-96 (pri-miR-96) using the targaprimir-96 probe shown in Figure 4.9 [113]. Mukherjee, Blain, Petter, and co-authors have used PEARL-seq to assess target engagement of an RNA binder against aptamer 21 (using the PEARL-seq probe illustrated in Figure 4.9) [23]. Schneekloth and co-authors used chem-CLIP to reveal a highly selective interaction between the PreQ1 riboswitch aptamer and a probe derived from a PreQ1 metabolite [116].

4.4.2 Competition with an Antisense Oligonucleotide (ASO)

In addition to covalent methods, target engagement may also be assessed through competition experiments with a gapmer ASO and an RNA binder that is complementary to the target. The ASO induces cleavage by recruitment of ribonuclease H (RNase H), resulting in lower abundance of the RNA. An RNA binder can compete with the gapmer ASO and increase the abundance of RNA as the binder is titrated in. Recently, Disney and co-authors employed this strategy by designing 6 ASOs that bind at different sites of the SNCA IRE hairpin structure and competed with the compound Synucleozid to ascertain the putative binding site (termed ASO-Bind-Map) [117]. An advantage ASOs have over covalent methods like PEARL-seq and Chem-CLIP is that the new chemical entities do not have to be derived; only the sequence of the target RNA is required. Using this method in combination with the above covalent methods, one can further validate an RNA binder's target engagement.

4.5 Defining SAR and Functional Assays

Compounds that bind to a target RNA and demonstrate target engagement should be tested in at least one functional assay (preferably more to mitigate false positives) to determine if the observed binding leads to a change in the level of protein expression. Once an RNA binder demonstrates on-target functional activity (as further demonstrated by in-cell target engagement, vide supra), the RNA binder is fully validated. By acquiring functional data in tandem with binding data, SAR can be developed and applied to new designs, thus propelling the design-make-test-analyze cycle [118]. Researchers may apply the same principles from protein target-based drug discovery to optimizing RNA binders by designing and making structural changes to the binder, gathering and analyzing data, and then formulating new structural changes to improve binding, drug-like properties [119], and functional activity. For RNA drug discovery, this is best exemplified by risdiplam [120] and branaplam [121], splice modulators that will be further discussed in Chapter 7. Further, Ernst and colleagues optimized [122] rocaglamide A and congeners, a class of natural products that inhibits protein synthesis by forming a stable ternary complex with polypurine rich messenger RNAs and eIF4A [123]. The authors made derivatives with improved drug-like properties and discovered eFT226 (zotatifin) that is currently in clinical development to treat cancer.

4.5.1 Functional Assays

A functional assay can be designed based on the RNA target of interest and the mechanistic hypothesis. Cellular gene-reporter assays are commonly employed, wherein the level of protein expression is assessed via a surrogate reporter. These can be tested in a cell-free environment first [124]. Fluorescent proteins and luciferases are examples of such reporters and can be introduced via methods such as viral transduction, transient transfection, or endogenous gene editing. A second reporter driven by an IRES in a bicistronic expression vector can help normalize signal [125]. For example, Todd and co-authors used a dual luciferase reporter assay to confirm if small molecule BIX01294 could inhibit +1CGG translation (as measured by NanoLuciferase luminescence) in HEK293 cells, and at 25 μM, +1CGG RNA translation was significantly reduced although the compound was found to be moderately toxic by measure of FireflyLuciferase luminescence and cell morphology [126]. A popular version of luciferase reporter called HiBiT utilizes a split luciferase concept, whereby a small *N*-terminal sequence of NanoLuciferase can be expressed at the endogenous locus of the target gene and reconstituted with the remainder of the NanoLuciferase in the form of a recombinant protein along with a substrate. This gives a bioluminescent readout for the tagged target protein [127].

Minigene splicing reporters are used to assess compounds that have an effect on mRNA splicing [128]. Precursors for risdiplam, a drug used to treat SMA [129], were identified using a high-throughput screen with a luciferase reporter minigene. Although the discovery was made via a cell-based screen, one could apply such an assay to assess functional activity from binding first approaches. Additional methods of assessing the function of RNA-binding small molecules include immunoassays, which are used to determine the protein levels of the target of interest. These types of assays include western blotting, Simple Westerns™ [130], and many forms of sandwich ELISA such as traditional ELISAs, electrochemiluminescence-based MSD [131], and bead-based (no-wash) AlphaLISA [132]. Mass spectrometry and proteomics are also used for assessing levels of protein coded by a target RNA [133]. These methods are important for confirming changes in the levels of proteins in endogenous settings of cells or animals. Emerging technologies are sure to make this evaluation more robust and easier.

4.5.2 Phenotypic Screens

Phenotypic screens [134] are functional assays that identify compounds based on an observed phenotype (biological effect) without knowledge of molecular target or mechanism (agnostic screening). These screens have also been used to discover RNA binders despite being agnostic to a small molecule's target. Phenotypic screens can be formatted to be high throughput, and in the cases of risdiplam [120] and branaplam [121], phenotypic screens identified hits that were further optimized to the respective lead series. After several rounds of optimization, risdiplam was approved for treatment of SMA (cf. Section 4.6 and Chapter 7). Careful target engagement and mechanism of action studies should be carried out to determine whether a molecule is acting through an RNA interaction mechanism. For example, didehydro-cortistatin A (dCA) inhibits production of new viral particles from HIV-1-infected cells, but Mousseau and coworkers demonstrated that dCA disrupts transcription of the integrated HIV-1 genome by binding to the TAR-binding domain of Tat, not to TAR RNA [135].

4.6 Identifying a Lead Series

For small molecules, it is well known what constitutes a good lead series [136]. A lead series is identified once RNA binding is confirmed by at least two orthogonal biophysical methods (cf. Section 4.3), has SAR that repeats across different methods, is selective for a target RNA, shows target engagement in cells connected to a cellular response (cf. Sections 4.4 and 4.5), and has reasonable pharmacokinetic properties. Figure 4.10 outlines the process for identifying a lead series with the goal of ultimately delivering a compound for clinical development.

Hit confirmation involves structure confirmation by resynthesis and purification, which is critical to ensure that the presumed structure is correct. Confirmed hits should also demonstrate binding to an RNA by at least two orthogonal biophysical methods. Further, SAR around similar analogs should be consistent across different biophysical methods. Hit optimization entails improvements in SAR regarding binding affinity and functional activity. Compounds in this stage should also demonstrate target engagement (cf. Sections 4.4 and 4.5) and should be screened

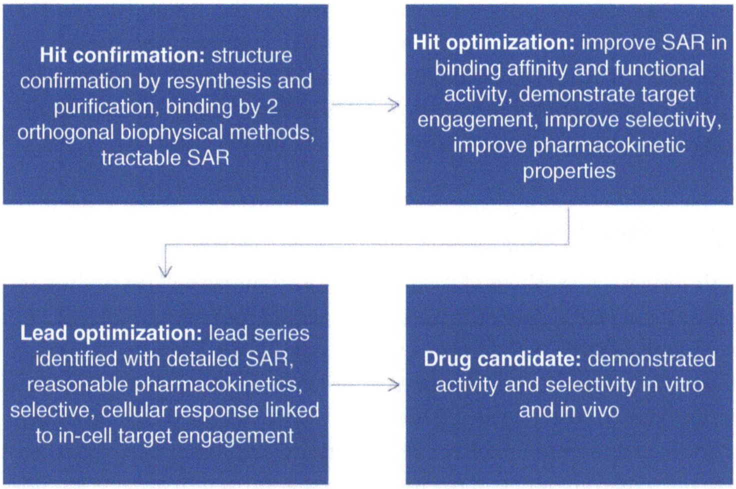

Figure 4.10 Process for identifying a lead series with the goal of making a compound for clinical development. First, a hit is found, confirmed, and optimized using methods discussed in Sections 4.1 through 4.5. The lead series is further optimized to a drug candidate that should demonstrate activity and selectivity in vitro and in vivo and have toxicological data acquired in multiple species.

for selectivity for the RNA of interest among other RNAs in the transcriptome. Pharmacokinetic properties should also be tested for and improved in this stage. A lead series is selected after gathering detailed SAR across binding and functional assays, reasonable pharmacokinetics, selectivity information regarding RNA targets and protein targets, and linking any cellular response to in-cell target engagement. Ultimately, the lead series can be further optimized to a drug candidate that should demonstrate activity and selectivity in vitro and in vivo and have toxicological data acquired in multiple species.

4.6.1 Hit Optimization

Also known as hit-to-lead [137], the goal of hit optimization is to improve an RNA binder's affinity, functional activity, selectivity, and pharmacokinetic properties with the eventual goal being to assess in vivo efficacy. Work in this phase consists of SAR investigations around an RNA binder, combining data gathered from binding and functional assays, and making new structural hypotheses to further improve a compound. If structural information about an RNA is known, structure-based drug design techniques can be applied to develop the SAR faster and in a more focused way.

Selectivity and toxicity should also be interrogated, optimized, and mitigated, respectively, at this point. Selectivity may be assessed through several methods. First, a selectivity panel of RNAs can be tested for binding by a hit analog using one of the biophysical methods previously mentioned in this chapter. Second, a PEARL-seq probe (or a similar probe mentioned in Section 4.4) may be developed for a hit analog that assesses target engagement across the transcriptome [23]. Third, RNA-seq [138] may be used to assess selectivity by measuring global gene expression changes induced by treatment with an RNA binder. Fourth, traditional methods may be used to interrogate selectivity and toxicity such as in vitro pharmacological profiling by using off-target screening panels [139].

4.6.2 Risdiplam Hit-to-Lead

SMA is a genetic disease caused by mutation or deletion of the survival motor neuron 1 (SMN1) gene and is a leading genetic cause of infant and toddler mortality [120b]. Survival motor neuron (SMN) protein is expressed in all body tissues and is essential for development and functional homeostasis in many species [140]. In humans, SMN protein is produced by two genes: SMN1 and SMN2, although the latter gene produces low levels of full-length mRNA due to alternative splicing of exon 7. Nusinersen, an RNA antisense oligonucleotide, was the first approved treatment for SMA and works by inhibiting a splicing silencer that allows for SMN2 exon 7 splicing, thus expressing SMN protein [141]. Although a breakthrough drug, nusinersen must be administered intrathecally, i.e. by injection in the cerebrospinal fluid of the spine.

Risdiplam, an FDA approved oral small-molecule splice modulator of SMN2 exon 7, was discovered first by using a high-throughput phenotypic screen designed to identify small-molecule compounds that increase the inclusion of exon 7 during SMN2 pre-mRNA splicing in an SMN2 minigene reporter assay (HEK293 cells) [120b]. Ratni and co-authors identified coumarin derivative R-1 as a promising hit (Figure 4.11). In parallel, SAR was started on both the coumarin and benzoxazole moieties of the molecule, along with scaffold hopping around the coumarin core. Isocoumarin SMN-C1, coumarin SMN-C2, and pyridopyrimidinone SMN-C3 were

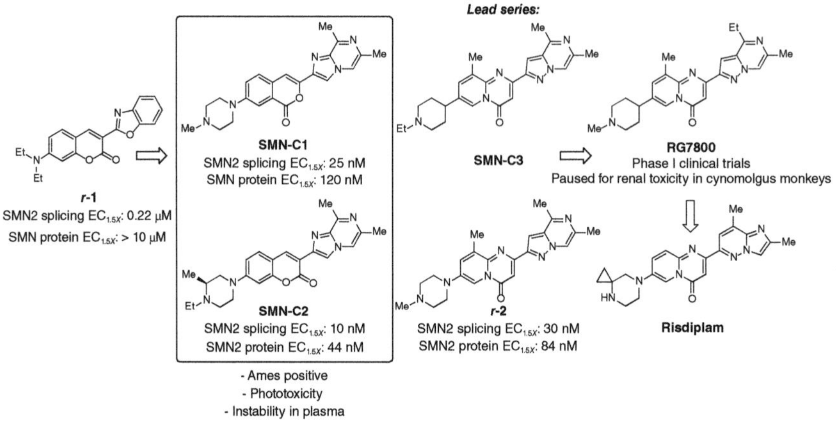

Figure 4.11 Initial coumarin hit R-1 and lead series containing a pyridopyrimidine core. Although potent, SMN-C1 and SMN-C2 possessed selectivity and chemical instability problems that the pyridopyrimidine core lead series did not have. The pyridopyrimidine series was further optimized to arrive at risdiplam, the first small molecule approved treatment for SMA that increases the inclusion of exon 7 during SMN2 pre-mRNA splicing.

identified as orally bioavailable and all three analogs modified SMN2 splicing in SMA patient-derived cells [142]. However, SMN-C1 and SMN-C2 exhibited Ames toxicity (genotoxicity), phototoxicity, and chemical instability in plasma and aqueous buffers. Further optimization of these series resulted in either potent compounds that still exhibited Ames toxicity or compounds that were ineffective in the in vitro SMN2 minigene reporter assay. Pyridopyrimidone core-containing compounds SMN-C3 and R-2 were free of the phototoxicity and plasma stability issues that halted progression of the SMN-C1 and 'C2 series. Further optimization of the series brought forth candidate RG7800, which was tested in Phase I clinical trials for spinal SMA. However, due to observed renal toxicity in cynomolgus monkeys, researchers paused further clinical trials involving RG7800. From RG7800, Ratni and co-workers further optimized the series to improve selectivity vs. off-target genes as measured through transcriptome-wide RNA-seq using type 1 SMA patient fibroblasts [143] and improved on-target potency, thus allowing clinicians to lower the efficacious dose in patients.

4.6.3 Branaplam Lead Generation

Like risdiplam, researchers at Novartis performed an HTS to identify small-molecule modulators that increase the SMN2 exon 7 inclusion using an NSC34 motor neuron cell line expressing an SMN2 minigene reporter [144]. Primary hits were confirmed, and among those hits identified was pyridazine B-1 (Figure 4.12) which possessed SMN EC_{50} of 600 nM (2.5 fold expression), but also suffered from high in vivo clearance, low brain exposure, and potent hERG inhibition [120a].

Cheung and co-authors improved the SMN Elisa potency (SMN Δ7 mouse myoblast assay) by replacing the benzothiophene with an ortho-phenol. Further,

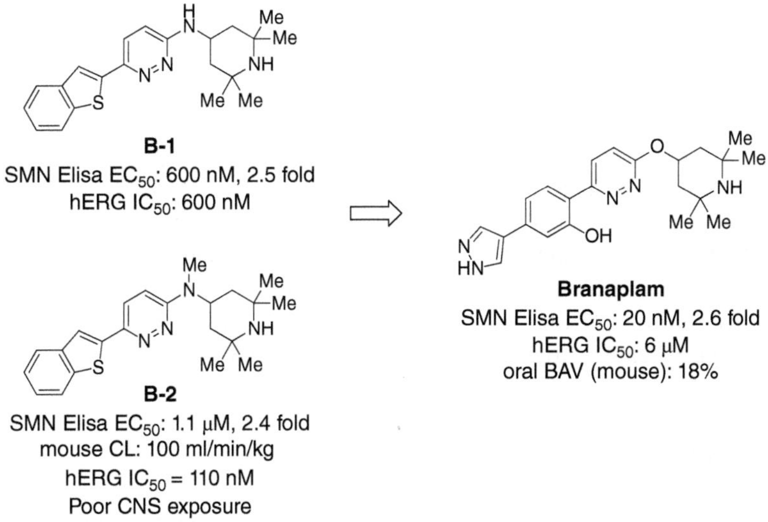

Figure 4.12 Initial pyridazine hit B-1 and derivative B-2 were targeted as the lead series resulting in the discovery of branaplam.

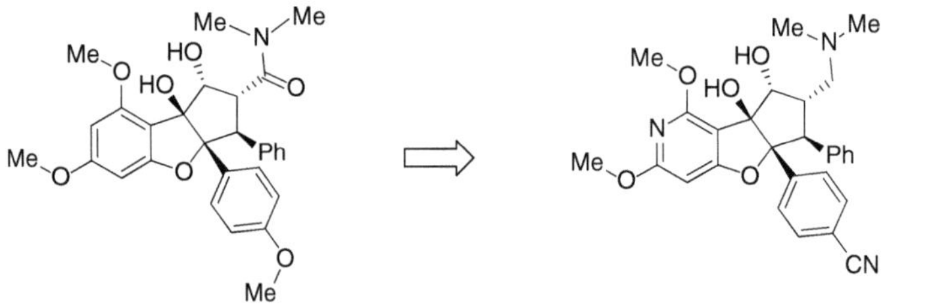

(−)-Rocaglamide A
Cell IC_{50}: 20 nM

Poor physicochemical properties
Poor metabolic stability

Zotatifin
Cell IC_{50}: 11 nM

>20 mg/ml aqueous solubility
CL (rat): 48 ml/min/kg

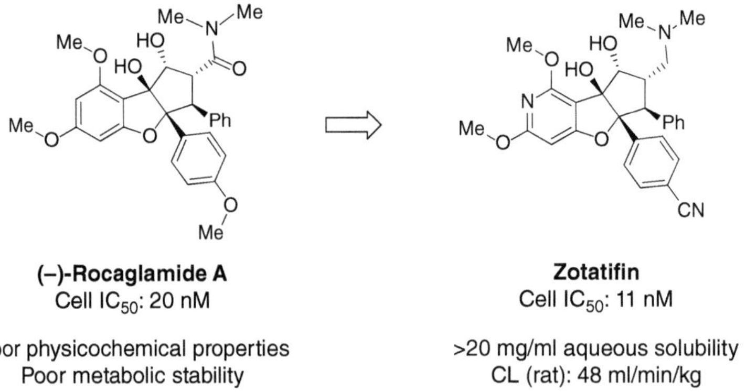

Figure 4.13 Rocaglamide natural product lead series (represented by (−)-rocaglamide A) was optimized to zotatifin (eFT226), an inhibitor of RNA helicase eIF4A, currently in clinical trials for cancer and SARS-CoV-2.

researchers at Novartis reduced hERG inhibition by adding electron withdrawing polar groups on the western aromatic side of the molecule. Lastly, changing the *N*-methylamine linker (cf. compound B-2, Figure 4.12) to an oxygen led to branaplam, which exhibited improved brain exposure and efficacy in the SMN Δ7 mouse model. Currently, clinical trials with branaplam as treatments for both SMA and Huntington's Disease are paused.

4.6.4 Zotatifin Lead Generation

(—)-Rocaglamide A and congeners, a class of natural products that inhibits protein synthesis by forming a stable ternary complex with polypurine-rich messenger RNAs and eIF4A [123b], have been shown to be potent antiproliferative and antiviral agents [145]. Researchers at eFFECTOR Therapeutics chose the rocaglamide scaffold as a lead series to further optimize resulting in the discovery of zotafitin, the first eIF4A inhibitor tested in human clinical trials (Figure 4.13) [122]. To optimize rocaglamide A, Ernst and co-authors focused on improving the poor solubility and metabolic stability by exploring new ways to decrease the lipophilicity of the molecule. Ultimately, the molecule was made to be more polar and soluble through changing the western dimethoxy phenyl to dimethoxy pyridine and converting the amide to a basic *N,N*-dimethyl amine. Further, the *p*-methoxyphenyl was changed to a *p*-cyanophenyl to simultaneously improve potency and lower lipophilicity, which has been previously explored by other research groups [146]. Zotatifin is currently in Phase II clinical trials for breast cancer and SARS-CoV-2.

4.7 Concluding Thoughts and Outlook

In this chapter, we outlined knowledge-based and agnostic screening approaches for the identification of RNA binders, including both virtual screening methods and high-throughput screening methods. Further, we have shown methods used to assess binding affinity, binding site(s) of an RNA ligand, target engagement, and functional activity – all of which are necessary in generating lead RNA binders to progress for lead optimization and eventually clinical development. The future of RNA drug discovery is promising as we continue to develop methods for generating and optimizing RNA binders.

Acknowledgments

We would like to thank Joel Dufour, Scott Gorman, Sarah Mahoney, Anthony Montibello, Herschel Mukherjee, Scott Rusin, and Yaqiang Wang for their suggestions and edits on various parts of the manuscript. We also want to thank Craig Blain, Nick Marsh, Lee Roberts, and Erik Spek for their review of the manuscript and suggested edits. Lastly, we would like to thank Nick Marsh and Lee Roberts for their guidance in organizing the manuscript.

References

1 Daldrop, P., Reyes, F.E., Robinson, D.A. et al. (2011). Novel ligands for a purine riboswitch discovered by RNA-ligand docking. *Chem. Biol.* 18 (3): https://doi.org/10.1016/j.chembiol.2010.12.020.
2 Gilbert, S.D., Stoddard, C.D., Wise, S.J., and Batey, R.T. (2006). Thermodynamic and kinetic characterization of ligand binding to the purine riboswitch aptamer domain. *J. Mol. Biol.* 359 (3): https://doi.org/10.1016/j.jmb.2006.04.003.
3 Pereira, D.A. and Williams, J.A. (2007). Origin and evolution of high throughput screening. *Br. J. Pharmacol.* 152 (1): 53–61. https://doi.org/10.1038/sj.bjp.0707373.
4 Fenn, J.B., Mann, M., Meng, C.K. et al. (1989). Electrospray ionization for mass spectrometry of large biomolecules. *Science* 246 (4926): 64–71. https://doi.org/10.1126/science.2675315.
5 Banerjee, S. and Mazumdar, S. (2012). Electrospray ionization mass spectrometry: a technique to access the information beyond the molecular weight of the analyte. *Int. J. Anal. Chem.* 2012: 1–40. https://doi.org/10.1155/2012/282574.
6 Ganem, B., Li, Y.T., and Henion, J.D. (1991). Detection of noncovalent receptor-ligand complexes by mass spectrometry. *JACS* 113 (16): 6294–6296. https://doi.org/10.1021/ja00016a069.
7 Cheng, X., Chen, R., Bruce, J.E. et al. (1995). Using electrospray ionization FTICR mass spectrometry to study competitive binding of inhibitors to carbonic anhydrase. *JACS* 117 (34): 8859–8860. https://doi.org/10.1021/ja00139a023.
8 Herschlag, D., Bonilla, S., and Bisaria, N. (2018). The story of RNA folding, as told in epochs. *Cold Spring Harbor Perspect. Biol.* 10 (10): https://doi.org/10.1101/cshperspect.a032433.
9 Sannes Lowery, K.A., Cummins, L.L., Chen, S. et al. (2005). *Integrated Strategies for Drug Discovery Using Mass Spectrometry*. Hoboken, NJ: Wiley.

10 Marshall, A.G., Hendrickson, C.L., and Jackson, G.S. (1998). Fourier transform ion cyclotron resonance mass spectrometry: a primer. *Mass Spectrom. Rev.* 17 (1): 1–35. https://doi.org/10.1002/(SICI)1098-2787(1998)17:1<1::AID-MAS1>3.0.CO;2-K.

11 Griffey, R.H., Sannes-Lowery, K.A., Drader, J.J. et al. (2000). Characterization of low-affinity complexes between RNA and small molecules using electrospray ionization mass spectrometry. *JACS* 122 (41): 9933–9938. https://doi.org/10.1021/ja0017108.

12 Loo, J.A., Holsworth, D.D., and Root-Bernstein, R.S. (1994). Use of electrospray ionization mass spectrometry to probe antisense peptide interactions. *Biol. Mass. Spectrom.* 23 (1): 6–12. https://doi.org/10.1002/bms.1200230103.

13 Hofstadler, S.A., Sannes-Lowery, K.A., Crooke, S.T. et al. (1999). Multiplexed screening of neutral mass-tagged RNA targets against ligand libraries with electrospray ionization FTICR MS: a paradigm for high- throughput affinity screening. *Anal. Chem.* 71 (16): 3436–3440. https://doi.org/10.1021/ac990262n.

14 Seth, P.P., Miyaji, A., Jefferson, E.A. et al. (2005). SAR by MS: discovery of a new class of RNA-binding small molecules for the hepatitis C virus: internal ribosome entry site IIA subdomain. *J. Med. Chem.* 48 (23): 7099–7102. https://doi.org/10.1021/jm050815o.

15 Sannes-Lowery, K.A., Griffey, R.H., and Hofstadler, S.A. (2000). Measuring dissociation constants of RNA and aminoglycoside antibiotics by electrospray ionization mass spectrometry. *Anal. Biochem.* 280 (2): 264–271. https://doi.org/10.1006/abio.2000.4550.

16 Annis, D.A., Athanasopoulos, J., Curran, P.J. et al. (2004). An affinity selection-mass spectrometry method for the identification of small molecule ligands from self-encoded combinatorial libraries: discovery of a novel antagonist of *E. coli* dihydrofolate reductase. *Int. J. Mass Spectrom.* 238 (2): 77–83. https://doi.org/10.1016/j.ijms.2003.11.022.

17 Rizvi, N.F., Howe, J.A., Nahvi, A. et al. (2018). Discovery of selective RNA-binding small molecules by affinity-selection mass spectrometry. *ACS Chem. Biol.* 13 (3): 820–831. https://doi.org/10.1021/acschembio.7b01013.

18 O'Connell, T.N., Ramsay, J., Rieth, S.F. et al. (2014). Solution-based indirect affinity selection mass spectrometry-A general tool for high-throughput screening of pharmaceutical compound libraries. *Anal. Chem.* 86 (15): 7413–7420. https://doi.org/10.1021/ac500938y.

19 Annis, D.A., Nazef, N., Chuang, C.C. et al. (2004). A general technique to rank protein-ligand binding affinities and determine allosteric versus direct binding site competition in compound mixtures. *JACS* 126 (47): 15495–15503. https://doi.org/10.1021/ja048365x.

20 Brenner, S. and Lerner, R.A. (1992). *Encoded combinatorial chemistry (chemical repertoire/encoded libraries/commaless code)* 89: https://www.pnas.org.

21 Litovchick, A., Tian, X., Monteiro, M.I. et al. (2019). Novel nucleic acid binding small molecules discovered using DNA-encoded chemistry. *Molecules* 24 (10): https://doi.org/10.3390/molecules24102026.Previous example of DEL to find ligands of DNA quartets:

22 Petersen, L.K., Blakskjær, P., Chaikuad, A. et al. (2016). Novel p38α MAP kinase inhibitors identified from yoctoReactor DNA-encoded small molecule library. *MedChemComm* 7 (7): 1332–1339. https://doi.org/10.1039/C6MD00241B.

23 Mukherjee, H., Blain, J.C., Vandivier, L.E. et al. (2020). PEARL-seq: a photoaffinity platform for the analysis of small molecule-RNA interactions. *ACS Chem. Biol.* 15 (9): 2374–2381. https://doi.org/10.1021/acschembio.0c00357.

24 Chen, Q., Li, Y., Lin, C. et al. (2022). Expanding the DNA-encoded library toolbox: identifying small molecules targeting RNA. *Nucleic Acids Res.* 50 (12): E67. https://doi.org/10.1093/nar/gkac173.

25 Benhamou, R.I., Suresh, B.M., Tong, Y. et al. (2022). DNA-encoded library versus RNA-encoded library selection enables design of an oncogenic noncoding RNA inhibitor. *Proc. Natl. Acad. Sci. U.S.A.* 119 (6): https://doi.org/10.1073/pnas.2114971119.

26 MacConnell, A.B., McEnaney, P.J., Cavett, V.J., and Paegel, B.M. (2015). DNA-encoded solid-phase synthesis: encoding language design and complex oligomer library synthesis. *ACS Comb. Sci.* 17 (9): 518–534. https://doi.org/10.1021/acscombsci.5b00106.

27 Gibaut, Q.M.R., Akahori, Y., Bush, J.A. et al. (2022). Study of an RNA-focused DNA-encoded library informs design of a degrader of a r(CUG) repeat expansion. *JACS* https://doi.org/10.1021/jacs.2c08883.

28 Connelly, C.M., Abulwerdi, F.A., and Schneekloth, J.S. (2017). Discovery of RNA binding small molecules using small molecule microarrays. In: *Methods in Molecular Biology*, vol. 1518, 157–175. Humana Press Inc. https://doi.org/10.1007/978-1-4939-6584-7_11.

29 Velagapudi, S.P., Costales, M.G., Vummidi, B.R. et al. (2018). Approved anti-cancer drugs target oncogenic non-coding RNAs. *Cell Chem. Biol.* 25 (9): 1086–1094.e7. https://doi.org/10.1016/j.chembiol.2018.05.015.

30 Disney, M.D. and Seeberger, P.H. (2004). Aminoglycoside microarrays to explore interactions of antibiotics 14th RNAs and proteins. *Chem. A Eur. J.* 10 (13): 3308–3314. https://doi.org/10.1002/chem.200306017.

31 Sztuba-Solinska, J., Shenoy, S.R., Gareiss, P. et al. (2014). Identification of biologically active, HIV TAR RNA-binding small molecules using small molecule microarrays. *JACS* 136 (23): 8402–8410. https://doi.org/10.1021/ja502754f.

32 Connelly, C.M., Boer, R.E., Moon, M.H. et al. (2017). Discovery of inhibitors of MicroRNA-21 processing using small molecule microarrays. *ACS Chem. Biol.* 12 (2): 435–443. https://doi.org/10.1021/acschembio.6b00945.

33 Connelly, C.M., Numata, T., Boer, R.E. et al. (2019). Synthetic ligands for PreQ 1 riboswitches provide structural and mechanistic insights into targeting RNA tertiary structure. *Nat. Commun.* 10 (1): https://doi.org/10.1038/s41467-019-09493-3.

34 Abulwerdi, F.A., Xu, W., Ageeli, A.A. et al. (2019). Selective small-molecule targeting of a triple helix encoded by the long noncoding RNA, MALAT1. *ACS Chem. Biol.* https://doi.org/10.1021/acschembio.8b00807.

35 Tran, B., Pichling, P., Tenney, L. et al. (2020). Parallel discovery strategies provide a basis for riboswitch ligand design. *Cell Chem. Biol.* 27 (10): 1241–1249.e4. https://doi.org/10.1016/j.chembiol.2020.07.021.

36 Suresh, B. M., Akahori, Y., Taghavi, A., Crynen, G., Gibaut, Q. M. R., Li, Y., & Disney, M. D. (2022). Low-molecular weight small molecules can potently bind RNA and affect oncogenic pathways in cells. *JACS*, 144(45), 20815–20824. doi:https://doi.org/10.1021/jacs.2c08770.

37 Ertl, P. (2003). Cheminformatics analysis of organic substituents: identification of the most common substituents, calculation of substituent properties, and automatic identification of drug-like bioisosteric groups. *ChemInform* 34 (21): https://doi.org/10.1002/chin.200321198.

38 Bohacek, R. S., McMartin, C., & Guida, W. C. (1996). The art and practice of structure-based drug design: A molecular modeling perspective. In *Medicinal Research Reviews* (Vol. 16, Issue 1). https://doi.org/10.1002/(SICI)1098-1128(199601)16:1<3::AID-MED1>3.0.CO;2-6.

39 Fink, T. and Raymond, J.L. (2007). Virtual exploration of the chemical universe up to 11 atoms of C, N, O, F: Assembly of 26.4 million structures (110.9 million stereoisomers) and analysis for new ring systems, stereochemistry, physicochemical properties, compound classes, and drug discovery. *JCIM* 47 (2): https://doi.org/10.1021/ci600423u.

40 Cressina, E., Chen, L., Abell, C. et al. (2011). Fragment screening against the thiamine pyrophosphate riboswitch thiM. *Chem. Sci.* 2 (1): https://doi.org/10.1039/c0sc00406e.

41 Warner, K.D., Homan, P., Weeks, K.M. et al. (2014). Validating fragment-based drug discovery for biological RNAs: lead fragments bind and remodel the TPP riboswitch specifically. *Chem. Biol.* 21 (5): 591–595. https://doi.org/10.1016/J.CHEMBIOL.2014.03.007.

42 Garavís, M., López-Méndez, B., Somoza, A. et al. (2014). Discovery of selective ligands for telomeric RNA G-quadruplexes (TERRA) through 19F-NMR based fragment screening. *ACS Chem. Biol.* 9 (7): https://doi.org/10.1021/cb500100z.

43 Zeiger, M., Stark, S., Kalden, E. et al. (2014). Fragment based search for small molecule inhibitors of HIV-1 Tat-TAR. *Bioorg. Med. Chem. Lett.* 24 (24): https://doi.org/10.1016/j.bmcl.2014.11.004.

44 Lee, M.K., Bottini, A., Kim, M. et al. (2014). A novel small-molecule binds to the influenza A virus RNA promoter and inhibits viral replication. *Chem. Commun.* 50 (3): https://doi.org/10.1039/c3cc46973e.

45 Congreve, M., Carr, R., Murray, C., and Jhoti, H. (2003). A “Rule of Three” for fragment-based lead discovery? *Drug Discovery Today* 8 (19): https://doi.org/10.1016/S1359-6446(03)02831-9.

46 Cox, O.B., Krojer, T., Collins, P. et al. (2016). A poised fragment library enables rapid synthetic expansion yielding the first reported inhibitors of PHIP(2), an atypical bromodomain. *Chem. Sci.* 7 (3): https://doi.org/10.1039/c5sc03115j.

47 Morgan, B.S., Sanaba, B.G., Donlic, A. et al. (2019). R-BIND: an interactive database for exploring and developing RNA-targeted chemical probes. *ACS Chem. Biol.* 14 (12): https://doi.org/10.1021/acschembio.9b00631.

48 Mehta, A., Sonam, S., Gouri, I. et al. (2014). SMMRNA: a database of small molecule modulators of RNA. *Nucleic Acids Res.* 42 (D1): https://doi.org/10.1093/nar/gkt976.

49 Bodoor, K., Boyapati, V., Gopu, V. et al. (2009). Design and implementation of an ribonucleic acid (RNA) directed fragment library. *J. Med. Chem.* 52 (12): https://doi.org/10.1021/jm9000659.

50 Padroni, G., Patwardhan, N.N., Schapira, M., and Hargrove, A.E. (2020). Systematic analysis of the interactions driving small molecule-RNA recognition. *RSC. Med. Chem.* 11 (7): https://doi.org/10.1039/d0md00167h.

51 Nasiri, H.R., Bell, N.M., Mc Luckie, K.I.E. et al. (2014). Targeting a c-MYC G-quadruplex DNA with a fragment library. *Chem. Commun.* 50 (14): https://doi.org/10.1039/c3cc48390h.

52 Kirsch, P., Hartman, A.M., Hirsch, A.K.H., and Empting, M. (2019). Concepts and core principles of fragment-based drug design. *Molecules* 24 (23): https://doi.org/10.3390/molecules24234309.

53 Barnwal, R.P., Yang, F., and Varani, G. (2017). Applications of NMR to structure determination of RNAs large and small. *Arch. Biochem. Biophys.* 628: https://doi.org/10.1016/j.abb.2017.06.003.

54 Sreeramulu, S., Richter, C., Berg, H. et al. (2021). Exploring the druggability of conserved RNA regulatory elements in the SARS-CoV-2 genome. *Angew. Chem. Int. Ed.* 60 (35): 19191–19200. https://doi.org/10.1002/anie.202103693.

55 Scott, D.E., Coyne, A.G., Hudson, S.A., and Abell, C. (2012). Fragment-based approaches in drug discovery and chemical biology. *Biochemistry* 51 (25): https://doi.org/10.1021/bi3005126.

56 Lundquist, K.P., Panchal, V., Gotfredsen, C.H. et al. (2021). Fragment-based drug discovery for RNA targets. *ChemMedChem* 16 (17): https://doi.org/10.1002/cmdc.202100324.

57 Lipfert, J. and Doniach, S. (2007). Small-angle X-ray scattering from RNA, proteins, and protein complexes. *Annu. Rev. Biophys. Biomol. Struct.* 36: https://doi.org/10.1146/annurev.biophys.36.040306.132655.

58 Fang, X., Stagno, J.R., Bhandari, Y.R. et al. (2015). Small-angle X-ray scattering: a bridge between RNA secondary structures and three-dimensional topological structures. *Curr. Opin. Struct. Biol.* 30: https://doi.org/10.1016/j.sbi.2015.02.010.

59 Menichelli, E., Lam, B.J., Wang, Y. et al. (2022). Discovery of small molecules that target a tertiary-structured RNA. *Proc. Natl. Acad. Sci. U.S.A.* 119 (48): https://doi.org/10.1073/pnas.2213117119.

60 Suresh, B.M., Li, W., Zhang, P. et al. (2020). A general fragment-based approach to identify and optimize bioactive ligands targeting RNA. *Proc. Natl. Acad. Sci. U.S.A.* 117 (52): 33197–33203. https://doi.org/10.1073/pnas.2012217117.

61 Hughes, S.J., Millan, D.S., Kilty, I.C. et al. (2011). Fragment based discovery of a novel and selective PI3 kinase inhibitor. *Bioorg. Med. Chem. Lett.* 21 (21): https://doi.org/10.1016/j.bmcl.2011.07.117.

62 (a) Smith, G.P. and Petrenko, V.A. (1997). Phage display. *Chem. Rev.* 97 (2): 391–410. https://doi.org/10.1021/cr960065d; (b) Frenzel, A., Kügler, J.,

Helmsing, S., Meier, D., Schirrmann, T., Hust, M., & Dübel, S. (2017). Designing human antibodies by phage display. In *Transf. Med. Hemother.* (Vol. 44, Issue 5, pp. 312–318). . https://doi.org/10.1159/000479633

63 Li, M., Duc, A.C.E., Klosi, E. et al. (2009). Selection of peptides that target the aminoacyl-tRNA site of bacterial 16S ribosomal RNA. *Biochemistry* 48 (35): 8299–8311. https://doi.org/10.1021/bi900982t.

64 Lamichhane, T.N., Abeydeera, N.D., Duc, A.C.E. et al. (2011). Selection of peptides targeting helix 31 of bacterial 16S ribosomal RNA by screening M13 phage-display libraries. *Molecules* 16 (2): 1211–1239. https://doi.org/10.3390/molecules16021211.

65 Cawez, F., Duray, E., Hu, Y. et al. (2018). Combinatorial design of a nanobody that specifically targets structured RNAs. *J. Mol. Biol.* 430 (11): 1652–1670. https://doi.org/10.1016/j.jmb.2018.03.032.

66 Yee, S.S. and nter Gauglitz, G. (1999). Surface plasmon resonance sensors: review. *Sens. Actuat. B* 54.

67 Davis, T.M. and Wilson, W.D. (2000). Determination of the refractive index increments of small molecules for correction of surface plasmon resonance data. *Anal. Biochem.* 284 (2): 348–353. https://doi.org/10.1006/abio.2000.4726.

68 Liu, Y. and Wilson, W.D. (2010). Quantitative analysis of small molecule-nucleic acid interactions with a biosensor surface and surface plasmon resonance detection. *Methods Mol. Biol.* N.J.), 613: 1–23. https://doi.org/10.1007/978-1-60327-418-0_1.

69 Biacore application guide 29368543 AA

70 Myszka, D.G. (2000). Kinetic, equilibrium, and thermodynamic analysis of macromolecular interactions with BIACORE. *Methods Enzymol.* 323: https://doi.org/10.1016/S0076-6879(00)23372-7323.

71 Arney, J.W. and Weeks, K.M. (2022). RNA-ligand interactions quantified by surface plasmon resonance with reference subtraction. *Biochemistry* 61 (15): 1625–1632. https://doi.org/10.1021/acs.biochem.2c00177.

72 Sahoo, H. (2011). Förster resonance energy transfer – a spectroscopic nanoruler: principle and applications. *J. Photochem. Photobiol., C* 12 (1): 20–30. https://doi.org/10.1016/j.jphotochemrev.2011.05.001.

73 . Grecco, H. E., & Verveer, P. J. (2011). FRET in cell biology: still shining in the age of super-resolution? In *ChemPhysChem* (Vol. 12, Issue 3, pp. 484–490). Wiley-VCH Verlag. https://doi.org/10.1002/cphc.201000795

74 Dibrov, S.M., Johnston-Cox, H., Weng, Y.H., and Hermann, T. (2007). Functional architecture of HCV IRES domain II stabilized by divalent metal ions in the crystal and in solution. *Angew. Chem. Int. Ed.* 46 (1–2): 226–229. https://doi.org/10.1002/anie.200603807.

75 Parsons, J., Castaldi, M.P., Dutta, S. et al. (2009). Conformational inhibition of the hepatitis C virus internal ribosome entry site RNA. *Nat. Chem. Biol.* 5 (11): 823–825. https://doi.org/10.1038/nchembio.217.

76 Chen, J.L., Zhang, P., Abe, M. et al. (2020). Design, optimization, and study of small molecules that target tau pre-mRNA and affect splicing. *JACS* 142 (19): 8706–8727. https://doi.org/10.1021/jacs.0c00768.

77 Chen, C.Z., Sobczak, K., Hoskins, J. et al. (2012). Two high-throughput screening assays for aberrant RNA-protein interactions in myotonic dystrophy type 1. *Anal. Bioanal.Chem.* 402 (5): 1889–1898. https://doi.org/10.1007/s00216-011-5604-0.

78 Jones, A.C. and Neely, R.K. (2015). 2-aminopurine as a fluorescent probe of DNA conformation and the DNA-enzyme interface. *Q. Rev. Biophys.* 48 (2): https://doi.org/10.1017/S0033583514000158.

79 Carnevali, M., Parsons, J., Wyles, D.L., and Hermann, T. (2010). A modular approach to synthetic RNA binders of the hepatitis C virus internal ribosome entry site. *ChemBioChem* 11 (10): 1364–1367. https://doi.org/10.1002/cbic.201000177.

80 Gaied, N.B., Glasser, N., Ramalanjaona, N. et al. (2005). 8-vinyl-deoxyadenosine, an alternative fluorescent nucleoside analog to 2′-deoxyribosyl-2-aminopurine with improved properties. *Nucleic Acids Res.* 33 (3): https://doi.org/10.1093/nar/gki253.

81 Nadler, A., Strohmeier, J., and Diederichsen, U. (2011). 8-vinyl-2′-deoxyguanosine as a fluorescent 2′-deoxyguanosine mimic for investigating DNA hybridization and topology. *Angew. Chem. Int. Ed.* 50 (23): https://doi.org/10.1002/anie.201100078.

82 Noé, M.S., Sinkeldam, R.W., and Tor, Y. (2013). Oligodeoxynucleotides containing multiple thiophene-modified isomorphic fluorescent nucleosides. *J. Org. Chem.* 78 (16): https://doi.org/10.1021/jo4008964.

83 Soulière, M.F., Haller, A., Rieder, R., and Micura, R. (2011). A powerful approach for the selection of 2-aminopurine substitution sites to investigate RNA folding. *JACS* 133 (40): 16161–16167. https://doi.org/10.1021/ja2063583.

84 Soulière, M.F. and Micura, R. (2014). Use of SHAPE to select 2AP substitution sites for RNA-ligand interactions and dynamics studies. *Methods Mol. Biol.* 1103: 227–239. https://doi.org/10.1007/978-1-62703-730-3_17.

85 Wicks, S.L. and Hargrove, A.E. (2019). Fluorescent indicator displacement assays to identify and characterize small molecule interactions with RNA. *Methods* 167: 3–14. https://doi.org/10.1016/j.ymeth.2019.04.018.

86 Shindy, H.A. (2017). Fundamentals in the chemistry of cyanine dyes: a review. *Dyes Pigm.* 145: https://doi.org/10.1016/j.dyepig.2017.06.029.

87 Dash, S., Panigrahi, M., Baliyarsingh, S. et al. (2011). Cyanine dyes – nucleic acids interactions. *Curr. Org. Chem.* 15 (15): https://doi.org/10.2174/138527211796367336.

88 Pei, R. and Stojanovic, M.N. (2008). Study of thiazole orange in aptamer-based dye-displacement assays. *Anal. Bioanal.Chem.* 390 (4): https://doi.org/10.1007/s00216-007-1773-2.

89 Sarpong, K. and Datta, B. (2012). Nucleic-acid-binding chromophores as efficient indicators of aptamer-target interactions. *J. Nucleic Acids* 2012: https://doi.org/10.1155/2012/247280.

90 Asare-Okai, P.N. and Chow, C.S. (2011). A modified fluorescent intercalator displacement assay for RNA ligand discovery. *Anal. Biochem.* 408 (2): 269–276. https://doi.org/10.1016/j.ab.2010.09.020.

91 Tran, T. and Disney, M.D. (2012). Identifying the preferred RNA motifs and chemotypes that interact by probing millions of combinations. *Nat. Commun.* https://doi.org/10.1038/ncomms2119.

92 Haniff, H.S., Graves, A., and Disney, M.D. (2018). Selective small molecule recognition of RNA base pairs. *ACS Comb. Sci.* 20 (8): https://doi.org/10.1021/acscombsci.8b00049.

93 Pinto, M.M.M., Sousa, M.E., and Nascimento, M.S.J. (2005). Xanthone derivatives: new insights in biological activities. *Curr. Med. Chem.* 12 (21): https://doi.org/10.2174/092986705774370691.

94 Pace, T.C.S., Monahan, S.L., MacRae, A.I. et al. (2006). Photophysics of aminoxanthone derivatives and their application as binding probes for DNA†. *Photochem. Photobiol.* 82 (1): https://doi.org/10.1562/2005-05-16-ra-529.

95 Zhang, J., Umemoto, S., and Nakatani, K. (2010). Fluorescent indicator displacement assay for ligand-RNA interactions. *JACS* 132 (11): 3660–3661. https://doi.org/10.1021/ja100089u.

96 Murata, A., Fukuzumi, T., Umemoto, S., and Nakatani, K. (2013). Xanthone derivatives as potential inhibitors of miRNA processing by human Dicer: targeting secondary structures of pre-miRNA by small molecules. *Bioorg. Med. Chem. Lett.* 23 (1): https://doi.org/10.1016/j.bmcl.2012.10.108.

97 Umemoto, S., Im, S., Zhang, J. et al. (2012). Structure-activity studies on the fluorescent indicator in a displacement assay for the screening of small molecules binding to RNA. *Chem. A Eur. J.* 18 (32): https://doi.org/10.1002/chem.201103932.

98 Murata, A., Harada, Y., Fukuzumi, T., and Nakatani, K. (2013). Fluorescent indicator displacement assay of ligands targeting 10 microRNA precursors. *Bioorg. Med. Chem.* 21 (22): https://doi.org/10.1016/j.bmc.2013.09.007.

99 Fukuzumi, T., Murata, A., Aikawa, H. et al. (2015). Exploratory study on the RNA-binding structural motifs by library screening targeting pre-miRNA-29 a. *Chem. A Eur. J.* 21 (47): https://doi.org/10.1002/chem.201502913.

100 Jerabek-Willemsen, M., André, T., Wanner, R. et al. (2014). MicroScale thermophoresis: Interaction analysis and beyond. *J. Mol. Struct.* 1077: 101–113. https://doi.org/10.1016/j.molstruc.2014.03.009.

101 Duhr, S. and Braun, D. (2006). Why molecules move along a temperature gradient. *PNAS* 103: 19678–19682. www.pnas.orgcgidoi10.1073pnas.0603873103.

102 Moon, M.H., Hilimire, T.A., Sanders, A.M., and Schneekloth, J.S. (2018). Measuring RNA-ligand interactions with microscale thermophoresis. *Biochemistry* 57 (31): 4638–4643. https://doi.org/10.1021/acs.biochem.7b01141.

103 Haniff, H.S., Tong, Y., Liu, X. et al. (2020). Targeting the SARS-COV-2 RNA genome with small molecule binders and ribonuclease targeting chimera (RiboTAC) degraders. *ACS Cent. Sci.* 6 (10): 1713–1721. https://doi.org/10.1021/acscentsci.0c00984.

104 Umuhire Juru, A., Patwardhan, N.N., and Hargrove, A.E. (2019). Understanding the contributions of conformational changes, thermodynamics, and kinetics of RNA-small molecule interactions. *ACS Chem. Biol.* 14 (5): https://doi.org/10.1021/acschembio.8b00945.

105 Sokoloski, J.E. and Bevilacqua, P.C. (2012). Analysis of RNA folding and ligand binding by conventional and high-throughput calorimetry. *Methods Mol. Biol.* 905: https://doi.org/10.1007/978-1-61779-949-5_10.

106 Salim, N.N. and Feig, A.L. (2009). Isothermal titration calorimetry of RNA. *Methods* 47 (3): https://doi.org/10.1016/j.ymeth.2008.09.003.

107 Wiseman, T., Williston, S., Brandts, J.F., and Lin, L.N. (1989). Rapid measurement of binding constants and heats of binding using a new titration calorimeter. *Anal. Biochem.* 179 (1): https://doi.org/10.1016/0003-2697(89)90213-3.

108 Tellinghuisen, J. (2005). Statistical error in isothermal titration calorimetry: variance function estimation from generalized least squares. *Anal. Biochem.* 343 (1): https://doi.org/10.1016/j.ab.2005.04.026.

109 Liberman, J.A., Bogue, J.T., Jenkins, J.L. et al. (2014). ITC analysis of ligand binding to PreQ1 riboswitches. *Methods Enzymol.* 549 (C): https://doi.org/10.1016/B978-0-12-801122-5.00018-0.

110 Hermann, T. and Westhof, E. (1998). Aminoglycoside binding to the hammerhead ribozyme: a general model for the interaction of cationic antibiotics with RNA. *J. Mol. Biol.* 276 (5): https://doi.org/10.1006/jmbi.1997.1590.

111 Lynch, S.R. and Puglisi, J.D. (2001). Structural origins of aminoglycoside specificity for prokaryotic ribosomes. *J. Mol. Biol.* 306 (5): https://doi.org/10.1006/jmbi.2000.4420.

112 Kaul, M. and Pilch, D.S. (2002). Thermodynamics of aminoglycoside-rRNA recognition: the binding of neomycin-class aminoglycosides to the A site of 16S rRNA. *Biochemistry* 41 (24): https://doi.org/10.1021/bi020130f.

113 (a) Velagapudi, S. P., Li, Y., & Disney, M. D. (2019). A cross-linking approach to map small molecule-RNA binding sites in cells. *Bioorg. Med. Chem. Lett.*, 29(12), 1532–1536. https://doi.org/10.1016/j.bmcl.2019.04.001; for other instances of chem-CLIP, see: (b) Tong, Y., Gibaut, Q.M.R., Rouse, W. et al. (2022). Transcriptome-Wide Mapping of Small-Molecule RNA-Binding Sites in Cells Informs an Isoform-Specific Degrader of QSOX1 mRNA. *JACS* 144 (26): 11620–11625. https://doi.org/10.1021/jacs.2c01929; c Bush, J.A., Aikawa, H., Fuerst, R. et al. (2021). Ribonuclease recruitment using a small molecule reduced c9ALS/FTD r(G4C2) repeat expansion in vitro and in vivo ALS models. *Sci. Transl. Med.* 13 (617): eabd5991. https://doi.org/10.1126/scitranslmed.abd5991.

114 Mortison, J.D., Schenone, M., Myers, J.A. et al. (2018). Tetracyclines modify translation by targeting key human rRNA substructures. *Cell Chem. Biol.* 25 (12): 1506–1518.e13. https://doi.org/10.1016/j.chembiol.2018.09.010.

115 Wang, J., Schultz, P.G., and Johnson, K.A. (2018). Mechanistic studies of a small-molecule modulator of SMN2 splicing. *Proc. Natl. Acad. Sci. U.S.A.* 115 (20): E4604–E4612. https://doi.org/10.1073/pnas.1800260115.

116 Balaratnam, S., Rhodes, C., Bume, D.D. et al. (2021). A chemical probe based on the PreQ1 metabolite enables transcriptome-wide mapping of binding sites. *Nat. Commun.* 12 (1): https://doi.org/10.1038/s41467-021-25973-x.

117 Zhang, P., Park, H.-J., Zhang, J. et al. (2020). Translation of the intrinsically disordered protein α-synuclein is inhibited by a small molecule targeting its structured mRNA. *Proc. Natl. Acad. Sci. U.S.A.* 117 (3): 1457–1467. https://doi.org/10.1073/pnas.1905057117.

118 Plowright, A.T., Johnstone, C., Kihlberg, J. et al. (2012). Hypothesis driven drug design: improving quality and effectiveness of the design-make-test-analyse cycle. *Drug Discovery Today* 17 (1–2): 56–62. https://doi.org/10.1016/j.drudis.2011.09.012.

119 Di, L. and Kerns, E.H. (2008). *Drug-Like Properties: Concepts, Structure Design and Methods: From ADME to Toxicity Optimization*. Burlington: Elsevier.

120 (a)Ratni, H., Ebeling, M., Baird, J. et al. (2018). Discovery of risdiplam, a selective survival of motor neuron-2 (SMN2) gene splicing modifier for the treatment of spinal muscular atrophy (SMA). *J. Med. Chem.* 61 (15): 6501–6517. https://doi.org/10.1021/acs.jmedchem.8b00741.For references on risdiplam, see: (b) Ratni, H., Scalco, R.S., and Stephan, A.H. (2021). Risdiplam, the first approved small molecule splicing modifier drug as a blueprint for future transformative medicines. *ACS Med. Chem. Lett.* 12 (6): 874–877. https://doi.org/10.1021/acsmedchemlett.0c00659.

121 Cheung, A.K., Hurley, B., Kerrigan, R. et al. (2018). Discovery of small molecule splicing modulators of survival motor neuron-2 (SMN2) for the treatment of spinal muscular atrophy (SMA). *J. Med. Chem.* 61 (24): 11021–11036. https://doi.org/10.1021/acs.jmedchem.8b01291.

122 Ernst, J.T., Thompson, P.A., Nilewski, C. et al. (2020). Design of development candidate eFT226, a first in class inhibitor of eukaryotic initiation factor 4A RNA helicase. *J. Med. Chem.* 63 (11): 5879–5955. https://doi.org/10.1021/acs.jmedchem.0c00182.

123 (a) Bordeleau, M.-E., Mori, A., Oberer, M. et al. (2006). Functional characterization of IRESes by an inhibitor of the RNA helicase eIF4A. *Nat. Chem. Biol.* 2 (4): 213–220. https://doi.org/10.1038/nchembio776. (b) Bordeleau, M.-E., Robert, F., Gerard, B. et al. (2008). Therapeutic suppression of translation initiation modulates chemosensitivity in a mouse lymphoma model. *J. Clin. Invest.* https://doi.org/10.1172/jci34753.

124 . Garenne, D., Haines, M. C., Romantseva, E. F., Freemont, P., Strychalski, E. A., & Noireaux, V. (2021). Cell-free gene expression. In *Nature Reviews Methods Primers* (Vol. 1, Issue 1). Springer Nature. https://doi.org/10.1038/s43586-021-00046-x

125 Gurtu, V., Yan, G., and Zhang, G. (1996). IRES bicistronic expression vectors for efficient creation of stable mammalian cell lines. *Biochem. Biophys. Res. Commun.* 229 (1): 295–298. https://doi.org/10.1006/bbrc.1996.1795.

126 Green, K.M., Sheth, U.J., Flores, B.N. et al. (2019). High-throughput screening yields several small-molecule inhibitors of repeat-associated non-AUG translation. *J. Biol. Chem.* 294 (49): 18624–18638. https://doi.org/10.1074/jbc.RA119.009951.

127 Schwinn, M.K., Steffen, L.S., Zimmerman, K. et al. (2020). A simple and scalable strategy for analysis of endogenous protein dynamics. *Sci. Rep.* 10 (1): https://doi.org/10.1038/s41598-020-65832-1.

128 (a)Singh, G. and Cooper, T.A. (2006). Minigene reporter for identification and analysis of cis elements and trans factors affecting pre-mRNA splicing. *BioTechniques* 41 (2): 177–181. 10.2144/000112208.For references on splicing reporters, see: (b) Nasim, M.T. and Eperon, I.C. (2006). A double-reporter splicing assay for determining splicing efficiency in mammalian cells. *Nat. Protoc.* 1 (2): 1022–1028. https://doi.org/10.1038/nprot.2006.148.

129 Kakazu, J., Walker, N.L., Babin, K.C. et al. (2021). Risdiplam for the use of spinal muscular atrophy. *Orthoped. Rev.* 13 (2): 10.52965/001c.25579.

130 Nguyen, U., Squaglia, N., Boge, A., and Fung, P.A. (2011). The simple western™: a gel-free, blot-free, hands-free Western blotting reinvention. *Nat. Methods* 8 (11): v–vi. https://doi.org/10.1038/nmeth.f.353.

131 Cohen, L. and Walt, D.R. (2019). Highly sensitive and multiplexed protein measurements. *Chem. Rev.* 119 (1): 293–321. https://doi.org/10.1021/acs.chemrev.8b00257.

132 Beaudet, L., Rodriguez-Suarez, R., Venne, M.-H. et al. (2008). AlphaLISA immunoassays: the no-wash alternative to ELISAs for research and drug discovery. *Nat. Methods* 5 (12): an8–an9. https://doi.org/10.1038/nmeth.f.230.

133 Zhang, G., Ueberheide, B.M., Waldemarson, S. et al. (2010). Protein quantitation using mass spectrometry. *Methods Mol. Biol.* 673: 211–222. https://doi.org/10.1007/978-1-60761-842-3_13.

134 (a)Vincent, F., Nueda, A., Lee, J. et al. (2022). Phenotypic drug discovery: recent successes, lessons learned and new directions. *Nat. Rev. Drug Discovery* https://doi.org/10.1038/s41573-022-00472-w.For reviews on phenotypic screens, see: (b) Eggert, U.S. (2013). The why and how of phenotypic small-molecule screens. *Nat. Chem. Biol.* 9 (4): 206–209. https://doi.org/10.1038/nchembio.1206.

135 Mousseau, G., Clementz, M.A., Bakeman, W.N. et al. (2012). An analog of the natural steroidal alkaloid cortistatin a potently suppresses tat-dependent HIV transcription. *Cell Host Microbe* 12 (1): 97–108. https://doi.org/10.1016/j.chom.2012.05.016.

136 (a) Rankovic, Z. and Morhpy, R. (2010). *Lead Generation Approaches in Drug Discovery*. Weinheim: Wiley. (b) Deprez-Poulain, R. and Deprez, B. (2004). Facts, figures and trends in lead generation. *Curr. Top. Med. Chem.* 4. (c) Meanwell, N.A. (2011). Improving drug candidates by design: a focus on physicochemical properties as a means of improving compound disposition and safety. *Chem. Res. Toxicol.* 24 (9): 1420–1456. https://doi.org/10.1021/tx200211v.

137 Hughes, J.P., Rees, S.S., Kalindjian, S.B., and Philpott, K.L. (2011). Principles of early drug discovery. *Br. J. Pharmacol.* 162 (6): 1239–1249. https://doi.org/10.1111/j.1476-5381.2010.01127.x.

138 Stark, R., Grzelak, M., and Hadfield, J. (2019). RNA sequencing: the teenage years. *Nat. Rev. Genet.* 20 (11): 631–656. https://doi.org/10.1038/s41576-019-0150-2.

139 (a) Bowes, J., Brown, A.J., Hamon, J. et al. (2012). Reducing safety-related drug attrition: The use of in vitro pharmacological profiling. *Nat. Rev. Drug Discovery* 11 (12): 909–922. https://doi.org/10.1038/nrd3845. (b) Bendels, S., Bissantz, C., Fasching, B. et al. (2019). Safety screening in early drug discovery: an optimized assay panel. *J. Pharmacol. Toxicol. Methods* 99: https://doi.org/10.1016/j.vascn.2019.106609.

140 Schrank, B., Gotz, R., Gunnersen, J.M. et al. (1997). Inactivation of the survival motor neuron gene, a candidate gene for human spinal muscular atrophy, leads to massive cell death in early mouse embryos. *PNAS* 94: 9920–9925.

141 Hua, Y., Vickers, T.A., Okunola, H.L. et al. (2008). Antisense masking of an hnRNP A1/A2 intronic splicing silencer corrects SMN2 splicing in transgenic mice. *Am. J. Hum. Genet.* 82 (4): 834–848.

142 Ratni, H., Mueller, L., and Ebeling, M. (2019). Rewriting the (tran)script: application to spinal muscular atrophy. *Prog. Med. Chem.* 58: 119–156. https://doi.org/10.1016/bs.pmch.2018.12.003.

143 Sivaramakrishnan, M., McCarthy, K.D., Campagne, S. et al. (2017). Binding to SMN2 pre-mRNA-protein complex elicits specificity for small molecule splicing modifiers. *Nat. Commun.* 8 (1): https://doi.org/10.1038/s41467-017-01559-4.

144 Palacino, J., Swalley, S.E., Song, C. et al. (2015). SMN2 splice modulators enhance U1–pre-mRNA association and rescue SMA mice. *Nat. Chem. Biol.* 11 (7): 511–517. https://doi.org/10.1038/nchembio.1837.

145 Schulz, G., Victoria, C., Kirschning, A., and Steinmann, E. (2021). Rocaglamide and silvestrol: a long story from anti-tumor to anti-coronavirus compounds. *Nat. Prod. Rep.* 38 (1): 18–23. https://doi.org/10.1039/D0NP00024H.

146 Liu, T., Nair, S.J., Lescarbeau, A. et al. (2012). Synthetic silvestrol analogues as potent and selective protein synthesis inhibitors. *J. Med. Chem.* 55 (20): 8859–8878. https://doi.org/10.1021/jm3011542.

5

Chemical Matter That Binds RNA

Emily G. Swanson Hay, Zhengguo Cai, and Amanda E. Hargrove

Duke University, Department of Chemistry, 124 Science Drive, Durham, NC 27705, USA

5.1 Introduction

Therapeutic drugs act on specific molecular targets to impact or alter the corresponding biological pathways, thus delivering pharmacological effects toward the disease phenotypes of interest. Most of the small-molecule drugs in clinical use target proteins. In total <700 proteins are currently targeted, representing merely 0.05% of the human genome [1]. In contrast, over 70% of the human genome is transcribed into RNA, and RNA-targeted therapies could greatly expand the range of drug development. Interest in RNAs as potential drug targets has been increasing in part due to the mounting evidence that non-coding RNAs (ncRNAs) pervasively regulate gene expression and protein function in cells, participating in disease development and viral infections. The feasibility of RNA-targeted therapies has been demonstrated by the successful deployment of multiple modalities, including antisense oligonucleotides, small interfering RNAs, and RNA aptamers [2].

There is also growing interest in developing small-molecule-based therapies because of improved oral administration and cell permeability, as well as to expand the number of targets to include highly structured RNAs that might not be readily targeted by antisense-based strategies. Many RNAs bear structural motifs that could form binding pockets or clefts suitable for selective small-molecule binding [1]. The chemical nature of RNA, including the dynamic structure and densely charged backbone, requires ligands with specific physiochemical properties that might be limited in current screening libraries. Many efforts have been made to understand what types of molecular design could favor RNA targeting based on cheminformatic analysis, which led to multiple collections of literature-reported ligands, such as the *R*NA-Targeting *BI*oactive Liga*N*d *D*atabase (R-BIND), [3–5], Nucleic Acid Ligand Database (NALDB) [6] and Small Molecule Modulators of RNA (SMMRNA) [7], as well as curated libraries to increase hit rates of screening, such as Inforna [8, 9] and the Duke RNA-Targeted Library (DRTL) [10]. The increasing pool of reported RNA-targeted small molecules with diverse chemical structures provides a reliable data source for such analysis and elicits a distinguished chemical space occupied

RNA as a Drug Target: The Next Frontier for Medicinal Chemistry, First Edition.
Edited by John Schneekloth and Martin Pettersson.

by ligands that are able to bind to RNA, which can be further refined by those demonstrating biological activity.

In this chapter, we focus on RNA ligands and discuss what type of chemical entities should be pursued for RNA targeting. We will first review common chemical scaffolds and their structural features with varied RNA-binding properties, from naturally discovered ligands to synthetic small molecules. Representative works on the construction of focused libraries will be introduced to explain library curation methods and the improved hit rates this strategy can achieve, followed by the discussion of methods to explore novel chemical space, a case study highlighting classes of ligands presented in this chapter, and future directions for the field of small-molecule RNA targeting.

5.2 Natural Ligands

Many of the early insights into RNA–small-molecule targeting came from exploring naturally occurring RNA–small-molecule interactions. From antibiotics to riboswitch ligands, there are many examples of how diverse and complex small molecules can bind RNA to regulate biological systems. Additionally, by utilizing the chemical diversity of ligands generated through complex biosynthetic pathways, new RNA-binding molecules can be identified. Disney and coworkers recently performed a screen with the Scripps Research Natural Products Discovery Center collections and identified a natural product, nocathiacin I, that selectively targeted pre-miR-18a and had bioactivity in a prostate cancer cell line [11]. This work exemplifies how the potential of natural products may be harnessed for targeting RNA, and how expanding beyond common antibiotic scaffolds may afford more selective ligands. Further examination of the functional binding interactions that have evolved for RNA and small molecules, alongside investigating novel RNA–natural product interactions, may help inform future ligand design for novel RNA targets.

5.2.1 Aminoglycosides

Aminoglycosides represent a major class of RNA-binding natural products consisting of oligosaccharides that contain amine groups, giving the molecules hydrogen-bonding capability as well as positive charge(s) that drive electrostatic interactions with RNA molecules [12–14]. In fact, aminoglycosides were among the first known small molecules to affect biology through RNA binding [15]. Extracted from various bacteria, aminoglycosides serve as antibiotics through a variety of mechanisms that result in the disruption of protein synthesis through binding to ribosomal RNA (rRNA), often in the aminoacyl-transfer RNA (tRNA) site (A-site), thereby interfering with bacterial function [12, 16]. Due to aminoglycosides containing oligosaccharide units, they often have much higher stereocenter and oxygen counts than other RNA-targeting ligands, while their positive charge can make them promiscuous RNA binders [3, 17]. Many naturally occurring aminoglycosides have

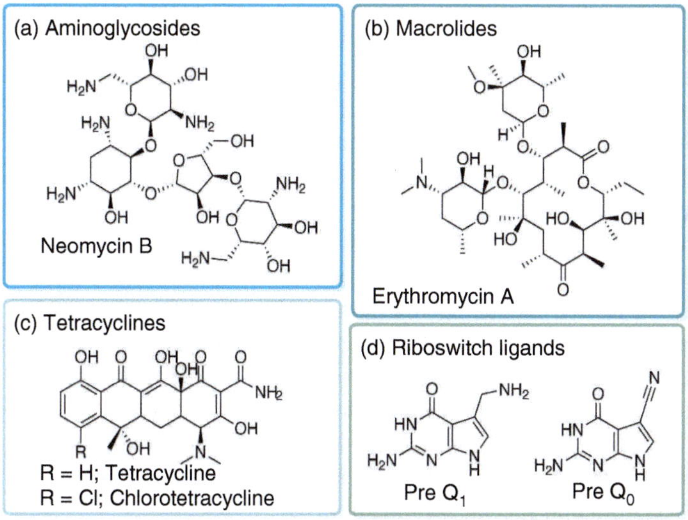

Figure 5.1 Examples of natural molecules from classes described in Section 5.2, including (a) aminoglycosides, (b) macrolides, (c) tetracyclines, and (d) native riboswitch ligands.

been investigated for use as broad-scale antibiotics, such as neomycin (Figure 5.1a); however these natural antibiotics often run into challenges with resistance [18]. Resistance can occur through modifications to the aminoglycoside itself by enzymes that cause it to become inactive, as well as through mutations or modifications in the rRNA sequence that prevent binding of the ligands [18, 19]. Despite these challenges, aminoglycosides remain a large class of antibiotics on market still today.

Besides targeting rRNA, aminoglycosides have been investigated as ligands against a variety of other RNA structures. As an example, in a study investigating the hammerhead ribozyme RNA, neomycin B was found to have an affinity on the same order of magnitude as rRNA–neomycin interactions [20]. This work demonstrated the non-specific nature of aminoglycosides showing that neomycin interacts with a variety of RNA structures with similar affinities. In another study investigating aminoglycoside targeting of human immunodeficiency virus (HIV) Rev response element (RRE) RNA, a critical structure in HIV replication, aminoglycosides were modified with acridine or made dimeric with the goal of increasing specificity for RRE [21]. While high-affinity aminoglycoside derivatives were identified, the novel ligands did not show high specificity when compared to transfer RNA (tRNA) and DNA [21]. While aminoglycosides have been critical in combatting bacterial infections, their propensity for developing resistance and lack of specificity make them challenging molecules to continue to develop. Nevertheless, understanding their complex recognition is still valuable to future RNA-targeting efforts.

5.2.2 Tetracyclines

Besides aminoglycosides, tetracyclines are another major class of rRNA-targeting natural product antibiotics on the market (Figure 5.1c). In 2020, tetracyclines were the 4th most prescribed antibiotic class in the United States, composing 15.5% of outpatient prescribed antibiotics [22]. Tetracycline functions through a similar mechanism as aminoglycosides by binding to the A-site in the ribosome and disrupting protein synthesis [23, 24]. Tetracyclines also face challenges similar to those of aminoglycosides, encountering antibiotic resistance through multiple mechanisms, including efflux [24]. While some synthetic derivatives have been successful at circumventing resistance in Gram-positive bacteria, it is not an effective treatment for all bacteria [24]. Tetracyclines are distinct from aminoglycosides in their structural features. They are composed of four fused rings and thus have a more linear structure overall. This structure may allow for intercalation in double-stranded RNA through stacking between RNA bases. Studies have shown that tetracyclines have activity against various RNA viruses including HIV and Japanese encephalitis virus (JEV), where minocycline was found to mitigate infection and reduce the viral titer respectively [25, 26]. Tetracyclines have the potential for broad applications, but as with aminoglycosides encounter difficulties with off-target effects from non-specific binding of RNA.

5.2.3 Macrolides

Macrolides are antibiotics that consist of 14-membered rings, with azithromycin, a synthetic derivative of the naturally occurring macrolide erythromycin (Figure 5.1b), being the second most prescribed antibiotic in 2020 [22, 27]. Macrolides have been found to bind near the exit tunnel of nascent peptide chains in rRNA, leveraging hydrogen-bonding and hydrophobic interactions to interfere with protein synthesis in bacteria [28]. However, these molecules again suffer similar challenges of antibiotic resistance, with the natural ligand erythromycin developing resistance through multiple mechanisms [28, 29]. To combat this resistance, similar strategies of synthesizing near derivatives that can circumvent resistance mechanisms were developed [28]. Additionally, macrolides were investigated for activity against non-ribosomal RNA. In a study to evaluate the ability of antibiotics to target microRNAs (miRNAs) and alter their processing, it was discovered that while the macrolides showed binding to the target miRNAs, they did not inhibit their processing while other antibiotics were potent inhibitors [30]. Together, macrolides and the previously described aminoglycosides and tetracyclines represent some of the most explored scaffolds for RNA targeting due to their activity against bacteria and high clinical usage.

5.2.4 Native Riboswitch Ligands

Bacteria have unique feedback mechanisms for biosynthetic pathways that involve metabolite binding to an RNA riboswitch molecule causing a conformational change that alters gene expression (see Chapter 8 for further discussion on riboswitches). Riboswitches consist of an aptamer domain that forms a ligand-binding pocket and an expression platform. Upon ligand binding to the aptamer domain, conformational changes alter the expression platform to switch gene expression on or off [31]. A recent survey identified over 50 functional riboswitch classes that have been experimentally validated [32]. Riboswitches may represent some of the most well-regulated and specific RNA-ligand interactions in nature. Precise interactions allow for distinguishing chemically similar ligands such that only one biomolecule can switch on or off a given pathway in a biological system.

An example of this precise recognition is the abundant prequenosine$_1$ (PreQ$_1$) riboswitch. Three distinct riboswitch classes have been identified and evaluated in bacteria for their recognition of PreQ$_1$ (Figure 5.1d), a chemical derivative of guanine, and similar analogues, such as PreQ$_0$ [33]. These varying classes have distinct RNA aptamer domains that specifically recognize the various guanine analogues with varying degrees of specificity [33]. In the case of the Class III PreQ$_1$ riboswitch there is a two order of magnitude preference for PreQ$_1$ over PreQ$_0$ where the ligands vary only by the reduction of a single nitrile to an amine in PreQ$_1$ [33]. Furthermore, there are a variety of riboswitch classes that target diverse molecular structures including cofactors, amino acids and sugars [32]. With such unique recognition properties and interactions there is much we can learn from understanding riboswitch recognition in targeting novel RNA structures.

Taking lessons from nature on selective RNA-ligand interactions may be the key to understanding how to selectively target other RNA structures in the future. While antibiotics may be prone to developing resistance and promiscuous RNA binding, their chemical properties and modes of RNA recognition lend critical insight into the design of more potent and selective ligands for novel RNA targets. Antibiotics and riboswitch ligands show complex recognition through a variety of interactions from intercalation to hydrogen-bonding or hydrophobic interactions. In addition to native riboswitch ligands, selective ligands from synthetic and high-throughput screening libraries have been discovered, including Ribocil-C targeting the flavin mononucleotide (FMN) riboswitch [34], and compounds targeting the PreQ$_1$ and ZTP riboswitches from high-throughput screening and synthetic optimization, respectively [35, 36]. By understanding how ligands achieve specific recognition of RNA sequence and structure we may find more selective chemical probes.

5.3 Commercial Ligands

With the limited number of proteins deemed druggable and the knowledge that a majority of the human genome does not encode for proteins, the market for identifying novel RNA-binding molecules has grown significantly in recent years [37–39]. The plethora of novel targets led to an increase in industry-curated libraries designed specifically to target RNA [40, 41]. In addition to large industrial libraries, many academic institutions have also designed and acquired drug-like libraries of compounds with increased propensities for RNA binding [10, 42]. While these libraries have been curated through a variety of methods, they have led to collections of molecules with similar properties as observed through statistical analysis, machine-learning models, and sub-structure searches, reinforcing the existence of a privileged space for RNA-targeting small molecules.

5.3.1 Industrial Libraries

The increasing demand for RNA therapeutics has led large companies to develop libraries designed for RNA targeting or screening. For example, Merck performed high-throughput screening of over 50,000 chemically diverse small molecules against 42 RNA structures [40]. They then used the chemical properties of molecules found to bind RNA in this preliminary screen to develop a smaller RNA-focused library (~3700 molecules). Within this focused library they observed higher hit rates across RNA targets in a secondary screen, scaffolds enriched in selective ligands (Figure 5.2a), and the properties of the library were similar to those of molecules previously published in R-BIND [40]. In a collaboration with AstraZeneca, Disney and coworkers also performed a high-throughput screen utilizing the properties of their Inforna database to develop a ~2000-member library from AstraZeneca's collection of greater than two million compounds [41]. Similar to the screen Merck performed, hit rates higher than those of general screening campaigns were observed, and the properties of these ligands were similar to those of both R-BIND and SMMRNA [3, 7, 41]. The mounting studies curating novel libraries continually show an overlap in properties of the resulting hits, supporting the existence of distinct properties that influence RNA binding. Academic institutions have been simultaneously curating similar libraries and observing similar trends.

5.3.2 Academic Libraries

While large industrial or pharmaceutical libraries are critical for understanding the properties of RNA-targeting molecules and providing large datasets, they can be inaccessible to academic institutions. Thus, some groups or institutions have started their own library collections for RNA targeting, making the screening and applications of these libraries more accessible to the field through collaborations. The Disney lab curated their Inforna database, which consists of a collection of RNA-targeting small molecules known to bind specific RNA secondary structures [8, 9, 41]. The Inforna library has continually grown with the addition of

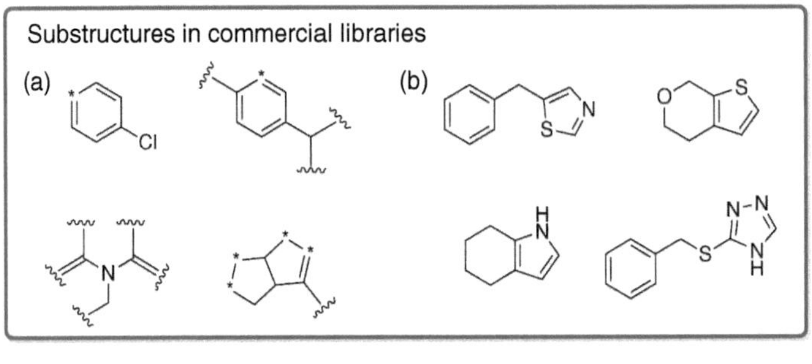

Figure 5.2 Examples of enriched substructures identified in selective ligands from (a) Rizvi and coworkers. Source: Rizvi et al. [40]/with permission of Elsevier; and (b) Yazdani and coworkers. Source: Yazdani et al. [42]/with permission of John Wiley & Sons.

new ligands upon screening of novel RNA-biased libraries, some of which come from large sets of commercial ligands [41]. After multiple rounds of curation through screening, the molecules within Inforna continue to show similar chemical properties to each other and those of other RNA-targeted small-molecule libraries. The Inforna database has been used to design selective and potent inhibitors of a variety of RNA targets, showing its utility and ability to identify RNA specific chemotypes in small-molecule ligands.

Recently, the Hargrove lab reported the design and application of the DRTL [10]. The DRTL was curated by using a nearest-neighbor algorithm to identify commercially available ligands that were similar in cheminformatic properties to the ligands within R-BIND. The library was screened against four RNA targets, and hit rates similar to other RNA-focused library screens were observed. While the majority of the properties of DRTL molecules were not significantly different from R-BIND ligands, the scaffolds or structures were unique as calculated by Tanimoto dissimilarity scores [10]. This work demonstrated that using chemical properties to define RNA-binding ligands can allow for the discovery of novel RNA-binding scaffolds.

Additionally, similar work was performed by the Schneekloth lab to curate a library of approximately 2000 RNA-binding molecules [42]. The Repository of RNA Binders to Nucleic acids, or ROBIN, was developed through screening 24,572 diverse ligands from commercial libraries against 36 unique nucleic acid targets [42]. In this work, machine-learning algorithms were used to identify properties of the ROBIN molecules that are unique or enriched compared to libraries of protein-binding molecules [42]. By comparing substructures of ROBIN RNA-binding and non-binding molecules, the authors identified enriched substructures that were consistent with previously identified functional groups and chemotypes (Figure 5.2b) [42]. This work allows for prediction of novel ligands while further defining the chemical space of RNA-targeting small molecules, giving the field a basis to continue exploring RNA-specific chemical space through an in-depth understanding of specific scaffolds or properties that can be expanded with further commercial mining or synthetic tuning.

5.4 Synthetic Ligands

Many efforts have been made to explore chemical space of RNA-targeted small molecules by scaffold-based synthesis, leading to a number of derivatives bearing specific core structures (Figure 5.3). Different from screening existing commercial libraries, which can lead to the identification of repeat hit molecules or promiscuous ligands, examination of synthetic ligands could greatly extend the chemical space being investigated and proactively modulate small-molecule-binding profiles (e.g. selectivity, cytotoxicity, pharmacokinetics) against specific RNA targets. There is a plethora of reviews for RNA targeting discussing different classes of RNA targets and various synthetic molecules that have been explored [43–47]. In this section, representative small-molecule scaffolds for RNA targeting will be introduced,

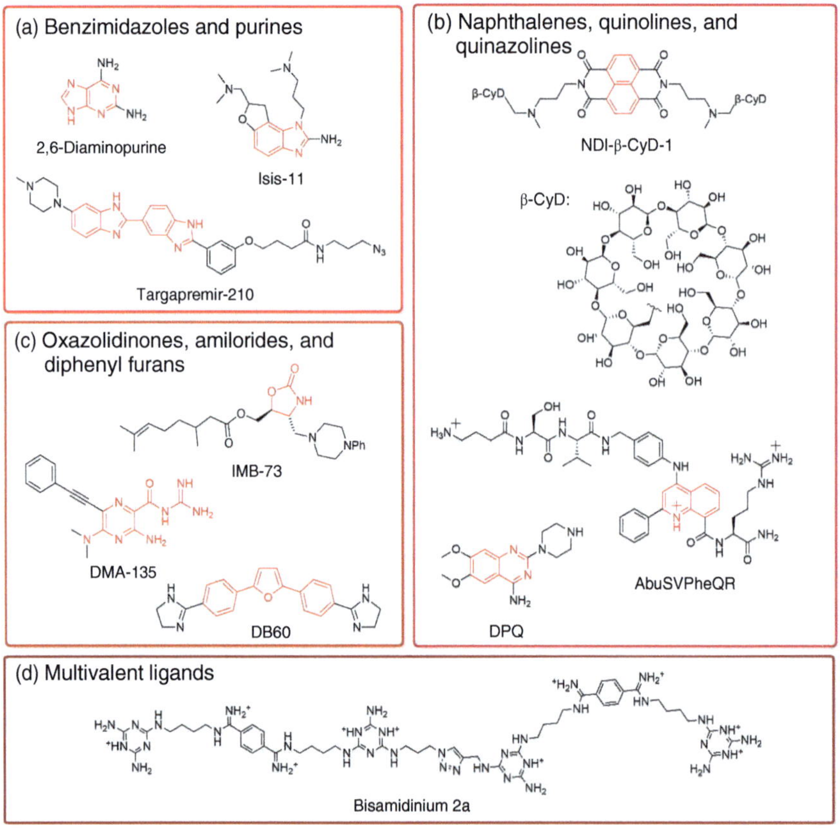

Figure 5.3 Examples of chemical ligands with core structures discussed in Section 5.4 highlighted in red, including, (a) benzimidazoles and purines; (b) naphthalenes, quinolines, and quinazolines; (c) oxazolidinones, amilorides, and diphenyl furans; and (d) multivalent ligands.

including multivalent ligands that assemble multiple modules into one structure to achieve enhanced RNA-targeting effects.

5.4.1 Benzimidazoles and Purines

Benzimidazole ring systems exist extensively in many natural products and clinical drugs, with structural similarity to purine bases (Figure 5.3a). The benzimidazole scaffold was first identified to target RNA in a mass spectroscopy (MS)-based high-throughput screening against the internal ribosomal entry site (IRES) IIa subdomain in hepatitis C virus (HCV) [48]. The binding mode of lead benzimidazoles was identified with multiple orthogonal methods [49–51], which revealed a significant ligand-induced conformational change from an unliganded bent shape to the linear conformation complexed with small molecules inhibiting viral translation. Relatedly, Hoechst dyes are nucleic-acid-staining molecules that contains a bis-benzimidazole scaffold. These molecules were found to afford high-affinity binding and bioactivity toward multiple RNA targets, including self-splicing group I intron as an antifungal [52, 53], repeat expansion RNAs in neurodegenerative disease models [54, 55], and miRNAs with diverse secondary motifs implicated in cancers [56, 57]. The MOA of these high-affinity bis-benzimidazoles includes interruption of essential folding pathways, restoration of functional proteins by competitive binding, and modulation of miRNA biogenesis via Drosha or Dicer ribonuclease-mediated processing [58].

Purine represents a frequently occurring nitrogen-containing heterocycle due to its presence in adenine and guanine nucleobases. Synthetic purine derivatives identified with RNA-targeting capabilities were mostly tested in recognition of bacterial riboswitches, mimicking the cognate purine ligands binding to the aptamer domain, such as the guanine- and adenine-specific riboswitches [59]. The advantages of adapting benzimidazoles and purines for RNA targeting might include pharmacological properties, such as superior membrane permeability and low cytotoxicity as they are structurally analogous to endogenous heterocycles.

5.4.2 Naphthalenes, Quinolines, and Quinazolines

The naphthalene-based RNA-targeting chemotype is usually found with naphthalene diimide (NDI), a type of known guanine-quadruplex (G4) binder (Figure 5.3b). NDI-based compounds have been documented with high-affinity and large planar surface favored for threading-type intercalation against G4s, as well as great potential for chemical variability on naphthalene rings and imide nitrogens. Zou et al. designed a di-substituted NDI with two conjugated β-cyclodextrins, which showed improved specificity for the recognition of the parallel RNA G4 topology over a hybrid G4 topology and double-stranded DNA (dsDNA) [60]. In this design, the bulky cyclodextrin group disrupts the binding with dsDNA due to steric hindrance. The preferred binding toward the parallel RNA G4 was explained by the orientation of side chain loops, which allowed nucleobases in the loops to bind the cyclodextrin. Loop nucleobases were not available for binding in the hybrid G4 topology, leading to weaker affinities.

Quinoline derivatives have been identified for antitumor, antiviral, and anti-inflammatory use and are also known as DNA intercalators. The application of such scaffolds in the early studies of RNA targeting involved the design of helix-threading peptides, where the intercalator module (e.g. quinoline) inserts into the base paired nucleic acid duplex and the other substituents locate in the opposite groove of the helix [61]. Gareiss and coworkers employed resin-bound dynamic combinatorial chemistry to identify the first compounds able to inhibit MBNL1 protein binding to (CUG) repeat RNA in myotonic dystrophy type 1 (DM1) treatment [62]. The hit compound with a quinoline moiety was further evolved into benzo[g]quinolines and showed improved binding properties *in vivo* [63].

Like quinoline, quinazoline has a bicyclic aromatic structure with fused benzene and pyrimidine rings (Figure 5.3b). The potential of this scaffold for RNA binding can be traced from many studies. For instance, Lee and coworkers identified an amino-quinazoline compound from NMR-based fragment screening that showed binding to influenza A virus promoter sequence with moderate affinity and inhibition of viral replication [64]. Inspired by the crystal structure of a 2-amino-benzimidazole inhibitor targeting the IRES of HCV, Charrette and coworkers designed several 2-amino-quinazoline compounds using a shape complementary strategy to increase pocket filling [65], indicating that structure-guided shape complementarity could be a useful approach in RNA ligand optimization.

5.4.3 Oxazolidinones

Many promiscuous binding interactions of small molecules to RNA originate from the densely charged RNA backbone, which can exert strong electrostatic interactions and intercalation. Oxazolidinones are a type molecule with low overall charge and a non-aromatic core that has shown binding to RNA, such as linezolid and tedizolid antibiotics interacting with bacterial rRNA (Figure 5.3c) [66, 67]. Besides rRNA, another well-studied RNA target recognized by oxazolidinones is the T-box riboswitch antiterminator RNA, which is an essential regulatory element found in many Gram-positive bacteria. Maciagiewicz and coworkers performed quantitative structure–activity relationship (QSAR) study to understand C-5-substituted oxazolidinone-induced fluorescence changes in Förster resonance energy transfer (FRET)-labeled antiterminator RNA [68]. The results further support that hydrogen-bonding and hydrophobic properties play significant roles in ligand binding within scaffolds lacking a strong positive charge.

5.4.4 Amilorides

The structure of an amiloride is characterized by a pyrazine ring combined with amino and acylguanidino groups that confer potential hydrogen-bonding capacities (Figure 5.3c). The early studies on amilorides for targeting nucleic acids were focused on the design of an abasic site (AP site) binder via pseudo-base pairing due to the enrichment of hydrogen bond donor and acceptor atoms in the structure [69]. Stelzer and coworkers first discovered 5′-(*N*,*N*)-dimethyl amiloride (DMA) as a novel binder for HIV-1 transactivation response element (TAR) from an ensemble-based virtual screening [70]. Following SAR studies on the C-5 and C-6 modifications led to a series of DMA compounds with improved binding affinities and specificities against HIV-1 TAR [71]. In later research, Hargrove and coworkers demonstrated the tunability of this scaffold by targeting many other RNAs with amiloride derivatives, including multiple HIV RNAs [72], enterovirus 71 (EV71) IRES stem-loop II subdomain [73, 74] and 5′-untranslated regions of severe acute respiratory syndrome coronavirus 2 (SARS-CoV-2) genome [75]. The latter studies further highlighted the potential of amiloride derivatives as biologically active, RNA-targeted antiviral compounds, specifically against EV71 and SARS-CoV-2. The compounds act by binding to RNA stem-loop motifs, altering their conformations and disrupting interactions or processes important for viral translation and replication.

5.4.5 Diphenyl Furan

Diphenyl furan (DPF) is generally functionalized with amidine-based side chains attached to the phenyl rings (Figure 5.3c). Wilson and coworkers performed extensive synthetic and biophysical studies on DPF's potential in binding genomic RNA of HIV, such as TAR and RRE [76–78]. The compounds displayed high affinity and selectivity against wild-type RRE or TAR, when compared to the poly(A•U) duplex control or other mutants, and inhibited Tat-mediated transactivation in HIV-infected cells [78]. Donlic and coworkers took a different perspective, investigating shape diversity of DPFs in the selective recognition of an RNA triple-helix structure by synthesizing a set of para-, meta-, and ortho-DPF regioisomers that occupy distinguished topological space [79, 80]. The synthetic ligands presented diverse binding affinities and selectivity against metastasis-associated lung adenocarcinoma transcript 1 (MALAT1) triple helix, from fluorescent titration, thermal stability, and exonucleolytic degradation assays. DPFs, with feasible tunability on multiple positions, also inspired other structures with amidine-functionalized unfused aromatic ring systems, such as diminazenes [81].

5.4.6 Multivalent Ligands

Multivalency is a prevalent strategy adopted by many biological interactions, including molecular recognition at cell surfaces. The application of multivalent ligands in RNA recognition can greatly enhance binding affinity and specificity by introducing multiple modules into one molecule to realize additive or cooperative effects. The design of multivalent ligands involves identification of monomeric recognition modules and optimization of the intervening linker (Figure 5.3d). Many of the multivalent ligands designed so far aimed to target RNAs with repeat expansions, as these targets have repeated secondary motifs that can be captured by specific monomeric chemical probes. In 2008, Miller et al. identified the first non-nucleic acid-based ligands that targeted r(CUG) repeat RNA via a dynamic combinatorial chemistry (DCC) method [62]. While optimization of the linker usually becomes the essential part of assembling multiple binding moieties into an effective chemical probe, the cell permeability of the multivalent ligands should also be considered during rational design. Zimmerman et al. incorporated bisamidinium groove binders into the linker of an oligomeric ligand to mimic polycationic and amphiphilic characteristics of the cell-penetrating peptide (CPP) structure [82]. The synthetic multivalent ligand showed good cell permeability and capacity to recognize U–U mismatches in r(CUG) repeat RNA with low toxicity in both cell and mice models.

5.5 Computational Tools for the Exploration of Chemical Space

Efforts to extend the currently known chemical space of RNA-targeted small molecules have used diverse approaches, often with a computational focus. Various

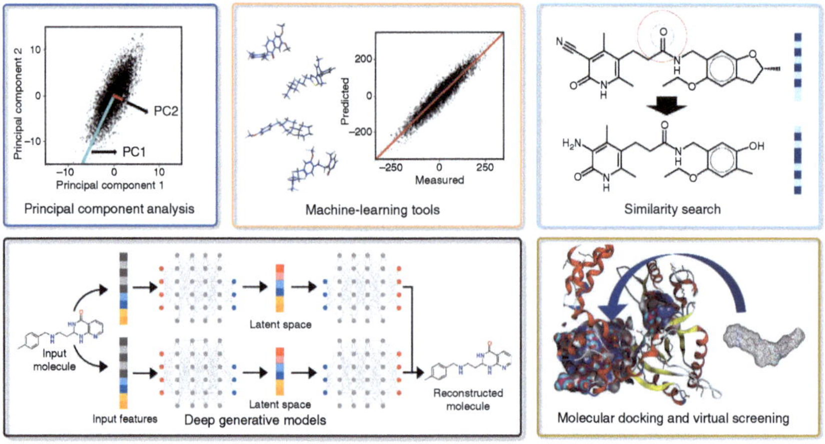

Figure 5.4 Potential tools to explore larger chemical space in the future: cheminformatics analysis (e.g. PCA), machine-learning tools, similarity search, deep generative models, and structure-based molecular docking and virtual screening.

cheminformatic approaches including similarity search, principal component analysis (PCA), and sophisticated machine-learning methods have been deployed for identifying more chemotypes (Figure 5.4). With high-resolution RNA structural data, molecular docking and virtual screening, a wider range of chemical space can be efficiently explored. By advancing HTS data in combination with high-performance computing units, *de novo* ligand design using generative chemistry methods may be achieved.

5.5.1 Similarity Searches and Principal Component Analysis

Chemical similarity search algorithms and metrics are computational methods used to identify and compare molecules based on their structures and properties. Collections of known RNA-binding molecules could provide valuable information and guide our search toward more potent compounds via various similarity metrics. Cheminformatic tools could help interpret such information and translate it into chemically readable formats. PCAs reveal the most relevant molecular features by decreasing the dimensionality of the chemical space being investigated, thus enabling similarity search of novel structures in a predefined feature space. Such chemical searches have proven successful in constructing an effective RNA-biased library [40, 83] starting with several known active structures. Multiple algorithms have been employed for searching similar compounds with a reference molecule or a library, including Tanimoto similarity, nearest neighbor search, and substructure search. Depending on what endpoint is being investigated, the similarity metrics used in such chemical searches can also vary, from molecular descriptors in distance-based metrics to molecular fingerprints in bit vector-based metrics and structural overlap in 3D space [84]. Often, the type of similarity metrics used impacts the quality of resulting compounds more strongly than the search algorithm itself [85]. Unfortunately, the exact features relevant to the activity of interest need to be elucidated from proximations, such as quantitative structure–activity relationship studies (QSAR), or more generalized rules identified from large data mining. With the breadth of tools available for similarity searches and dimensionality reduction, a deep understanding of existing chemical space can be gained with the goal of informing the next generation of RNA-targeting small molecules.

5.5.2 Additional Machine-Learning Tools

Machine-learning-assisted drug discovery is a valuable tool in understanding RNA:small-molecule recognition, particularly because of the inherent RNA dynamics that make characterizing small-molecule-binding modes a challenge [40, 42, 86, 87]. Indeed, machine-learning approaches have been increasingly utilized to facilitate ligand discovery for targeting RNA. These methods aim to model the complex structure–activity relationships between small molecules and RNA to enable more efficient identification of active compounds. One general strategy is to train classification/regression models to distinguish RNA-binding molecules from non-binders based on calculated molecular features. For example, naive Bayesian models have been applied to determine key chemical properties of molecules likely to interact with RNA [40]. The knowledge from such models can then guide the design of focused screening libraries enriched in putative RNA-binding molecules. QSAR models can also guide the design of new RNA-targeting molecules. To expand the applicability domain of conventional QSAR models beyond a single scaffold, a set of structurally diverse RNA-binding molecules was incorporated [88]. With representative sampling, QSAR models effectively predicted affinity and kinetics for novel chemotypes binding to a target RNA. Beyond learning information from the experimental readout, predictive modeling of RNA–ligand interactions directly from RNA structure has been explored. Graph-based representations of RNA-binding sites in known structures were used as input for graph neural networks or other machine-learning architectures to predict suitable interacting ligands [89, 90]. By learning from atomic details of known RNA–ligand complexes, such computational methods can suggest likely binders without performing a screen. Overall, machine-learning strategies have demonstrated significant promise to enhance the discovery of RNA-targeted ligands.

It is worth noting that recent advances in deep learning (DL) have triggered several seminal works using generative models for *de novo* molecular design, where deep neural networks are employed to resemble the molecular generation process and fulfil property optimization [91–94]. Though current efforts are made to target protein structures, these approaches could be easily extended to target RNAs. Commonly used generative DL architectures include recurrent neural networks, generative adversarial networks, and autoencoders [91]. Using various types of molecular representations from simple 1D sequences to the 2D molecular graph, and even 3D spatial points as the input, the molecular generating process can be learned efficiently, and novel molecules are continuously sampled. The automatic chemical design combined with machine-learning models mapping the structure–activity landscape has great potential for efficient generation of RNA-targeted small molecules, speeding up the discovery of small-molecule-based chemical probes.

5.5.3 Structure-Based Ligand Design

Structure-based ligand design such as molecular docking is hindered by a lack of determined RNA structures and appropriate scoring functions, though research interests keep growing in the field [95]. The scarcity of high- or even low-resolution RNA 3D structures deposited in the Protein Data Bank (PDB) database when compared to the tremendous number of protein:ligand structures poses a significant limitation. In 2020 there were nearly 300× more unique high resolution protein:small-molecule structures deposited in the PDB than RNA:small-molecule structures [96, 97]. Despite this limited number of RNA:ligand structures, these data have become a valuable source for modeling RNA-ligand binding. One challenge in RNA docking is the dynamic nature of RNA structures, which can lead to different bound state conformations with different small molecules. To account for RNA dynamics in docking, Stelzer et al. generated an ensemble of experimentally informed RNA conformers via NMR and molecular dynamics and found that the binding energies of small-molecule interactions could be predicted with comparable results to when the bound structure was available [70]. Such ensemble-based docking further identified several novel TAR binders, including DMA, which evolved as an important RNA-binding scaffold as previously mentioned. The knowledge from protein-based docking and scoring can be transferred to RNA targets after addressing some common pitfalls, including target dynamics, ligand protomer, and tautomer correction, and solvation effect upon ligand binding. Kallert and coworkers transferred protein-based docking protocols to preQ1-riboswitch virtual screening and successfully identified six active compounds [98]. These hit molecules re-capitulated most of the important interactions based on generated docking poses, though with confined structural diversity and novelty, suggesting the utility of such protein-centric docking methods in the evaluation of RNA-binding ligands. It is anticipated that future progress requires continued advancement of computational techniques as well as growth of structural databases and measurement data for RNA–ligand complexes. Physics-based and knowledge-based scoring functions have shown promising success for modeling RNA–ligand binding, but machine-learning methods, though still new in this field, hold great potential to further improve prediction performance [99].

5.6 Case Studies in Examining and Expanding RNA-Targeted Chemical Space

With the ever-growing number of discovered RNA-targeting ligands and libraries designed around RNA-privileged chemical space or scaffolds, and the advancement of tools such as those described in this chapter, there is an opportunity to leverage the existing knowledge to better guide future design or studies. Here we present a few case studies for how information on the similarities and differences between libraries can be examined, and how this may help to inform future efforts.

5.6.1 Using QSAR to Probe RNA-Targeting Small-Molecule Properties

QSAR can be used to bridge ligand structural parameters and bioactivity or binding profiles. The application of QSAR models can be employed from early hit identification stages to the later-stage lead optimization. Due to the statistical nature of the approach, the quality and size of the modeling data directly determines the ability of the model to accurately reveal the underlying distribution of the structure–activity landscape, i.e. the propensity for overtraining a model with insufficient or low-quality data is high, while the algorithm used to build the model impacts the outcome slightly due to different inherent assumptions.

The use of QSAR studies for RNA targets is in its infancy, and few examples in the field directly fulfil the goal of ligand discovery. More often, the QSAR model provides a lens to help chemists decipher the molecular descriptors that contribute to RNA binding. For instance, Maciagiewicz et al. synthesized 53 oxazolidinone ligands and tested their binding to T-box riboswitch antiterminator RNA via a FRET assay. The ligand-induced fluorescence change was correlated with ligand descriptors to afford the QSAR model, which revealed several key physicochemical properties that contributed mostly to the fitting. The study provided quantitative evidence that dipole moment, hydrogen-bonding capacity, and hydrophobicity played important roles in oxazolidinones recognizing T-box antiterminator RNA [68].

Additionally, QSAR models could provide an efficient tool that allows fast evaluation of the virtual library within its applicable domain before any experiment is done. For instance, Patwardhan and coworkers prioritized synthesis of one DMA compound out of many others from a virtual library, based on the QSAR predictions [72]. The compound was discovered to be one of the tightest binders in their DMA library against HIV-1 exonic splicing silencer of Vpr (ESSV). Many QSAR studies struggle with limited applicable domain, which means only a specific subset of compounds can be used for predictions. To establish a broadly applicable framework for RNA-targeted ligand discovery, Cai and coworkers developed QSAR models that connect the molecular properties of structurally diverse small molecules to their binding behaviors against HIV-1 TAR [88]. In this study, the authors applied multiple linear regression with feature selection to build predictive and interpretable models that quantitatively correlate physicochemical and structural descriptors of ligands across multiple chemical scaffolds with their experimentally determined binding parameters. Through rigorous validation on new molecules, the study revealed accurate prediction of binding strength and kinetic rate constants [88]. Overall, this work puts forth a generalizable approach leveraging QSAR modeling to elucidate structure–activity relationships and rationally guide the design of RNA-targeted ligands. With the number of small-molecule–RNA interactions being annotated from experiments, QSAR will be increasingly important to discover more bioactive RNA-targeted ligands and assist decision-making during hit-to-lead triage.

5.6.2 Evaluating the Chemical Space of Natural, Synthetic, and Commercial Ligands

In this chapter, we have described the types of ligands developed from nature, synthetic efforts and those existing in commercial libraries. To better understand the commonalities and diversity between these groups, we performed a PCA on 3 datasets. The natural ligands were composed of natural products with no synthetic modifications from the data set of RNA targeted ligands reported by Aboul-Ela, originally collected by Bodoor and coworkers [13, 100]. The synthetic ligands are represented by molecules from R-BIND small molecules reported to be a part of synthetic libraries, and the commercial ligands are a subset of 80 molecules from the DRTL that were selected using a Kennard–Stone algorithm as previously reported [5, 10, 88, 101]. There was no duplication among the selected ligands. With these three libraries a PCA was performed on 20 normalized cheminformatic parameters, following previously reported procedures [3]. Along PCs 1 and 2, there is a strong separation between commercial and natural ligands, and we see synthetic ligands covering space in both of the natural and commercial libraries (Figure 5.5a). There is a bit more separation for synthetic ligands when looking along PCs 1 and 3, as well as PCs 2 and 3 (Figure 5.5b,c). Polar surface area and hydrogen bond donors and acceptors strongly contribute to spread along PC1, while ring parameters contribute to PC2, and nitrogen and oxygen account for a significant portion of the spread along PC3 (Figure 5.5d,e, key parameters in bold). The spread along PC 3 for synthetics may be explained by large nitrogen counts compared to low oxygen counts observed in R-BIND [5] compared to natural ligands, which are enriched with alcohols from aminoglycosides.

In addition to the PCA we evaluated the shape of the molecules in the various libraries through calculating principal moments of inertia (PMI). As one may expect, natural ligands were the most sphere-like due to the inclusion of aminoglycosides and other large flexible ring systems, while commercial ligands were the most rod-like, although this was not a statistically significant difference when compared to the synthetic ligands, as evaluated by a Kolmogorov–Smirnov test (Figure 5.6). For all analyses in the Kolmogorov–Smirnov test the commercial and natural libraries were statistically significant, while the only other difference observed was between commercial and synthetic ligands in the distance to sphere. This data appears consistent with the results from PCA with the largest spread between commercial and natural ligands and synthetics sharing some similarities with both libraries. Understanding the differences between these libraries and the propensities of different classes of molecules to bind RNA more promiscuously or selectively can inform future ligand design by biasing new libraries toward the properties of a specific class, such as natural products where we know a high degree of selectivity has often been evolved.

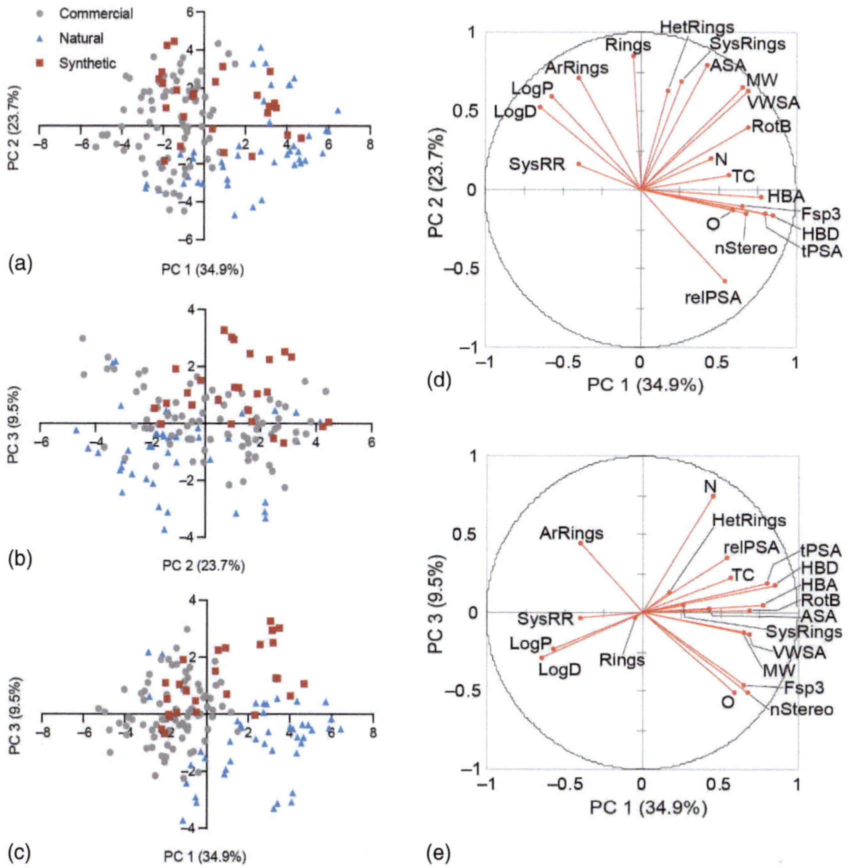

Figure 5.5 Principal component analysis (PCA) of libraries. (a) Graph of PC 1 and 2. (b) Graph of PC 2 and 3. (c) Graph of PC 1 and 3. (d) Loading plot depicting contribution of cheminformatic parameters to PC 1 and 2. (e) Loading plot depicting contribution of cheminformatic parameters to PC 2 and 3. PCA performed in XLStat-Student (version 2021.4.1.1209) and PCA graphs generated in GraphPad Prism (version 9.4.1 for Mac). Cheminformatic parameters were calculated using ChemAxon (Marvin version 21.4.6, 2021) as previously described. Source: Adapted from Morgan et al. [3]. MW = Molecular Weight, HBA = Hydrogen Bond Acceptors, HBD = Hydrogen Bond Donors, Log P = n-Octanol/Water Partition Coefficient, RotB = Number of Rotatable Bonds, tPSA = Topological Polar Surface Area, log D = n-Octanol/Water Partition Coefficient, N = Number of Nitrogen Atoms, O = Number of Oxygen Atoms, Rings = Number of Rings, ArRings = Number of Aromatic Rings, HetRings = Number of Heteroatom-Containing Rings, SysRings = Number of Ring Systems, SysRR = Ring Complexity, Fsp^3 = Fraction of sp^3-Hybridized Carbons, nStereo = Number of Stereocenters, ASA = Accessible Surface Area, RelPSA = Relative Polar Surface Area, TC = Total Charge, VWSA = Van der Waals Surface Area.

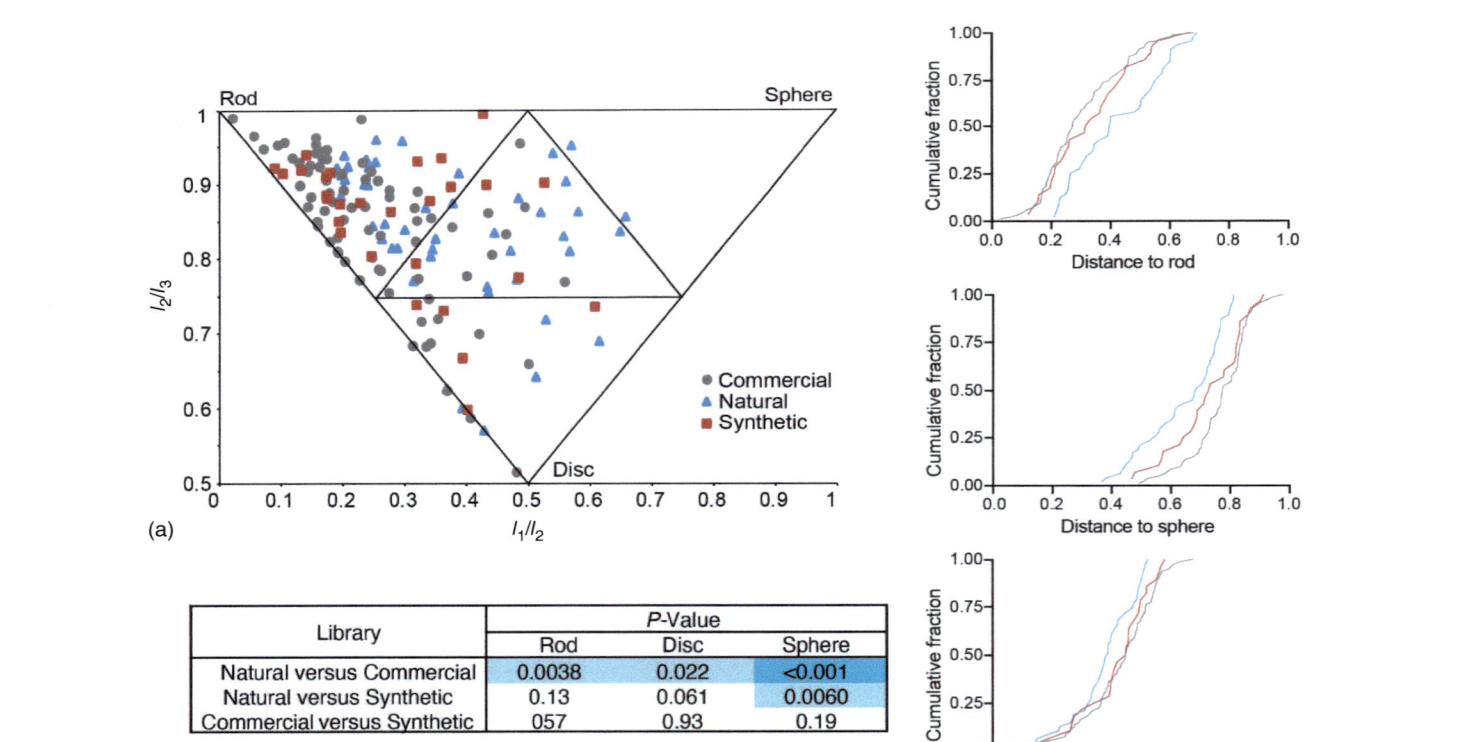

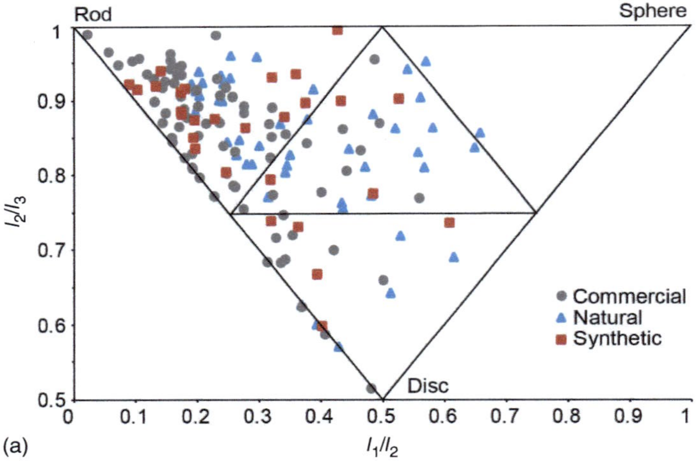

(a)

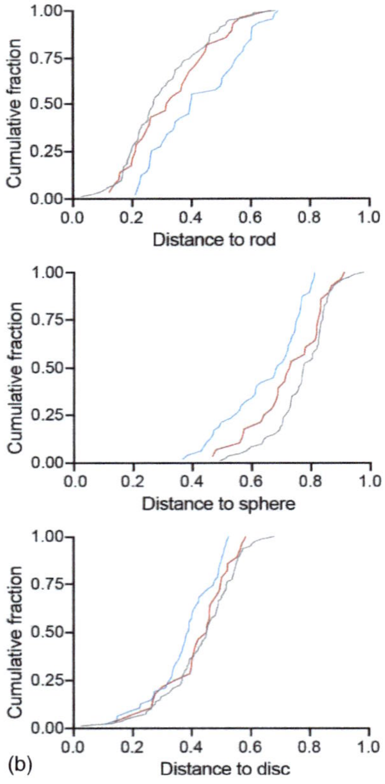

(b)

Library	*P*-Value		
	Rod	Disc	Sphere
Natural versus Commercial	0.0038	0.022	<0.001
Natural versus Synthetic	0.13	0.061	0.0060
Commercial versus Synthetic	057	0.93	0.19

(c)

Figure 5.6 Shape analysis of natural, commercial, and synthetic ligands. (a) Principal Moments of Inertia (PMI) analysis for natural, commercial, and synthetic ligands. (b) Cumulative distributions for distances from rod, disc, and sphere vertices. PMI was calculated as previously reported. Source: Adapted from Morgan et al. [4]. (c) Statistical comparison from Kolmogorov–Smirnov Test between libraries performed as previously reported [4]. Light blue = *P*-value <0.05; Dark blue = *P*-value <0.001. Performed in R (version 4.1.2) Graphs were created in GraphPad Prism (version 9.4.1 for Mac).

5.7 Conclusions and Outlook

In this chapter we have presented diverse ligands known to target RNA as well as tools to evaluate libraries and further our understanding of chemical matter that binds to RNA. Through investigating existing data and ligands, the field has identified trends in properties of RNA targeted ligands and through the use of machine-learning techniques presented here, a deeper understanding of how ligands recognize RNA may be achieved. By examining natural, commercial, and synthetic ligands that target RNA in the case study presented here, we identified significant diversity in chemical space, showing the range of molecules and by extension interactions that can be formed between ligands and RNA. With the continuing adaptation of machine-learning algorithms to RNA targeting, we look forward to a deep understanding of RNA recognition by small molecules and the rational design of novel RNA-targeted probes.

Acknowledgments

The authors thank Dr. Greta Bagnolini and TinTin Luu for their help in editing this chapter. Funding was provided by NSF CAREER (1750375).

References

1 Warner, K.D., Hajdin, C.E., and Weeks, K.M. (2018). Principles for targeting RNA with drug-like small molecules. *Nat. Rev. Drug Discovery* 17 (8): 547–558.

2 Yu, A.-M. and Tu, M.-J. (2022). Deliver the promise: RNAs as a new class of molecular entities for therapy and vaccination. *Pharmacol. Ther.* 230: 107967.

3 Morgan, B.S., Forte, J.E., Culver, R.N. et al. (2017). Discovery of key physicochemical, structural, and spatial properties of RNA-targeted bioactive ligands. *Angew. Chem. Int. Ed.* 56 (43): 13498–13502.

4 Morgan, B.S., Sanaba, B.G., Donlic, A. et al. (2019). R-BIND: an interactive database for exploring and developing RNA-targeted chemical probes. *ACS Chem. Biol.* 14 (12): 2691–2700.

5 Donlic, A., Swanson, E.G., Chiu, L.-Y. et al. (2022). R-BIND 2.0: an updated database of bioactive RNA-targeting small molecules and associated RNA secondary structures. *ACS Chem. Biol.* 17 (6): 1556–1566.

6 Kumar Mishra, S. and Kumar, A. (2016). NALDB: nucleic acid ligand database for small molecules targeting nucleic acid. *Database* 2016: baw002.

7 Mehta, A., Sonam, S., Gouri, I. et al. (2014). SMMRNA: a database of small molecule modulators of RNA. *Nucleic Acids Res.* 42 (D1): D132–D141.

8 Disney, M.D., Winkelsas, A.M., Velagapudi, S.P. et al. (2016). Inforna 2.0: a platform for the sequence-based design of small molecules targeting structured RNAs. *ACS Chem. Biol.* 11 (6): 1720–1728.

9 Velagapudi, S.P., Gallo, S.M., and Disney, M.D. (2014). Sequence-based design of bioactive small molecules that target precursor microRNAs. *Nat. Chem. Biol.* 10 (4): 291–297.
10 Wicks, S.L., Morgan, B.S., Wilson, A.W., and Hargrove, A.E. (2023). Probing bioactive chemical space to discover RNA-targeted small molecules. bioRxiv. 2023:2023.07.31.551350.
11 Ye, F., Haniff, H.S., Suresh, B.M. et al. (2022). Rational approach to identify RNA targets of natural products enables identification of nocathiacin as an inhibitor of an oncogenic RNA. *ACS Chem. Biol.* 17 (2): 474–482.
12 Vicens, Q. and Westhof, E. (2003). RNA as a drug target: the case of aminoglycosides. *ChemBioChem* 4 (10): 1018–1023.
13 Aboul-ela, F. (2010). Strategies for the design of RNA-binding small molecules. *Future Med. Chem.* 2 (1): 93–119.
14 Zhou, J., Wang, G., Zhang, L.-H., and Ye, X.-S. (2007). Modifications of aminoglycoside antibiotics targeting RNA. *Med. Res. Rev.* 27 (3): 279–316.
15 Disney, M.D. (2019). Targeting RNA with small molecules to capture opportunities at the intersection of chemistry, biology, and medicine. *JACS* 141 (17): 6776–6790.
16 Krause, K.M., Serio, A.W., Kane, T.R., and Connolly, L.E. (2016). Aminoglycosides: an overview. *Cold Spring Harbor Perspect. Med.* 6 (6).
17 Thomas, J.R. and Hergenrother, P.J. (2008). Targeting RNA with small molecules. *Chem. Rev.* 108 (4): 1171–1224.
18 Doi, Y., Wachino, J.I., and Arakawa, Y. (2016). Aminoglycoside resistance: the emergence of acquired 16S ribosomal RNA methyltransferases. *Infect. Dis. Clin. North Am.* 30 (2): 523–537.
19 Garneau-Tsodikova, S. and Labby, K.J. (2016). Mechanisms of resistance to aminoglycoside antibiotics: overview and perspectives. *Medchemcomm* 7 (1): 11–27.
20 Llano-Sotelo, B. and Chow, C.S. (1999). RNA-aminoglycoside antibiotic interactions: fluorescence detection of binding and conformational change. *Bioorg. Med. Chem. Lett.* 9 (2): 213–216.
21 Luedtke, N.W., Liu, Q., and Tor, Y. (2003). RNA–ligand interactions: affinity and specificity of aminoglycoside dimers and acridine conjugates to the HIV-1 rev response element. *Biochemistry* 42 (39): 11391–11403.
22 The Centers for Disease Control and Prevention (2020). Outpatient antibiotic prescriptions — United States.
23 Brodersen, D.E., Clemons, W.M., Carter, A.P. et al. (2000). The structural basis for the action of the antibiotics tetracycline, pactamycin, and hygromycin b on the 30S ribosomal subunit. *Cell* 103 (7): 1143–1154.
24 Zhanel, G.G., Homenuik, K., Nichol, K. et al. (2004). The glycylcyclines. *Drugs* 64 (1): 63–88.
25 Szeto, G.L., Brice, A.K., Yang, H.-C. et al. (2010). Minocycline attenuates HIV infection and reactivation by suppressing cellular activation in human CD4+ T cells. *J. Infect. Dis.* 201 (8): 1132–1140.

26 Mishra, M.K. and Basu, A. (2008). Minocycline neuroprotects, reduces microglial activation, inhibits caspase 3 induction, and viral replication following Japanese encephalitis. *J. Neurochem.* 105 (5): 1582–1595.

27 Douthwaite, S. and Champney, W.S. (2001). Structures of ketolides and macrolides determine their mode of interaction with the ribosomal target site. *J. Antimicrob. Chemother.* 48 (suppl_2): 1–8.

28 Dinos, G.P. (2017). The macrolide antibiotic renaissance. *Br. J. Pharmacol.* 174 (18): 2967–2983.

29 Vázquez-Laslop, N. and Mankin, A.S. (2018). How macrolide antibiotics work. *Trends Biochem. Sci.* 43 (9): 668–684.

30 Tran, T.P.A., Vo, D.D., Di Giorgio, A., and Duca, M. (2015). Ribosome-targeting antibiotics as inhibitors of oncogenic microRNAs biogenesis: old scaffolds for new perspectives in RNA targeting. *Bioorg. Med. Chem.* 23 (17): 5334–5344.

31 Garst, A.D., Edwards, A.L., and Batey, R.T. (2011). Riboswitches: structures and mechanisms. *Cold Spring Harbor Perspect. Biol.* 3 (6).

32 Breaker, R.R. (2022). The biochemical landscape of riboswitch ligands. *Biochemistry* 61 (3): 137–149.

33 McCown Phillip, J., Liang Jonathan, J., Weinberg, Z., and Breaker, R.R. (2014). Structural, functional, and taxonomic diversity of three PreQ1 riboswitch classes. *Chem. Biol.* 21 (7): 880–889.

34 Howe, J.A., Wang, H., Fischmann, T.O. et al. (2015). Selective small-molecule inhibition of an RNA structural element. *Nature* 526 (7575): 672–677.

35 Connelly, C.M., Numata, T., Boer, R.E. et al. (2019). Synthetic ligands for PreQ1 riboswitches provide structural and mechanistic insights into targeting RNA tertiary structure. *Nat. Commun.* 10 (1): 1501.

36 Tran, B., Pichling, P., Tenney, L. et al. (2020). Parallel discovery strategies provide a basis for riboswitch ligand design. *Cell Chem. Biol.* 27 (10): 1241–1249.e4.

37 Hangauer, M.J., Vaughn, I.W., and McManus, M.T. (2013). Pervasive transcription of the human genome produces thousands of previously unidentified long intergenic noncoding RNAs. *PLos Genet.* 9 (6): e1003569.

38 Hopkins, A.L. and Groom, C.R. (2002). The druggable genome. *Nat. Rev. Drug Discovery* 1 (9): 727–730.

39 Wang, F., Zuroske, T., and Watts, J.K. (2020). RNA therapeutics on the rise. *Nat. Rev. Drug Discovery* 19 (7): 441–442.

40 Rizvi, N.F., Santa Maria, J.P., Nahvi, A. et al. (2020). Targeting RNA with small molecules: identification of selective, RNA-binding small molecules occupying drug-like chemical space. *SLAS Discovery* 25 (4): 384–396.

41 Haniff, H.S., Knerr, L., Liu, X. et al. (2020). Design of a small molecule that stimulates vascular endothelial growth factor A enabled by screening RNA fold–small molecule interactions. *Nat. Chem.* 12 (10): 952–961.

42 Yazdani, K., Jordan, D., Yang, M. et al. (2023). Machine learning informs RNA-binding chemical space. *Angew. Chem. Int. Ed.* 62 (11): e202211358.

43 Rizvi, N.F. and Smith, G.F. (2017). RNA as a small molecule druggable target. *Bioorg. Med. Chem. Lett.* 27 (23): 5083–5088.

44 Di Giorgio, A. and Duca, M. (2019). Synthetic small-molecule RNA ligands: future prospects as therapeutic agents. *MedChemComm* 10 (8): 1242–1255.

45 Sztuba-Solinska, J., Chavez-Calvillo, G., and Cline, S.E. (2019). Unveiling the druggable RNA targets and small molecule therapeutics. *Bioorg. Med. Chem.* 27 (10): 2149–2165.

46 Yu, A.-M., Choi, Y.H., and Tu, M.-J. (2020). RNA drugs and RNA targets for small molecules: principles, progress, and challenges. *Pharmacol. Rev.* 72 (4): 862.

47 Zamani, F. and Suzuki, T. (2021). Synthetic RNA modulators in drug discovery. *J. Med. Chem.* 64 (11): 7110–7155.

48 Seth, P.P., Miyaji, A., Jefferson, E.A. et al. (2005). SAR by MS: discovery of a new class of RNA-binding small molecules for the hepatitis C virus: internal ribosome entry site IIA subdomain. *J. Med. Chem.* 48 (23): 7099–7102.

49 Parsons, J., Castaldi, M.P., Dutta, S. et al. (2009). Conformational inhibition of the hepatitis C virus internal ribosome entry site RNA. *Nat. Chem. Biol.* 5 (11): 823–825.

50 Paulsen, R.B., Seth, P.P., Swayze, E.E. et al. (2010). Inhibitor-induced structural change in the HCV IRES domain IIa RNA. *Proc. Natl. Acad. Sci. U.S.A.* 107 (16): 7263–7268.

51 Dibrov, S.M., Ding, K., Brunn, N.D. et al. (2012). Structure of a hepatitis C virus RNA domain in complex with a translation inhibitor reveals a binding mode reminiscent of riboswitches. *Proc. Natl. Acad. Sci. U.S.A.* 109 (14): 5223–5228.

52 Disney, M.D., Childs, J.L., and Turner, D.H. (2004). Hoechst 33258 selectively inhibits group I intron self-splicing by affecting RNA folding. *ChemBioChem* 5 (12): 1647–1652.

53 Disney, M.D., Stephenson, R., Wright, T.W. et al. (2005). Activity of Hoechst 33258 against *Pneumocystis carinii* f. sp. *muris*, *Candida albicans*, and *Candida dubliniensis*. *Antimicrob. Agents Chemother.* 49 (4): 1326–1330.

54 Rzuczek, S.G., Colgan, L.A., Nakai, Y. et al. (2016). Precise small-molecule recognition of a toxic CUG RNA repeat expansion. *Nat. Chem. Biol.* 13: 188.

55 Childs-Disney, J.L., Hoskins, J., Rzuczek, S.G. et al. (2012). Rationally designed small molecules targeting the RNA that causes myotonic dystrophy type 1 are potently bioactive. *ACS Chem. Biol.* 7 (5): 856–862.

56 Costales, M.G., Haga, C.L., Velagapudi, S.P. et al. (2017). Small molecule inhibition of microRNA-210 reprograms an oncogenic hypoxic circuit. *JACS* 139 (9): 3446–3455.

57 Velagapudi, S.P., Cameron, M.D., Haga, C.L. et al. (2016). Design of a small molecule against an oncogenic noncoding RNA. *Proc. Natl. Acad. Sci. U.S.A.* 113 (21): 5898–5903.

58 Costales, M.G., Childs-Disney, J.L., Haniff, H.S., and Disney, M.D. (2020). How we think about targeting RNA with small molecules. *J. Med. Chem.* 63 (17): 8880–8900.

59 Kim, J.N. and Breaker, R.R. (2008). Purine sensing by riboswitches. *Biol. Cell* 100 (1): 1–11.

60 Zou, T., Sato, Y., Kaneyoshi, S. et al. (2022). Naphthalene diimides carrying two β-cyclodextrins prefer telomere RNA G-quadruplex recognition. *Molecules* 27 (13).

61 Krishnamurthy, M., Gooch, B.D., and Beal, P.A. (2004). Peptide quinoline conjugates: a new class of RNA-binding molecules. *Org. Lett.* 6 (1): 63–66.

62 Gareiss, P.C., Sobczak, K., McNaughton, B.R. et al. (2008). Dynamic combinatorial selection of molecules capable of inhibiting the (CUG) repeat RNA–MBNL1 interaction in vitro: discovery of lead compounds targeting myotonic dystrophy (DM1). *JACS* 130 (48): 16254–16261.

63 Ofori, L.O., Hoskins, J., Nakamori, M. et al. (2012). From dynamic combinatorial 'hit' to lead: in vitro and in vivo activity of compounds targeting the pathogenic RNAs that cause myotonic dystrophy. *Nucleic Acids Res.* 40 (13): 6380–6390.

64 Lee, M.-K., Bottini, A., Kim, M. et al. (2014). A novel small-molecule binds to the influenza A virus RNA promoter and inhibits viral replication. *Chem. Commun.* 50 (3): 368–370.

65 Charrette, B.P., Boerneke, M.A., and Hermann, T. (2016). Ligand optimization by improving shape complementarity at a hepatitis C virus RNA target. *ACS Chem. Biol.* 11 (12): 3263–3267.

66 Hashemian, S.M.R., Farhadi, T., and Ganjparvar, M. (2018). Linezolid: a review of its properties, function, and use in critical care. *Drug Des. Dev. Ther.* 12: 1759–1767.

67 Burdette, S.D. and Trotman, R. (2015). Tedizolid: the first once-daily oxazolidinone class antibiotic. *Clin. Infect. Dis.* 61 (8): 1315–1321.

68 Maciagiewicz, I., Zhou, S., Bergmeier, S.C., and Hines, J.V. (2011). Structure-activity studies of RNA-binding oxazolidinone derivatives. *Bioorg. Med. Chem. Lett.* 21 (15): 4524–4527.

69 Sato, Y., Ichihashi, T., Nishizawa, S., and Teramae, N. (2012). Strong and selective binding of amiloride to an abasic site in RNA duplexes: thermodynamic characterization and MicroRNA detection. *Angew. Chem. Int. Ed.* 51 (26): 6369–6372.

70 Stelzer, A.C., Frank, A.T., Kratz, J.D. et al. (2011). Discovery of selective bioactive small molecules by targeting an RNA dynamic ensemble. *Nat. Chem. Biol.* 7 (8): 553–559.

71 Patwardhan, N.N., Ganser, L.R., Kapral, G.J. et al. (2017). Amiloride as a new RNA-binding scaffold with activity against HIV-1 TAR. *MedChemComm* 8 (5): 1022–1036.

72 Patwardhan, N.N., Cai, Z., Umuhire Juru, A., and Hargrove, A.E. (2019). Driving factors in amiloride recognition of HIV RNA targets. *Org. Biomol. Chem.* 17 (42): 9313–9320.

73 Davila-Calderon, J., Patwardhan, N.N., Chiu, L.-Y. et al. (2020). IRES-targeting small molecule inhibits enterovirus 71 replication via allosteric stabilization of a ternary complex. *Nat. Commun.* 11 (1): 4775.

74 Davila-Calderon, J., Li, M.-L., Penumutchu, S.R., et al. Enterovirus evolution reveals the mechanism of an RNA-targeted antiviral and determinants of viral replication. bioRxiv. 2023:2023.02.20.529064.

75 Zafferani, M., Haddad, C., Luo, L. et al. Amilorides inhibit SARS-CoV-2 replication in vitro by targeting RNA structures. *Sci. Adv.* 7 (48): eabl6096.

76 Wilson, W.D., Ratmeyer, L., Zhao, M. et al. (1996). Design and analysis of RNA structure-specific agents as potential antivirals. *J. Mol. Recognit.* 9 (2): 187–196.

77 Ratmeyer, L., Zapp, M.L., Green, M.R. et al. (1996). Inhibition of HIV-1 Rev–RRE interaction by diphenylfuran derivatives. *Biochemistry* 35 (42): 13689–13696.

78 Gelus, N., Bailly, C., Hamy, F. et al. (1999). Inhibition of HIV-1 Tat-TAR interaction by diphenylfuran derivatives: effects of the terminal basic side chains. *Bioorg. Med. Chem.* 7 (6): 1089–1096.

79 Donlic, A., Morgan, B.S., Xu, J.L. et al. (2018). Discovery of small molecule ligands for MALAT1 by tuning an RNA-binding Scaffold. *Angew. Chem.* 130 (40): 13426–13431.

80 Donlic, A., Zafferani, M., Padroni, G. et al. (2020). Regulation of MALAT1 triple helix stability and in vitro degradation by diphenylfurans. *Nucleic Acids Res.* 48 (14): 7653–7664.

81 Zafferani, M., Martyr, J.G., Muralidharan, D. et al. (2022). Multiassay profiling of a focused small molecule library reveals predictive bidirectional modulation of the lncRNA MALAT1 triplex stability in vitro. *ACS Chem. Biol.*

82 Lee, J., Bai, Y., Chembazhi, U.V. et al. (2019). Intrinsically cell-penetrating multivalent and multitargeting ligands for myotonic dystrophy type 1. *Proc. Natl. Acad. Sci. U.S.A.* 116 (18): 8709–8714.

83 Childs-Disney, J.L., Tran, T., Vummidi, B.R. et al. (2018). A massively parallel selection of small molecule-RNA motif binding partners informs design of an antiviral from sequence. *Chem* 4 (10): 2384–2404.

84 Sousa, T., Correia, J., Pereira, V., and Rocha, M. (2021). Generative deep learning for targeted compound design. *JCIM* 61 (11): 5343–5361.

85 Bajorath, J., Peltason, L., Wawer, M. et al. (2009). Navigating structure–activity landscapes. *Drug Discovery Today* 14 (13): 698–705.

86 Xu, Z. and Frank, A.T. (2022). AI-generated virtual libraries could help uncover RNA-specific regions of chemical space. bioRxiv.

87 Grimberg, H., Tiwari, V.S., Tam, B. et al. (2022). Machine learning approaches to optimize small-molecule inhibitors for RNA targeting. *J. Cheminf.* 14 (1): 4.

88 Cai, Z., Zafferani, M., Akande, O.M., and Hargrove, A.E. (2022). Quantitative structure–activity relationship (QSAR) study predicts small-molecule binding to RNA structure. *J. Med. Chem.* 65 (10): 7262–7277.

89 Oliver, C., Mallet, V., Gendron, R.S. et al. (2020). Augmented base pairing networks encode RNA-small molecule binding preferences. *Nucleic Acids Res.* 48 (14): 7690–7699.

90 Deng, Z., Gu, R., Bi, H., et al. (2022). Predicting ligand-RNA binding using E3 equivariant network and pretraining.

91 Bian, Y. and Xie, X.-Q. (2021). Generative chemistry: drug discovery with deep learning generative models. *J. Mol. Model.* 27 (3): 71.

92 Gómez-Bombarelli, R., Wei, J.N., Duvenaud, D. et al. (2018). Automatic chemical design using a data-driven continuous representation of molecules. *ACS Cent. Sci.* 4 (2): 268–276.

93 Zhavoronkov, A., Ivanenkov, Y.A., Aliper, A. et al. (2019). Deep learning enables rapid identification of potent DDR1 kinase inhibitors. *Nat. Biotechnol.* 37 (9): 1038–1040.

94 Godinez, W.J., Ma, E.J., Chao, A.T. et al. (2022). Design of potent antimalarials with generative chemistry. *Nat. Mach. Intell.* 4 (2): 180–186.

95 Manigrasso, J., Marcia, M., and De Vivo, M. (2021). Computer-aided design of RNA-targeted small molecules: a growing need in drug discovery. *Chem.* 7 (11): 2965–2988.

96 Padroni, G., Patwardhan, N.N., Schapira, M., and Hargrove, A.E. (2020). Systematic analysis of the interactions driving small molecule–RNA recognition. *RSC Med. Chem.* 11 (7): 802–813.

97 Ferreira de Freitas, R. and Schapira, M. (2017). A systematic analysis of atomic protein–ligand interactions in the PDB. *MedChemComm* 8 (10): 1970–1981.

98 Kallert, E., Fischer, T.R., Schneider, S. et al. (2022). Protein-based virtual screening tools applied for RNA–ligand docking identify new binders of the preQ1-riboswitch. *JCIM*.

99 Zhou, Y., Jiang, Y., and Chen, S.-J. (2022). RNA–ligand molecular docking: advances and challenges. *WIREs Comput. Mol. Sci.* 12 (3): e1571.

100 Bodoor, K., Boyapati, V., Gopu, V. et al. (2009). Design and implementation of an ribonucleic acid (RNA) directed fragment library. *J. Med. Chem.* 52 (12): 3753–3761.

101 Kennard, R.W. and Stone, L.A. (1969). Computer aided design of experiments. *Technometrics* 11 (1): 137–148.

6

MicroRNAs as Targets for Small-Molecule Binders

Maria Duca

Université Côte d'Azur, CNRS, Institute of Chemistry of Nice, 28 avenue Valrose, 06100 Nice, France

6.1 Introduction

Among the various therapeutic targets exploited by currently marketed drugs, proteins represent the large majority and are also the most studied for the development of new therapies. However, it is known that a large majority of the human genome is transcribed into RNA and that only 1.5% of this RNA is then translated into proteins [1]. Moreover, among these proteins only a very small percentage is correlated with a pathology and many of them are qualified as "undruggable," because these proteins do not contain suitable binding sites in which small molecules can bind with good affinity and specificity. The remaining part of the genome produces non-coding RNAs (ncRNAs), which represent major players for the regulation of many cellular processes, such as transcription, translation, or the regulation of gene expression. The discovery, characterization, and in-depth study of these RNAs have led to the discovery that these structures may represent valid therapeutic targets [2]. This allows for a much broader spectrum of therapies than is currently available and offers hope for a number of diseases that have no existing or effective treatment to date.

Over the last 20 years, several strategies have been developed to target RNA [3]. Among these approaches, the use of oligonucleotides is the most common method and involves short nucleotide sequences capable of specifically recognizing the target RNA. Antisense oligonucleotides (ASOs) and small interfering RNAs (siRNAs), for example, are two classes of oligonucleotides that inhibit a particular RNA by complementary recognition of RNA sequences [4]. To date, many oligonucleotides are in clinical trials and several have been marketed. It should be noted, however, that there are a number of limitations to the use of oligonucleotides as therapeutics, such as cost, biodistribution to the site of action, and metabolic stability. The use of peptides represents a second strategy to target RNA [5]. These compounds of intermediate molecular weight can provide a large surface area for interaction with RNA and have good potential to form complexes with high affinity and specificity. More easily modified and optimized than oligonucleotides, peptides still present

RNA as a Drug Target: The Next Frontier for Medicinal Chemistry, First Edition.
Edited by John Schneekloth and Martin Pettersson.

limitations for *in vivo* applications due to stability and biodistribution. The third approach for targeting RNA is the use of small molecules that are able to interact with the target RNA through the recognition of RNA tertiary structural features rather than the primary sequence [6]. Indeed, the association of single- and double-stranded regions of most biologically relevant RNAs induces the formation of three-dimensional structures that are more similar to the structures of a protein than that of a DNA double helix [7]. These structures can thus be targeted by small molecules with the advantage that they can in principle overcome the constraints of oligonucleotides and peptides thanks to much more favorable pharmacological properties. The use of small molecules to target RNA for chemical biology and medicinal chemistry studies is thus a particularly promising approach although many challenges still need to be addressed. Among the most studied targets, one can cite ribosomal RNAs (rRNAs) and riboswitches in bacteria; genomic RNAs in viruses; extended RNA repeats, splicing of precursor messenger RNAs (pre-mRNAs) and microRNAs (miRNAs) in eukaryotes.

The main issue in all these studies is the identification of ligands able to bind specifically to the targeted RNA with high affinity. Nevertheless, several successful examples are already in the literature and, even more importantly, on the market (Figure 6.1). Indeed antibiotics, such as aminoglycosides, chloramphenicols, lincosamides, macrolides, oxazolidinones, or tetracyclines are known to bind to specific sites on the RNA of the prokaryotic ribosome and inhibit protein synthesis in bacteria [8]. These compounds were the first to demonstrate the feasibility of using small molecules to target RNA. More recently, risdiplam has been approved by the FDA for the treatment of spinal muscular atrophy (SMA) [9]. This drug is able to modify splicing upon binding to a pre-mRNA and thereby correct the expression of SMN protein that is altered in this pathology. These efforts have also led the way to the discovery of other splicing modulators [10].

Among the most exploited RNA targets in the literature, miRNAs, belonging to the class of ncRNAs, have been widely studied. Beside ribosomal RNA (rRNA) and transfer RNA (tRNA), both of which are linked to the translation of mRNAs into proteins, many classes of ncRNAs exist and are generally divided into two families: long non-coding RNAs (lncRNAs) and small non-coding RNAs including miRNAs.

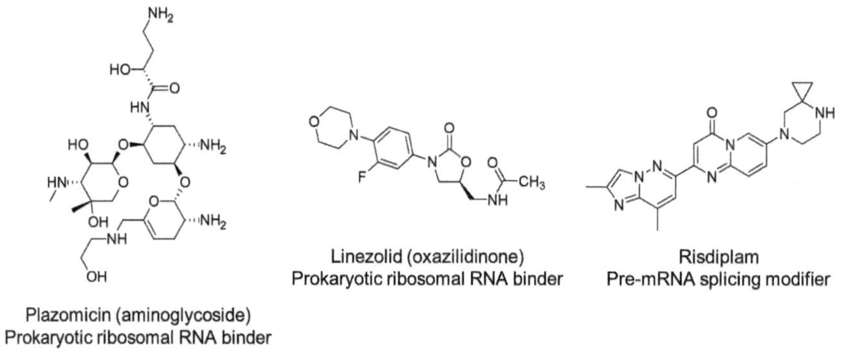

Figure 6.1 Examples of marketed drugs acting as RNA binders as the main molecular mechanism of action.

The discovery and identification of miRNAs and of their functions in the regulation of gene expression is one of the most important discoveries of the last decades. In particular, the deregulation of miRNAs has been associated with the initiation and development of a large number of diseases including cancers. As a consequence, miRNAs represent a new class of therapeutic targets for the development of anti-cancer therapies. Given the recent success of small molecules targeting RNA, targeting miRNAs is currently of high interest to the scientific community and could represent a particularly effective strategy in the treatment of cancers or other miRNA-associated pathologies. Furthermore, chemical probes able to interfere with the miRNA network are important tools to elucidate intracellular pathways that have not yet been completely understood. In this chapter, we will illustrate in detail how miRNAs have been targeted by small molecules and which strategies can be employed to efficiently and specifically inhibit therapeutically relevant miRNAs.

6.2 MicroRNAs

As mentioned above, miRNAs are small ncRNAs consisting of short oligonucleotides of 18–25 nucleotides. MiRNAs are involved in the regulation of gene expression through selective interaction with one or more mRNAs to induce their degradation and inhibit translation. The first miRNA, Lin-4, was discovered in 1993 in the worm species *Caenorhabditis elegans* [11]. Lin 4 regulates lin-14 messenger RNA leading to a decrease in production of its associated proteins. This research led to characterization of a new mechanism of regulation of gene expression and revolutionized the understanding of molecular biology. Seven years separate this discovery from that of a second miRNA, let-7, again in *C. elegans*, but also found in animals and humans [12]. Since then, many miRNAs have been identified in animals, plants, and viruses, some of which are present in all of these species [13]. Numerous studies have been undertaken to precisely link each miRNA to the genes it regulates. Some miRNAs have high levels of expression, others very low, and all vary from species to species. Aided by increasingly sophisticated biotechnologies, the discovery of these new players in living organisms has grown exponentially since the early 2000s.

In each species, miRNAs can be grouped into families. Members of these families are transcribed by adjacent genes and have the same core sequence (called the "seed sequence"), i.e. the sequence responsible for the recognition of targeted mRNAs [14]. The number of miRNAs varies within these families and also varies from species to species. Regarding nomenclature, several suffixes can be found in miRNA names. When two miRNAs have an identical sequence but come from a different precursor, the suffixes added are numbers (e.g. miR-1-1 and miR-1-2). When two miRNAs come from the same precursor but not from the same strand, they are annotated with a suffix "-3p" or "-5p" depending on the strand where they are located if they are found in similar proportions in the cell (e.g. miR-146b-3p and miR-146b-5p). If one of these two miRNAs is much more abundant than the other form, an asterisk will follow the name of the less abundant one (e.g. miR 146*). Finally, the suffix will be a letter if the miRNAs have identical sequences except for one or two nucleotides (e.g. miR-146a and miR146b). In order to understand the strategies that are being used to target miRNAs, it is important to understand how they are formed and how they function, and this will be the subject of the following section.

6.3 MicroRNAs Biogenesis

MiRNA biogenesis is a multistep process involving key enzymes that begins in the nucleus with the transcription of a miRNA gene into primary miRNAs (pri-miRNAs) consisting of 500 to 3000 nucleotides (Figure 6.2, Step 1) [15]. Once produced and structured in the nucleus, the pri-miRNA is cleaved by the microprocessor, a protein complex formed by Drosha and DCGR8 [16]. Drosha is a nuclear ribonuclease III (RNAse III) that interacts specifically with double-stranded RNAs (Figure 6.2, Step 2) [17]. This cleavage induces the formation of a sequence consisting of 70 nucleotides called pre-miRNA. Pri-miRNA and pre-miRNA have a stem–loop structure, characteristic of many biologically relevant non-coding RNAs, inducing the formation of particular binding pockets and offering the possibility for small-molecule RNA ligands to bind. The pre-miRNA is then recognized by the Exportin 5 (Exp5)–RanGTP complex, which is a transporter that transfers molecules and macromolecules from the nucleus to the cytoplasm (Figure 6.2, Step 3) [18].

Once in the cytoplasm, the pre-miRNA is cleaved by another RNAse III called Dicer (Figure 6.2, Step 4) that begins recognition by binding to the 3′-end of

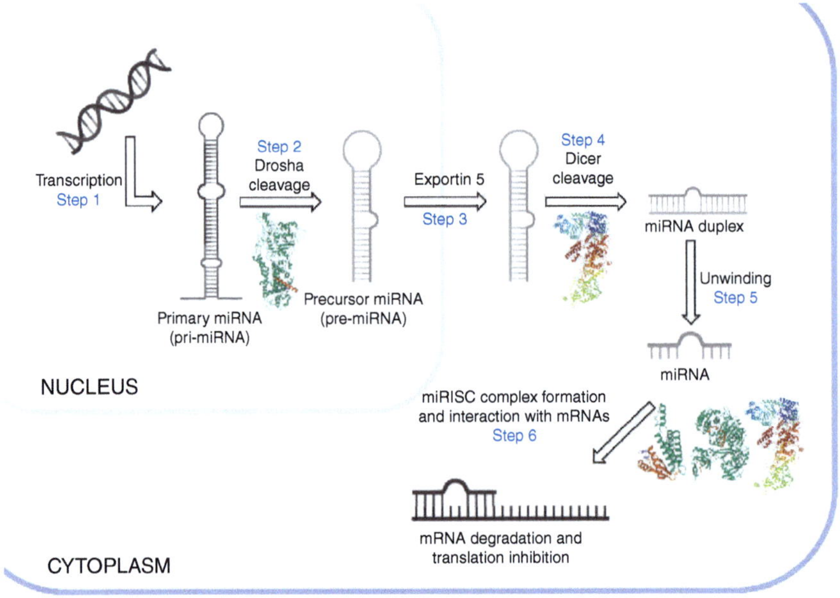

Figure 6.2 Biogenesis of miRNAs inside human cells. The most important proteins and enzymes involved in the process are Drosha (PDB:6LXE), Dicer (PDB:7XW3), TRBP (PDB:4WYQ), and Argonaute2 (PDB:4OLA).

the substrate [19]. The catalytic domain of the enzyme will then cleave the 5′ and 3′ strands of the double-stranded RNA (dsRNA) within about 20–25 base pairs of their ends. Unlike Drosha, Dicer is able to cleave pre-miRNA alone. However, its activity has been shown to be modulated by associated proteins, particularly the TAR RNA-binding protein (TRBP). The resulting sequence is a double-stranded RNA, 18–25 nucleotides long, called miRNA duplex, or miRNA/miRNA*, these two strands being guide and passenger, respectively. After cleavage, the Dicer–TRBP–miRNA duplex complex is able to interact with a protein of the Argonaut family (Ago). The guide strand is then loaded onto Ago, while the passenger strand is unwound and detached from the duplex before being degraded (Figure 6.2, Step 5). Thus, the RNA-induced silencing complex (RISC) [20] ready to interact with the target mRNA(s) is formed, containing Dicer, TRBP, and Ago which carries the mature single-stranded miRNA. Once formed, the RISC complex guides the miRNA to its target mRNA to bind to the 3′-untranslated regions (3′-UTR) and regulate the expression of one or more proteins by inhibiting translation or inducing degradation of the corresponding mRNA (Figure 6.2, Step 6).

It has been shown that each miRNA can regulate hundreds of mRNAs and that the production of the majority of protein-coding genes is under the control of miRNAs and therefore many, if not all, biological processes. Given their degree of involvement in the regulation of gene expression, it is not surprising that a small deregulation of miRNA expression levels can lead to a destabilization of the cellular machinery [21]. Thus, the complex intracellular miRNA network is essential for cellular homeostasis, but it also represents a very delicate equilibrium that can be deregulated by the overexpression or the underexpression of one or more miRNAs. Several pathologies such as cancers, cardiovascular or neurodegenerative diseases have been correlated with a deregulation of certain miRNAs [22].

6.4 Targeting MicroRNAs with Small-Molecule RNA Binders

Given the pivotal role of miRNAs in various pathologies, many studies have been devoted to the search for small molecules able to interfere with the miRNA network by either inducing or inhibiting the production and function of deregulated miRNAs [23]. The role of miRNAs in cancer has been particularly studied since miRNAs represent important biomarkers but also promising anticancer targets [24]. As mentioned above, in cancers some miRNAs are overexpressed, inhibit the synthesis of tumor suppressor proteins, and are called oncogenes. Other miRNAs are underexpressed, inhibit the synthesis of oncogenic proteins, and are called tumor suppressors [24, 25]. These deregulation processes tend to promote oncogenesis and tumor maintenance. However, the classification of miRNAs as oncogenes or tumor suppressors cannot be generalized since some of them can be oncogenic in one type of cancer and tumor suppressors in others. It is therefore important to identify the biological functions and targets of miRNAs involved in the cancer under study before considering these miRNAs as potential drug targets.

Several strategies have been proposed both for the activation of tumor suppressor miRNAs and for the inhibition of oncogenic miRNAs. Oligonucleotides have largely been applied to this aim [26]. Indeed, these high-molecular-weight molecules can increase expression of tumor suppressor miRNA or directly inhibit the function of an oncogenic one. This approach is very effective and specific, but limitations remain in its clinical application. Small molecules are now considered a viable and similarly specific approach based on structure recognition of one of the precursors in the biogenesis process (indirect mechanism) instead of the miRNAs themselves (direct mechanism). In the following sections, we will detail some of the main examples of small molecules discovered to interfere with the miRNAs network with a particular attention to their application in cancer.

6.4.1 Induction of miRNAs Expression: Tackling the Decrease of Tumor Suppressor miRNAs

A few examples of small molecules have been reported as inducers of expression of under-expressed tumor suppressor miRNAs in cancer cells. The basis for this approach is the observation that a large number of miRNAs are under-expressed in cancer cells and that a non-specific activation of their expression could have a positive outcome in inhibiting cancer cell proliferation [27]. One of the first reported examples is enoxacin (compound **1**, Figure 6.3), a fluoroquinolone antibiotic, reported by Shan and co-workers after screening 2000 US FDA-approved drugs using an intracellular reporter system based on enhanced green fluorescent protein (EGFP) [28]. Enoxacin was able to selectively increase the expression levels of some miRNAs. The reported studies suggested that enoxacin could facilitate the interaction between TAR RNA binding protein (TRBP) and RNAs inside cells and promote the loading of miRNAs onto RISC. This enhancement is largely dependent on the levels of expression of miRNAs inside cells rather than on specific RNA sequences. Compound **1** is thus a non-specific activator of miRNAs function. Further studies demonstrated that enoxacin has a powerful cancer-specific growth inhibitory effect in human cell cultures and in *in vivo* mouse models [29]. This biological activity is due to the binding of enoxacin to TRBP, a protein essential for

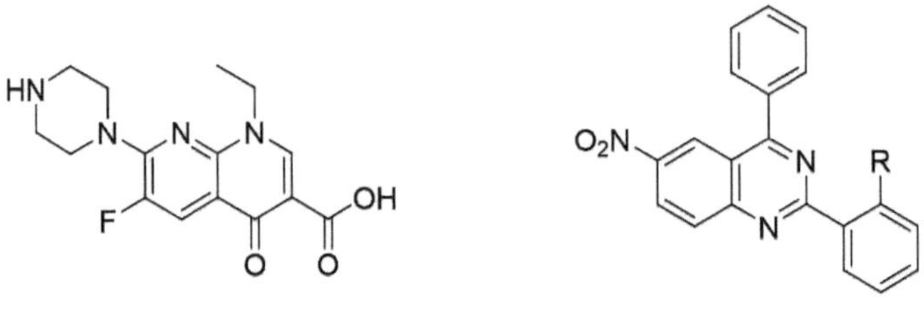

1 (Enoxacin) **2** (R = H, OH, NO_2)

Figure 6.3 Chemical structure of compounds able to activate miRNAs biogenesis and function: enoxacin (**1**) and quinoxalines (**2**).

miRNAs function, thus increasing miRNAs effects and restoring the expression of tumor suppressor miRNAs.

Maiti and co-workers also reported the screening of different classes of small molecules for their miRNome modulation potential. Noteworthy, three quinazoline compounds, such as compound **2** (Figure 6.3), were shown to non-specifically upregulate tumor suppressor miRNAs in MCF-7 cancer cells and to inhibit cancer cells proliferation with an EC_{50} of 20 µM [30]. The authors demonstrated that these compounds act by inducing apoptosis or cell cycle arrest. As for enoxacin, the effect is non-specific and not related to a direct RNA binding.

As illustrated by these examples, activation of miRNAs expression by small molecules cannot represent a specific approach, and it is proposed as a general method to increase miRNAs levels without discriminating which miRNAs are affected. After these few examples, there were no further developments, and the research in the field focused on the specific inhibition of oncogenic miRNAs as will be described in the following sections.

6.4.2 Inhibition of miRNAs Production: Pre- and Pri-miRNA Binders

The strategy of inhibiting overexpressed miRNAs has been focused on inhibiting their biogenesis. For example, interaction with the mature miRNA to prevent interactions with mRNA (Step 6 in Figure 6.2), or inhibiting enzymes involved in the different steps of miRNA biogenesis and maturation (Steps 2–5 in Figure 6.2). This approach is thus based on the hypothesis that a molecule that is able to bind efficiently and specifically to a miRNA precursor could inhibit its biogenesis [23]. MiRNA precursors (pre-miRNAs and pri-miRNAs) bear a particular secondary and tertiary structure that associates single-stranded and double-stranded regions and induces the formation of three-dimensional structures favorable to specific interaction with small molecules. The interaction of a small molecule with one of the oncogenic miRNA precursors can thus inhibit the corresponding biogenesis step, such as the cleavage of the pri-miRNA by Drosha or of the pre-miRNA by Dicer and thus block the synthesis of the overexpressed oncogenic miRNA [31]. It is also possible to interfere with RNA–protein interactions such as miRNA-Ago or miRNA-Lin28, the latter being an essential protein for miRNA function.

The examples reported in the literature so far concern molecules identified by high-throughput screening of large collections of compounds (>500 molecules), by screening focused libraries of compounds known to interact with RNA or by designing selective ligands based on the structure of the targeted RNA. In the following section we will discuss key examples of miRNA-inhibiting agents and the methodologies used to discover them.

6.4.2.1 Discovery of miRNAs Inhibitors by Intracellular Assays

High-throughput screening (HTS) allows the identification of molecules able to bind to miRNAs or their precursors in order to inhibit their functions. Various screening methods have been developed over time based on the use of fluorescence and/or luminescence, with cellular, *in vitro* or *in silico* assays. Intracellular assays have

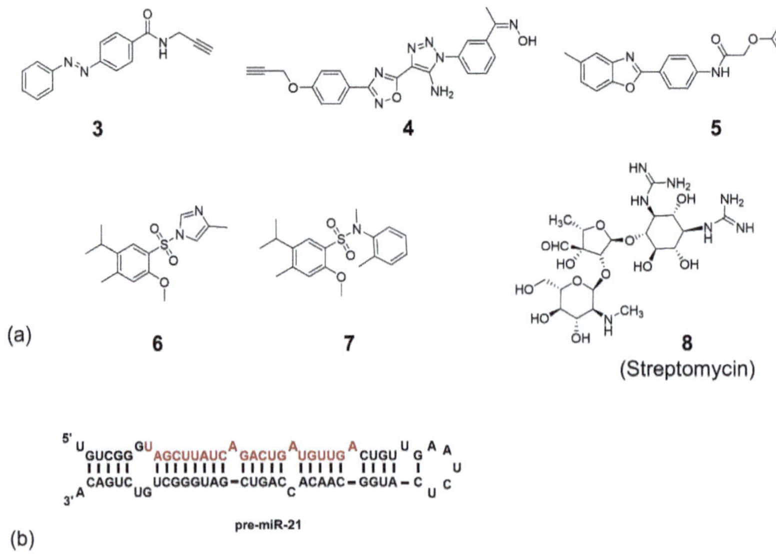

Figure 6.4 (a) Inhibitors of miRNAs biogenesis **3–8** discovered by intracellular assays. (b) Primary and secondary structure of pre-miR-21.

been widely employed to screen compound libraries because they allow for the fast evaluation of the phenotype as well as for the quantification of the targeted miRNA.

The first library screen for the identification of oncogenic miRNA inhibitors was performed by Deiters' team in 2008 with an intracellular assay based on a luciferase reporter system [32]. Screening of more than 1000 compounds against miR-21, a widely studied oncogenic miRNA in a large number of cancers, followed by structure–activity relationship studies led to the identification of the derivative diazobenzene **3** (Figure 6.4a), capable of inhibiting miR-21 production. The study of the mode of action of this analogue suggests that this compound inhibits the transcription of the miR-21 gene into pri-miR-21. It should be noted that this compound does not affect the expression of other miRNAs at the intracellular level, suggesting specificity of action. Deiters' team continued to exploit library screening to find small molecules that inhibit the production and/or action of oncogenic miRNAs. Using the same type of intracellular assay, they screened more than 300,000 compounds, and structure–activity relationship studies led in 2018 to the identification of compound **4** (Figure 6.4a) and of ether-amide **5** (Figure 6.4a), both highly effective and selective inhibitors of miR-21 production [23, 33]. However, studies regarding the mechanism of action show that **4** does not affect either gene transcription or pri-miR-21 formation in cells, whereas the ether-amide compound family to which **5** belongs inhibits miR-21 biogenesis at the level of the transcription step with a similar action to the azobenzene molecule **3**. Cellular assays have also demonstrated the ability of compound **4** to restore the sensitivity of kidney carcinoma cells to chemotherapy and the inhibition by treatment with molecule **5** of proliferation and microtumor formation in cervical cancer cells. These cellular proof-of-concept studies make these two anti-cancer molecules particularly promising. Using a similar reporter system, the same authors have also screened compounds that could inhibit miR-122 that is directly involved in the proliferation of hepatitis C virus (HCV) [34]. A primary screen of more than 300,000 compounds was followed by various steps of selection led to the identification of compound **6** as the most promising for further development. Medicinal chemistry optimization of this compound led to improved analogs such as compound **7**, which shows similar potency to that of **6** (IC_{50} = 12.5 μM in an intracellular assay for the measurement of miR-122 inhibition) but also a high specificity to inhibit the production of miR-122 without affecting the expression of other miRNAs. The study of the mechanism of action showed that these compounds are likely to interact with HNF4α transcription factor directly instead of with a nucleic acid involved in the biogenesis pathway. These compounds are thus not acting as specific RNA binders.

An alternative strategy to HTS is to screen focused libraries that are enriched with compounds known to have the ability to bind RNA. In this context, an intracellular screening approach was used to test 15 aminoglycosides using a luciferase assay to identify inhibitors of miR-21 activity [35]. Streptomycin (compound **8**, Figure 6.4a) was identified as the most effective inhibitor with a level of inhibition comparable to that of a specific antisense oligonucleotide. Also tested on various other miRNAs, **8** showed only partial selectivity, proving that the molecule does not inhibit Dicer which would result in non-selective and therefore probably toxic inhibitors. Docking and footprinting studies have shown that streptomycin binds efficiently to pre-miR-21 (Figure 6.4b), near the apical loop, which blocks the access, and therefore the cleavage, of Dicer. To finalize the study, cell-based assays in Jurkat lines were conducted. The level of miR-21 is well repressed and an increase in apoptosis is observed, the latter being linked to an increase in the level of PDCD4, an apoptosis-inducing protein and one of the main targets of miR-21.

Intracellular assays proved to be effective in the discovery of specific miRNA inhibitors, but it is clear that the mechanism of action of hits derived from screens needs to be verified. As noted above, in some cases the mechanism did not involve direct binding to RNA but rather involved inhibition of transcription. *In vitro* assays that will be described in the following sections are more suitable to discover RNA binders able to inhibit miRNA processing in a specific manner.

6.4.2.2 Target-Based *In Vitro* Assays

A large number of RNA binders have been discovered thanks to target-based assays mimicking the intracellular context. Some of these ligands have subsequently been tested in cells to verify their biological activity with very successful results, and target-based *in vitro* assays proved to be particularly efficient for the discovery of specific ligands. Fluorescence-based biochemical assays are the most common approaches that have been employed for screening. In this context, Nakatani's team has developed an HTS screen via a fluorescent indicator displacement (FID) assay where a fluorescent intercalator can be displaced by a ligand, thus inducing a decrease of fluorescence upon binding [36]. While this assay format is particularly suited for identifying compounds that bind RNA via a non-selective intercalation mode, some promising compounds have been identified. Indeed, these studies have allowed for the screening of several thousand compounds on different pre-miRNAs for the identification of compounds inhibiting Dicer cleavage. As an example, after an initial screen and structure–activity relationship studies, compound **9** (Figure 6.5) could be identified as an inhibitor of pre-miR-29a cleavage by Dicer [37]. This tricyclic compound containing a central isoxazole linked to a phenyl and an oxadiazole shows binding to pre-miR-29a in SPR studies. Even though the binding affinity was not precisely quantified, this kind of chemical structure could be a starting point for the search for new pre-miRNA ligands.

Using a similar approach, Herdewijin and co-workers screened 22 molecules as potential inhibitors of Dicer-mediated cleavage of pre-miR-155, which is known to be involved in normal and oncogenic immune functions [38]. Among these molecules, intercalating agents such as ethidium bromide **10** and Hoechst 33258 **11** as well as the aminoglycosides kanamycin B **12b** and neomycin B **13** (Figure 6.5) showed the best affinity for the target. Aminoglycosides are well-known RNA ligands that bind to the RNA of the prokaryotic ribosome and inhibit protein synthesis in bacteria [39]. They are therefore used clinically as antibiotics [8]. However, only the intercalating agents were able to inhibit Dicer cleavage. Another screen of 14 commercial aminoglycosides for their ability to inhibit Dicer cleavage on pre-miR-27a, an oncogenic miRNA overexpressed in various cancers led to the identification of streptomycin **8**, neomycin **13**, and tobramycin as efficient inhibitors [40]. These compounds were then studied in MCF-7 cells that overexpress miR-27a with a luciferase assay to confirm the inhibitory activities in cells. All three molecules decreased miR-27a expression by 35–50%.

In order to identify inhibitors of pre-miR-21 cleavage by Dicer, a fluorescence resonance energy transfer (FRET) assay was developed by Davies and Arenz in 2006 against miR-21 [41]. A first study thus led to the identification of an aminoglycoside, kanamycin A **12a** (Figure 6.5), as an inhibitor of pre-miRNA cleavage by Dicer. Arenz's team also worked on the synthesis of aminoglycoside mimetics and identified compound **14** (Figure 6.5) as an inhibitor of Dicer cleavage of pre-let-7 [42]. Aminoglycosides have thus been extensively studied for their ability to interfere with oncogenic miRNA biogenesis.

A screen of several classes of antibiotics (aminoglycosides, tetracyclines, macrolides, lincosamides, linezolid, chloramphenicol, and puromycin) to identify inhibitors of Dicer cleavage was performed on four pre-miRNAs involved in various cancers (−372, −373, −17, and −21) [43]. Neomycin B **13** was identified as the most active molecule for the different pre-miRNAs as well as the best ligand for the precursors of these miRNAs. Minocycline **15**, which belongs to the tetracycline family, also showed interesting activity. Tetracyclines, like aminoglycosides, bind to the prokaryotic ribosome and are used clinically as antibiotics. Compounds **13** and **15** bind to pre-miRNAs at the Dicer binding site which prevents Dicer from binding to its target and inhibits cleavage.

Another screen based on the FRET technique was conducted using 640 compounds to identify inhibitors of miR-372 biogenesis. Specifically, the goal was to find molecules capable of binding to pre-miR-372 and, in turn, inhibit the biogenesis of this oncogenic miRNA [44]. The miR-372 is oncogenic in several cancers such as

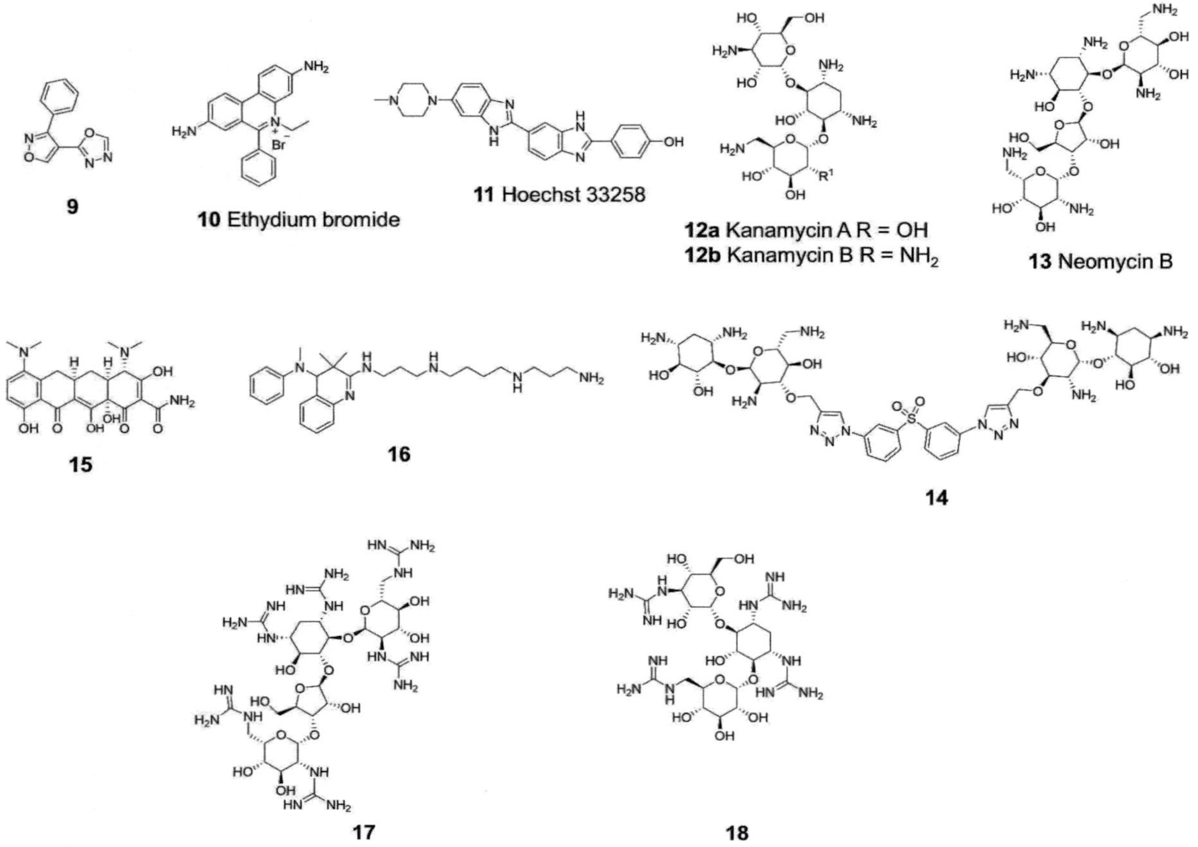

Figure 6.5 Chemical structures of compounds **9–18** discovered with *in vitro* target-based assays able to detect inhibition of the biogenesis of miRNAs.

gastric adenocarcinoma [45], esophageal cancer [46], and thyroid cancer [47]. This screen identified three active compounds, among which the spermine-amidine compound **16** (Figure 6.5) was the most promising. Indeed, compound **16** inhibits the biogenesis of miR-372 *in vitro* as well as in cancer cells. This compound showed excellent specificity in the presence of other nucleic acids such as transfer RNA or DNA. Moreover, the antiproliferative activity on gastric adenocarcinoma cells overexpressing miR-372 is highly specific since no activity is observed on other gastric epithelial cell lines. The miRnome study revealed that this compound acts only on a small number of miRNAs with a similar interaction site. The set of inhibited miRNAs also share a protein target: the tumor suppressor protein LATS2. The latter is the target of miR-372, and its expression is restored at the cellular level in the presence of the miR-372 inhibitor.

Disney's team has also been heavily involved in the identification of oncogenic miRNA inhibitors using a very efficient screening methodology based on two-dimensional combinatorial screening (2DCS) [48]. In a first study, two guanidinylated aminoglycosides (G-NeoB **17** and G-KanA **18**, Figure 6.5) were identified by screening a library of compounds bound to an agarose surface against a large library of labeled RNAs containing 6-nucleotide internal loops [49]. Amplification and sequencing of compound-bound RNAs allowed the identification of specific interactions between guanidinylated compounds and one (or more) loop(s). The miRNA precursors containing these loops were then identified, and indeed G-NeoB **17** (Figure 6.5) selectively recognizes an internal loop located on the pri-miR-10a which corresponds to the catalytic site of Drosha. Noteworthy, miR-10a is involved in many cancers and represents an interesting biological target [50]. The study of the cellular activity on HeLa cells confirmed the inhibition activity of compound **17**; the biogenesis of miR-10a is specifically inhibited at the level of pri-miRNA cleavage, as proven by the accumulation of pri-miR-10a in the studied cells.

In the search for new assays suitable for the discovery of compounds inhibiting the production of miRNAs, a technique known as catalytic enzyme-linked click chemistry assay (cat-ELCCA) was developed. This assay is based on the combination of click chemistry-based assays with catalytic signal amplification [51]. When performing cat-ELCCA, a biotinylated biomolecule is initially immobilized in the wells of a microtiter plate coated with streptavidin. A click chemistry handle may already be present in this substrate or may be added by an enzymatic or biomolecular interaction. An initial click reaction with labeled horseradish peroxidase (HRP) is used to start the detection process. This is followed by the addition of a pro-absorbent, -fluorescent, or -chemiluminescent HRP substrate. The assay was created to check the presence of the terminal loop of the immobilized pre-miRNA in the case of Dicer cat-ELCCA. In the presence of Dicer, the loop is cleaved, yielding no signal; while in the presence of an inhibitor, the loop remains intact resulting in signal production. This provides a turn-on assay for inhibition detection [52]. Pre-miR-21 was chosen as an initial RNA target for screening ~50,000 small molecules and ~33,000 natural product extracts (NPEs) leading to the identification of known but non-specific RNA binders, tetracyclines being the strongest inhibitors. Despite the difficulties in

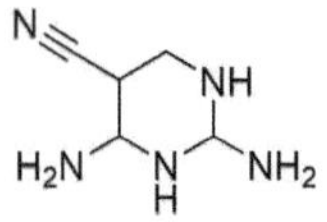

19 AC1MMYR2

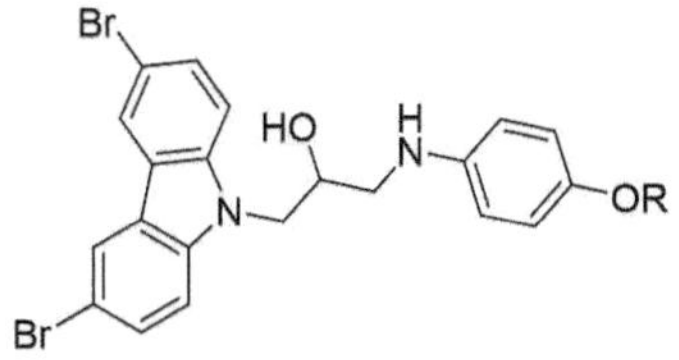

20a R = Me
20b R = Et

Figure 6.6 Compounds **19, 20a**, and **20b** able to bind precursors of miRNAs and discovered upon in silico screenings. The compounds have been reported as racemic structures.

the identification of specific binders and inhibitors, this assay proved to be extremely efficient for screening large HTS of compound libraries.

Beside intracellular and *in vitro* assays, *in silico* methodologies also showed to be promising for the discovery of compounds able to interfere with miRNA biogenesis. Kang et al. screened 1990 molecules *in silico* based on the three-dimensional structure of pre-miR-21 [53]. Five molecules were studied in more detail on epithelial cancer cells (glioblastoma, breast cancer, and gastric cancer) and compound **19** (AC1MMYR2, Figure 6.6) showed the best activity on different cell lines.

However, this compound also indirectly targets other miRNAs such as miR-181 and miR 200a/b. Despite this lack of specificity, AC1MMYR2 showed very good antitumor results in preclinical *in vivo* studies of glioblastoma and breast cancer [54]. Recently, 20,000 compounds were screened by the small-molecule microarray (SMM) method for pre-miR-21 ligands [55]. After screening and optimization, two molecules **20a** and **20b** (Figure 6.6) were identified as promising. The study of their mechanism of action showed that these molecules bind to the apical loop of pre-miR-21 and prevent the proper function of Dicer.

These examples demonstrate that despite the implicit theoretical results obtained by in silico studies, experimental applications of the compounds discovered by means of docking can be successful. Altogether, the target-based *in vitro* assays described above have proven to be particularly promising for the discovery of inhibitors of miRNAs biogenesis with the discovery of strong inhibitors *in vitro* and in some cases in cells.

6.4.2.3 Design of Specific Ligands of Pre- and Pri-miRNAs

Although screening assays have identified very promising inhibitors, the rational design of ligands specific for a particular miRNA would be the ideal methodology to obtain efficient inhibition and also be able to modulate the activity of the compounds and avoid toxic effects. To date, it remains extremely difficult to design RNA ligands specific for a certain sequence/structure, but some examples have been reported in the literature. Lu et al. were inspired by the first structure identified by HTS (compound **3**, Figure 6.4) and synthesized several analogues considering that the diphenylazene structure could be replaced by the more synthetically accessible *N*-phenylbenzamide structure [56]. These analogues were first tested for their ability to inhibit miR-21 biogenesis and function in HeLa and U-87 cells. Compound **21**

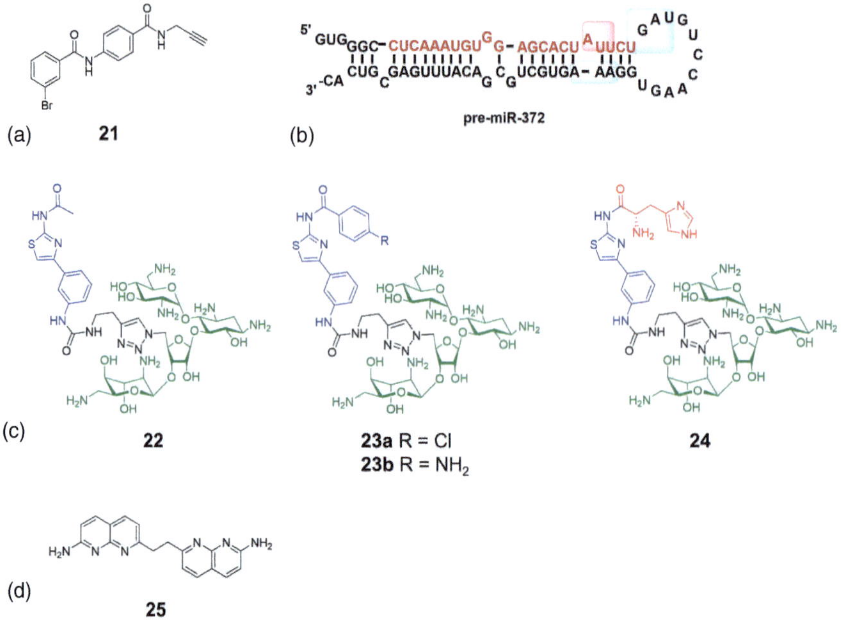

Figure 6.7 Chemical structure of RNA ligands designed to bind to pre-miRNAs. (a) Compound **21**. (b) Primary and secondary structures of pre-miR-372. Colored squares indicate the binding sites of compounds **22–24** with the colors corresponding to the moiety interacting at the indicated site. (c) Compounds **22–24** designed to target pre-miR-372. Colors indicate the different moieties and their site of interaction on the target. (d) Naphthyridine **25**.

(Figure 6.7a) was identified as the most effective, showing inhibition of miR-21 production at 10 μM. In order to evaluate the specificity of this compound, 12 other miRNAs were tested and showed that the inhibition was specific for miR-21. This study confirmed that chemical optimization of a known ligand can lead to better inhibitors.

Multifunctional ligands have also been designed as conjugates between different RNA binding domains bringing both affinity and selectivity for the target. In this context, multifunctional compounds in which several motifs known to interact with RNA in an affine and/or specific manner were conjugated on the same molecule. The aim of our studies was initially to target the production of the oncogenic miR-372 upon binding to pre-miR-372 (Figure 6.7b). As mentioned above, this miRNA has a protein target called LATS2 which is a tumor suppressor protein whose expression is inhibited by miR-372. The first ligands studied consisted of two interaction motifs: an aminoglycoside (neomycin) and an artificial nucleobase [57]. A screen that had been performed previously identified neomycin as the most favorable compound of this family for inhibiting miR-372 production [43]. It was therefore chosen for the preparation of a first set of ligands and was conjugated to several natural and artificial nucleobases. The latter have been previously described in the context of the triple-helix strategy for interaction with DNA base pairs [58].

Indeed, these compounds form specific hydrogen bonds, known as Hoogsteen bonds, as opposed to Watson–Crick bonds with DNA base pairs. These nucleobases have therefore been diverted to form specific bonds with the base pairs of miRNA precursors and in particular with pre-miR-372 (Figure 6.7b). This type of conjugate is thus designed to interact at the single-strand/double-strand junctions of the target.

Among the compounds synthesized and tested as inhibitors of miR-372 production, compound **22** (Figure 6.7c) showed very promising results [57]. Indeed, this compound inhibits pre-miR-372 cleavage *in vitro*, and the proliferation of gastric adenocarcinoma (AGS) cells that specifically overexpress miR-372 as the same compound has no effect on the proliferation of other gastric epithelium cells that do not express the targeted miRNA. Quantification of miRNAs at the intracellular level showed that miR-372 production is inhibited in a dose-dependent manner but also that other miRNAs are affected. The study of the target protein LATS2 showed that its translation is restored in the presence of ligand **22**.

Medicinal chemistry optimization of compound **22** was performed in order to better describe the pharmacophore essential for activity and to design more active compounds [59]. By varying both the nucleobase, the aminoglycoside, and the spacer used to link these two parts, it was possible to identify the analogues **23a** and **23b** in which the nucleobase moiety was extended by addition of another aromatic ring [59]. These two molecules retain the same intracellular specificity and have better inhibitory activities against AGS cell proliferation. The study of the binding site on the pre-miR-372 target has clarified the formed interactions and enabled design of more effective ligands. In this context, new ligands containing neomycin, nucleobase, and also an amino acid were designed [60]. Being known to interact efficiently with RNA as they are the main constituents of natural RNA ligands, i.e., peptides, three basic amino acids (lysine, histidine, and arginine) were chosen. This study resulted in the discovery of compound **24** that was selective for miR-372 and -373 (Figure 6.7c). In addition to the previously obtained interactions with the neomycin and artificial nucleobase moiety, the histidine side chain allows selective interaction with the stem–loop junction, which enhances affinity and increases selectivity toward pre-miR-372 (Figure 6.7b). At the intracellular level, compound **24** maintains its specific antiproliferative activity on gastric adenocarcinoma cells overexpressing miR-372.

The team of Nakatani and coworkers recently developed a chemical tool to specifically inhibit Dicer processing of pre-miRNAs upon stabilization of pre-miRNAs dimers. To this aim, they employed a cytosine-binding compound, naphthyridine **25** (Figure 6.7d), to interfere with Dicer cleavage of pre-miR-29a. The latter contains a C-bulge close to the cleavage site of Dicer, and the authors demonstrated that binding to this bulge effectively inhibited Dicer cleavage with a specific mechanism of action [61]. Indeed, **24** binds to the loop residues of pre-miR-29a and induces the dimerization of these RNA structures. The dimerization is responsible for the eventual inhibition of Dicer processing.

In order to improve the design of ligands specific to a particular sequence/structure, the team of Disney and co-workers also developed an efficient and original methodology called Inforna [62]. This approach is based on the 2-DCS methodology previously described above, and it is applied to a small-molecule library in the presence of a large collection of RNA motifs (internal loops, bulges, apical loops). Second, RNA sequences capable of binding to one or more ligands are analyzed with structure–activity relationships through sequencing (StARTS) [63]. The latter is a statistical tool that compiles the characteristics of RNA motifs that are responsible for interaction with ligands identified by 2-DCS and thus predicts the affinities and selectivities of a ligand/RNA interaction. This analysis indicates the probability that a ligand binds and is specific for a particular RNA structure. Finally, the combination of the results obtained by 2-DCS and StARTS with structural information of the potential RNA targets leads to the identification of particularly efficient and highly specific ligands for the RNA containing the targeted structure.

Inforna was initially applied to the precursors of 1024 miRNAs, and particularly active ligands were identified for 22 oncogenic pre-miRNAs. Compounds **26**, **27**, and **28** (Figure 6.8a) were identified as ligands for pri-miR-182, pri-miR-96, and pre-miR-210, all of which are oncogenic and overexpressed in different cancers [64]. While compound **26** is a derivative of kanamycin A, the other two molecules contain benzimidazole and methylpiperazine moieties that therefore appear to be preferred motifs for interactions with the internal loops of miRNA precursors. Additional studies were performed on compound **27**, identifying it as more specific for miR-96 than a complementary LNA oligonucleotide sequence. This compound induced cell apoptosis at micromolar concentrations in breast cancer cells by binding to the pri-miR-96 at the level of a U-U internal loop (green region in Figure 6.8b). Following development of the Inforna approach, it was applied to a large number of small molecules. Similar to **27**, compound **28** was identified as a specific binder of the G-G internal loop of pri-miR-96 (blue region in Figure 6.8b). The two molecules were thus conjugated to form a dimer (compound **29**, TargaprimiR-96) in Figure 6.8a) optimally designed to have each monomer at its binding site on the pri-miRNA [65]. This molecule binds with greater affinity to pri-miR-96 and inhibits pri-miR-96 biogenesis 400-fold over **26** in breast cancer cells. In addition, studies in *in vivo* models of triple negative breast cancer (TNBC) show that the dimer specifically inhibits tumor growth and induces apoptosis. Pharmacokinetic studies evaluating the concentration of the dimer in the plasma of mice after 48h show a concentration much higher than that required to obtain a biological effect, proving the bioactive potential of TargaprimiR-96 *in vivo*.

A few years later, compound **28**, called TargapremiR-210, was studied as a ligand for pre-miR-210 (Figure 6.8b) and an inhibitor of Dicer-mediated cleavage [66]. Although cellular target engagement was not established, the study identified the C–C internal loop (blue circle, Figure 6.8b) as the primary target of TargapremiR-210 with an affinity constant of 165 nM compared to more than 2 μM for any other loop. This internal loop is located close to the catalytic site of Dicer in pre-miR-210 which makes this molecule active against pre-miR-210 cleavage at a nanomolar level. This study established a correlation between activity and affinity when a ligand binds to a functional site of a miRNA precursor. MiR-210 is of therapeutic interest because it is highly expressed in cancer cells under hypoxic conditions, such as in MDA-MB-231 triple-negative breast cancer cells. TargapremiR-210 was therefore tested *in vitro* and

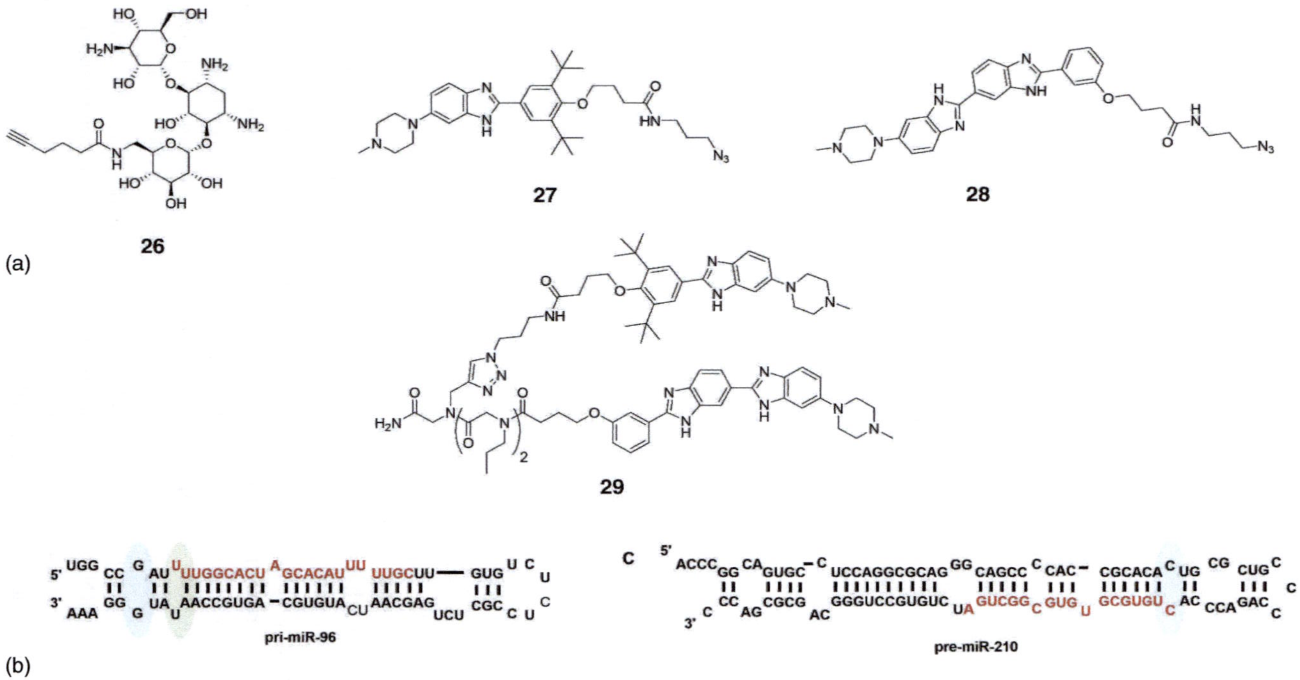

Figure 6.8 (a) Chemical structures of ligands 26–28 identified with InfoRNA. (b) Primary and secondary structures of pre-miR-210 and part of pri-miR-96.

in vivo to evaluate its therapeutic potential. This molecule selectively recognizes pre-miR-210 in both cases and showed biological activity inducing cell apoptosis in vitro and tumor growth reduction *in vivo*.

Using the same kind of approach, a compound specific for the inhibition of the production of miR-18a, a miRNA belonging to the miR-17-92 cluster and overexpressed in prostate cancer, was identified. This compound (**30**, Figure 6.9) strongly and specifically interacts with pre miR-17, -18a, and -20 in a U, G, or A bulge regions, all three located in the catalytic site of Dicer [67]. Treatment of prostate cancer cells with this ligand, called Targapremir-18a, showed inhibition of miR-18a production, restoration of the expression of the tumor suppressor protein serine/threonine kinase 4 (STK4), and induction of apoptosis. The study of the cellular targets of Targapremir-18a was pursued using the Chem-CLIP (Chemical Cross-Linking and Isolation by Pull Down) technique [68]. This approach is based on the combination of a specific RNA ligand with a chemical scaffold capable of covalently binding to RNA (most common are chlorambucil or diazirines [highlighted in green in compound **31**, Figure 6.9]). Furthermore, a chemical handle allowing the subsequent isolation of the complex is added to the compound and is generally represented by biotin (highlighted in orange in compound **31**, Figure 6.9). The resulting probe molecule will bind to the RNA target followed by covalent bond formation whereupon the ligand/target complex can be isolated with magnetic beads coated with streptavidin. The RNA target can subsequently be isolated and identified by RT-qPCR. In the case of TargapremiR-18a **31**, specific binding to the miR-18a precursor could be confirmed as the primary target, with pre-miR-17 and -20a as secondary targets.

Other oncogenic miRNAs have been targeted using the same approach. After demonstrating both in vitro and in vivo that it is possible to inhibit miRNA biogenesis by using small molecules to target the Drosha or Dicer cleavage sites, the Disney group studied additional miRNAs including miR-544, which is upregulated in tumor cells in response to hypoxia [69]. Compound **32** bearing a naphthyridine scaffold substituted with amines, pyrrolidines, and a cyano group, was identified by Inforna as the most effective against this target. This compound inhibits the action of Dicer and has similar effects to ASOs at 25-fold lower concentrations. This inhibitor also confirmed a biological role for miR-544 in apoptosis resistance, tumor growth, and chemotherapy resistance, making it a prime target for cancer therapy [69]. Compound **33**, consisting of an azido-neomycin, decreases the level of miR-525 *in vivo* through action on the pri-miR-525, and by binding to the Drosha catalytic site [70]. This miRNA is particularly overexpressed in liver cancers indicating its therapeutic importance as it inhibits the invasive properties of a hepatocellular carcinoma cell line. Although this molecule can bind to a large number of cellular RNAs, only binding to sites such as the Drosha catalytic site for miR-525 allows a biological response. A relevant example of the potential of the InfoRNA approach in the design of miRNAs inhibitors is the discovery of compound **34** that specifically interacts with a UA double base pair of pre-miR-200c and of compound **35** that interacts with an internal UU loop adjacent to the UA base pairs [71]. MiR-200 family associated with type 2 diabetes includes five distinct

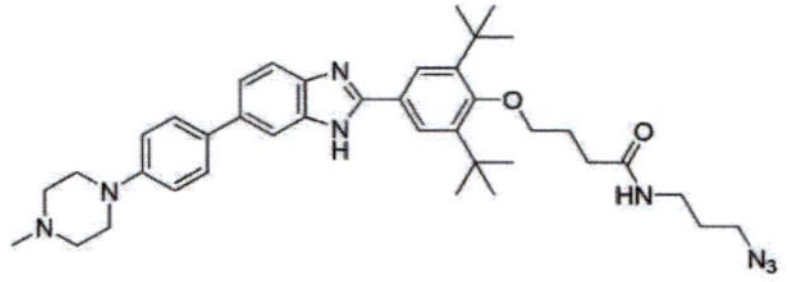

30

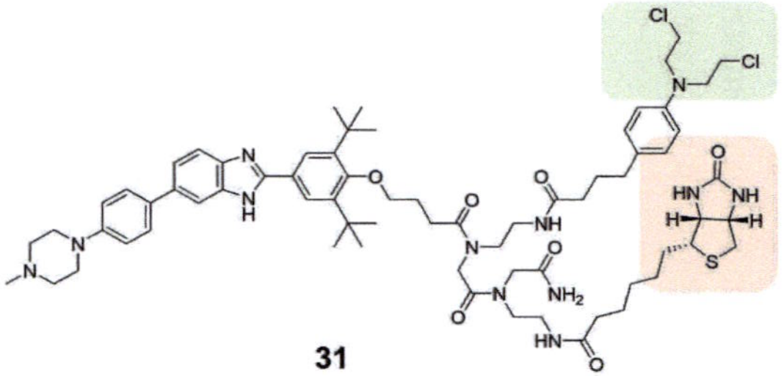

31

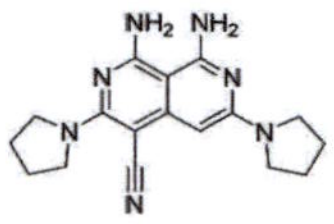

32

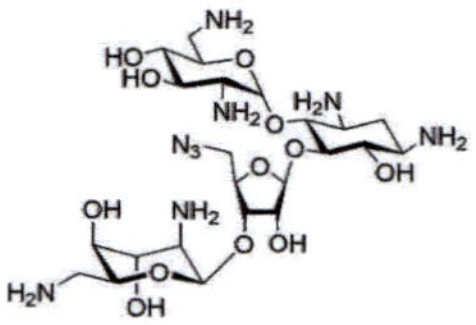

33

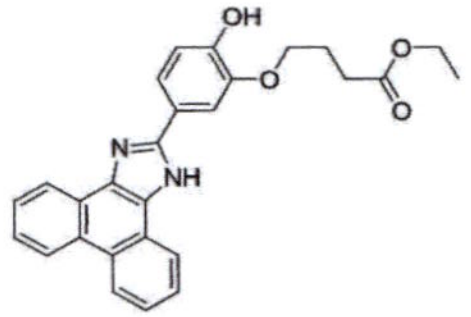

34

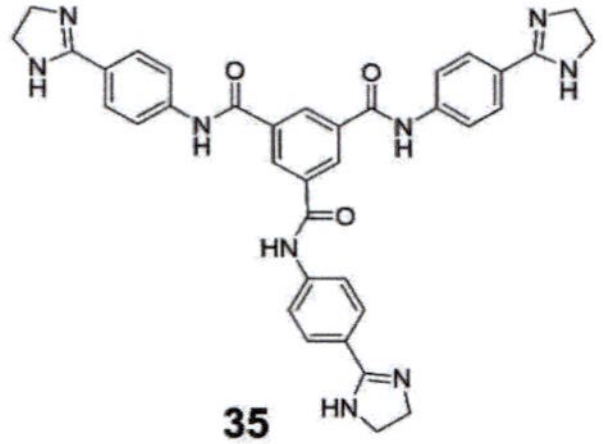

35

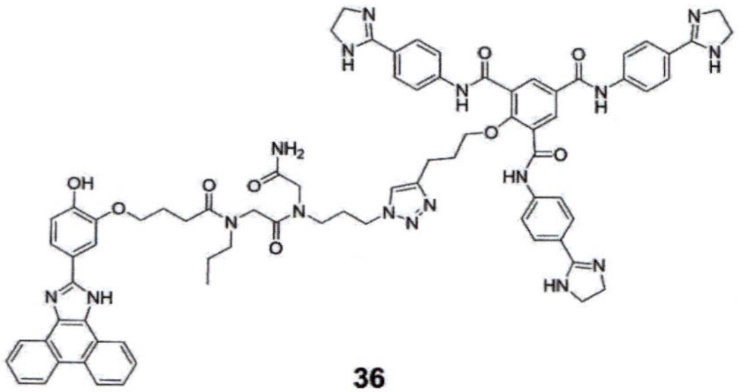

36

Figure 6.9 Chemical structure of ligands **30–36** discovered by InfoRNA and specific for a particular structure of pre-miRNA. The conjugation of **34** and **35** led to new ligand **36**, highly specific for pre-miR-200c.

members, but overexpression of miR-200c is sufficient to induce β-cell apoptosis. The combination of **34** and **35** resulted in ligand **36** that is highly specific for miR-200c compared to the other members of the same family.

Collectively, these examples illustrate that while pure rational design remains a challenge, tools are available to facilitate design of specific compounds. Furthermore, these tools are continually evolving to further enable design of efficient binders. Compounds exhibiting high specificity for a chosen miRNA precursor induced the desired biological effect. Furthermore, such compounds also represent important chemical tools to elucidate the role of miRNAs in cancer and other related pathologies. Based on these considerations, other classical medicinal chemistry strategies have been developed for the targeting of miRNAs with small molecules as it will be described in the following sections.

6.4.2.4 Fragment-Based Drug Design

The same medicinal chemistry approaches commonly used for the discovery of compounds targeting proteins can be employed for the identification of RNA binders specific for a particular structure. In this context, fragment-based drug design (FBDD) has recently been utilized to find RNA binders that target miRNA precursors such as those illustrated in the previous sections [72]. FBDD involves screening of libraries of fragments, which are compounds with low molecular weight (generally <300 Da) and with low number of functionalities. The aim is to identify small chemical scaffolds that can bind to a target of interest, often with low affinity and/or activity. Following validation of target binding through orthogonal biophysical techniques, these fragment hits are subsequently optimized by addition of substituents (fragment growing) or linking two fragments with a close binding site on the target (fragment linking) leading compounds with high affinities and activities. NMR is a frequently employed technique for fragment-based screening since it allows for assessment of affinity and identification of the binding sites. NMR was recently applied to the search for fragments that inhibit the biogenesis of miR-21 upon binding to pre-miR-21 [73]. A screen of 420 compounds led to the identification of 18 hits. After refining the screen and validating the identified hits, thiadiazole fragment **37** (Figure 6.10) was demonstrated to bind in close proximity

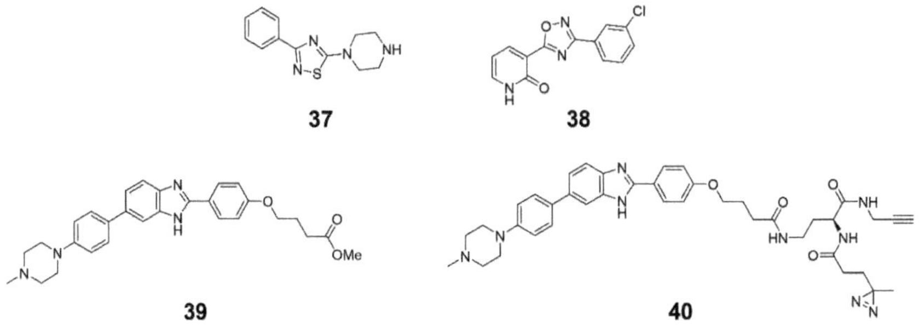

Figure 6.10 Compounds **37**, **38** discovered using a fragment-based drug design approach, and compounds **39**, **40** discovered using InfoRNA as probes for the development of fragment screening.

to the Dicer cleavage site on pre-miR-21. Further assays would be needed to assess the actual biological activity of this kind of compound, but it represents a starting point for the development of new ligands targeting this oncogenic miRNA.

Advanced FBDD was then performed combining this approach with InfoRNA. This latter approach, described in the previous section, has been applied to the screening of fragment libraries [74]. The largest collection of RNA-focused small-molecule fragments to date ($n = 2500$) was created by examining features in all published compounds that bind RNA. The most relevant interactions between fragments and RNA were identified. Approximately 12.8 million interactions were found by examining the RNA-binding landscape for each fragment following a library-versus-library selection using an RNA library displaying a discrete structural feature. Mining of this dataset across the human transcriptome led to the identification of a drug-like fragment (compound **38** in Figure 6.10) as a potent and specific inhibitor of miR-372 biogenesis, thus alleviating invasive and proliferative oncogenic phenotypes in gastric cancer cells. Noteworthy, **38** has favorable properties, including favorable affinity for the RNA target of 300 ± 130 nM, a molecular weight of 273 Da, and quantitative estimate of drug-likeness (QED) score of 0.8. Thus, these studies demonstrate that a low-molecular-weight, fragment-like compound can specifically and potently modulate RNA targets.

InfoRNA allowed for the identification of compound **39** that binds in the Dicer cleavage site of pre-miR-21 [75]. To develop a methodology for fragment screening, compound **40** was prepared by addition of a diazirine group for the photoactivated capture of bound RNA targets and a terminal alkyne handle that can be bioorthogonally coupled to an azide-containing purification tag through click chemistry. Evaluation of pre-miR-21 binding by **40** was performed using the ChemCLIP approach confirming that the binding site was similar to **39**. A fragment library of compounds containing the diazirine and the alkyne moieties were then generated, and the application of the same strategy allowed for the identification of several fragments able to bind pre-miR-21. The combination of these fragments produced a particular active compound with increased potency to inhibit pre-miR-21 processing and to decrease the levels of mature miR-21. In triple-negative breast cancer cells, the substance had selective effects on the transcriptome and reduced an invasive phenotype linked to miR-21.

6.4.2.5 DNA-Encoded Libraries (DELs)

The use of DNA-encoded libraries (DELs) in drug discovery has already led to successful results and led to the discovery of new drug candidates currently in clinical trials. However, only recently has this technology been applied to the search for RNA binders. In a relevant example, a screen of a DNA-encoded library against a library of RNA structures enabled the evaluation of 300 million interactions in total and resulted in identification of numerous ligand/target pairs [76]. Among them, ligands specific for the 5′-GAG/3′-CCC internal loop present in an oncogenic primary miRNA (pri-miR-27a) were identified. Compound **41** (Figure 6.11) has nanomolar binding affinity for the target, decreased miR-27a expression in four different cancer cell lines at nanomolar concentrations, and exhibits high selectivity across miRnome in triple-negative breast cancer cells.

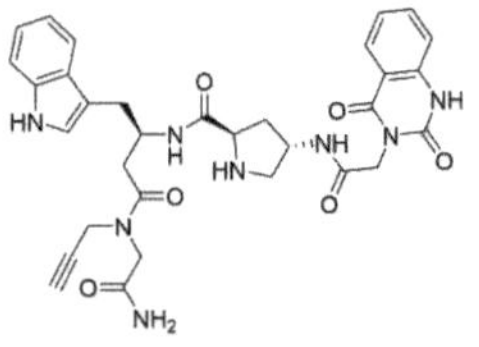

41

Figure 6.11 Chemical structure of ligand **41** identified using DELs.

Similar to FBDD, DEL screening approaches have high potential for the identification of novel RNA binders that exhibit the desired specificity. While only few examples have been reported to date, these techniques are surely extremely promising and will probably lead to bioactive compounds in the near future.

6.5 Inhibition of RNA–Protein Interactions in miRNAs Pathways

Beside direct binding of RNA binders to one of the miRNAs precursors, it is also possible to target the interactions formed between miRNAs and miRNA precursors with the partner proteins essential for miRNA functions. Abell et al. designed oligonucleotide-small-molecule conjugates to inhibit the interaction between the miRNA–Ago2 complex and mRNA [77]. The goal of such conjugates is the specific recognition of the miRNA target by the oligonucleotide moiety, which will guide the small-molecule inhibitor of Ago2 close to the targeted protein. The designed compounds contain a short oligonucleotide sequence (tetramer) complementary to miR-122 linked to an Ago2 inhibitor (compound **42**, Figure 6.12) that was identified by an *in silico* screen of 627,000 compounds. Optimization of these conjugates led to the synthesis of compounds **43** and **44** containing a miR-122-specific 5′-TCAC-3′ peptide nucleic acid (PNA) tetramer. Fluorescence assays to evaluate the ability of

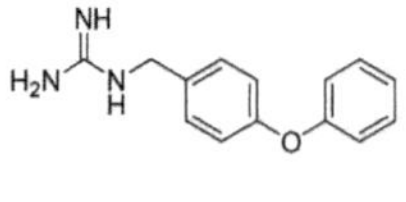

42

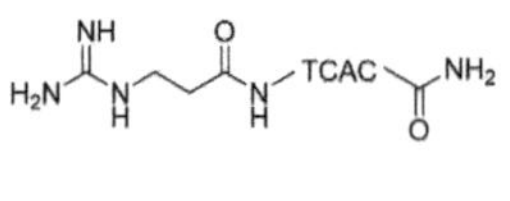

43

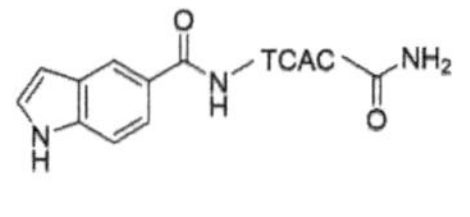

44

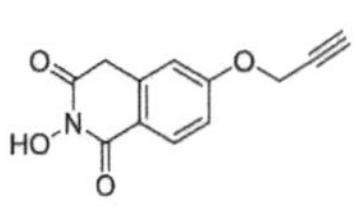

45

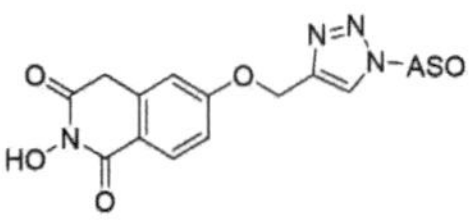

46

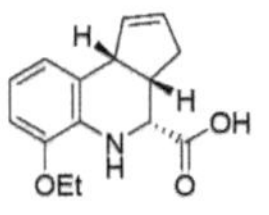

47

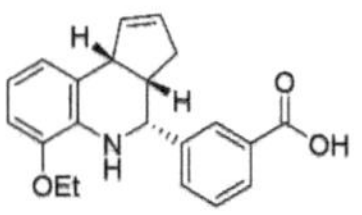

48

Figure 6.12 Compounds inhibiting the interaction between Ago2 and miRNA (**42–46**) and between Lin28 and pre-Let-7 (**47, 48**).

the conjugates to inhibit miRNA–Ago2 interaction with mRNA as well as its cleavage were performed. These conjugates thus revealed a ten-fold higher IC_{50} than the PNA tetramer sequence alone, demonstrating the potential of such a strategy to inhibit miRNA functions. Liang et al. employed a conjugation strategy to inhibit pre-miR-21 cleavage by Dicer [78, 79]. In this study, the compounds were obtained by conjugation of two types of oligonucleotides (morpholino or PNA) of different lengths and a 2-hydroxy-isoiquinoline-1,3-dione motif (molecule 45, Figure 6.12), previously identified as a weak inhibitor of Dicer [79]. Such molecules can be used because oligonucleotides allow vectorization and provide an increase in local effective concentration. Biological evaluation of the different conjugates was performed by electrophoresis and led to the identification of the bifunctional molecule **46** containing an 11-mer PNA with a GAGATTCAACA sequence specific to the apical loop of pre-miR-21. This conjugate inhibits pre-miR-21 cleavage by Dicer with an IC_{50} of 0.5 μM compared to 100 μM for the Dicer inhibitor alone. Although the use of shorter ASOs compared to oligonucleotides may provide benefits in terms of specificity and cellular distribution, the bifunctional molecules in this study are not cell permeable and require further optimization.

Another important interaction that has been considered in miRNA-targeting studies is the one between the miRNA-binding proteins LIN28 and let-7 [80]. Let-7 miRNAs function as a tumor suppressor by downregulating the expression of oncogenes including RAS, c-MYC, HMGA2 [81]. LIN28 is a post-transcriptional regulator protein that binds to pri- and pre-let7, thus blocking let-7 maturation and inducing its degradation. Many primary human tumor cells overexpress LIN28, and this has been connected to poor clinical prognosis. Inhibition of LIN28/pre-let-7 interaction is thus considered a potential anticancer approach, and various studies reported small-molecule inhibitors of this interaction [82]. Recently, Wu and coworkers identified tetrahydroquinoline (THQ) as a weak inhibitor of LIN28 and decided to perform the medicinal chemistry optimization of this scaffold [83]. This led to compounds **45**, **46** having low micromolar IC_{50} for LIN28 inhibition but devoid of intracellular activity. Despite this drawback, only few examples of LIN28 inhibitors have been reported so far and these remain promising scaffolds for future medicinal chemistry improvements.

Recently, new specific assays are being developed to identify novel compounds that inhibit RNA/protein interactions. The field includes RNA interaction with protein-mediated complementation assay, or RiPCA [84]. In this assay, cells are engineered to express the small subunit of the split luciferase, NanoLuc, fused to HT, an engineered dehalogenase that covalently binds to chloroalkane-containing ligands leading to a fusion protein SmHT. The cells are then transiently co-transfected with a plasmid encoding the RBP-of-interest fused to the large subunit of NanoLuc and a chloroalkane-modified RNA probe, which allows covalent conjugation to SmHT. Subsequent interaction between the RBP and RNA drives reconstitution of NanoLuc, generating chemiluminescence upon treatment of cells with the NanoLuc luciferase substrate. This assay was used to prove the interaction of a pre-miRNA, pre-let-7, with Lin28 and was particularly useful to detect this interaction intracellularly. This methodology could thus be employed in the future to screen for inhibitors of this interaction.

6.6 Adding Cleavage Properties to miRNAs Interfering Agents

As illustrated by all the examples above, small-molecule binders of miRNA precursors proved to be efficient tools to inhibit the intracellular expression of pathological miRNAs and sometimes also to induce the desired effect *in vivo*. A step further in the search for efficient miRNA inhibitors is to introduce additional properties to ligands that not only bind to the target, but also induce its degradation and cleavage in cells and eventually *in vivo*. In a first attempt to find compounds able to bind an RNA target and induce its cleavage, bleomycin A5 (compound **49**, Figure 6.13), a natural product known to induce DNA and RNA strand breaks and used as an anticancer agent, was studied as a binder and cleaving agent on different RNA motifs and structures [85]. It was shown that bleomycin A5 preferentially cleaves motifs containing A-U base pairs as well as purine-rich sequences. *In vitro* and *in vivo* assays were carried out on pre-miR-10b, which contains these motifs and is an oncogenic miRNA that is overexpressed in many cancers and involved in invasion and metastasis. All assays confirmed the action of the compound on the intended target. Bleomycin was then employed to introduce cleavage properties to other specific pre-miRNA ligands. As a typical example, targaprimir-96 (conjugate **29**, Figure 6.8) was coupled to bleomycin A5 (conjugate **50**, Figure 6.13) by introducing an azido group on the spermidine side chain and coupling using 1,3-dipolar cycloaddition reaction. This led to very efficient inhibition of Drosha processing and to the cleavage of pri-miR-96 in intracellular assays [86].

A major advance in the field of RNA ligands in general and miRNA inhibitors in particular has been made recently with the design of chimeric compounds called RIBOTACs capable of targeting a miRNA precursor and inducing its degradation by recruitment of a ribonuclease in a manner similar to that performed on protein targets by PROTACs (described in further detail in Chapter 9) [87]. As an example, compound **29** was conjugated to a 2′-5′-poly(A) oligonucleotide capable of recruiting an endogenous RNase L inducing degradation of pri-miR-96 at the intracellular level and in sub-stoichiometric amounts (conjugate **51**, Figure 6.13). This strategy was applied successfully to other pre-miRNAs ligands. In a relevant example, a specific ligand of pre-miR-21 (compound **52**, Figure 6.13) identified with Inforna was optimized by the preparation of dimer **53** and then coupled to bleomycin or to a small-molecule compound able to recruit RNase L, leading to conjugate **54** [88]. The latter induces the degradation of pre-miR-21 at the intracellular level and in sub-stoichiometric amounts. It has 20-fold higher activity than the corresponding dimer in reducing the intracellular level of miR-21 and 10-fold higher than the bleomycin conjugate. Finally, the *in vivo* study of this molecule showed that cleavage of pre-miR 21 leads to inhibition of breast cancer metastasis to the lung.

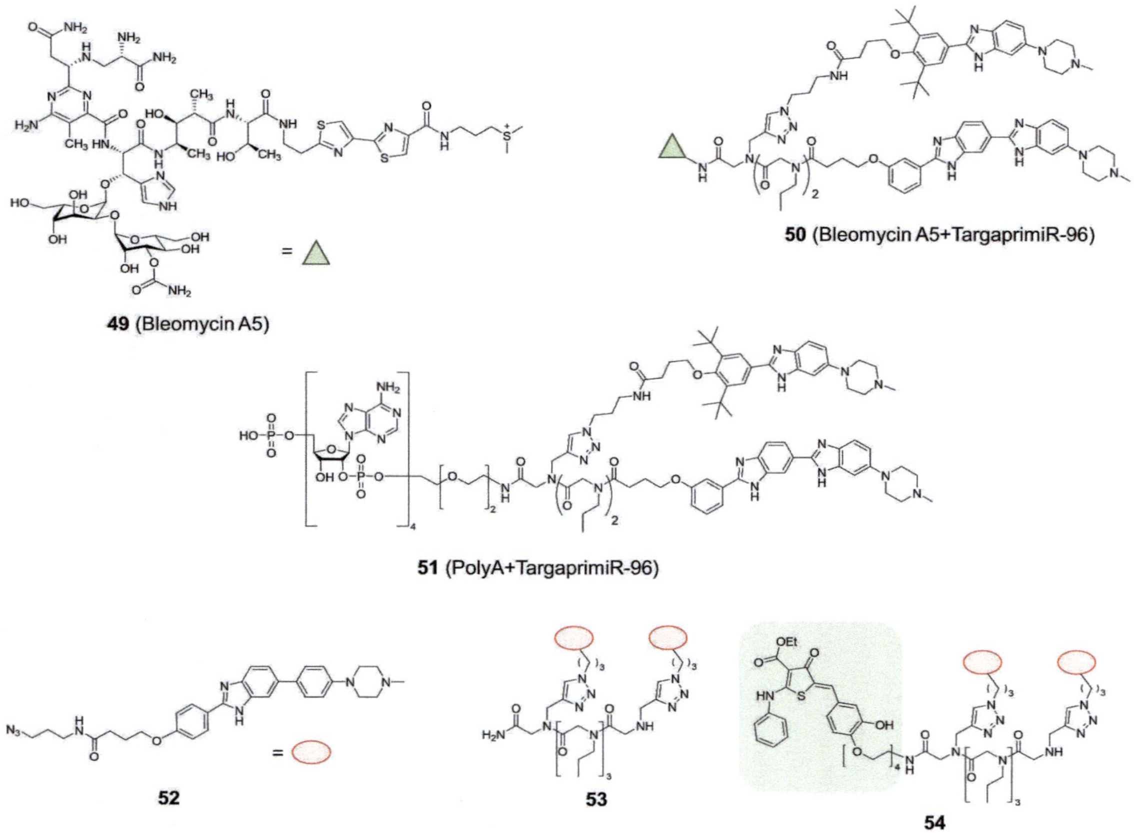

49 (Bleomycin A5)

50 (Bleomycin A5+TargaprimiR-96)

51 (PolyA+TargaprimiR-96)

52

53

54

Figure 6.13 Examples of conjugates able to induce the cleavage of the targeted RNA thanks to the presence of bleomycin (compounds **49**, **50**) or to the presence of a RNase L recruiter (compounds **51–54**).

The addition of cleavage properties to specific RNA binders thus showed to be particularly promising to induce the desired biological effect thanks to the degradation of the RNA target. The synthesized conjugates may still have to be optimized for therapeutic application, but in vivo studies clearly demonstrated the potential of this strategy.

6.7 Conclusions

In conclusion, the examples of RNA ligands described in this chapter illustrate the feasibility of the approach and the possibility of obtaining specificity of action *in vitro* as well as at the cellular level and *in vivo*. miRNAs represent particularly promising targets not only for anticancer therapies, which are currently the most studied, but also for other pathologies in which these short non-coding RNAs are involved as well as for antiviral approaches. However, the miRNA network is extremely rich and complex since thousands of miRNAs have been identified, and each one controls the expression of hundreds of proteins. Modulation of this network may have important effects on the biology of the cell, and toxicity could be a major limitation of the approach based on the targeting of these RNAs. Furthermore, the miRNA precursors that usually represent the target of small-molecule miRNA inhibitors have very similar three-dimensional structures, thus limiting the possibilities for selective binding. Despite this limitation, very specific ligands have been identified showing biological activity in cells and *in vivo*, which encourages the scientific community to pursue this strategy. Finally, the field of RNA ligands for therapeutic applications is broad and rapidly expanding for targeting a large number of targets such as viral, bacterial, and other eukaryotic non-coding RNAs. Altogether, the gathered results will play a major role in defining the main features for RNA binders and in opening the possibility for the rational design of efficient and specific inhibitors.

References

1 Warner, K.D., Hajdin, C.E., and Weeks, K.M. (2018). Principles for targeting RNA with drug-like small molecules. *Nat. Rev. Drug Discovery* 17 (8): 547–558.

2 Falese, J.P., Donlic, A., and Hargrove, A.E. (2021). Targeting RNA with small molecules: from fundamental principles towards the clinic. *Chem. Soc. Rev.* 50 (4): 2224–2243.

3 Childs-Disney, J.L., Yang, X., Gibaut, Q.M.R. et al. (2022). Targeting RNA structures with small molecules. *Nat. Rev. Drug Discovery* 21: 736–762.

4 Crooke, S.T., Baker, B.F., Crooke, R.M., and Liang, X.H. (2021). Antisense technology: an overview and prospectus. *Nat. Rev. Drug Discovery* 20 (6): 427–453.

5 Battiste, J.L., Mao, H., Rao, N.S. et al. (1996). Alpha helix-RNA major groove recognition in an HIV-1 rev peptide-RRE RNA complex. *Science* 273 (5281):

1547–1551; Pai, J., Yoon, T., Kim, N.D. et al. (2012). High-throughput profiling of peptide-RNA interactions using peptide microarrays. *JACS* 134 (46): 19287–19296; Puglisi, J.D., Chen, L., Blanchard, S., and Frankel, A.D. (1995). Solution structure of a bovine immunodeficiency virus Tat-TAR peptide-RNA complex. *Science* 270 (5239): 1200–1203.

6 Meyer, S.M., Williams, C.C., Akahori, Y. et al. (2020). Small molecule recognition of disease-relevant RNA structures. *Chem. Soc. Rev.* 49 (19): 7167–7199.

7 Ursu, A., Childs-Disney, J.L., Andrews, R.J. et al. (2020). Design of small molecules targeting RNA structure from sequence. *Chem. Soc. Rev.* 49 (20): 7252–7270.

8 Wilson, D.N. (2014). Ribosome-targeting antibiotics and mechanisms of bacterial resistance. *Nat. Rev. Microbiol.* 12 (1): 35–48.

9 Ratni, H., Scalco, R.S., and Stephan, A.H. (2021). Risdiplam, the first approved small molecule splicing modifier drug as a blueprint for future transformative medicines. *ACS Med. Chem. Lett.* 12 (6): 874–877.

10 Krach, F., Stemick, J., Boerstler, T. et al. (2022). An alternative splicing modulator decreases mutant HTT and improves the molecular fingerprint in Huntington's disease patient neurons. *Nat. Commun.* 13 (1): 6797.

11 Lee, R.C., Feinbaum, R.L., and Ambros, V. (1993). The *C. elegans* heterochronic gene lin-4 encodes small RNAs with antisense complementarity to lin-14. *Cell* 75 (5): 843–854.

12 Slack, F.J., Basson, M., Liu, Z. et al. (2000). The lin-41 RBCC gene acts in the C. elegans heterochronic pathway between the let-7 regulatory RNA and the LIN-29 transcription factor. *Mol. Cell* 5 (4): 659–669.

13 Li, S.C., Chan, W.C., Hu, L.Y. et al. (2010). Identification of homologous microRNAs in 56 animal genomes. *Genomics* 96 (1): 1–9.

14 Bartel, D.P. (2009). MicroRNAs: target recognition and regulatory functions. *Cell* 136 (2): 215–233.

15 Kim, V.N., Han, J., and Siomi, M.C. (2009). Biogenesis of small RNAs in animals. *Nat. Rev. Mol. Cell Biol.* 10 (2): 126–139.

16 Han, J., Lee, Y., Yeom, K.H. et al. (2004). The Drosha-DGCR8 complex in primary microRNA processing. *Genes Dev.* 18 (24): 3016–3027.

17 Lee, Y., Ahn, C., Han, J. et al. (2003). The nuclear RNase III Drosha initiates microRNA processing. *Nature* 425 (6956): 415–419.

18 Yi, R., Qin, Y., Macara, I.G., and Cullen, B.R. (2003). Exportin-5 mediates the nuclear export of pre-microRNAs and short hairpin RNAs. *Genes Dev.* 17 (24): 3011–3016.

19 Ma, J.B., Ye, K., and Patel, D.J. (2004). Structural basis for overhang-specific small interfering RNA recognition by the PAZ domain. *Nature* 429 (6989): 318–322.

20 Hutvagner, G. and Simard, M.J. (2008). Argonaute proteins: key players in RNA silencing. *Nat. Rev. Mol. Cell Biol.* 9 (1): 22–32.

21 Selbach, M., Schwanhausser, B., Thierfelder, N. et al. (2008). Widespread changes in protein synthesis induced by microRNAs. *Nature* 455 (7209): 58–63.

22 Paul, P., Chakraborty, A., Sarkar, D. et al. (2018). Interplay between miRNAs and human diseases. *J. Cell. Physiol.* 233 (3): 2007–2018.

23 Naro, Y., Ankenbruck, N., Thomas, M. et al. (2018). Small molecule inhibition of MicroRNA miR-21 rescues chemosensitivity of renal-cell carcinoma to topotecan. *J. Med. Chem.* 61 (14): 5900–5909.

24 Calin, G.A. and Croce, C.M. (2006). MicroRNA signatures in human cancers. *Nat. Rev. Cancer* 6 (11): 857–866.

25 Esquela-Kerscher, A. and Slack, F.J. (2006). Oncomirs - microRNAs with a role in cancer. *Nat. Rev. Cancer* 6 (4): 259–269.

26 Li, Z. and Rana, T.M. (2014). Therapeutic targeting of microRNAs: current status and future challenges. *Nat. Rev. Drug Discovery* 13 (8): 622–638.

27 Lu, J., Getz, G., Miska, E.A. et al. (2005). MicroRNA expression profiles classify human cancers. *Nature* 435 (7043): 834–838.

28 Shan, G., Li, Y., Zhang, J. et al. (2008). A small molecule enhances RNA interference and promotes microRNA processing. *Nat. Biotechnol.* 26 (8): 933–940.

29 Melo, S., Villanueva, A., Moutinho, C. et al. (2011). Small molecule enoxacin is a cancer-specific growth inhibitor that acts by enhancing TAR RNA-binding protein 2-mediated microRNA processing. *PNAS* 108 (11): 4394–4399.

30 Nahar, S., Bose, D., Kumar Panja, S. et al. (2014). Anti-cancer therapeutic potential of quinazoline based small molecules via global upregulation of miRNAs. *Chem. Commun. (Camb).* 50 (35): 4639–4642.

31 Di Giorgio, A., Tran, T.P., and Duca, M. (2016). Small-molecule approaches toward the targeting of oncogenic miRNAs: roadmap for the discovery of RNA modulators. *Future Med. Chem.* 8 (7): 803–816.

32 Gumireddy, K., Young, D.D., Xiong, X. et al. (2008). Small-molecule inhibitors of microrna miR-21 function. *Angew. Chem. Int. Ed.* 47 (39): 7482–7484.

33 Ankenbruck, N., Kumbhare, R., Naro, Y. et al. (2019). Small molecule inhibition of microRNA-21 expression reduces cell viability and microtumor formation. *Bioorg. Med. Chem.* 27 (16): 3735–3743.

34 Emanuelson, C., Ankerbruck, N., Kumbhare, R. et al. (2022). Transcriptional inhibition of MicroRNA miR-122 by small molecules reduces hepatitis C virus replication in liver cells. *J. Med. Chem.* 65 (24): 16338–16352.

35 Bose, D., Jayaraj, G., Suryawanshi, H. et al. (2012). The tuberculosis drug streptomycin as a potential cancer therapeutic: inhibition of miR-21 function by directly targeting its precursor. *Angew. Chem. Int. Ed.* 51 (4): 1019–1023.

36 Murata, A., Harada, Y., Fukuzumi, T., and Nakatani, K. (2013). Fluorescent indicator displacement assay of ligands targeting 10 microRNA precursors. *Bioorg. Med. Chem.* 21 (22): 7101–7106.

37 Fukuzumi, T., Murata, A., Aikawa, H. et al. (2015). Exploratory study on the RNA-binding structural motifs by library screening targeting pre-miRNA-29 a. *Chem. Eur. J.* 21 (47): 16859–16867.

38 Maiti, M., Nauwelaerts, K., and Herdewijn, P. (2012). Pre-microRNA binding aminoglycosides and antitumor drugs as inhibitors of Dicer catalyzed microRNA processing. *Bioorg. Med. Chem. Lett.* 22 (4): 1709–1711.

39 Magnet, S. and Blanchard, J.S. (2005). Molecular insights into aminoglycoside action and resistance. *Chem. Rev.* 105 (2): 477–498.

40 Bose, D., Jayaraj, G.G., Kumar, S., and Maiti, S. (2013). A molecular-beacon-based screen for small molecule inhibitors of miRNA maturation. *ACS Chem. Biol.* 8 (5): 930–938.

41 Davies, B.P. and Arenz, C. (2006). A homogenous assay for micro RNA maturation. *Angew. Chem. Int. Ed.* 45 (33): 5550–5552.

42 Klemm, C.M., Berthelmann, A., Neubacher, S., and Arenz, C. (2009). Short and efficient synthesis of alkyne-modified amino glycoside building blocks. *Eur. J. Org. Chem.* 2009: 2788–2794.

43 Tran, T.P., Vo, D.D., Di Giorgio, A., and Duca, M. (2015). Ribosome-targeting antibiotics as inhibitors of oncogenic microRNAs biogenesis: old scaffolds for new perspectives in RNA targeting. *Bioorg. Med. Chem.* 23 (17): 5334–5344.

44 Staedel, C., Tran, T.P.A., Giraud, J. et al. (2018). Modulation of oncogenic miRNA biogenesis using functionalized polyamines. *Sci. Rep.* 8 (1): 1667.

45 Cho, W.J., Shin, J.M., Kim, J.S. et al. (2009). miR-372 regulates cell cycle and apoptosis of ags human gastric cancer cell line through direct regulation of LATS2. *Mol. Cell* 28 (6): 521–527.

46 Lee, K.H., Goan, Y.G., Hsiao, M. et al. (2009). MicroRNA-373 (miR-373) post-transcriptionally regulates large tumor suppressor, homolog 2 (LATS2) and stimulates proliferation in human esophageal cancer. *Exp. Cell. Res.* 315 (15): 2529–2538.

47 Rippe, V., Dittberner, L., Lorenz, V.N. et al. (2010). The two stem cell microRNA gene clusters C19MC and miR-371-3 are activated by specific chromosomal rearrangements in a subgroup of thyroid adenomas. *PLoS One* 5 (3): e9485.

48 Disney, M.D., Labuda, L.P., Paul, D.J. et al. (2008). Two-dimensional combinatorial screening identifies specific aminoglycoside-RNA internal loop partners. *JACS* 130 (33): 11185–11194.

49 Velagapudi, S.P. and Disney, M.D. (2014). Two-dimensional combinatorial screening enables the bottom-up design of a microRNA-10b inhibitor. *Chem. Commun. (Camb).* 50 (23): 3027–3029.

50 Liu, F., Shi, Y., Liu, Z. et al. (2021). The emerging role of miR-10 family in gastric cancer. *Cell Cycle* 20 (15): 1468–1476.

51 Lorenz, D.A. and Garner, A.L. (2016). A click chemistry-based microRNA maturation assay optimized for high-throughput screening. *Chem. Commun. (Camb).* 52 (53): 8267–8270.

52 Lorenz, D.A., Vander Roest, S., Larsen, M.J., and Garner, A.L. (2018). Development and implementation of an HTS-compatible assay for the discovery of selective small-molecule ligands for pre-microRNAs. *SLAS Discov.* 23 (1): 47–54.

53 Shi, Z., Zhang, J., Qian, X. et al. (2013). AC1MMYR2, an inhibitor of dicer-mediated biogenesis of Oncomir miR-21, reverses epithelial-mesenchymal transition and suppresses tumor growth and progression. *Cancer Res.* 73 (17): 5519–5531.

54 Ren, Y., Zhou, X., Yang, J.J. et al. (2015). AC1MMYR2 impairs high dose paclitaxel-induced tumor metastasis by targeting miR-21/CDK5 axis. *Cancer Lett.* 362 (2): 174–182.
55 Connelly, C.M., Boer, R.E., Moon, M.H. et al. (2017). Discovery of inhibitors of MicroRNA-21 processing using small molecule microarrays. *ACS Chem. Biol.* 12 (2): 435–443.
56 Jiang, C.S., Wang, X.M., Zhang, S.Q. et al. (2015). Discovery of 4-benzoylamino-N-(prop-2-yn-1-yl)benzamides as novel microRNA-21 inhibitors. *Bioorg. Med. Chem.* 23 (19): 6510–6519.
57 Vo, D.D., Staedel, C., Zehnacker, L. et al. (2014). Targeting the production of oncogenic microRNAs with multimodal synthetic small molecules. *ACS Chem. Biol.* 9 (3): 711–721.
58 Malnuit, V., Duca, M., and Benhida, R. (2011). Targeting DNA base pair mismatch with artificial nucleobases. Advances and perspectives in triple helix strategy. *Org. Biomol. Chem.* 9 (2): 326–336.
59 Vo, D.D., Tran, T.P., Staedel, C. et al. (2016). Oncogenic MicroRNAs biogenesis as a drug target: structure-activity relationship studies on new aminoglycoside conjugates. *Chem. Eur. J.* 22 (15): 5350–5362.
60 Maucort, C., Vo, D.D., Aouad, S. et al. (2021). Design and implementation of synthetic RNA binders for the inhibition of miR-21 biogenesis. *ACS Med. Chem. Lett.* 12 (6): 899–906; Vo, D.D., Becquart, C., Tran, T.P.A. et al. (2018). Building of neomycin-nucleobase-amino acid conjugates for the inhibition of oncogenic miRNAs biogenesis. *Org. Biomol. Chem.* 16 (34): 6262–6274.
61 Murata, A., Mori, Y., Di, Y. et al. (2021). Small molecule-induced dimerization of hairpin RNA interfered with the Dicer cleavage reaction. *Biochemistry* 60 (4): 245–249.
62 Disney, M.D., Winkelsas, A.M., Velagapudi, S.P. et al. (2016). Inforna 2.0: a platform for the sequence-based design of small molecules targeting structured RNAs. *ACS Chem. Biol.* 11 (6): 1720–1728.
63 Velagapudi, S.P., Seedhouse, S.J., and Disney, M.D. (2010). Structure-activity relationships through sequencing (StARTS) defines optimal and suboptimal RNA motif targets for small molecules. *Angew. Chem. Int. Ed.* 49 (22): 3816–3818.
64 Velagapudi, S.P., Gallo, S.M., and Disney, M.D. (2014). Sequence-based design of bioactive small molecules that target precursor microRNAs. *Nat. Chem. Biol.* 10 (4): 291–297.
65 Velagapudi, S.P., Cameron, M.D., Haga, C.L. et al. (2016). Design of a small molecule against an oncogenic noncoding RNA. *PNAS* 113 (21): 5898–5903.
66 Costales, M.G., Haga, C.L., Velagapudi, S.P. et al. (2017). Small molecule inhibition of microRNA-210 reprograms an oncogenic hypoxic circuit. *JACS* 139 (9): 3446–3455.
67 Velagapudi, S.P., Luo, Y., Tran, T. et al. (2017). Defining RNA-small molecule affinity landscapes enables design of a small molecule inhibitor of an oncogenic noncoding RNA. *ACS Cent. Sci.* 3 (3): 205–216.

68 Guan, L. and Disney, M.D. (2013). Covalent small-molecule-RNA complex formation enables cellular profiling of small-molecule-RNA interactions. *Angew. Chem. Int. Ed.* 52 (38): 10010–10013.

69 Haga, C.L., Velagapudi, S.P., Strivelli, J.R. et al. (2015). Small molecule inhibition of miR-544 biogenesis disrupts adaptive responses to hypoxia by modulating ATM-mTOR signaling. *ACS Chem. Biol.* 10 (10): 2267–2276.

70 Childs-Disney, J.L. and Disney, M.D. (2016). Small molecule targeting of a MicroRNA associated with hepatocellular carcinoma. *ACS Chem. Biol.* 11 (2): 375–380.

71 Haniff, H.S., Liu, X., Tong, Y. et al. (2022). A structure-specific small molecule inhibits a miRNA-200 family member precursor and reverses a type 2 diabetes phenotype. *Cell Chem. Biol.* 29 (2): 300–311. e310.

72 Lundquist, K.P., Panchal, V., Gotfredsen, C.H. et al. (2021). Fragment-based drug discovery for RNA targets. *ChemMedChem* 16 (17): 2588–2603.

73 Shortridge, M.D. and Varani, G. (2021). Efficient NMR screening approach to discover small molecule fragments binding structured RNA. *ACS Med. Chem. Lett.* 12 (8): 1253–1260.

74 Suresh, B.M., Akahori, Y., Taghavi, A. et al. (2022). Low-molecular weight small molecules can potently bind RNA and affect oncogenic pathways in cells. *JACS* 144 (45): 20815–20824.

75 Suresh, B.M., Lia, Zhanga, P., Wang, K.W. et al. (2020). A general fragment-based approach to identify and optimize bioactive ligands targeting RNA. *Proc. Natl. Acad. Sci.* 117 (52): 33197–33203.

76 Benhamou, R.I., Suresh, B.M., Tong, Y. et al. (2022). DNA-encoded library versus RNA-encoded library selection enables design of an oncogenic noncoding RNA inhibitor. *PNAS* 119 (6).

77 Schmidt, M.F., Korb, O., and Abell, C. (2013). MicroRNA-specific argonaute 2 protein inhibitors. *ACS Chem. Biol.* 8 (10): 2122–2126.

78 Bhattarai, U., Hsieh, W.C., Yan, H. et al. (2020). Bifunctional small molecule-oligonucleotide hybrid as microRNA inhibitor. *Bioorg. Med. Chem.* 28 (7): 115394. Yan, H.; Bhattarai, U.; Song, Y.; Liang, F. S. Design, synthesis and activity of light deactivatable microRNA inhibitor *Bioorg. Chem.* 2018, 80, 492–497. Yan, H.; Liang, F. S. miRNA inhibition by proximity-enabled Dicer inactivation *Methods.* 2019, 167, 117–123.

79 Yan, H., Bhattarai, U., Guo, Z.F., and Liang, F.S. (2017). Regulating miRNA-21 biogenesis by bifunctional small molecules. *JACS* 139 (14): 4987–4990.

80 Piskounova, E., Polytarchou, C., Thornton, J.E. et al. (2011). Lin28A and Lin28B inhibit let-7 microRNA biogenesis by distinct mechanisms. *Cell* 147 (5): 1066–1079.

81 Balzeau, J., Menezes, M.R., Cao, S., and Hagan, J.P. (2017). The LIN28/let-7 pathway in cancer. *Front. Genet.* 8: 31.

82 Borgelt, L., Li, F., Hommen, P. et al. (2021). Trisubstituted pyrrolinones as small-molecule inhibitors disrupting the protein-RNA interaction of LIN28 and Let-7. *ACS Med. Chem. Lett.* 12 (6): 893–898; Lim, D., Byun, W.G., Koo, J.Y. et al.

(2016). Discovery of a small-molecule inhibitor of protein-microRNA interaction using binding assay with a site-specifically labeled Lin28. *JACS* 138 (41): 13630–13638. Lorenz, D.A., Kaur, T., Kerk, S.A. et al. (2018). Expansion of cat-ELCCA for the discovery of small molecule inhibitors of the Pre-let-7-Lin28 RNA-protein interaction. *ACS Med. Chem. Lett.* 9 (6): 517–521.

83 Goebel, G.L., Hohnen, L., Borgelt, L. et al. (2022). Small molecules with tetrahydroquinoline-containing Povarov scaffolds as inhibitors disrupting the protein-RNA interaction of LIN28-let-7. *Eur. J. Med. Chem.* 228: 114014.

84 Rosenblum, S.L., Lorenz, D.A., and Garner, A.L. (2021). A live-cell assay for the detection of pre-microRNA-protein interactions. *RSC Chem. Biol.* 2 (1): 241–247.

85 Angelbello, A.J. and Disney, M.D. (2018). Bleomycin can cleave an oncogenic noncoding RNA. *ChemBioChem* 19 (1): 43–47.

86 Li, Y. and Disney, M.D. (2018). Precise small molecule degradation of a noncoding RNA identifies cellular binding sites and modulates an oncogenic phenotype. *ACS Chem. Biol.* 13 (11): 3065–3071.

87 Costales, M.G., Matsumoto, Y., Velagapudi, S.P., and Disney, M.D. (2018). Small molecule targeted recruitment of a nuclease to RNA. *JACS* 140 (22): 6741–6744.

88 Costales, M.G., Aikawa, H., Li, Y. et al. (2020). Small-molecule targeted recruitment of a nuclease to cleave an oncogenic RNA in a mouse model of metastatic cancer. *PNAS* 117 (5): 2406–2411.

7

Pre-mRNA Splicing Modulation

Scott J. Barraza and Matthew G. Woll

Chemistry Department, PTC Therapeutics, Inc., South Plainfield, NJ, USA

7.1 Introduction

One of the most startling surprises of the Human Genome Project was the discovery that humans possessed fewer genes than was predicted; until 2001, estimates had placed the number between 40,000 and 100,000 genes – roughly consistent with the number of proteins – but the actual value appeared to be ~30,000! [1, 2] Yet, even this was too high, and has since been downwardly revised to a total of ~19,000 genes [3] – a value lower than many "simple" animals and well below that of plants [4]. The question of how so few genes could encode so many proteins had an answer, however. The mechanism underlying protein diversity had been reported as early as 1977 from pioneering research in the laboratories of Richard Roberts (then at Cold Spring Harbor Laboratory) and Phillip Sharp (at the Massachusetts Institute of Technology), for which both received the 1993 Nobel Prize in Physiology or Medicine [5]. Originally working with virus models – and later higher organisms – the researchers revealed that genes were segmented and could encode many protein variations through inclusion or exclusion of different segments at the pre-mRNA level. This surprising diversity-generating mechanism was termed "alternative splicing". From the perspective of drug development, pre-mRNA alternative splicing presents an attractive approach to the pharmacological intervention of human disease and may offer an effective solution to indirectly drugging proteins traditionally considered "undruggable" through direct manipulation of their pre-mRNA transcripts [6, 7].

Pharmacological modulation of alternative splicing was first demonstrated with antisense oligonucleotides (ASOs) in the 1980s [8–10], years before the landmark publications from the human genome project. This feat would eventually culminate in the 2016 FDA approval of the first splicing-modifying drug, nusinersen (Spinraza®), for the treatment of spinal muscular atrophy (SMA) [11]. Though trailing, small molecules were not far behind. The first small-molecule splicing modulators were kinase and phosphatase inhibitors reported in the early 1990s; since then, many classes and mechanisms of small molecules have been discovered

RNA as a Drug Target: The Next Frontier for Medicinal Chemistry, First Edition.
Edited by John Schneekloth and Martin Pettersson.

[12, 13]. Most successful of these is **risdiplam** (Evrysdi®), the first small molecule FDA-approved splicing-modulating drug, approved for use in SMA in 2020.

This chapter seeks to illustrate the mechanisms of pre-mRNA alternative splicing and highlight the various points in which small molecules may intervene with curated examples. Larger molecules, such as oligonucleotides, will not be covered in depth. Finally, several drug discovery case studies will be discussed – including that of **H3B-8800** and **risdiplam** – that will integrate splicing modulator development with lessons from other chapters in this book.

7.2 Overview of Splicing Biology

7.2.1 The Spliceosome

The complex responsible for pre-mRNA splicing is the spliceosome, which is composed of six core snRNPs (small nuclear ribonucleoproteins) (Figure 7.1), each containing an snRNA (small nuclear RNA) and a defined set of proteins. Two types of spliceosomes are recognized in humans: (i) the major spliceosome and (ii) the minor spliceosome, which differs from the former in protein and RNA identity [14–16]. Furthermore, the major spliceosome resides solely in the nucleus, whereas cellular localization of the minor spliceosome remains contentious [17, 18]. This chapter will focus on the major spliceosome as it is responsible for >99% of all pre-mRNA splicing events [19]; however, it is worth noting that the minor spliceosome may be a valid therapeutic target in a small set of diseases [20]. There also exist a handful of protein-catalyzed splicing processes, such as the IRE1-mediated splicing of the *XBP1* transcript [21], but these are rare regulatory mechanisms acting on transcripts that have already been mostly processed by the major spliceosome. These special cases will not be covered here.

The major spliceosome does not exist as a discrete entity in the nucleus; instead, it is assembled in precise locations along the pre-mRNA transcript in a stepwise manner (Figure 7.2). It is important to note that the illustrated overview is characteristic of "intron definition," in which the growing spliceosome spans the intron to identify the exon-intron borders; this form of definition predominates when introns are shorter than flanking exons and is particularly common in lower eukaryotes (among which yeast splicing has been extensively studied). In humans, however, introns tend to be substantially longer than exons and the major mode of splice site recognition is consequently "exon definition" in which the spliceosome spans the exon from the 3′ss of one intron to the 5′ss of the next. Because many details of exon definition remain unsettled, and because it adds a great deal of complexity, it is omitted from the splicing overview.

In the first step of assembly, U1 snRNP "defines" the 5′-splice site (5′ss) – the border that distinguishes the 3′ end of one exon from the 5′ end of the adjacent intron – by binding a nucleotide sequence unique to the 5′ss. The result is *complex E* and is followed by ATP-dependent formation of *complex A*, in which U2 snRNP binds and defines the 3′-splice site (3′ss). In the subsequent and pinnacle step of spliceosome assembly, U4/U5/U6 tri-snRNP is recruited to the 5′-ss to form

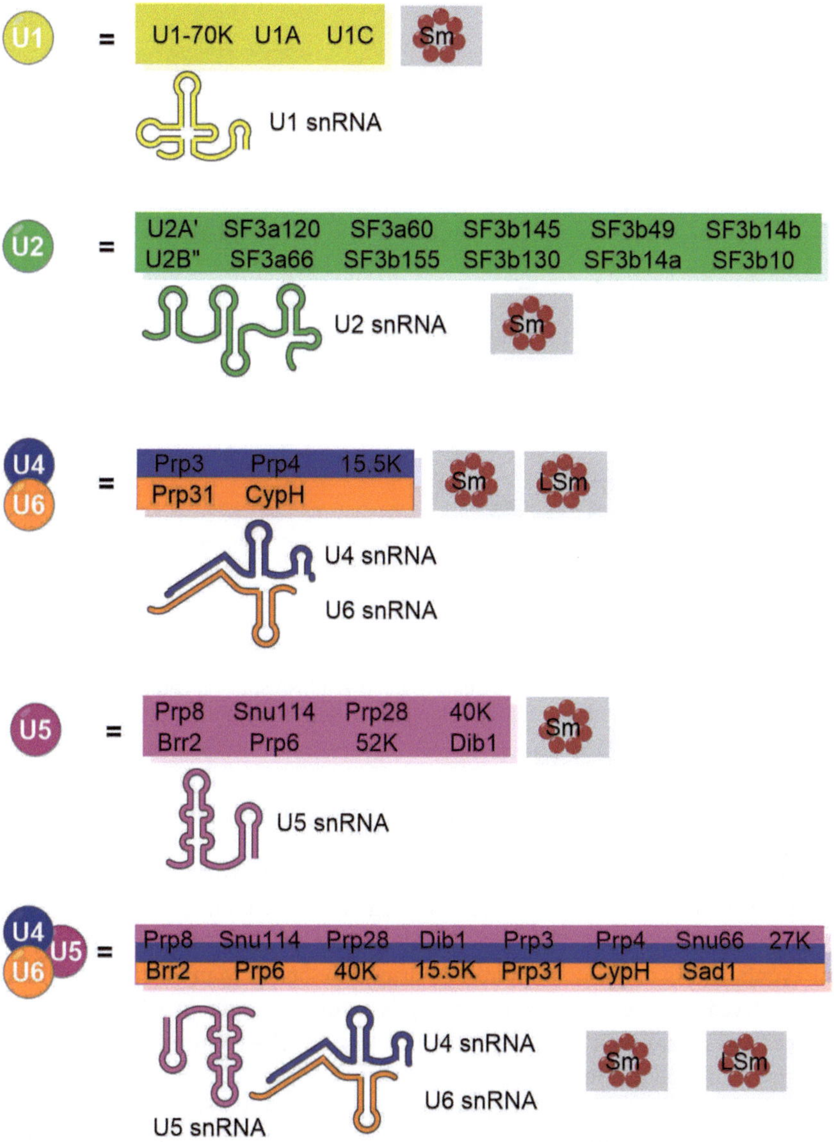

Figure 7.1 Core snRNPs (small nuclear ribonucleoproteins) of the human major spliceosome. Each snRNP is composed of an snRNA (small nuclear RNA) and a defined set of proteins.

precatalytic *complex B* – the system is ready to enter the catalysis phase. Transition to the catalytically competent intermediate *complex B** requires ATP-dependent structural rearrangement followed by dissociation of U1 and U4 snRNP, after which *complex B** catalyzes intron-exon cleavage of the 5′ss and fusion to the 3′ss, forming an RNA lariat-containing intermediate called *complex C*. The complex subsequently severs the 3′ss, joins the exons, and releases the lariat, after which the spliceosome is disassembled for additional cycles of pre-mRNA splicing.

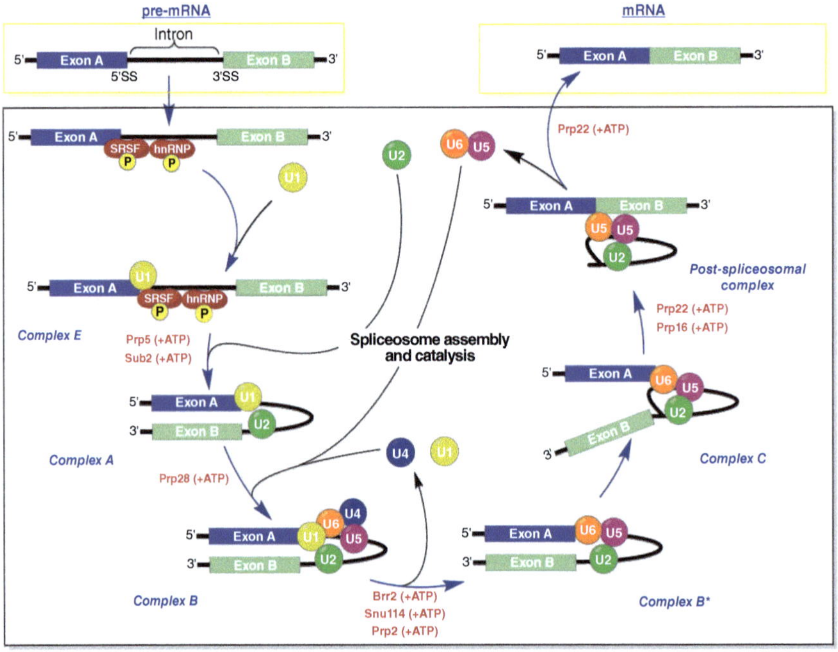

Figure 7.2 Overview of spliceosome assembly and pre-mRNA splicing catalysis. For clarity, the intron definition mode of splice site recognition is illustrated, and splicing factors have been omitted after Complex E.

7.2.2 Classes of Alternative Splicing

There are two major types of pre-mRNA splicing. The first – *constitutive splicing* – is the default condition in which exons are ligated in their linear order following sequential intron removal. The second – *alternative splicing* – encompasses divergent events and is of greatest interest to drug developers. Many varieties of have been observed (Figure 7.3). Exon skipping is a common type in which the exon is spliced out of the final mRNA and usually occurs when splice site recognition is disrupted, or spliceosome function is depressed. Mutually exclusive skipping is related, in which if one exon is included the other must be skipped. Intron retention is the inclusion of an intron in the final transcript and, like exon skipping, is often associated with disturbed splice site recognition. A special regulatory case of intron retention called intron *detention* will be explored later, in which nuclear pools of partially-matured mRNA containing a single detained intron are available for activation by intron excision in response to cellular stimuli [22]. Alternative 5′-splicing often occurs when an intronic sequence resembling a 5′-splice site is recognized instead of the consensus site at the canonical exon-intron junction. Similarly, alternative 3′-splicing occurs when an intronic 3′-splice site-like sequence is recognized. Pseudoexon (or cryptic exon) inclusion shares properties of alternative 5′- and 3′-splicing. In this case, the intronic pseudoexons contain most but not all features characteristic of a true exon.

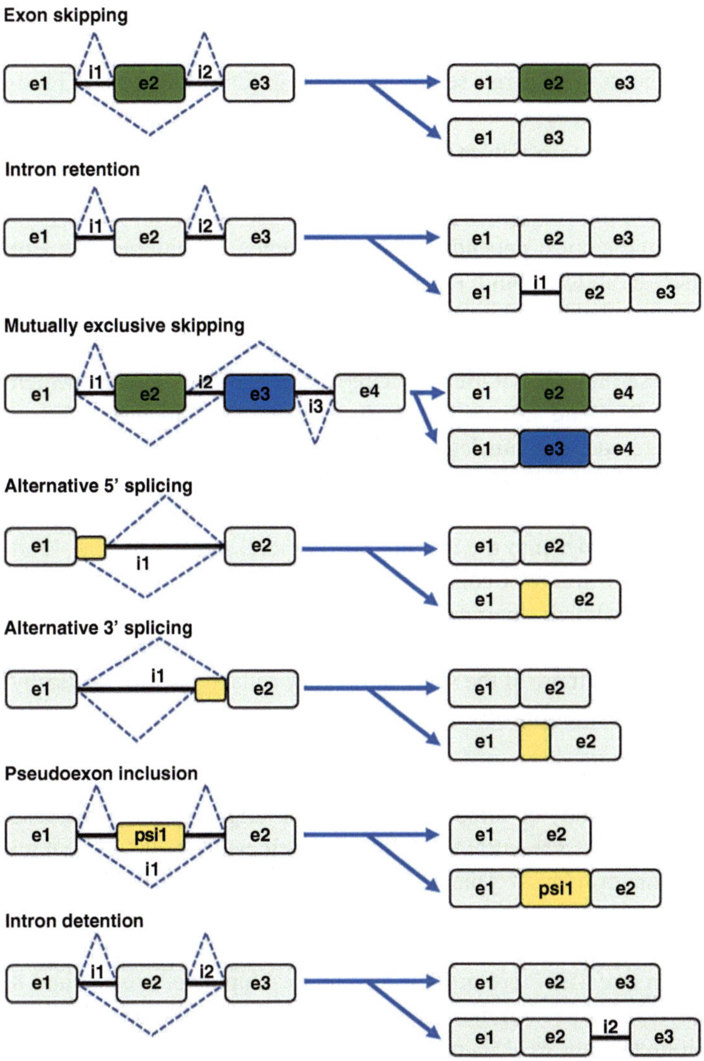

Figure 7.3 Classes of pre-mRNA alternative splicing.

7.3 Pharmacological Mechanisms of Splicing Modulation

7.3.1 *Cis*- and *Trans*-Regulatory Elements (Splicing Factors)

Many genomic sequences falsely resemble *bona fide* 5′- and 3′-splice sites but evade splicing; conversely, many constitutive exon-intron junctions are composed of 5′ss and 3′ss sequences divergent from the canonical form but are nonetheless recognized by the spliceosome [23]. Clearly more control is involved in defining exons and introns than that provided by U1 and U2 snRNP alone. Chief among splicing governors are *cis*-regulatory elements and *trans*-regulatory elements (splicing factors), both of which are localized around splice sites to enhance or suppress spliceosome recognition of exon-intron junctions.

Cis-regulatory elements are discrete sequences on pre-mRNA that serve as binding sites for *trans*-regulatory elements and may be as long as a dozen nucleotides or as short as four. They are classified according to location and function: (i) exonic splicing enhancers (ESE), (ii) exonic splicing silencers (ESS), (iii) intronic splicing enhancers (ISE), or (iv) intronic splicing silencers (ISS). However, this categorization is complicated and context-dependent – e.g. the same *cis*-regulatory element may be an enhancer in an exon but a silencer in an intron [24]. *Trans*-regulatory elements – most often called RNA-binding proteins or *splicing factors* – are proteins recruited to *cis*-regulatory sequences on pre-mRNA. The two most abundant families include (i) serine/arginine-rich splicing factor (SRSF) proteins, which predominantly bind ESE and ISE sequences to enhance exon inclusion/intron exclusion and (ii) heterogeneous nuclear riboproteins (hnRNPs), which preferentially interact with ESS and ISS sequences to suppress splicing activity [25, 26]. The majority of these splicing factors bind exons within 50 nucleotides of the splice site and up to 500 nucleotides into the intron. Furthermore, splicing factors – and hnRNPs in particular – form diverse combinatorial complexes with pre-mRNA containing hundreds of individuals, their arrangement dictated by relative abundance and distribution of specific *cis*-regulatory sequences [27]. It is important to note that splicing factors – even those of the same type – may collaborate synergistically in one combination or antagonistically in another.

7.3.1.1 Stabilization of *Cis*-Regulatory Elements

Perhaps due to the availability of compounds developed originally for telomerase inhibition [28–32], the first pre-mRNA *cis*-regulatory elements probed by small molecules were G-quadruplexes. That G-quadruplexes were valid targets for splicing modulation was seminally demonstrated by Riou et al. in 2004, in which a **bisquinolinium triazine** (Figure 7.4a) bound and stabilized a quadruplex located within intron 6 of *TERT* pre-mRNA, leading to skipping of exons 7 and 8 [33, 34]. A quadruplex stabilization mechanism was consistent with the prevailing telomerase inhibition hypothesis [35] and was further supported by the first unambiguous demonstration of ligand-induced G-quadruplex stabilization by Hurley et al. in 1999 [36]. Since then, drug discovery efforts have grown to target other *cis*-regulatory elements (e.g. stem loops and hairpins, Figure 7.4a).

The stabilization strategy finds current application in frontotemporal dementia with parkinsonism (FTDP), a disease characterized by disturbed behavior, cognition, and motor function believed to originate in part from toxic tau aggregates encoded by the *MAPT* gene [37, 38]. In healthy adults, two tau isoforms are expressed in equal levels – 4R-tau (*MAPT* exon 10 inclusion) and 3R-tau (*MAPT* exon 10 skipping). In FTDP, however, mutations destabilize a *cis*-regulatory stem loop near the 5′ss in intron 10, compromising the loop's ability to engage silencing splicing factors leading to greater exon 10 inclusion and thus higher levels of pathogenic 4R-tau (Figure 7.4c). Seeking stem loop stabilizers, Disney et al. modeled a *MAPT* stem loop mutant and virtually mined an in-house database of

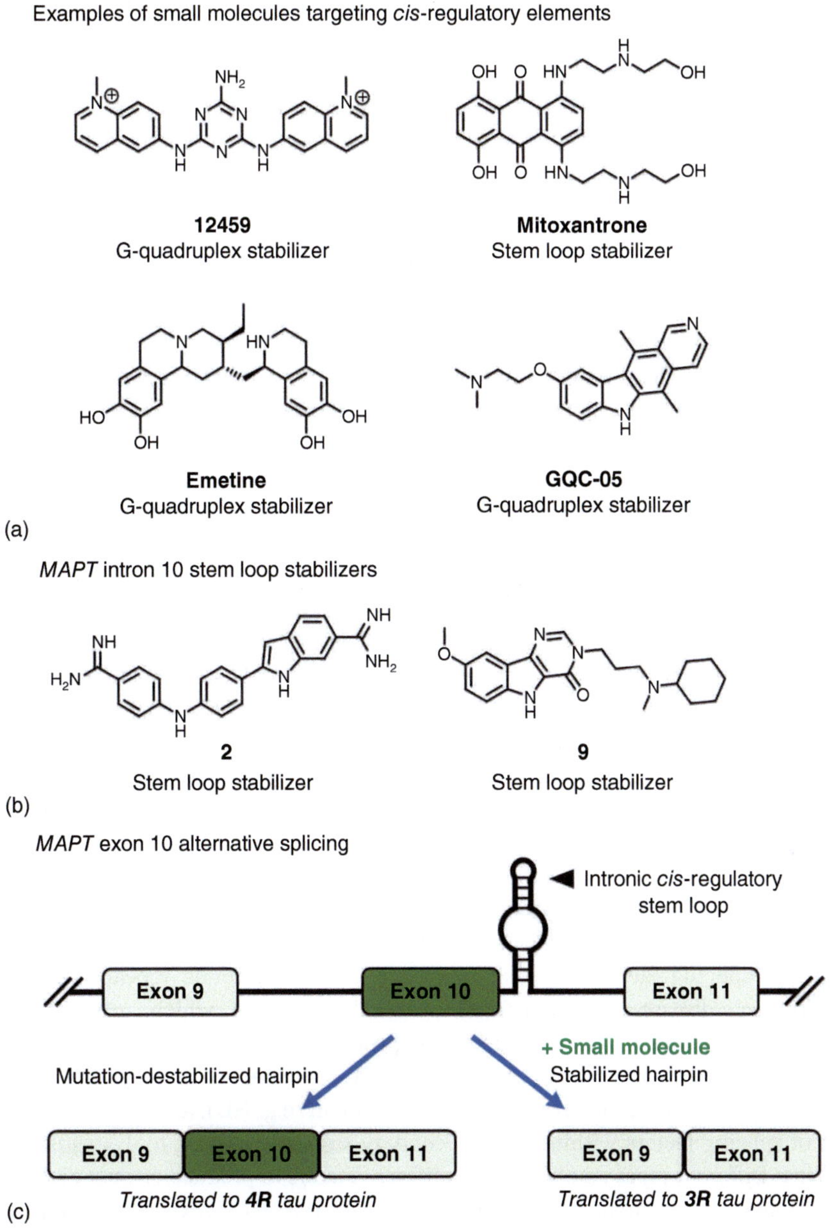

Figure 7.4 (a) Examples of *cis*-regulatory element stabilizers. (b) MAPT intron 10 stem loop stabilizers. (c) Illustration of MAPT exon 10 alternative splicing.

small molecule–RNA interactions called Inforna [39]. **Compound 2** was identified, which selectively bound and stabilized the mutant stem loop (K_D = 10 μM, −1.4 kcal/mol optical melting assessment). Splicing activity was confirmed in whole cells by RT-PCR, consistent with the stabilization hypothesis. Disney et al. then partnered with Pfizer and explored ligand- and structure-based hit expansion strategies around **Compound 2** to optimize potency and drug-likeness [40]. The latter approach was more successful and rendered **Cmpd 9** (Figure 7.4b), which possessed similar stem-loop affinity to the original hit (K_D = 5 μM) but improved drug-like properties. More importantly, **Cmpd 9** suppressed endogenous *MAPT* exon 10 inclusion and reduced pathogenic 4R-tau expression in primary neurons cultured from human-transgenic mice (50% 4R reduction at 40 μM).

7.3.1.2 Destabilization of *Cis*-Regulatory Elements

An alternative strategy to stabilization is *destabilization* of *cis*-regulatory elements; however, few splice-modulating small molecules have been conclusively shown to do this – indeed, disrupters are rare even among nonsplicing G-quadruplex ligands [41]. Nonetheless, in 2018, Scapozza et al. reported compelling evidence of a small-molecule stem loop destabilizer [42]. A single C-to-U mutation in *SMN2* pre-mRNA leads to pathological exon 7 skipping, but it was reasoned that inclusion might be rescued if a critical stem loop – TSL2 – was destabilized (Figure 7.5b). TSL2 bridges the exon-intron junction and traps the 5′ss in a base-paired stem, disruption of which should render the 5′ss more accessible to spliceosomal machinery. A fluorophore/ligand competition assay was developed to identify binders of a model TSL2 RNA oligonucleotide (Figure 7.5c), and an RNA-focused library of 304 compounds was screened. Several hits were identified, among them **PK4C9** (EC_{50} = 16 μM, Figure 7.5a), which demonstrated functional increase of full-length SMN protein in SMA patient cells (3-fold at 30 μM). Evidence from NMR, oligonucleotide mutants, and *in silico* studies supported a mechanism in which **PK4C9** destabilized a suppressive TSL2 pentaloop conformer and reinforced an accessible triloop (Figure 7.5d).

7.3.1.3 Inhibition of *Cis*-Regulatory RNA–Protein Interactions

Although not formally *cis*-regulatory elements, nucleotide repeat motifs nonetheless bind splicing factors. Diseases associated with nucleotide repeats include Huntington's disease (HD) and fragile X syndrome (FXS), which, respectively, suffer $r(CAG)_n$ and $r(CGG)_n$ triplets that progressively expand into dozens or hundreds of repeats over patient lifetimes [43–45]. There are two major pathologies: (i) translation of nucleotide repeats into toxic protein (e.g. HD), and (ii) sequestration of splicing factors within repeat secondary structure leading to dysregulated splicing. Different repeat motifs entrap different factors to produce distinct disease phenotypes – for example, spinocerebellar ataxia type 31 $r(UGGAA)_n$ binds SRSF1 and SRSF9 [46], while fragile X-associated tremor-ataxia syndrome $r(CGG)_n$ binds Sam68 and hNRNP A [47, 48]. However, the essential function of splicing factors precludes their direct targeting, restricting drug discovery programs to the liberation of splicing factors from repeat secondary structure through the development of sequence-specific, RNA-binding, protein–RNA interaction inhibitors.

The most prominent splicing-linked nucleotide repeat disorder is myotonic dystrophy type 1 (DM1). Excessive $r(CUG)_n$ motifs in the 3′-untranslated region of the *DMPK* gene form hairpin loops that sequester splicing factor MBNL1, resulting in

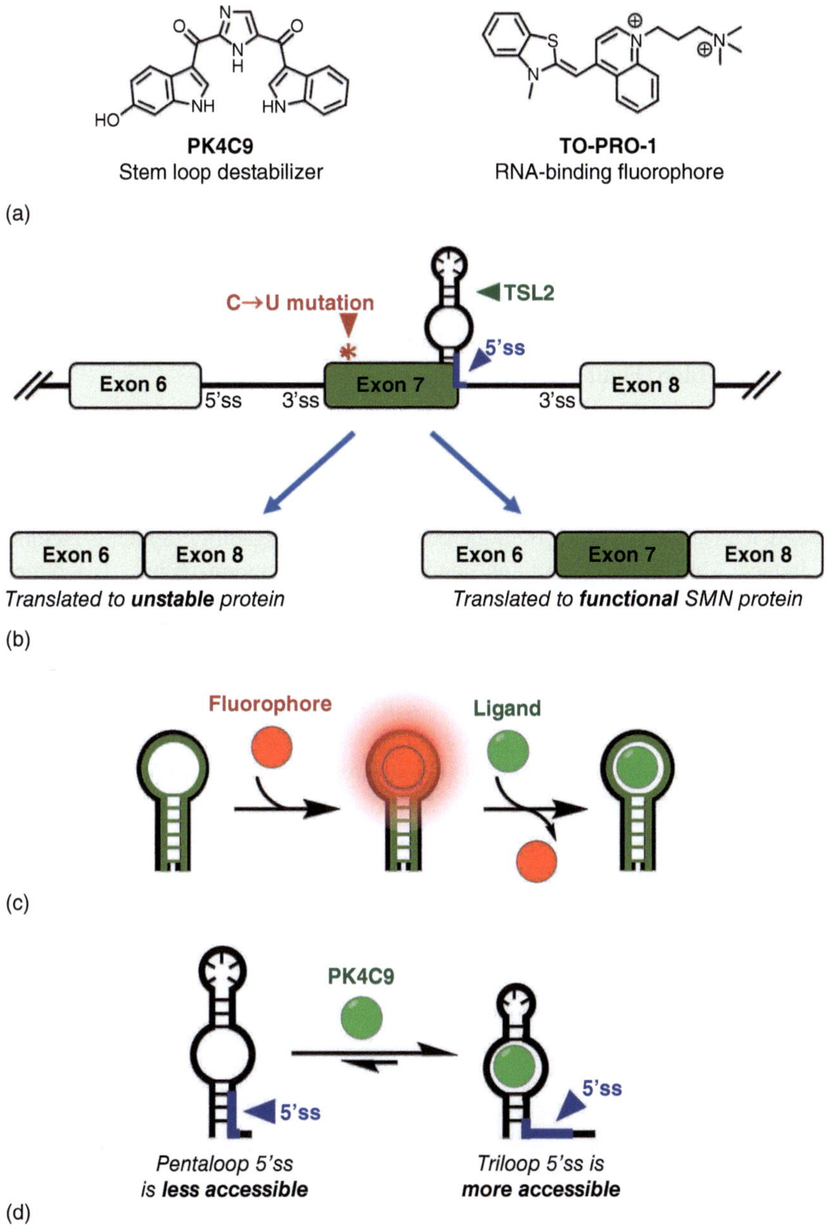

Figure 7.5 Destabilization of cis-regulatory elements. (a) Stem loop destabilizer **PK4C9** and RNA-binding fluorophore TO-PRO-1. (b) Illustration of SMN2 alternative splicing. (c) Schematic of the discovery competition assay. (d) **PK4C9** destabilizes a pentaloop conformation of TSL2 in exon 7, rendering the 5′ss more accessible to the spliceosome.

genome-wide dysregulation of critical MBNL1-regulated genes [49, 50]. Moreover, MBNL1 autoregulates its own alternative splicing, and localization to r(CUG)$_n$ RNA reduces functional isoform expression through aberrant inclusion of exon 5 [51]. In a twist on the traditional protein–RNA interaction inhibitor strategy, Disney et al. designed small molecules that released MBNL1 by *binding* and *degrading* r(CUG)$_n$ RNA [52]. First, a DNA-encoded library composed of >12,000 compounds with properties complementary to RNA–small molecule interactions was screened for binding to r(CUG)$_{12}$ RNA. Among sixteen hits, **Cmpd 1** (Figure 7.6) bound endogenous *DMPK* r(CUG)$_n$ but only modestly improved splicing phenotype in DM1-afflicted cells (~25% reduced *MBNL1* exon 5 inclusion at 5 μM). However, conjugation to bleomycin transformed **Cmpd 1** into an r(CUG)$_n$-specific RNA degrader, **DEL-Bleo** (Figure 7.6).

7.3.1.4 Inhibition of *Trans*-Regulatory Elements

Until recently, the *direct* targeting of splicing factors by small molecules received little attention (although they may be *indirectly* targeted through regulatory kinases, discussed later) likely due to their perceived poor druggability. Splicing factors (and indeed RNA-binding proteins generally) are (i) nonenzymatic, (ii) often highly disordered, and (iii) lack deep pockets for binding [53]. Nonetheless, the first small molecule recognized to interact with a splicing factor was **quercetin** in 2014 (Figure 7.7a), whose binding partner was identified as hnRNP A1 by photoaffinity pulldown [54]. *In vitro* studies indicated **quercetin** simultaneously inhibited hnRNP A1 function and downregulated expression, accounting for the compound's anti-tumor properties (e.g. androgen receptor AR-V7 alternative splicing, Figure 7.7b) [55]. However, it is worth remarking that **quercetin** also promiscuously interacts with many other biological targets, which may also contribute to the observed splicing profile [56–58]. For example, in 2022, Maiti et al.

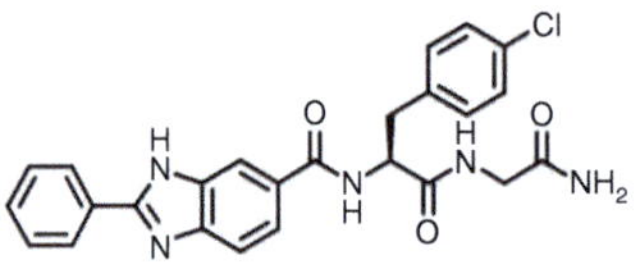

Cmpd1
r(CUG)$_n$ RPI inhibitor
MBNL1 Δ5 rescue (5 μM): 25%

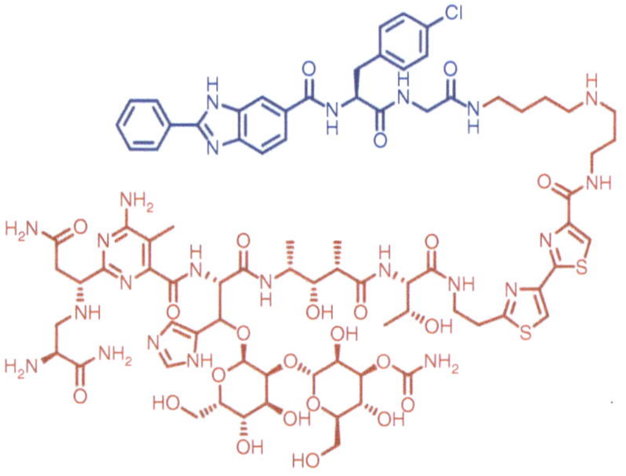

Del-Bleo
r(CUG)$_n$ RNA degrader
MBNL1 Δ5 rescue (5 μM): 40%

Figure 7.6 Structures of DMPK r(CUG)$_n$ nucleotide repeat RNA–protein interaction inhibitors and degraders.

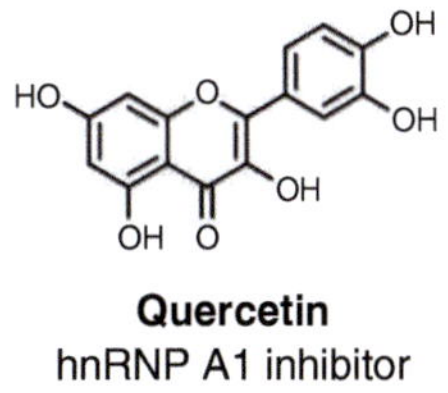

(a)

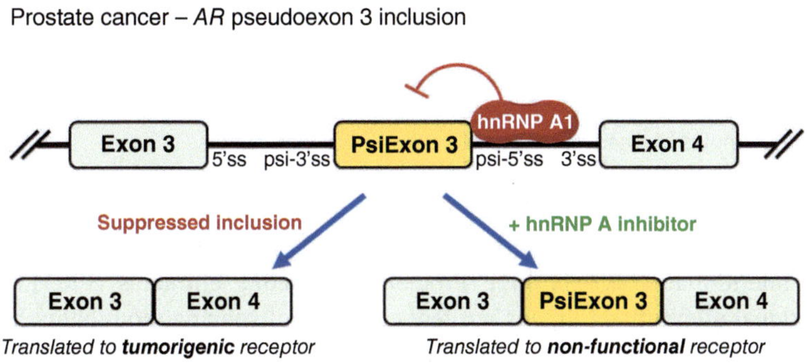

(b)

Figure 7.7 (a) Structure quercetin. (b) Illustration of AR pre-mRNA splicing. Splicing factor hnRNP A1 suppresses inclusion of a pseudoexon in intron 3, leading to mRNA encoding tumorigenic androgen receptor-V7. Quercetin promotes inclusion, leading to mRNA encoding a nonfunctional protein.

reported that **quercetin** can bind and modulate *MALAT1*, a long noncoding RNA (lncRNA) implicated in alternative splicing regulation [59].

7.3.1.5 Degradation of *Trans*-Regulatory Elements

A complementary strategy to the inhibition of splicing factor function is induced proteasome-mediated degradation. Unshackled from the traditional limitations of mass action pharmacology, small-molecule degraders may act catalytically and substoichiometrically to deplete their target proteins [60]. Furthermore, molecular glue-type mechanisms may overcome challenges associated with splicing factor druggability as there is no requirement for potent binding between degrader and target. Originally disclosed in 1999 as an anticancer agent, the first splicing factor degrader was Eisai's **indisulam**, although it was not recognized as such at the time [61]. In fact, the splicing modulatory mechanism was not elucidated until 2017 – long after clinical trials were discontinued due to underwhelming results in both combination and single agent therapy [62, 63]. Nijhawan et al. demonstrated that **indisulam** behaved as a molecular glue that promoted *selective* recognition and degradation of the splicing factor RBM39 by the CRL4-DCAF15 E3 ligase complex [64]. However, unlike Celgene's CelMods/IMiDs – which bind and modulate only the CRL4 adaptor, cereblon – **indisulam** and related aryl sulfonamides exhibit little affinity for either RBM39 or DCAF15 alone but instead discriminatingly recognize and stabilize the RBM39/CRL4-DCAF15 complex, accounting for the remarkable

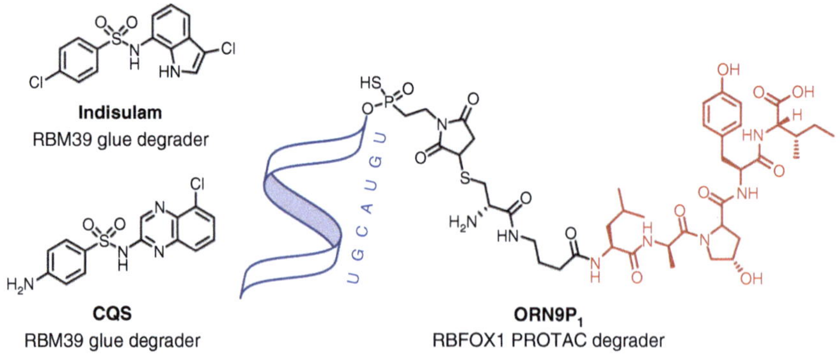

Figure 7.8 Examples of small-molecule degraders of splicing factors.

substrate selectivity [65, 66]. Unfortunately, the identification of molecular glues remains relegated to serendipity, although current efforts seek to develop screening tools for intentional discovery [67]. Proteolysis targeting chimeras (PROTACs) offer a rational alternative to glues but few examples of splicing modulators have been reported to-date. One example, **ORN9P$_1$** (Figure 7.8), was designed to recruit E3 ligases to splicing factor RBFOX1; however, in order to achieve high potency engagement, it was necessary to engage RBFOX1 with a seven-nucleotide oligomer resembling its natural *cis*-regulatory element [68].

7.3.1.6 Inhibition of *Trans*-Regulatory Element Protein–Protein Interactions (PPIs)

Although recognition of the 5′ss by U1 snRNP is mediated by an assortment of general splicing factors (e.g. SRSFs and hnRNPs), recognition of the 3′ss by U2 snRNP requires additional *specialized* factors, including: (i) SF1, which binds the branch point sequence (BPS) *cis*-regulatory element, (ii) U2AF2, which binds the polypyrimidine tract (PYT) *cis*-regulatory element, and (iii) U2AF1, which interacts with the 3′ss intron-exon junction (Figure 7.9) [69]. From the standpoint of on-target toxicity, these specialized splicing factors present attractive drug discovery targets over their multifunctional cousins. For example, hnRNPs perform numerous important regulatory duties independent of pre-mRNA splicing, including mRNA stabilization and nuclear transport, cytoplasmic translation regulation, and chromatin remodeling [70–72]; in contrast, U2AF1 performs a very minor noncanonical role in translation [73].

Advances in splicing factor biology have identified structural features of U2AF1 and U2AF2 amenable to small-molecule binding, among which the U2AF homology motif (UHM) domain – an RNA recognition motif (RRM) repurposed for protein–protein interactions (PPIs) – has found the most traction. In 2020, Bach et al. reported the discovery of UHM PPI inhibitor **7,8-dihydroxyperphenazine** (EC_{50} = 10 μM) from a screen of >42,000 compounds (Figure 7.10a) [74]. *In vitro* splicing confirmation demonstrated complete splicing inhibition of the sentinel pre-mRNA *MINX* at 50 μM, although hit expansion failed to identify more potent

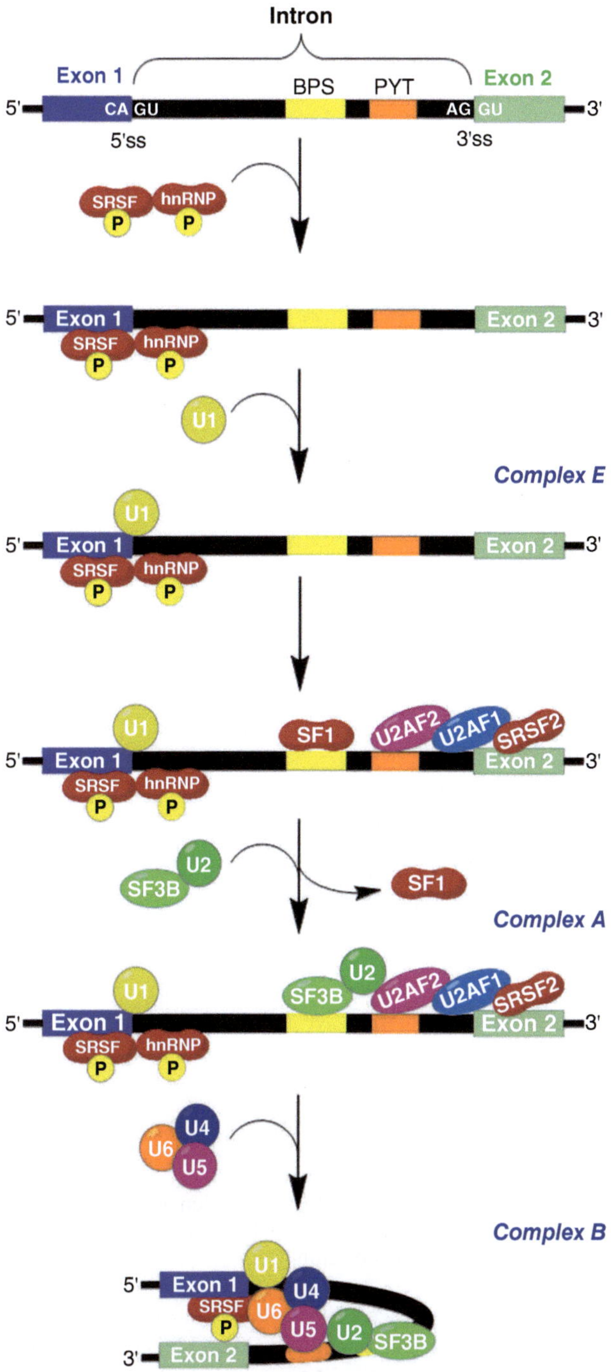

Figure 7.9 General regulation of 5′- and 3′-splice site recognition by splicing factors. Branch point sequence (BPS); polypyrimidine tract (PYT).

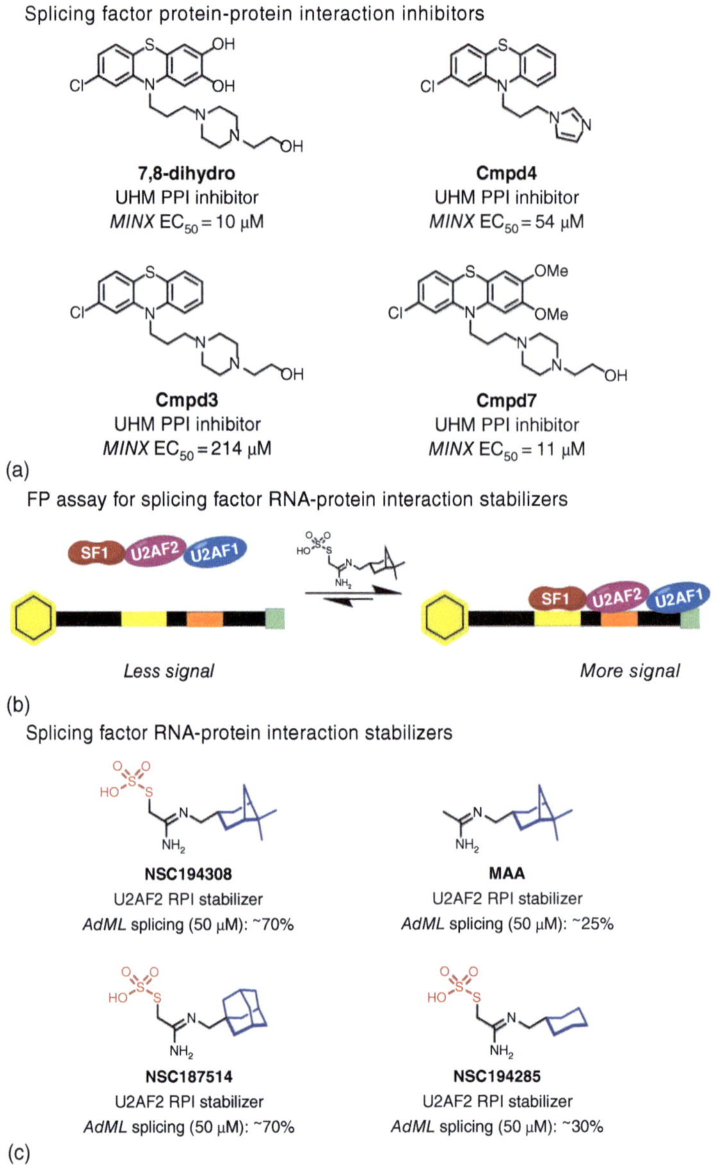

Figure 7.10 (a) U2AF homology motif (UHM) protein–protein interaction inhibitors. (b) Fluorescence polarization assay illustration used to discovery RNA–protein interaction stabilizers. (c) U2AF2-targeting RNA–protein interaction stabilizers.

analogs. Unexpectedly, however, **7,8-dihydroxyperphenazine** blocked assembly of spliceosomal Complex B, whereas its analog **Cmpd 7** interfered with Complex A. One explanation for this mechanism break may be structure-based preferences by these compounds for different UHM-containing splicing factors, which in addition to U2AF2 include PUF60, RBM39, SPF45, and SF1 [75].

7.3.1.7 Stabilization of *Trans*-Regulatory Element RNA–Protein Interactions (RPIs)

An alternative strategy to inhibition of splicing factor protein–protein interactions is stabilization of splicing factor *RNA–protein interactions* (RPIs). Spliceosome assembly is a dynamic process that requires not only the orderly association of components for proper progression through the assembly steps but also their eventual dissociation. Cancers bearing mutations in splicing factor and spliceosomal genes may be particularly vulnerable to association/dissociation imbalance as these malignancies are wholly dependent on the remaining wild-type machinery to fulfill their pre-mRNA splicing needs [76]. Cognizant of this therapeutic connection, Kielkopf et al. developed a fluorescent polarization screening assay to identify small-molecule stabilizers of a U2AF2/SF1/U2AF1^{S34F} ternary complex with a fluorophore-labeled RNA containing a minimal 3′ss (Figure 7.10b) [77]. The choice incorporation of mutant U2AF1^{S34F} was based on the frequency of this mutation in myelodysplastic syndromes and lung adenocarcinomas. Nearly 1500 compounds from the NCI Developmental Therapeutics Program were screened and one hit was identified – **NSC194308** (EC_{50} ~100 μM, Figure 7.10c), which was subject to *in vitro* splicing validation in HeLa cells where it inhibited splicing of the *AdML* minigene transcript (~70% intron retention at 50 μM) and eliminated spliceosomal complexes B and C as expected for U2AF2/SF1/U2AF1–RNA interaction stabilization. Furthermore, **NSC194308** exhibited modest selectivity for K562 leukemia cells with the U2AF1^{S34F} mutation over wild-type U2AF1 (CC_{50} = 5 μM vs. 18 μM, respectively), which was attributed to sequence specificity for canonical polypyrimidine tracts – U2AF2's *cis*-regulatory sequence – over degenerate tracts. Structural studies concluded **NSC194308** bound an open-form U2AF2 conformation in a pocket at the interface of two RNA-interacting domains. Limited hit expansion established the importance of hydrophobic groups occupying a protein pocket (**NSC194308** pinane and **NSC187514** adamantane compared **NSC194285** cyclohexane, Figure 7.10c) and an anionic thiosulfate in the vicinity of the pre-mRNA (**NSC194308** compared to **MAA**). The amidine would be expectedly cationic and potentially interactive with the negatively charged RNA phosphate backbone but was not scrutinized.

7.3.2 Kinases and Phosphatases

Kinases regulate all aspects of pre-mRNA splicing, including (i) splice site recognition, (ii) spliceosome assembly, and (iii) spliceosome function. The most prominent kinase families belong to the CDK-MAPK-GSK3-CLK (CMGC) group and notably include CDC2-like kinases (CLKs), dual-specificity tyrosine-regulated kinases (DYRKs), serine-arginine protein kinases (SRPKs), and Prp kinases. Many nontraditional kinases have been implicated as well, such as topoisomerase I [78]. The primary substrates of these kinases are splicing factors through which most pre-mRNA splicing modulation is mediated. The first FDA-approved drug targeting a kinase was imatinib in 2001 (albeit not for splicing), since then, a remarkable number of tools were established that expedite kinase drug discovery and development [79]. However, despite the great advances in the field, only one kinase inhibitor has entered clinical trials for which pre-mRNA splicing is a claimed mechanistic feature – **cirtuvivint** (from Biosplice Therapeutics, formerly Samumed), a pan-CLK/DYRK family inhibitor currently under Phase I anticancer investigation (Figure 7.11a) [80, 81]. This clinical paucity is noteworthy considering

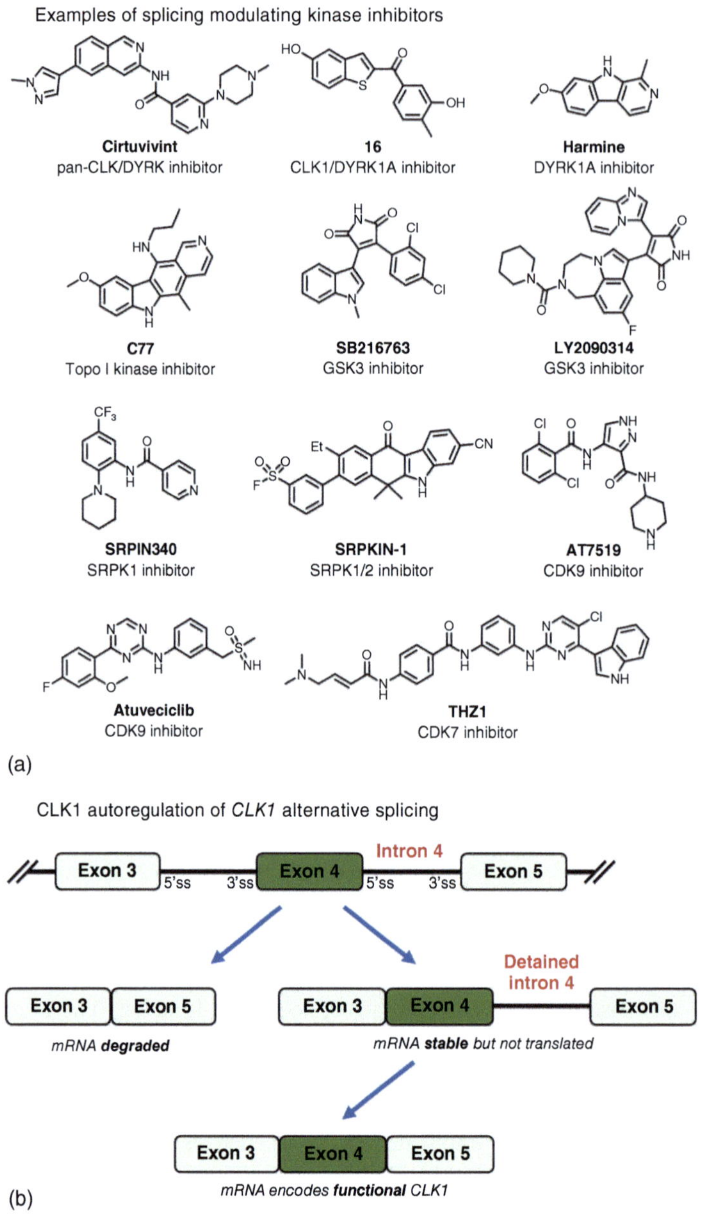

Figure 7.11 (a) Examples of kinase inhibitors that modulate splicing. (b) CLK1 autoregulation of CLK1 pre-mRNA alternative splicing. Exon 4 skipped isoform is rapidly degraded, whereas the intron 4 detained isoform is stable but cannot leave the nucleus and cannot be translated.

the huge number of splicing modulating kinase inhibitors discovered to-date, but, as it turns out, kinase regulatory biology presents certain development challenges.

7.3.2.1 Challenges in Targeting Kinases

Leaving aside the traditional issue of kinase specificity, the first challenge to modulating splicing through kinases is substrate selectivity. Although splicing factors are major targets of phosphorylation by CMGC kinases, they are not the only ones. For example, CLK1 – perhaps the most studied splicing-relevant kinase – regulates 5′ss recognition through phosphorylation of SRSFs. Incredibly, it also regulates 5′ss recognition through U1 snRNP; recent evidence suggests that the U1-70K protein component of U1 must be phosphorylated by CLK1 to trigger pre-mRNA recruitment and integration with SRSFs already present at the 5′ss [82]. Second, CMGC kinases are highly redundant, although the extent to which each can compensate for the loss of another is still a topic of active research. In 2014, Engel et al. presented evidence that DYRK1A can compensate for CLK1 inhibition to moderate splicing efficacy, necessitating the development of dual CLK1/DYRK1A inhibitors to achieve pre-mRNA splicing modulation [83]. Substrate overlap is probably not perfect, however. SRPK1 and SRPK2 have been reported to act at different spliceosome assembly steps [84], and Cochrane et al. have demonstrated that CLK1 and CLK2 regulate distinct steps and exhibit opposing roles in HIV-1 expression [85].

A third challenge concerns the poorly understood interactome of these kinases. Studies on cancer-relevant kinases have revealed regulatory roles for nonsubstrate proteins that modify catalytic activity [86–88]. Perhaps the most striking example of this in the context of splicing is the relationship between CLK1 and SRPK1. Although SRPK1 is broadly distributed throughout the cell, CLK1 is localized entirely to the nucleus where it maintains the SRPK1 nuclear pool via formation of a stable equimolar complex [89]. The affiliation is reciprocal; SRPK1 stimulates release of CLK1 from its phosphorylated SRSF substrates – a critical step that permits unobstructed binding of U1 snRNP to the 5′ss.

A fourth challenge in the development of kinase modulators is autoregulation. CLKs [90], DYRKS [91], and SRPKS [92] all self-regulate their catalytic activity via autophosphorylation, although not always through the same mechanism. DYRK self-phosphorylation, for example, is restricted to translation just prior to ribosomal release, whereas CLKs and SRPKs can phosphorylate themselves at any time [93]. More remarkable is the ability of these kinases to autoregulate their own pre-mRNA splicing. For instance, catalytically competent full-length CLK1 contains all 13 *CLK1* exons, but alternative splicing affords two inactive isoform options: (i) an exon 4 skipped transcript that is rapidly degraded through nonsense-mediated decay (NMD) and (ii) a stable intron 4 detention transcript [94, 95]. Under normal conditions, CLK1 *suppresses* its own efficient splicing and detained-intron *CLK1* transcripts pool in the nucleus. However, to compensate for small-molecule blockade, CLK1 promotes excision of intron 4 and upregulates formation of full-length *CLK1* mRNA (Figure 7.11b).

Finally, RNA transcription and pre-mRNA splicing are intrinsically intertwined and difficult to selectively modulate because both processes (i) occur contemporaneously and (ii) are regulated by CMGC family kinases [96]. In fact, the RNA polymerase II (RNAP II) transcription complex recruits splicing factors to the elongating pre-mRNA transcript to initiate splicing before transcription is even complete [97, 98]. Furthermore, RNAP II activity is regulated by cyclin-dependent kinases (CDKs), which are CMGC family members and closely related to splicing kinases [96]. It should be noted that some CDKs perform double duty; for example, proper interaction between U2 snRNP and the U5/U6 snRNPs requires phosphorylation of SF3B1 by CDK11 [99].

7.3.2.2 Inhibition of Kinases

Perhaps the most effective strategy in the discovery of kinase inhibitors is focused library screening [100, 101]. In contrast to traditional library design schemes – which favor broad chemical diversity for maximum generality – focused libraries are tailored to specific biological targets. Two classes are recognized: (i) *ligand-based* libraries use known compounds with desirable biological activity as templates and (ii) *structure-based* libraries utilize structural and physicochemical properties of the biological target to inform compound selection.

Despite the maturity of the kinase drug development field, the design of highly specific single-kinase inhibitors remains nearly impossible as compounds invariably possess unintended activity with unexpected kinases [102]. However, those unexpected kinases possibly include those which regulate pre-mRNA splicing, and it is this consideration that underlies the design of ligand-based focused libraries constructed from known kinase inhibitors. Webb et al. screened 2035 characterized kinase inhibitors for promoters of exon skipping in a whole-cell, MDM2-based, luciferase reporter model and identified hits **milciclib**, **PF-3758309**, and **PF-562271** (Figure 7.12) [102, 103]. Ostensibly, these compounds were CDK, PAK, and FAK inhibitors, respectively, but closer examination discovered all three to be inhibitors of splicing-associated CLK-family kinases. As expected, these compounds reduced phosphorylation of splicing factor SR proteins. Interestingly, **PF-562271** also suppressed phosphorylation of SF3B1, a known substrate of both DYRK1A and CDK-family kinases; however, **PF-562271** does not inhibit these, suggesting SF3B1 may be regulated by another as-yet unknown kinase.

7.3.2.3 Activation and Degradation of Kinases

The relative lack of success with kinase inhibition urges investigation into unconventional mechanisms of kinase modulation – agonism and degradation. Although

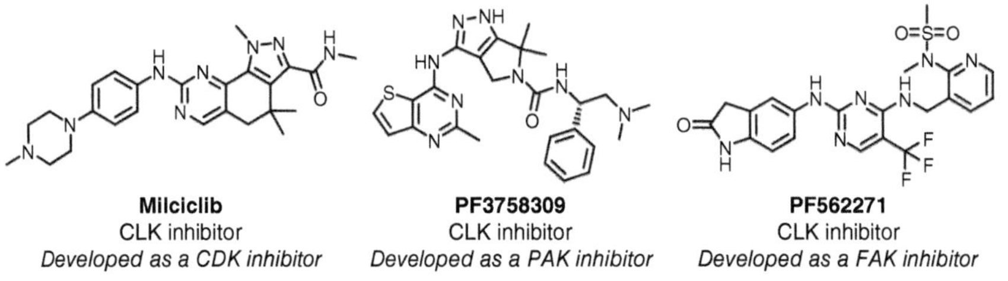

Figure 7.12 (a) Kinase inhibitors with previously unrecognized splicing activity discovered through ligand-focused library screening.

the following small molecules represent novel approaches to modulating splicing, both were identified serendipitously. Unfortunately, principles in the deliberate discovery of kinase agonists and degraders remain underdeveloped; until they mature, these mechanisms will be difficult to advance. Moreover, the advantages of these mechanisms over traditional kinase inhibition have not been methodically assessed.

In 2015, a dual-reporter minigene-based high-throughput screen from Hagiwara et al. discovered a small-molecule kinase *activator* that rescued inclusion of *ELP1* exon 20 (**RECTAS,** Figure 7.13a) [104]. Aberrant *ELP1* splicing is hallmark of familial dysautonomia: a single U-to-C mutation in the +6 position of intron 20 induces exon 20 skipping, the protein product of which is dysfunctional (Figure 7.13b). Several observations established **RECTAS'** mechanism of action: (i) intron 20 contained several ISE *cis*-regulatory binding sites for SRSF6, (ii) pulldown experiments identified CLK1 as **RECTAS'** biological target, (iii) SRSF6 phosphorylation/activation was enhanced by **RECTAS**, and (4) SRSF6 is a known substrate of CLK1. Furthermore, CLK inhibitors induced the opposite effect; suppression of SRSF6 phosphorylation and greater exon 20 skipping [105].

Another unusual kinase modulation mechanism is protein degradation. Expressly interested in discovering novel DYRK1A inhibitors, Hagiwara et al. developed a cell-based screening assay and identified **CaNDY** (Figure 7.13a), which was initially believed to be a classic ATP-competitive kinase inhibitor [106]. However, expression studies revealed selective depletion of DYRKs and CLKs (but no other kinases) reversible upon co-treatment with proteasome inhibitors. These results suggested that **CaNDY** functioned as a selective degrader of DYRKs and CLKs, and the compound was advanced for evaluation in splicing-associated cystic fibrosis. The origin of the disease in 60% of Class V cystic fibrosis patients can be traced to an intronic C-to-U mutation in *CFTR* that generates a false 5′ss that – when paired with a 3′ss-like sequence upstream – leads to pseudoexon inclusion (Figure 7.13c) [107]. The pseudo-3′ss is regulated by exonic SRSFs that enhance an otherwise weak U2 snRNP interaction, but the SRSFs are themselves regulated by CLK kinases; consequently, degradation of CLKs by **CaNDY** promoted pseudoexon skipping and restored functional *CFTR* expression.

7.3.2.4 Inhibition and Activation of Protein Phosphatases

Phosphatases perform regulatory roles complementary to those of kinases: where kinases *phosphorylate* splicing factors and activate them toward pre-mRNA binding, phosphatases *dephosphorylate* splicing factors and deactivate them [108, 109]. Additional substrates include the SF3B2 protein component of U2 snRNP, which must be dephosphorylated by protein phosphatase 2C (PP2C) to facilitate spliceosomal assembly of Complex A [110, 111]. It is therefore unsurprising that phosphatases were of great interest in the early history of splicing modulation by small molecules; by 1992, there were more examples of phosphatase inhibitors than there were of kinase inhibitors (although these were predominantly structurally complex secondary metabolites, Figure 7.14a) [13]. However, interest in phosphatases withered during the kinase drug development explosion and has not since recovered. To date, the only noteworthy discovery was that of **homoharringtonine** (Figure 7.14a),

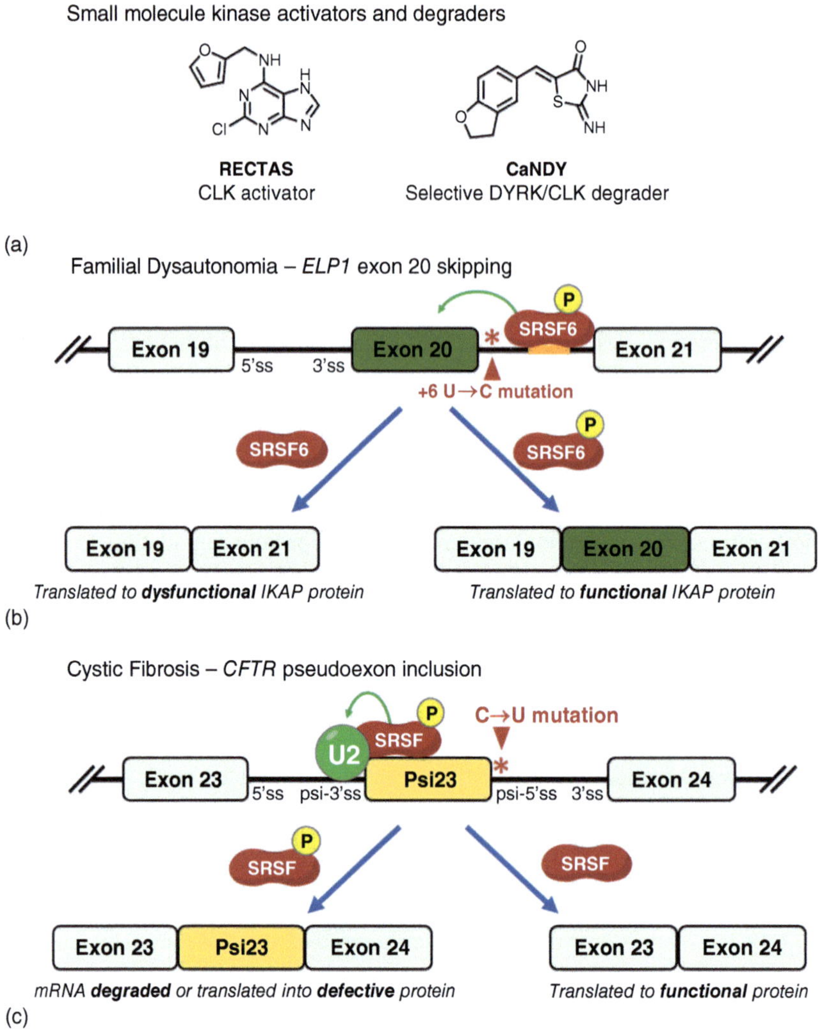

Figure 7.13 (a) Kinase activator RECTAS and kinase degrader CaNDY. (b) ELP1 exon 20 is skipped due to a U-to-C intronic mutation, resulting in dysfunctional IKAP protein and familial dysautonomia; **RECTAS** enhanced SRSF6 phosphorylation and promoted exon 20 inclusion. (c) A C-to-U intronic mutation in CFTR leads to pseudoexon inclusion and loss of functional protein; **CaNDY** degraded CLK kinases responsible for SRSF phosphorylation/activation and suppressed pseudoexon inclusion.

an anticancer drug approved in 2012 under the tradename omacetaxine. A 2018 mechanistic investigation by Lu et al. uncovered a splicing connection through which **homoharringtonine** promoted alternative 5′ss usage favoring formation of the proapoptotic short Bcl-xS transcript over the tumorigenic long Bcl-xL transcript (Figure 7.14b) [112, 113]. Overexpression, knockdown, and chemical genomic studies implicated phosphatase PP1 *activation* (not inhibition) as the primary mediator of **homoharringtonine**'s splicing activity.

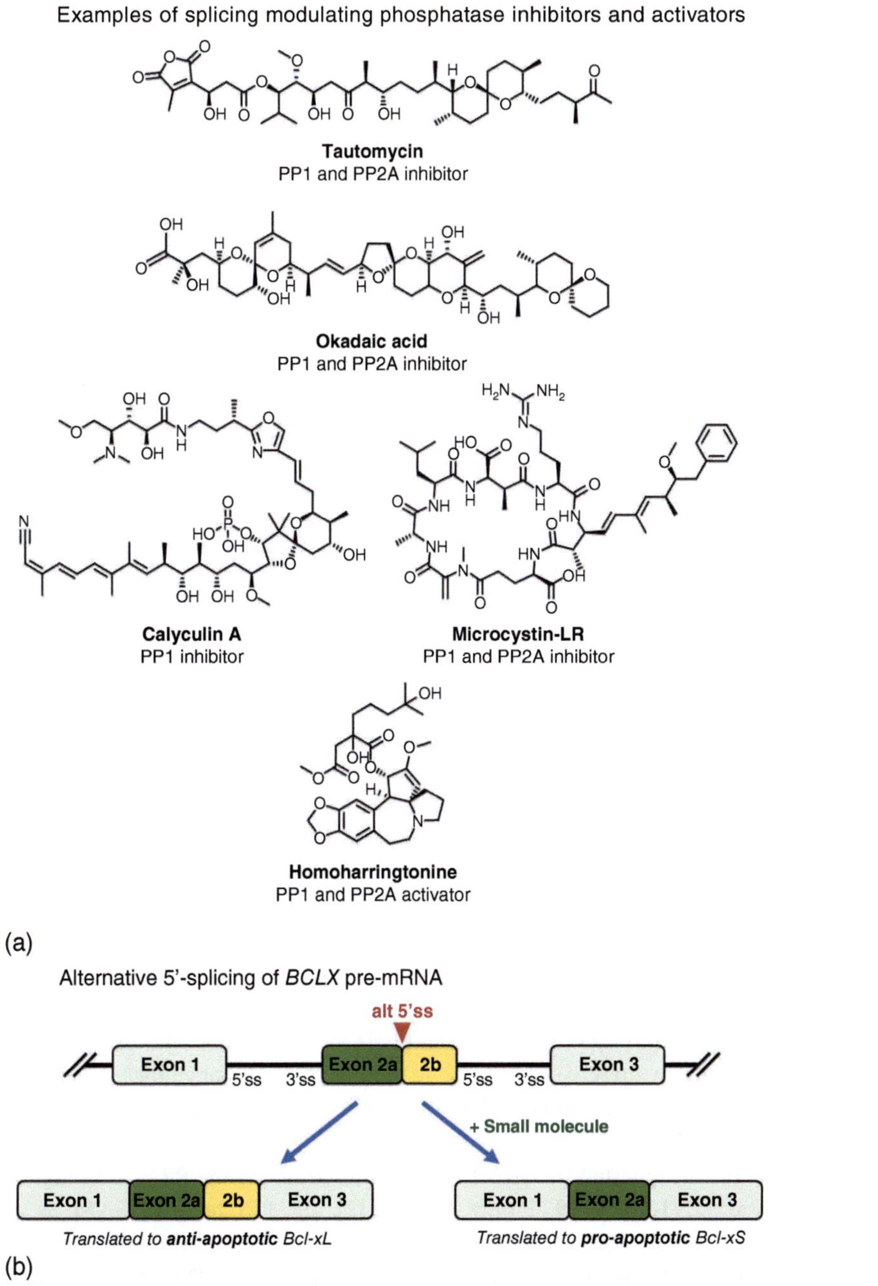

Figure 7.14 (a) Examples of phosphatase inhibitors and activators that modulate pre-mRNA splicing. (b) Illustration of BCLX alternative 5′-splicing. Use of an alternative 5′ss truncates exon 2, afforded short transcript encoding the proapoptosis factor Bcl-xS.

7.3.3 Epigenetic Writers and Erasers

Epigenetic tools – readers, writers, and erasers – regulate gene transcription through the post-translational modification of histones by either transferring (i.e. writing), removing (i.e. erasing), or recognizing (i.e. reading) so-called "marks," of which the most common marks are acetyl and methyl groups [114]. Because epigenetic tools control transcription, and transcription is contemporaneous with pre-mRNA splicing, small-molecule targeting of epigenetic tools may lead to splicing modulation. However, as with many previous examples, the regulatory roles of epigenetic tools are complex, and the distinction is blurred between transcriptional control and splicing control. For instance, some RNA-binding proteins are directly regulated by epigenetic writers; the acetyltransferase CBP directly acetylates splicing factor Sam68, in addition to histones [115]. U6 snRNP activity is also dependent on writers; adenosine 43 of the U6 snRNA must be *N*-methylated by methyltransferase METTL16 for 5′ss recognition [116, 117]. Nevertheless, the first epigenetic tools targeted by small-molecule splicing modulators were histone deacetylases (HDACs) as inhibition arrests spliceosome assembly [118–121]. Structurally, HDAC inhibitors (e.g. **SAHA**, **LBH589**, and **M344**; Figure 7.15) are recognizable by their shared hydroxamic acid functionality, a key pharmacophore element that coordinates and inactivates a catalytically required metal ion – usually zinc – in the HDAC active site [122]. Histone acetyl transferase (HAT) inhibitors, such as **anacardic acid,** affect splicing as well; in some cases, the molecular mechanism of inhibition involves catalytically noncompetitive occlusion of substrate binding [123, 124].

7.3.3.1 Inhibition of Epigenetic Writers

Methyl transferase inhibitors also modulate splicing – the first of which was **RG3039**, an inhibitor of DcpS discovered in 2005 [121, 125, 126] – and today receive greater attention than HDACs and HATs. The most popular methyl transferase is PRMT5, an oncogene whose dysregulation leads to epigenetic inactivation of tumor suppressor expression and promotion of androgen receptor expression [127, 128]; however, PRMT5 has additional roles, including an obligation to methylate spliceosomal Sm proteins for proper snRNP assembly [129–131]. These dual duties make PRMT5 inhibition an attractive target for the treatment of splicing-addicted cancers, which are dependent on protumorigenic alternatively spliced isoforms arising from dysregulated splicing.

In 2021, Janssen reported the structure-based discovery of the PRMT5 inhibitor **onametostat** (**JNJ-64619178,** Figure 7.16) [132]. PRMT5 requires **SAM** as a methyl source, and it was reasoned that adenosine-based small molecules might compete with **SAM** and thus antagonize transferase activity. The company first constructed a focused chemical library composed of small molecules whose design was based on Eli Lilly's 2012 ternary co-crystal structure of PRMT5 in complex with (i) MEP50 – an adaptor protein, (ii) a peptide model of a histone substrate, and (iii) a natural inhibitor (**A9145C**) [133]. The focused library was screened in a biochemical assay for inhibition of **SAM** consumption, and hits were triaged in a whole-cell assay monitoring methylation of spliceosomal Sm proteins [134]. Hit expansion

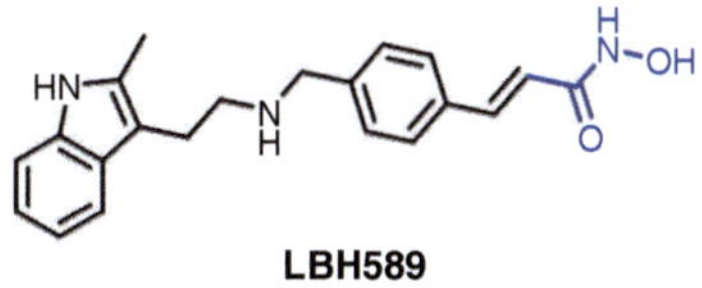

LBH589
HDAC inhibitor

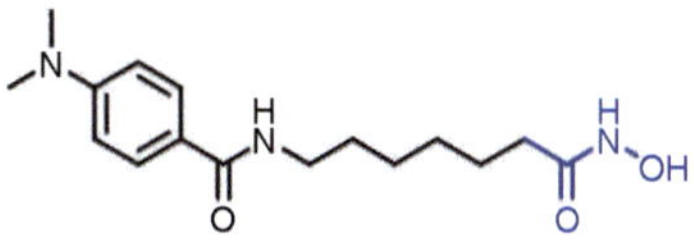

M344
HDAC inhibitor

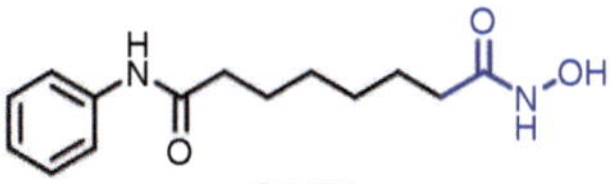

SAHA
HDAC inhibitor

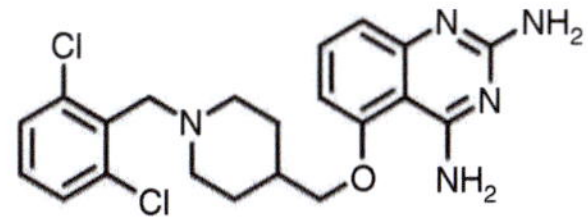

RG3039
DcpS inhibitor

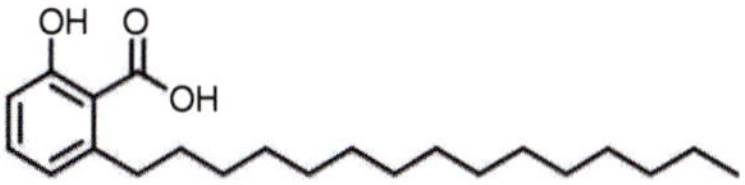

Anacardic acid
HAT inhibitor

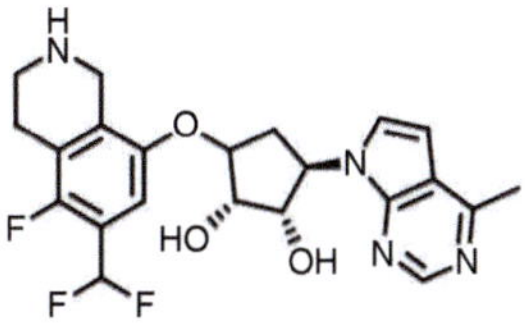

PF06939999
Selective PRMT5 inhibitor

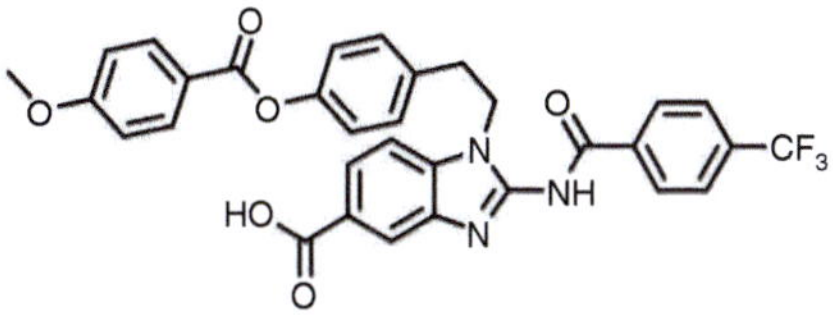

BIX01338
HMT inhibitor

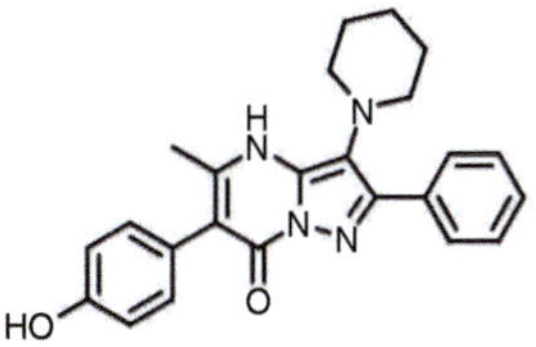

AGI24512
Indirect PRMT5 inhibitor

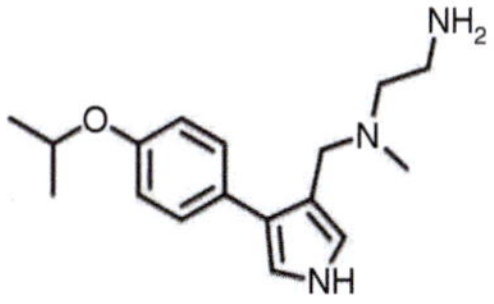

MS023
PRMT1 inhibitor

Figure 7.15 Examples of epigenetic tool inhibitors. The key pharmacophore feature of HDAC inhibitors (hydroxamic acid, top row) is colored blue.

underscored the critical and stereo-discriminating influence of a basic amine – a structural feature that, for undisclosed reasons, was abandoned during lead optimization. **Onametostat** is a potent Sm methylation inhibitor compared to its early analogs ($IC_{50}{}^{cell} = 0.2$ nM; analogs in Figure 7.16), but long assay incubation times are required for complete reduction of methylated Sm proteins (original = 48 hours, long = 96 hours), suggesting that prolonged and continuous exposures are necessary for maximum effect. An explanation for this time-dependent phenomenon came from kinetic studies, which indicated a very long PRMT5 residence time for **onametostat**. From a splicing perspective, RNA-seq showed greater splicing

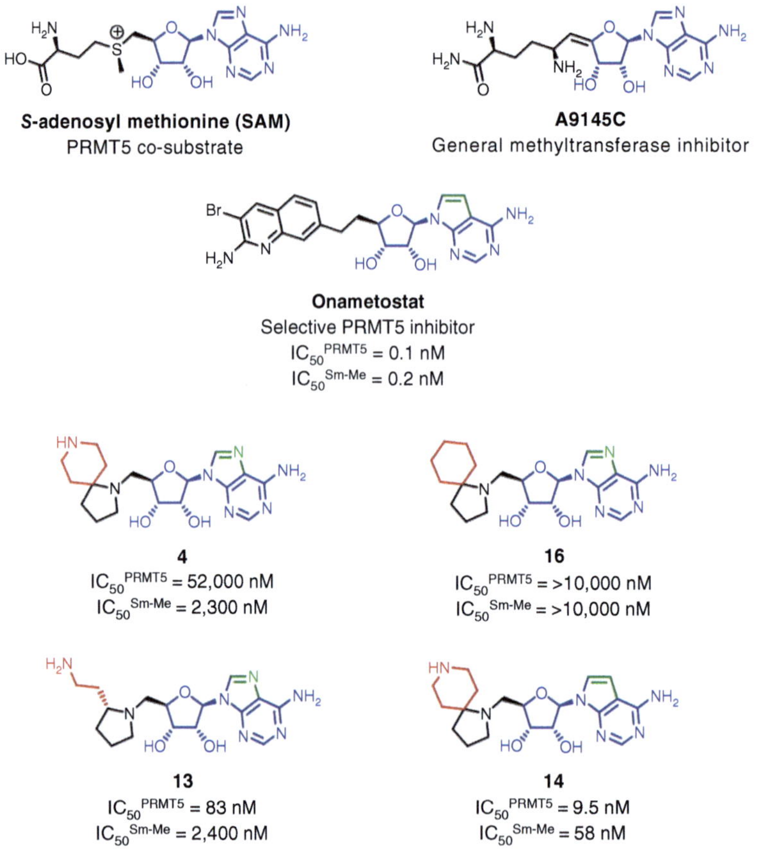

Figure 7.16 PRMT5 inhibitor onametostat, PRMT5 cosubstrate SAM, natural secondary metabolite A914C, and early onametostat analogs. IC_{50}^{PRMT5} is an enzymatic assessment of PRMT5 catalytic inhibition; $IC_{50}^{Sm\text{-}Me}$ is a whole cell assay measuring methylation of spliceosome Sm proteins.

disruption in liquid tumor lines sensitive to PRMT5 inhibition than in insensitive lines, with a significant increase in exon skipping, intron retention, and alternative splice site usage; however, no such correlation was observed in solid tumor lines carrying splicing factor mutations. Nonetheless, **onametostat** entered Phase I trials in 2018 for both cancer types, but patient enrollment was discontinued in 2021 due to disappointing clinical endpoints despite demonstration of robust PRMT5 target engagement [135].

7.3.4 RNA Helicases

RNA helicases regulate pre-mRNA splicing by remodeling pre-mRNA *cis*-regulatory structures and therefore represent plausible drug discovery targets; some special cases are also essential for proper spliceosome assembly [136–139]. However, this

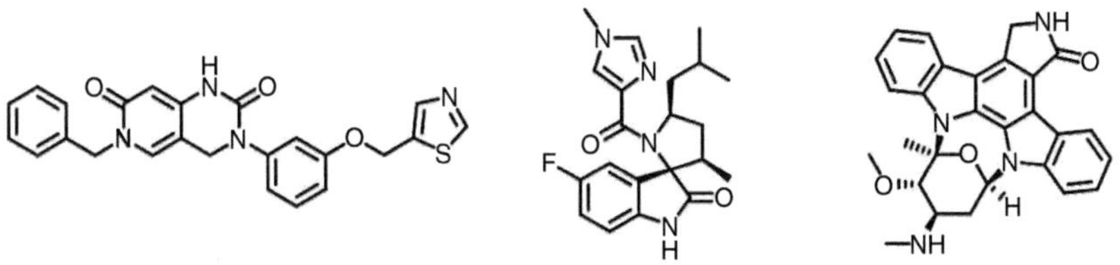

Cmpd 9
Brr2 inhibitor
ATPase IC_{50}: 79 nM
Helicase IC_{50}: 1,300 nM

Cmpd 32a
Brr2 inhibitor
ATPase IC_{50}: 21 nM
Helicase IC_{50}: 480 nM

Staurosporine
Posited helicase inhibitor

Figure 7.17 Examples of inhibitors of splicing-associated RNA helicases.

target class has been severely neglected. To-date, only two examples of small-molecule inhibitors of splicing-related RNA helicases have been described – both targeting the ATPase domain of Brr2, a key driver of U4 snRNP dissociation – but the applicability of this strategy remains unconfirmed as neither compound was assessed for splicing modulatory activity (**Cmpd 9** and **Cmpd 32a**, Figure 7.17) [140, 141]. Nonetheless, RNA helicases are highly homologous, so **Cmpd 9** and **Cmpd 32a** are noteworthy for their excellent inhibitory selectivity for Brr2 over closely related helicases. Both compounds were developed from hits originally identified in high-throughput screening for recombinant Brr2 ATPase activity – not helicase activity – as it is well documented in the DNA helicase field that assays measuring helicase activity are exceptionally susceptible to false positivity arising from interactions of small molecules with the DNA substrate [142]. An additional advantage of the ATPase tactic is that it affords an opportunity for focused library screening around kinase inhibitors. Indeed, it has been posited that the splicing activity of **staurosporine** (a nonselective kinase inhibitor) in *yeast* may be due to RNA helicase ATPase inhibition [143].

7.3.5 Drugging the Spliceosome

An assortment of small molecules has been found to inhibit spliceosome assembly: **Madrasin**, discovered in 2014, appeared to stall assembly at complex A [144], and **isoginkgetin** was reported in 2008 to interfere with recruitment of the U4/U5/U6 tri-snRNP complex, resulting in complex A accumulation (Figure 7.18) [145]. The mechanisms of these and other compounds are not well understood, but direct interaction with the spliceosome is unlikely for most. For example, quinone-containing inhibitors – e.g. **NSC659999** – and other redox-active small molecules indirectly inhibit assembly through reactive oxygen species [146, 147]. Compound-induced oxidative stress has also been implicated in inhibition of splicing catalysis (**BN82685**, Figure 7.18) [148]. Nevertheless, there exist well-characterized small molecules that specifically target the spliceosome, and they represent the most successful modulators of pre-mRNA splicing to-date, with multiple disclosed clinical agents and one FDA-approved drug as of 2023.

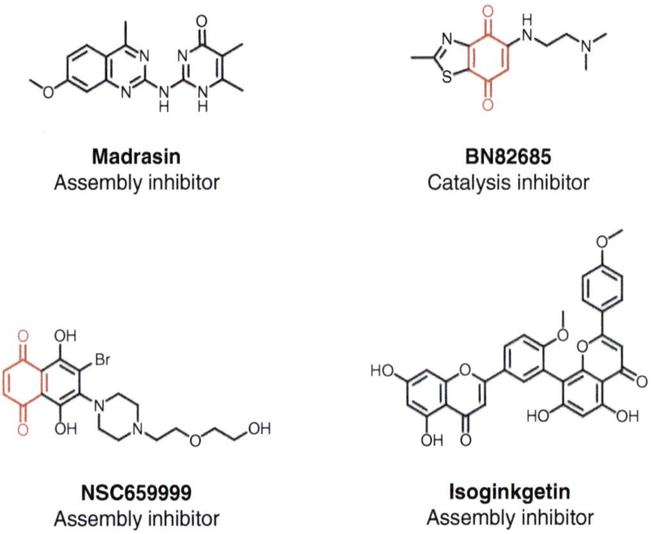

Figure 7.18 Examples of spliceosome assembly and splicing catalysis inhibitors. Redox-active quinone functionality highlighted in red.

7.3.5.1 Inhibition of U2 snRNP Recognition of the 3′-Splice Site

The first spliceosome-directed splicing modulator was discovered in 1996 but was not recognized as such until 2007 – **FR901464**, a natural secondary metabolite isolated from bacteria [149]. This was followed by **herboxidiene** in 2002 and **spliceostatin A** in 2007 [150, 151], and today many families are known, including the **meayamycins**, **sudemycins**, **thailanstatins**, and **pladienolides** (Figure 7.19) [152–154]. All of these compounds bind the interface of SF3B1 and PHF5A – two protein components of U2 snRNP – in a pocket that recognizes the branch point adenosine and facilitates recruitment of U2 snRNP to the pre-mRNA [155]. Compound binding simultaneously locks SF3B1 in an inactive conformation and physically blocks pre-mRNA binding, arresting early spliceosome assembly [153, 156–158].

7.3.5.2 E7107

The first recognized small-molecule splicing modulator to enter clinical trials was the SF3B1 inhibitor **E7107**, a semi-synthetic macrolide derived from the pladienolide family of secondary metabolites (Figure 7.20) noted for potent antitumor activities [159–162]. In 2007, **E7107** entered two Phase I, open-label, single-arm clinical trials for patients with solid tumors. The decision to pursue cancer indications was based not only on the excellent growth inhibition potency of **E7107** but also on selectivity for cancer cells over normal cells. The mechanistic basis of this preferential killing is still not fully understood, but several hypotheses have been proposed. First, many cancers suffer function-compromising spliceosomal mutations that render them exceptionally dependent on remaining wild-type spliceosomes [163]. Second, SF3B1 splicing modulators suppress expression of some tumorigenic genes and enhance expression of apoptotic factors; sudemycin, for example, inhibits *MDM2* oncogene expression via exon skipping [152, 164].

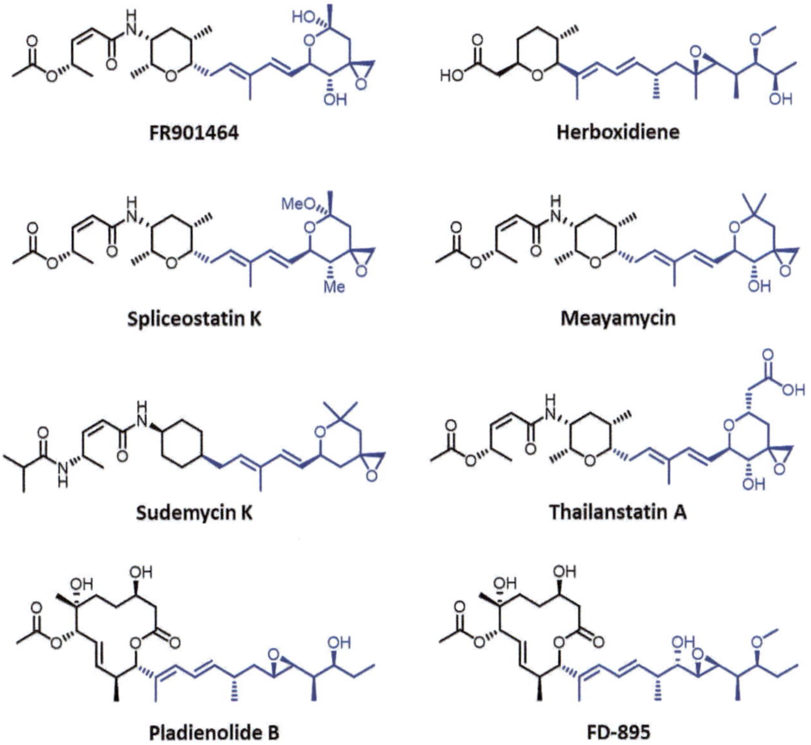

Figure 7.19 Examples of SF3B1 inhibitors. The shared pharmacophore (polyketide tail) is colored blue.

Finally, this compound class has been shown to enhance immune response to cancer cells through several mechanisms, including (i) expression of immunogenic alternatively spliced neoantigens and (ii) activation of antiviral signaling due to accumulation of mis-spliced double-stranded RNA [165, 166]. Unfortunately, **E7107** human trials were discontinued in 2009 due to dose-limiting adverse events [167], but interest in pladienolide-derived splicing modulators continued. In 2010, Eisai established H3 Biomedicine, who developed a remarkable successor to **E7107** called **H3B-8800** (Figure 7.20).

7.3.5.3 H3B-8800

The most notable feature distinguishing **H3B-8800** from **E7107** is the tail, which is distinctly synthetic in the former. All natural SF3B1 splicing modulators share a highly variable polyketide "tail" pharmacophore, excision of which affords analogs completely lacking in binding affinity, cytotoxic activity, and splicing ability (Figure 7.19) [168, 169]. The tolerance for diversely substituted tails is consistent with cryo-EM models in which the tail is disordered and solvent exposed, particularly near the tip (Figure 7.21); even the conspicuous oxirane is an unreactive and dispensable component [170]. However, all SF3B1 inhibitors require a notably conserved diene; consistent with this, **H3B-8800** retains the diene but substitutes

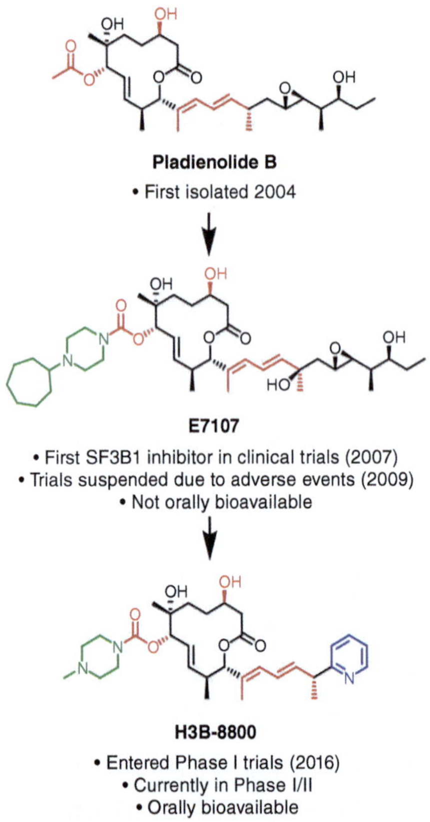

Figure 7.20 Development and evolution of pladienolide-derived SF3B1 inhibitors. Critical pharmacophore features (red); potency-enhancing substitutions colored (green); feature essential for sequence-specificity/gene selectivity (blue).

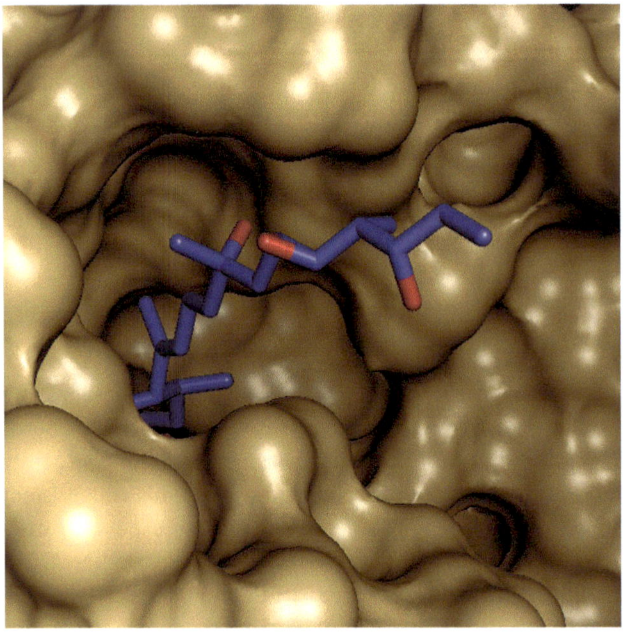

Figure 7.21 Cryo-EM model of E7107 bound to a SF3B1-PHF5A complex. Solvent-exposed polyketide tail depicted. PDB code 5ZYA.

the lenient tail tip with pyridine. H3 Biomedicine has not explicitly disclosed the reason for this substitution, but one explanation may be stability as many naturally occurring pladienolides are susceptible to tail-promoted enolide hydrolysis [171]. However – whatever the original reason – the pyridyl tail was discovered to confer sequence specificity toward weak branch points (i.e. weak splicing events), rendering **H3B-8800** a more selective (and potentially safer) splicing modulator than **E7107**.

In a panel of variable-3′ss minigenes, **H3B-8800** not only enhanced intron retention at weak 3′-splice sites relative to **E7107** but it also exhibited reduced splicing activity at canonical sites (Table 7.1) [172]. Transcriptome-wide RNA-sequencing revealed that weak branch point preference was not the only factor contributing to **H3B-8800**'s selectivity; retained introns were generally (i) short, (ii) GC-rich at the 3′-ss, and (iii) adjacent to a GC-enriched exon. (In contrast, the spliceosome itself conventionally prefers long introns with pronounced differences between intron and exon GC content.) [173] These properties of **H3B-8800** were manifest in cellular and mouse xenograft models, where it preferentially killed cancer lines carrying splicing mutations over wildtype cells; **E7107**, on the other hand, killed both cell lines equally.

Table 7.1 Splicing selectivity and sequence specificity of **H3B-8800** vs. **E7107**. Splicing was measured in HeLa nuclear extracts.

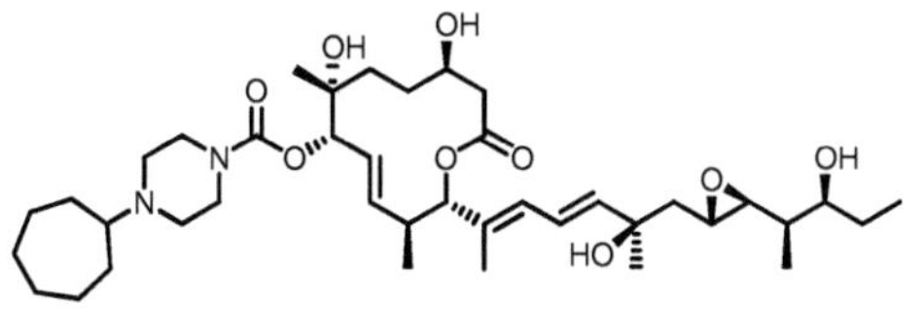

E7107

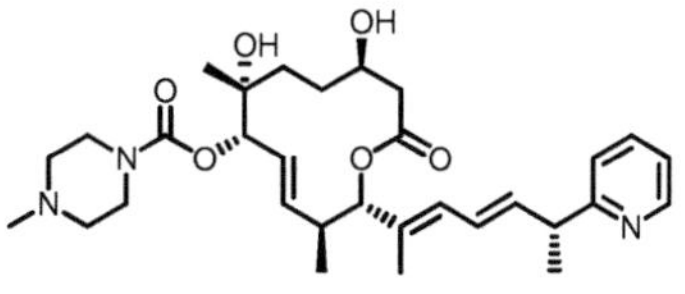

H3B-8800

Ad2[a)]	BPS[b)c)]	PYT[d)]	3′ss Type	E7107 IC_{50} (nM)	H3B-8800 IC_{50} (nM)
Ad2.1	UACU**AA**UCC	CCCUUUUUUUUCCA	Strong	9.1	>25,000
Ad2.2	UACU**AC**UC**A**	CCCUUUUUUUUCCA	Weak	9.9	NA
Ad2.14	UA**C**UU**A**UCC	CCCUUUUUCCCCCA	Strong	12.2	1,000
Ad2.17	UA**G**UU**A**UCC	CCCUUUUUCCCCCA	Weak	4.7	30
Ad2.12	UA**C**UU**A**UCC	CCCCCCCCCCCCCA	Strong	3.8	1,838
Ad2.15	UA**G**UU**A**UCC	CCCCCCCCCCCCCA	Weak	4.8	55
Ad2.13	UA**C**UU**A**UCC	CCCCCCCCCCCCCA	Strong	5.1	347.2
Ad2.16	UA**G**UU**A**UCC	CCCCCCCCUUUUUA	Weak	3	37.3

a) Adenovirus Ad2-derived mini-mRNA.
b) BPS, branch point sequence.
c) Branch point adenosine is bold and underlined, while noncanonical point mutation is bold only.
d) PYT, polypyrimidine tract.
Source: Adapted from Buonamici et al. [172]

In 2016, **H3B-8800** entered open-label Phase I clinical studies in patients with myeloid and myelomonocytic leukemias, and, in stark contrast to **E7107**, presented no to mild adverse effects. Although clinical responses did not meet threshold criteria (despite the presence of splicing mutations in 88% of the enrolled patients), the results helped identify potentially responsive patients for future studies. In 2022, **H3B-8800** was expanded into Phase II for a select patient cohort, where it remains under parallel assessment with the ongoing Phase I study. These achievements teach that (i) it is possible to develop sequence-specific, gene-selective splicing modulators and (ii) these selectivity properties are critical to drug safety.

7.3.5.4 Stabilizers of U1 snRNP Recognition of the 5′-Splice Site

The most lucrative class of spliceosome splicing modulators are the U1 snRNP stabilizers, which promote splicing by strengthening the interaction of U1 snRNP with weak, noncanonical 5′-splice sites (Figures 7.22 and 7.23). Examples include (i) PTC Therapeutic's and Hoffman-La Roche's **risdiplam** – Evrysdi® – the first FDA-approved small-molecule splicing modulator, indicated for SMA; (2) Novartis' **branaplam** – a clinical agent which achieved Phase II clinical trials for SMA and Huntington's disease; and (3) PTC Therapeutic's **PTC518** – an undisclosed agent in Phase II clinical trials for Huntington's disease.

Both **risdiplam** and **branaplam** were discovered during target-agnostic high-throughput screening for *SMN2* splicing modulators; consequently, their mechanisms of action were initially unknown [174, 175]. Evidence for U1 snRNP/5′ss stabilization was first inferred from RNA-seq, in which *SMN2* exon 7-like 5′ss sequences were observed enriched among modulated genes [176]. Both compounds favor weak, noncanonical −2G/−1A 5′ss (the canonical 5′ss is −2A/−1G, Figure 7.23b), and it has been proposed on the basis of NMR modeling that this specificity results from compound-mediated stabilization of a bulged register; the noncanonical U1 snRNA/pre-mRNA duplex is deformed by base-pair exclusion of −1A, a situation rectified by compound binding (Figure 7.24) [177]. Interestingly, despite ostensibly similar splicing profiles, deeper inspection revealed that the two compounds in fact selectively influence different gene subpopulations. To explain this, Allain et al. proposed a two-site binding model in which **risdiplam**'s selectivity arises from a dual requirement for both a *cis*-regulatory ESE sequence and an *SMN2*-like 5′ss, whereas **branaplam**'s only precondition is the latter [178]. However, comprehensive whole-genome RNA-seq investigations from PTC Therapeutics discerned discrete sequence specificities at the 5′ss itself: (i) **risdiplam** exhibits an additional pronounced preference for −4A (Figure 7.23c), (ii) but **branaplam** has a strong preference for −3A (Figure 7.23d) [179]. Unfortunately, the molecular etiology underlying these specificities is as yet unknown.

7.3.5.5 Introduction to Spinal Muscular Atrophy (SMA)

SMA is an often-lethal genetic disorder affecting 1 in 10,000 live births in the United States and 1 in 100,000 worldwide [180]. It is caused by mutation-linked loss of function of the *SMN1* gene and consequent deficiency of the protein SMN (*survival of motor neurons*), which normally mediates the assembly and biogenesis

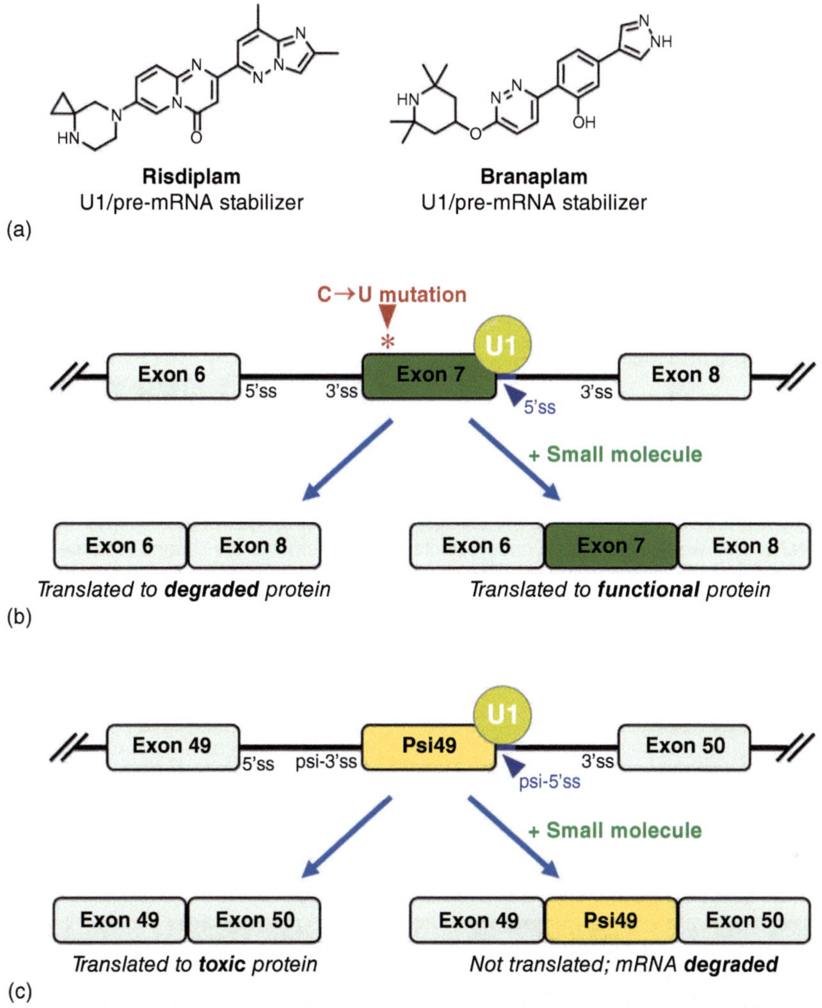

Figure 7.22 (a) Structures of **risdiplam** and **branaplam.** (b) Illustration of SMN2 alternative splicing. A single C-to-U mutation promotes exon 7 skipping. The Δ7 isoform mRNA encodes SMN protein that is rapidly degraded. The full-length isoform mRNA encodes stable, functional SMN protein. (c) Illustration of HTT-induced splicing. Small-molecule stabilization of U1 snRNP and pre-mRNA at pseudo-5′ss promotes inclusion of a pseudoexon, psi49. The inclusion mRNA is rapidly degraded by nonsense-mediated decay.

of nuclear ribonucleoproteins [181, 182]. SMA is categorized by severity from most severe (Type 0, prenatal) to least (Type IV, adult) and is defined by the age of symptom onset. Type I is the most prevalent (~60%); diagnosed within the first six months of birth, it is marked by a survival probability of 18% by 20 years of age [183]. Symptoms include neurodegeneration and loss of muscle function, including muscles that regulate essential functions like breathing.

Most humans have two to three copies of a homologous gene called *SMN2* that could compensate for the loss of *SMN1* if not for one flaw: a single C-to-U nucleotide

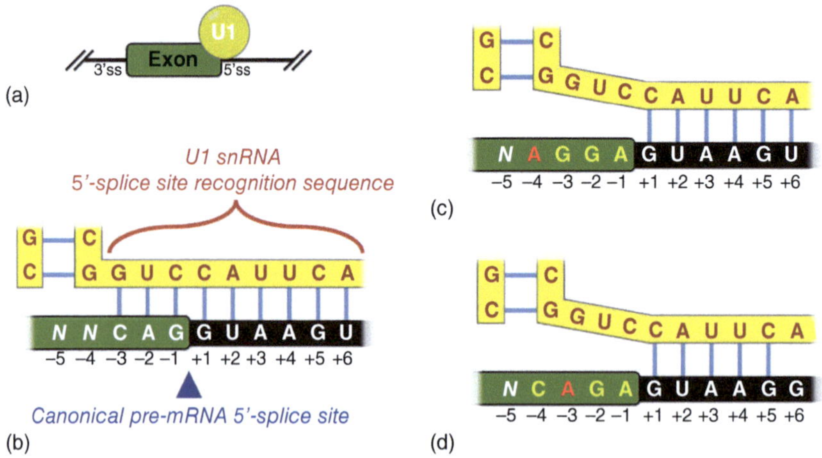

Figure 7.23 (a) Illustration of U1 snRNP interacting with the 5′-splice site. (b) The snRNA component of U1 snRNP recognizes the conserved 5′ss via a complementary sequence. (c) SMN2 exon 7 weak 5′ss; several exonic nucleotides differ from the canonical sequence. **Risdiplam** exhibits a strong preference for −4A (red). (d) HTT exon pseudoexon 49 weak 5′ss; exonic nucleotides differ from the canonical sequence. **Branaplam** displays a strong preference for −3A (red).

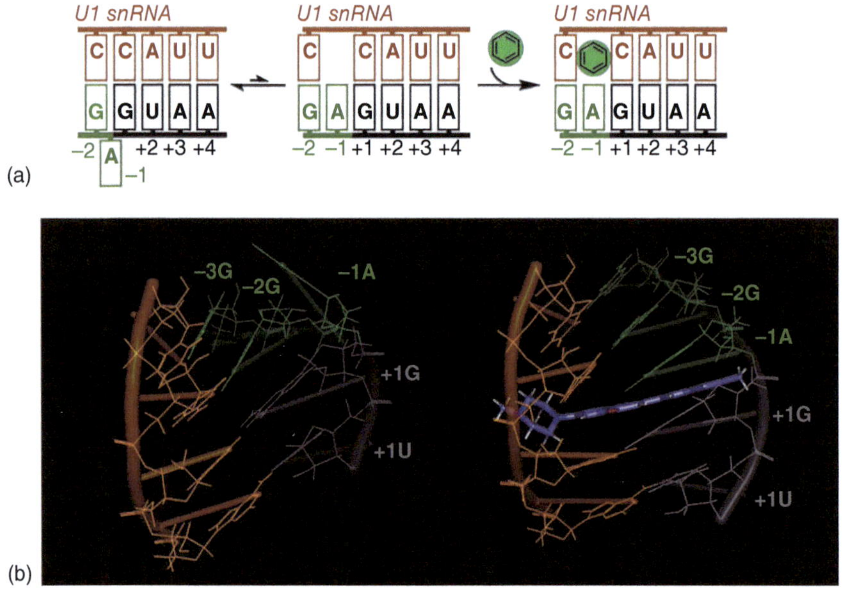

Figure 7.24 SMN2 weak 5′ss stabilization model. (a) −1A adenosine bulges out of register due to absence of a complementary base (PDB: 6HMI); **risdiplam** binds the U1 snRNA/pre-mRNA interface to permit −1A incorporation (PDB: 6HMO).

difference near the 3′ss of exon 7 (Figure 7.22b). This point mutation renders *SMN2* pre-mRNA susceptible to exon 7 skipping, resulting in translation of an unstable, truncated SMN protein [184]. However, the *SMN2* gene is not completely disabled, and low level inclusion produces a small quantity of full-length SMN. Clearly, there is some degree of spliceosome recognition, and 1990s researchers recognized the opportunity this presented – that splicing might be rescued by small molecules capable of strengthening the existing interaction between the spliceosome and *SMN2* pre-mRNA [185]. A burst of SMN splicing modulators were reported between 2001 and 2010, but few were drug-like and none were particularly potent [186–192].

With the underwhelming performance of small molecules, this was a popular time for anti-sense oligonucleotides (ASOs) [193–195]. Though optimization can be complicated, ASO design is conceptually straightforward: (i) identify a pre-mRNA sequence and (ii) synthesize a complementary ASO. Although there are several mechanisms through which ASOs may alter splicing, the most popular approach to *SMN2* involved physically blocking splicing suppressor *cis*-regulatory sequences. Many varieties featuring stabilized carbohydrate backbones were developed; Krainer et al., for example, spearheaded ASOs that obstructed binding of hnRNPs A1 and A2 to splicing silencer sequences in *SMN2* intron 7 [196]. These efforts would culminate in 2016 in the FDA approval of Biogen and Ionis Pharmaceutical's nusinersen (Spinraza®) for the treatment of SMA [197]. However, ASOs have several disadvantages compared to small molecules. First, they are generally not orally bioavailable; nusinersen, for instance, is administered to the central nervous system by intrathecal injection into the spine (known also as a lumbar puncture or spinal tap) [198]. Second, they do not exhibit the same broad systemic distribution of small molecules; ASOs delivered to the central nervous system do not readily proportionate to peripheral tissues (and vice versa), which is of consequence to diseases like SMA that suffer both central and peripheral neurodegeneration [199].

7.3.5.6 Risdiplam (Evrysdi®)

Attentive to ASO deficiencies in the treatment of SMA, PTC Therapeutics launched a discovery program in 2007 to identify and develop small-molecule splicing modulators with support from the SMA Foundation. Aiming for (i) excellent signal-to-noise and (ii) dynamic range for the detection of weak hits, a target-agnostic minigene-based reporter assay was developed suitable for high-throughput screening [175]. The minigene contained all of *SMN2* exon 7, downsized exons 6 and 8, and a firefly luciferase region (Figure 7.25). Exon 7 skipping afforded an out-of-frame sequence and therefore no translation of the luciferase reporter, whereas exon 7 inclusion produced an in-frame luciferase gene encoding photocatalytically competent luciferase. However, firefly luciferase reporters suffer a well-documented susceptibility to false positivity, so a quantitative PCR (qPCR) analysis of minigene transcripts was incorporated into the screening triage [200].

>200,000 compounds were screened and the weak hit **21** was identified and confirmed, after which hit expansion quickly established a strict requirement for a basic amine, although no structural or mechanistic insight was yet available at the time, this is consistent with NMR models in which the amine is

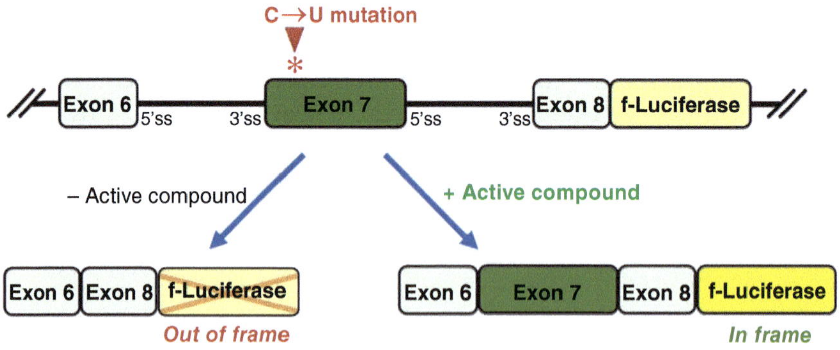

Figure 7.25 SMN2 minigene construct for high-throughput screening.

observed near the negatively charged phosphate backbone (Figure 7.24b). Major development milestones are illustrated in Figure 7.26. Lead optimization was primarily driven by minigene assay qPCR quantitation, but – as compound potency improved – an HTRF-based assay was included to assess full-length SMN protein in disease-relevant cells.

Select compounds were promoted into advanced studies to determine their functional disposition. Motor neuron cultures (prepared from SMA patient-derived induced pluripotent stem cells – IPSCs) produced >2-fold more protein when treated with **RG7800** ($EC_{1.5x}^{mini}$ = 23 nM, $EC_{1.5X}^{SMN}$ = 87 nM) and >3-fold more full-length SMN from an SMA mouse model following oral administration [201]. Importantly, increased protein was apparent in both CNS and peripheral tissue as expected from a broadly distributable small molecule. Cross-section immunohistological assessment of SMA mouse muscle and spine revealed dose-dependent arrest of both neurodegeneration and muscle atrophy. It is particularly noteworthy that while SMA model mice do not typically survive beyond 20 days after birth, once-daily **RG7800** administration enhanced survival and fitness such that the animals were nearly indistinguishable from healthy wild-type mice.

By this time, PTC Therapeutics and Hoffmann-La Roche were collaboratively joined and together launched **RG7800** into human clinical trials in 2014, where it demonstrated a clinically significant increase of full-length SMN in SMA patients [202]. Unfortunately, **RG7800** was discontinued due to unacceptable risks, including (i) hERG inhibition, (ii) phospholipidosis, and (iii) photoxicity. However, these specific events were not inherent to splicing activity, although scaffold hopping programs were ultimately unsuccessful, **RG7800** itself proved receptive to physicochemical tuning [203]. Incorporation of a cyclopropyl group sufficiently lowered amine pKa such that hERG inhibition and phospholipidosis were simultaneously eliminated (but not so low that potency was impaired), and substitution of 2-pyrazolpyrazine with 6-imidazopyridazine cleared phototoxicity risk (Figure 7.26). This new compound, **risdiplam** ($EC_{1.5x}^{mini}$ = 4 nM, $EC_{1.5X}^{SMN}$ = 29 nM), entered clinical trials in 2015 and exited in 2020 as the FDA-approved Evrysdi®.

It is noteworthy that **risdiplam** continues to exhibit outstanding long-term clinical safety [204–206]. This has been attributed in part to its sequence specificity

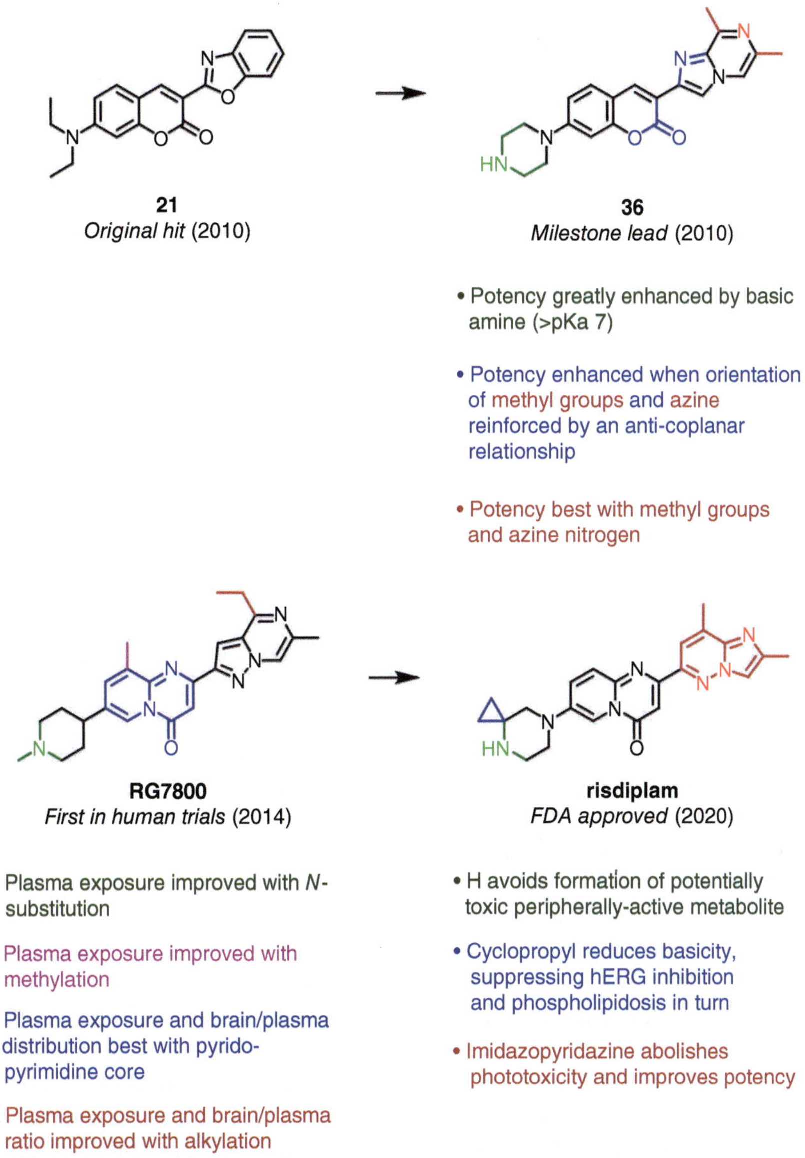

21
Original hit (2010)
36
Milestone lead (2010)
• Potency greatly enhanced by basic amine (>pKa 7)
• Potency enhanced when orientation of methyl groups and azine reinforced by an anti-coplanar relationship
• Potency best with methyl groups and azine nitrogen
RG7800
First in human trials (2014)
risdiplam
FDA approved (2020)
• Plasma exposure improved with N-substitution
• Plasma exposure improved with methylation
• Plasma exposure and brain/plasma distribution best with pyrido-pyrimidine core
• Plasma exposure and brain/plasma ratio improved with alkylation
• H avoids formation of potentially toxic peripherally-active metabolite
• Cyclopropyl reduces basicity, suppressing hERG inhibition and phospholipidosis in turn
• Imidazopyridazine abolishes phototoxicity and improves potency

Figure 7.26 Development evolution of risdiplam. Major structure–activity, structure–toxicity, and structure–pharmacokinetic relationships highlighted.

for noncanonical −2G/−1A 5′-splice sites – which enforces an inherent limitation on the number of potential on-mechanism/off-target splicing events – and the fact that *SMN2* is the most responsive gene to **risdiplam** treatment. However, toxicity is evident at *high* doses in animals – an observation around which two competing interpretations have evolved. The first claims toxicity is a consequence of compound-induced splicing of specific key regulatory genes (e.g. FOXM1 and MADD) [207], whereas the second ascribes toxicity to the absolute number of genes dysregulated at a given concentration (i.e. the "splicing burden") [208]. At this time, however, no systematic study exists that resolves these perspectives or provides conclusive guidance on the topic of splicing-related toxicity in the design of future splicing modulators.

Ultimately, **risdiplam** teaches that (i) the genesis of new programs may still be found in target-agnostic high-throughput screening and (ii) medicinal chemists may continue to rely on their traditional phenotypic tools of the art; detailed mechanistic insight is not required. Perhaps most importantly, **risdiplam's** approval is validation that therapeutic manipulation of splicing can be a safe and effective strategy in the correction of human disease.

7.4 Future Outlook

It should be evident that not all mechanisms of pre-mRNA splicing modulation are equal, and that some present greater challenges than others. However, the discovery and development of small-molecule splicing modulators has unmistakably matured since the crude seminal demonstrations of the 1990s – from weak and nonselective kinase inhibitors to potent and selective spliceosome modulators. Where then is splicing modulation heading? What new technologies will enable small-molecule discovery?

Until very recently, splicing drug discovery was focused on modulation of naturally regulated exons and introns, but considerable activity is now concentrated in the development of small-molecule inducers of unnatural *pseudoexons* – intronic sequences not normally found in mRNA despite ostensible possession of requisite splicing features (Figure 7.3). Among the different types of pseudoexons, those that introduce premature stop codons (PTCs) into mRNA are of greatest interest because PTC-containing mRNAs are susceptible to degradation through a protective cellular process called NMD (Figures 7.27a,b) [209, 210]. Therefore, small-molecule promoters of PTC pseudoexon inclusion are expected to downregulate target gene expression. An example leveraging this mechanism can be found in PTC Therapeutic's Huntington Disease program, for which their clinical candidate **PTC518** is undergoing Phase II trials. Huntington disease is a nucleotide repeat disorder originating from a $(CAG)_n$ triplet repeat expansion in exon 1 of the *HTT* gene because this mutant *HTT* encodes a toxic protein that accounts for much of the pathology, it is beneficial to minimize its expression [211, 212]. In 2021, researchers at PTC Therapeutics demonstrated that pseudoexons handicapped by noncanonical 5′ss sequences but otherwise resembling true exons could be activated by complementary variant U1 snRNAs, allowing the researchers to map potentially druggable targets in the genome [179]. Among these, a PTC-containing pseudoexon in *HTT* intron 49 was discovered whose inclusion (i) was induced by branaplam- and risdiplam-type splicing modulators and (ii) lead to *HTT* mRNA degradation and – most importantly – therapeutically meaningful *in vivo* protein reduction (Figure 7.27c). Since then, many new companies platformed on inducible pseudoexon alternative splicing have emerged [213], and although outlook is optimistic,

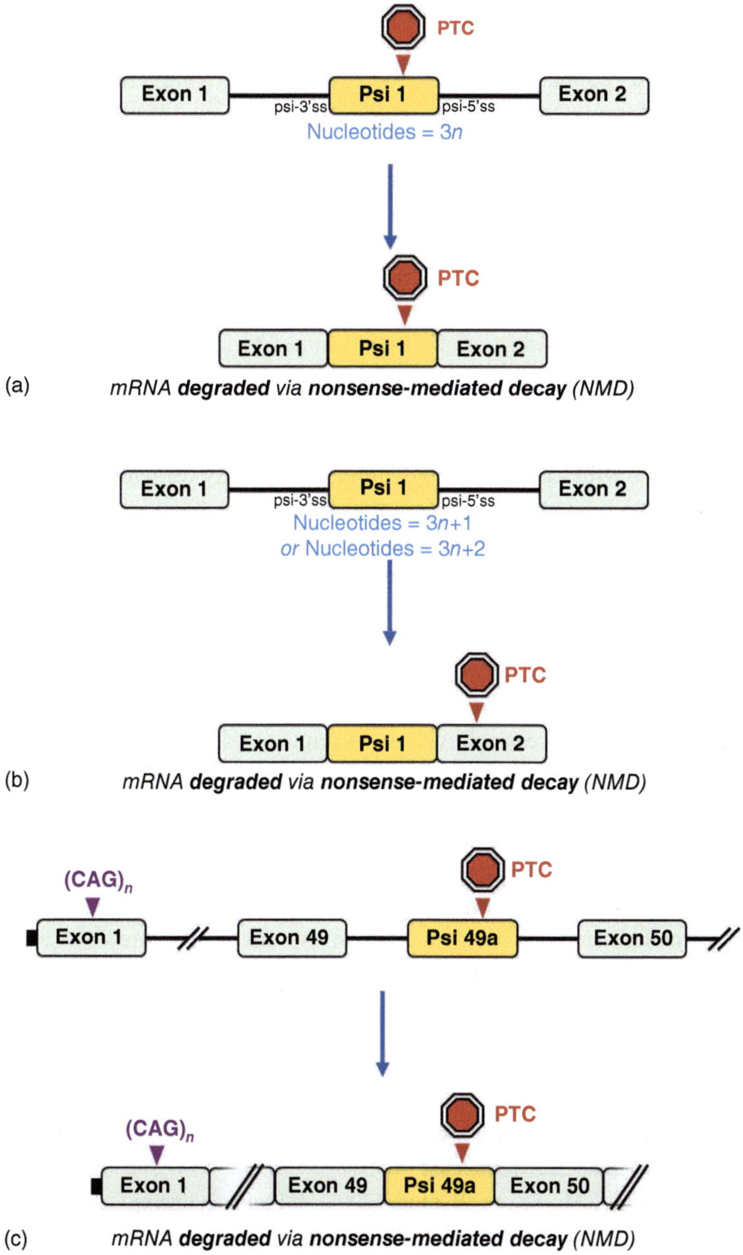

Figure 7.27 Two common modes of pseudoexon-induced nonsense-mediated decay. (a) The pseudoexon can contain a premature stop codon (PTC); (b) pseudoexon sequences composed of a number of nucleotides not divisible by three ($nt = 3n+1$, $nt = 3n+2$) may introduce premature stop codons due to frameshift of downstream exons; (c) compound-induced inclusion of pseudoexon 49a in the $(CAG)_n$ mutant HTT gene introduces a premature stop codon into the final mRNA transcript, which is then degraded through nonsense-mediated decay.

it must be said that the state of the art is currently restricted to noncanonical 5′-ss pseudoexons and derivatives of branaplam and risdiplam [214, 215].

Another area of exceptional interest is the design of RNA-targeted focused libraries composed of compounds complementary to the unique physicochemical properties of RNA [216–218]. Evidence supporting this strategy is illustrated by Pfizer's discovery of CD33 splicing modulators [219]. CD33 is a protein for which exon 2 skipping affords a beneficial variant associated with protection in late-onset Alzheimer's disease. Seeking small-molecule effectors of CD33 pre-mRNA alternative splicing, the company screened >3 million compounds and uncovered a cluster of hits originating from an older (albeit nonsplicing) RNA-targeting program [220, 221]. These compounds were originally optimized to inhibit translation of PCSK9 – a protein regulator of plasma cholesterol levels – by binding a ribosomal RNA–protein interface [177, 222, 223]. Although the mechanism of CD33 exon 2 skipping remains unreported, it is nonetheless remarkable that among millions of compounds, only those with established RNA-interacting ability were identified as developable splicing modulators.

Finally, the application of RNA sequencing (RNA-seq) to small-molecule discovery finds alluring prospect. Originally developed in 2007 for the analysis of differential gene expression, RNA-seq provides a multidimensional, high-content strategy for screening chemical libraries. A major disadvantage, however, is price. Although much more affordable now than 15 years ago, the technique still demands costs-per-compound well above traditional high-throughput screening, but recent adaptations have improved accessibility. For example, RASL-seq is a focused technique with excellent sensitivity but limited gene coverage [224, 225], BRB-seq and Tru-seq reduce the number of sequencing analyses through use of barcoding strategies that permit unambiguous deconvolution of multiplexed samples [226], and Novartis' DRUG-seq is a higher throughput modification of BRB-seq that obviates the need for RNA purification [227, 228]. Although these unconventional screening platforms have not yet been reported in the discovery of new splicing modulators, they are auspicious portents of an exciting and innovative future.

References

1 Venter, J.C., Adams, M.D., Myers, E.W. et al. (2001). The sequence of the human genome. *Science* 291: 1304–1351.
2 Lander, E.S., Linton, L.M., Birren, B. et al. (2001). Initial sequencing and analysis of the human genome. *Nature* 409: 860–921.
3 Ezkurdia, I., Juan, D., Rodriguez, J.M. et al. (2014). Multiple evidence strands suggest that there may be as few as 19 000 human protein-coding genes. *Hum. Mol. Genet.* 23: 5866–5878.
4 Pertea, M. and Salzberg, S.L. (2010). Between a chicken and a grape: estimating the number of human genes. *Genome Biol.* 11: 206.
5 Berget, S.M., Moore, C., and Sharp, P.A. (1977). Spliced segments at the 5′ terminus of adenovirus 2 late mRNA*. *Proc. Natl. Acad. Sci. U.S.A.* 74: 3171–3175.

6 Dang, C.V., Reddy, E.P., Shokat, K.M., and Soucek, L. (2017). Drugging the 'undruggable' cancer targets. *Nat. Rev. Cancer* 17: 502–508.

7 Zhang, G., Zhang, J., Gao, Y. et al. (2022). Strategies for targeting undruggable targets. *Expert Opin. Drug Discovery* 17: 55–69.

8 Mayeda, A., Hayase, Y., Inoue, H. et al. (1990). Surveying cis-acting sequences of pre-mRNA by adding antisense 2′-O-methyl oligoribonucleotides to a splicing reaction. *J. Biochem.* 108: 399–405.

9 Munroe, S.H. (1988). Antisense RNA inhibits splicing of pre-mRNA in vitro. *EMBO J.* 7: 2523–2532.

10 Ruskin, B. and Green, M.R. (1985). Specific and stable intron-factor interactions are established early during in vitro pre-mRNA splicing. *Cell* 43: 131–142.

11 Neil, E.E. and Bisaccia, E.K. (2019). Nusinersen: a novel antisense oligonucleotide for the treatment of spinal muscular atrophy. *J. Pediatr. Pharmacol. Therap.* 24: 194–203.

12 Harbers, M. and Hilz, H. (1991). Suppression of c-fos precursor RNA splicing by the protein kinase C inhibitor H7 [1-(5-isoquinolinesulphonyl)-2-methylpiperazine]. *Biochem. J.* 278: 305–308.

13 Mermoud, J.E., Cohen, P., and Lamond, A.I. (1992). Ser/Thr-specific protein phosphatases are required for both catalytic steps of pre-mRNA splicing. *Nucleic Acids Res.* 20: 5263–5269.

14 Will, C.L. and Lührmann, R. (2005). Splicing of a rare class of introns by the U12-dependent spliceosome. *Biol. Chem.* 386: 713–724.

15 Patel, A.A. and Steitz, J.A. (2003). Splicing double: insights from the second spliceosome. *Nat. Rev. Mol. Cell Biol.* 4: 960–970.

16 Patel, A.A., McCarthy, M., and Steitz, J.A. (2002). The splicing of U12-type introns can be a rate-limiting step in gene expression. *Embo J.* 21: 3804–3815.

17 König, H., Matter, N., Bader, R. et al. (2007). Splicing segregation: the minor spliceosome acts outside the nucleus and controls cell proliferation. *Cell* 131: 718–729.

18 Pessa, H.K.J., Will, C.L., Meng, X. et al. (2008). Minor spliceosome components are predominantly localized in the nucleus. *Proc. Natl. Acad. Sci. U.S.A* 105: 8655–8660.

19 Turunen, J.J., Niemelä, E.H., Verma, B., and Frilander, M.J. (2013). The significant other: splicing by the minor spliceosome. *WIREs RNA* 4: 61–76.

20 Jutzi, D., Akinyi, M.V., Mechtersheimer, J. et al. (2018). The emerging role of minor intron splicing in neurological disorders. *Cell Stress* 2: 40–54.

21 Lee, K., Tirasophon, W., Shen, X. et al. (2002). IRE1-mediated unconventional mRNA splicing and S2P-mediated ATF6 cleavage merge to regulate XBP1 in signaling the unfolded protein response. *Genes Dev.* 16: 452–466.

22 Boutz, P.L., Bhutkar, A., and Sharp, P.A. (2015). Detained introns are a novel, widespread class of post-transcriptionally spliced introns. *Genes Dev.* 29: 63–80.

23 Zhang, C., Li, W.-H., Krainer, A.R., and Zhang, M.Q. (2008). RNA landscape of evolution for optimal exon and intron discrimination. *Proc. Natl. Acad. Sci. U.S.A* 105: 5797–5802.

24 Ibrahim, E.C., Schaal, T.D., Hertel, K.J. et al. (2005). Serine/arginine-rich protein-dependent suppression of exon skipping by exonic splicing enhancers. *PNAS* 102: 5002–5007.

25 Busch, A. and Hertel, K.J. (2012). Evolution of SR protein and hnRNP splicing regulatory factors. *WIREs RNA* 3: 1–12.

26 Graveley, B.R. (2000). Sorting out the complexity of SR protein functions. *RNA* 6: 1197–1211.

27 Huelga, S.C., Vu, A.Q., Arnold, J.D. et al. (2012). Integrative genome-wide analysis reveals cooperative regulation of alternative splicing by hnRNP proteins. *Cell Rep.* 1: 167–178.

28 Perry, P.J. and Kelland, L.R. (1998). Telomeres and telomerase: targets for cancer chemotherapy? *Expert Opin. Ther. Pat.* 8: 1567–1586.

29 Rezler, E.M., Bearss, D.J., and Hurley, L.H. (2002). Telomeres and telomerases as drug targets. *Curr. Opin. Pharmacol.* 2: 415–423.

30 Read, M., Harrison, R.J., Romagnoli, B. et al. (2001). Structure-based design of selective and potent G quadruplex-mediated telomerase inhibitors. *Proc. Natl. Acad. Sci. U.S.A.* 98: 4844–4849.

31 Perry, P.J., Reszka, A.P., Wood, A.A. et al. (1998). Human telomerase inhibition by regioisomeric disubstituted amidoanthracene-9,10-diones. *J. Med. Chem.* 41: 4873–4884.

32 Perry, P.J., Gowan, S.M., Reszka, A.P. et al. (1998). 1,4- and 2,6-disubstituted amidoanthracene-9,10-dione derivatives as inhibitors of human telomerase. *J. Med. Chem.* 41: 3253–3260.

33 Ludlow, A.T., Slusher, A.L., and Sayed, M.E. (2019). Insights into telomerase/hTERT alternative splicing regulation using bioinformatics and network analysis in cancer. *Cancers (Basel)* 11.

34 Gomez, D., Lemarteleur, T., Lacroix, L. et al. (2004). Telomerase downregulation induced by the G-quadruplex ligand 12459 in A549 cells is mediated by hTERT RNA alternative splicing. *Nucleic Acids Res.* 32: 371–379.

35 Moye, A.L., Porter, K.C., Cohen, S.B. et al. (2015). Telomeric G-quadruplexes are a substrate and site of localization for human telomerase. *Nat. Commun.* 6: 7643.

36 Han, H., Cliff, C.L., and Hurley, L.H. (1999). Accelerated assembly of G-quadruplex structures by a small molecule. *Biochemistry* 38: 6981–6986.

37 von Bergen, M., Barghorn, S., Li, L. et al. (2001). Mutations of tau protein in frontotemporal dementia promote aggregation of paired helical filaments by enhancing local β-structure*. *J. Biol. Chem.* 276: 48165–48174.

38 VandeVrede, L., Ljubenkov, P.A., Rojas, J.C. et al. (2020). Four-repeat tauopathies: current management and future treatments. *Neurotherapeutics* 17: 1563–1581.

39 Luo, Y. and Disney, M.D. (2014). Bottom-up design of small molecules that stimulate exon 10 skipping in mutant MAPT pre-mRNA. *ChemBioChem* 15: 2041–2044.

40 Chen, J.L., Zhang, P., Abe, M. et al. (2020). Design, optimization, and study of small molecules that target tau pre-mRNA and affect splicing. *JACS* 142: 8706–8727.

41 Mitteaux, J., Lejault, P., Wojciechowski, F. et al. (2021). Identifying G-quadruplex-DNA-disrupting small molecules. *JACS* 143: 12567–12577.

42 Garcia-Lopez, A., Tessaro, F., Jonker, H.R.A. et al. (2018). Targeting RNA structure in SMN2 reverses spinal muscular atrophy molecular phenotypes. *Nat. Commun.* 9: 2032.

43 Tabrizi, S.J., Flower, M.D., Ross, C.A., and Wild, E.J. (2020). Huntington disease: new insights into molecular pathogenesis and therapeutic opportunities. *Nat. Rev. Neurol.* 16: 529–546.

44 Schmidt, M.H.M. and Pearson, C.E. (2016). Disease-associated repeat instability and mismatch repair. *DNA Repair* 38: 117–126.

45 Malik, I., Kelley, C.P., Wang, E.T., and Todd, P.K. (2021). Molecular mechanisms underlying nucleotide repeat expansion disorders. *Nat. Rev. Mol. Cell Biol.* 22: 589–607.

46 Ishiguro, T., Nagai, Y., and Ishikawa, K. (2021). Insight into *Spinocerebellar Ataxia* Type 31 (SCA31) from Drosophila model. *Front. Neurosci.* 15: 648133–648133.

47 Sofola, O.A., Jin, P., Qin, Y. et al. (2007). RNA-binding proteins hnRNP A2/B1 and CUGBP1 suppress fragile X CGG premutation repeat-induced neurodegeneration in a Drosophila model of FXTAS. *Neuron* 55: 565–571.

48 Sellier, C., Rau, F., Liu, Y. et al. (2010). Sam68 sequestration and partial loss of function are associated with splicing alterations in FXTAS patients. *Embo J.* 29: 1248–1261.

49 Taylor, K., Sznajder, L.J., Cywoniuk, P. et al. (2018). MBNL splicing activity depends on RNA binding site structural context. *Nucleic Acids Res.* 46: 9119–9133.

50 Itskovich, S.S., Gurunathan, A., Clark, J. et al. (2020). MBNL1 regulates essential alternative RNA splicing patterns in MLL-rearranged leukemia. *Nat. Commun.* 11: 2369.

51 Gates, D.P., Coonrod, L.A., and Berglund, J.A. (2011). Autoregulated splicing of muscleblind-like 1 (MBNL1) pre-mRNA*. *J. Biol. Chem.* 286: 34224–34233.

52 Gibaut, Q.M.R., Akahori, Y., Bush, J.A. et al. (2022). Study of an RNA-focused DNA-encoded library informs design of a degrader of a r(CUG) repeat expansion. *JACS* .

53 D'Agostino, V.G., Sighel, D., Zucal, C. et al. (2019). Screening approaches for targeting ribonucleoprotein complexes: a new dimension for drug discovery. *SLAS Discovery* 24: 314–331.

54 Ko, C.C., Chen, Y.J., Chen, C.T. et al. (2014). Chemical proteomics identifies heterogeneous nuclear ribonucleoprotein (hnRNP) A1 as the molecular target of quercetin in its anti-cancer effects in PC-3 cells. *J. Biol. Chem.* 289: 22078–22089.

55 Tummala, R., Lou, W., Gao, A.C., and Nadiminty, N. (2017). Quercetin targets hnRNPA1 to overcome enzalutamide resistance in prostate cancer cells. *Mol. Cancer Ther.* 16: 2770–2779.

56 Lee, K.W., Kang, N.J., Heo, Y.S. et al. (2008). Raf and MEK protein kinases are direct molecular targets for the chemopreventive effect of quercetin, a major flavonol in red wine. *Cancer Res.* 68: 946–955.

57 Wang, R.E., Hunt, C.R., Chen, J., and Taylor, J.S. (2011). Biotinylated quercetin as an intrinsic photoaffinity proteomics probe for the identification of quercetin target proteins. *Bioorg. Med. Chem.* 19: 4710–4720.

58 Wiseman, R.L., Zhang, Y., Lee, K.P. et al. (2010). Flavonol activation defines an unanticipated ligand-binding site in the kinase-RNase domain of IRE1. *Mol. Cell* 38: 291–304.

59 Rakheja, I., Ansari, A.H., Ray, A. et al. (2022). Small molecule quercetin binds MALAT1 triplex and modulates its cellular function. *Mol. Ther. Nucleic Acids* 30: 241–256.

60 Gao, H., Sun, X., and Rao, Y. (2020). PROTAC technology: opportunities and challenges. *ACS Med. Chem. Lett.* 11: 237–240.

61 Owa, T., Yoshino, H., Okauchi, T. et al. (1999). Discovery of novel antitumor sulfonamides targeting G1 phase of the cell cycle. *J. Med. Chem.* 42: 3789–3799.

62 Assi, R., Kantarjian, H.M., Kadia, T.M. et al. (2018). Final results of a phase 2, open-label study of indisulam, idarubicin, and cytarabine in patients with relapsed or refractory acute myeloid leukemia and high-risk myelodysplastic syndrome. *Cancer* 124: 2758–2765.

63 Talbot, D.C., von Pawel, J., Cattell, E. et al. (2007). A randomized phase II pharmacokinetic and pharmacodynamic study of indisulam as second-line therapy in patients with advanced non–small cell lung cancer. *Clin. Cancer Res.* 13: 1816–1822.

64 Han, T., Goralski, M., Gaskill, N. et al. (2017). Anticancer sulfonamides target splicing by inducing RBM39 degradation via recruitment to DCAF15. *Science* 356: eaal3755.

65 Ting, T.C., Goralski, M., Klein, K. et al. (2019). Aryl sulfonamides degrade RBM39 and RBM23 by recruitment to CRL4-DCAF15. *Cell Rep.* 29: 1499–1510.e6.

66 Bussiere, D.E., Xie, L., Srinivas, H. et al. (2020). Structural basis of indisulam-mediated RBM39 recruitment to DCAF15 E3 ligase complex. *Nat. Chem. Biol.* 16: 15–23.

67 Domostegui, A., Nieto-Barrado, L., Perez-Lopez, C., and Mayor-Ruiz, C. (2022). Chasing molecular glue degraders: screening approaches. *Chem. Soc. Rev.* 51: 5498–5517.

68 Ghidini, A., Cléry, A., Halloy, F. et al. (2021). RNA-PROTACs: degraders of RNA-binding proteins. *Angew. Chem. Int. Ed. Engl.* 60: 3163–3169.

69 Kielkopf, C.L., Lücke, S., and Green, M.R. (2004). U2AF homology motifs: protein recognition in the RRM world. *Genes Dev.* 18: 1513–1526.

70 Bomsztyk, K., Denisenko, O., and Ostrowski, J. (2004). hnRNP K: one protein multiple processes. *Bioessays* 26: 629–638.

71 Loflin, P., Chen, C.Y., and Shyu, A.B. (1999). Unraveling a cytoplasmic role for hnRNP D in the in vivo mRNA destabilization directed by the AU-rich element. *Genes Dev.* 13: 1884–1897.

72 Chaudhury, A., Chander, P., and Howe, P.H. (2010). Heterogeneous nuclear ribonucleoproteins (hnRNPs) in cellular processes: Focus on hnRNP E1's multifunctional regulatory roles. *RNA* 16: 1449–1462.

73 Palangat, M., Anastasakis, D.G., Fei, D.L. et al. (2019). The splicing factor U2AF1 contributes to cancer progression through a noncanonical role in translation regulation. *Genes Dev.* 33: 482–497.

74 Jagtap, P.K.A., Kubelka, T., Soni, K. et al. (2020). Identification of phenothiazine derivatives as UHM-binding inhibitors of early spliceosome assembly. *Nat. Commun.* 11: 5621.

75 Loerch, S. and Kielkopf, C.L. (2016). Unmasking the U2AF homology motif family: a bona fide protein-protein interaction motif in disguise. *RNA* 22: 1795–1807.

76 Eymin, B. (2021). Targeting the spliceosome machinery: a new therapeutic axis in cancer? *Biochem. Pharmacol.* 189: 114039.

77 Chatrikhi, R., Feeney, C.F., Pulvino, M.J. et al. (2021). A synthetic small molecule stalls pre-mRNA splicing by promoting an early-stage U2AF2-RNA complex. *Cell Chem. Biol.* 28: 1145–1157.e6.

78 Rossi, F., Labourier, E., Forné, T. et al. (1996). Specific phosphorylation of SR proteins by mammalian DNA topoisomerase I. *Nature* 381: 80–82.

79 Attwood, M.M., Fabbro, D., Sokolov, A.V. et al. (2021). Trends in kinase drug discovery: targets, indications and inhibitor design. *Nat. Rev. Drug Discovery* 20: 839–861.

80 Tam, B.Y., Chiu, K., Chung, H. et al. (2020). The CLK inhibitor SM08502 induces anti-tumor activity and reduces Wnt pathway gene expression in gastrointestinal cancer models. *Cancer Lett.* 473: 186–197.

81 Bossard, C., McMillan, E.A., Creger, E. et al. (2021). The Pan-Clk/Dyrk inhibitor cirtuvivint (SM08502) exposes mechanistic underpinnings of alternative splicing as a therapeutic vulnerability in heme malignancies. *Blood* 138: 2950.

82 Aubol Brandon, E., Wozniak Jacob, M., Fattet, L. et al. (2021). CLK1 reorganizes the splicing factor U1-70K for early spliceosomal protein assembly. *Proc. Natl. Acad. Sci. U.S.A.* 118: e2018251118.

83 Schmitt, C., Miralinaghi, P., Mariano, M. et al. (2014). Hydroxybenzothiophene ketones are efficient pre-mRNA splicing modulators due to dual inhibition of Dyrk1A and Clk1/4. *ACS Med. Chem. Lett.* 5: 963–967.

84 Mathew, R., Hartmuth, K., Möhlmann, S. et al. (2008). Phosphorylation of human PRP28 by SRPK2 is required for integration of the U4/U6-U5 tri-snRNP into the spliceosome. *Nat. Struct. Mol. Biol.* 15: 435–443.

85 Dahal, S., Clayton, K., Been, T. et al. (2022). Opposing roles of CLK SR kinases in controlling HIV-1 gene expression and latency. *Retrovirology* 19: 18.

86 Bialik, S. and Kimchi, A. (2014). The DAP-kinase interactome. *Apoptosis* 19: 316–328.

87 Seo, G., Han, H., Vargas, R.E. et al. (2020). MAP4K interactome reveals STRN4 as a key STRIPAK complex component in hippo pathway regulation. *Cell Rep.* 32: 107860.

88 Lindberg, M.F. and Meijer, L. (2021). Dual-specificity, tyrosine phosphorylation-regulated kinases (DYRKs) and cdc2-like kinases (CLKs) in human disease, an overview. *Int. J. Mol. Sci.* 22.

89 Aubol, B.E., Wu, G., Keshwani, M.M. et al. (2016). Release of SR proteins from CLK1 by SRPK1: a symbiotic kinase system for phosphorylation control of pre-mRNA splicing. *Mol. Cell* 63: 218–228.

90 Prasad, J. and James, L.M. (2003). Regulation and substrate specificity of the SR protein kinase Clk/Sty. *Mol. Cell. Biol.* 23: 4139–4149.

91 Lochhead, P.A. (2009). Protein kinase activation loop autophosphorylation in cis: overcoming a Catch-22 situation. *Sci. Signaling* 2: pe4.

92 Andrianantoandro, E. (2012). How growth factors govern alternative splicing. *Sci. Signaling* 5: ec220-ec220.

93 Lochhead, P.A., Sibbet, G., Morrice, N., and Cleghon, V. (2005). Activation-loop autophosphorylation is mediated by a novel transitional intermediate form of DYRKs. *Cell* 121: 925–936.

94 Sako, Y., Ninomiya, K., Okuno, Y. et al. (2017). Development of an orally available inhibitor of CLK1 for skipping a mutated dystrophin exon in Duchenne muscular dystrophy. *Sci. Rep.* 7: 46126.

95 Uzor, S., Zorzou, P., Bowler, E. et al. (2018). Autoregulation of the human splice factor kinase CLK1 through exon skipping and intron retention. *Gene* 670: 46–54.

96 Loyer, P., Trembley, J.H., Katona, R. et al. (2005). Role of CDK/cyclin complexes in transcription and RNA splicing. *Cell. Signalling* 17: 1033–1051.

97 Saldi, T., Cortazar, M.A., Sheridan, R.M., and Bentley, D.L. (2016). Coupling of RNA polymerase II transcription elongation with pre-mRNA splicing. *J. Mol. Biol.* 428: 2623–2635.

98 Bentley, D.L. (2014). Coupling mRNA processing with transcription in time and space. *Nat. Rev. Genet.* 15: 163–175.

99 Hluchý, M., Gajdušková, P., de los Ruiz, Mozos, I. et al. (2022). CDK11 regulates pre-mRNA splicing by phosphorylation of SF3B1. *Nature* 609: 829–834.

100 Lipkin, M.J., Stevens, A.P., Livingstone, D.J., and Harris, C.J. (2008). How large does a compound screening collection need to be? *Comb. Chem. High Throughput Screening* 11: 482–493.

101 Miller, J.L. (2006). Recent developments in focused library design: targeting gene-families. *Curr. Top. Med. Chem.* 6: 19–29.

102 Shi, Y., Bray, W., Smith, A.J. et al. (2020). An exon skipping screen identifies antitumor drugs that are potent modulators of pre-mRNA splicing, suggesting new therapeutic applications. *PLoS One* 15: e0233672.

103 Shi, Y., Joyner, A.S., Shadrick, W. et al. (2015). Pharmacodynamic assays to facilitate preclinical and clinical development of pre-mRNA splicing modulatory drug candidates. *Pharmacol. Res. Perspect.* 3: e00158.

104 Yoshida, M., Kataoka, N., Miyauchi, K. et al. (2015). Rectifier of aberrant mRNA splicing recovers tRNA modification in familial dysautonomia. *PNAS* 112: 2764–2769.

105 Ajiro, M., Awaya, T., Kim, Y.J. et al. (2021). Therapeutic manipulation of IKBKAP mis-splicing with a small molecule to cure familial dysautonomia. *Nat. Commun.* 12: 4507.

106 Sonamoto, R., Kii, I., Koike, Y. et al. (2015). Identification of a DYRK1A inhibitor that induces degradation of the target kinase using co-chaperone CDC37 fused with luciferase nanoKAZ. *Sci. Rep.* 5: 12728.

107 Shibata, S., Ajiro, M., and Hagiwara, M. (2020). Mechanism-based personalized medicine for cystic fibrosis by suppressing pseudo exon inclusion. *Cell Chem. Biol.* 27: 1472–1482.e6.

108 Mermoud, J.E., Cohen, P.T., and Lamond, A.I. (1994). Regulation of mammalian spliceosome assembly by a protein phosphorylation mechanism. *Embo J.* 13: 5679–5688.

109 Gu, J., Wang, W., Miao, S. et al. (2018). Protein Phosphatase 1 dephosphorylates TDP-43 and suppresses its function in tau exon 10 inclusion. *FEBS Lett.* 592: 402–410.

110 Murray, M.V., Kobayashi, R., and Krainer, A.R. (1999). The type 2C Ser/Thr phosphatase PP2Cgamma is a pre-mRNA splicing factor. *Genes Dev.* 13: 87–97.

111 Wang, C., Chua, K., Seghezzi, W. et al. (1998). Phosphorylation of spliceosomal protein SAP 155 coupled with splicing catalysis. *Genes Dev.* 12: 1409–1414.

112 Stevens, M. and Oltean, S. (2019). Modulation of the apoptosis gene Bcl-x function through alternative splicing. *Front. Genet.* 10: 804.

113 Sun, Q., Li, S., Li, J. et al. (2018). Homoharringtonine regulates the alternative splicing of Bcl-x and caspase 9 through a protein phosphatase 1-dependent mechanism. *BMC Complement. Altern. Med.* 18: 164.

114 Biswas, S. and Rao, C.M. (2018). Epigenetic tools (The Writers, The Readers and The Erasers) and their implications in cancer therapy. *Eur. J. Pharmacol.* 837: 8–24.

115 Babic, I., Jakymiw, A., and Fujita, D.J. (2004). The RNA binding protein Sam68 is acetylated in tumor cell lines, and its acetylation correlates with enhanced RNA binding activity. *Onco Ther.* 23: 3781–3789.

116 Parker, M.T., Soanes, B.K., Kusakina, J. et al. (2022). m6A modification of U6 snRNA modulates usage of two major classes of pre-mRNA 5' splice site. *eLife* 11: e78808.

117 Aoyama, T., Yamashita, S., and Tomita, K. (2020). Mechanistic insights into m6A modification of U6 snRNA by human METTL16. *Nucleic Acids Res.* 48: 5157–5168.

118 Kuhn, A.N., van Santen, M.A., Schwienhorst, A. et al. (2009). Stalling of spliceosome assembly at distinct stages by small-molecule inhibitors of protein acetylation and deacetylation. *RNA* 15: 153–175.

119 Pagliarini, V., Guerra, M., Di Rosa, V. et al. (2020). Combined treatment with the histone deacetylase inhibitor LBH589 and a splice-switch antisense oligonucleotide enhances SMN2 splicing and SMN expression in spinal muscular atrophy cells. *J. Neurochem.* 153: e14935.

120 Riessland, M., Brichta, L., Hahnen, E., and Wirth, B. (2006). The benzamide M344, a novel histone deacetylase inhibitor, significantly increases SMN2 RNA/protein levels in spinal muscular atrophy cells. *Hum. Genet.* 120: 101–110.

121 Jarecki, J., Chen, X., Bernardino, A. et al. (2005). Diverse small-molecule modulators of SMN expression found by high-throughput compound screening: early leads towards a therapeutic for spinal muscular atrophy. *Hum. Mol. Genet.* 14: 2003–2018.

122 Codd, R., Braich, N., Liu, J. et al. (2009). Zn(II)-dependent histone deacetylase inhibitors: suberoylanilide hydroxamic acid and trichostatin A. *Int. J. Biochem. Cell Biol.* 41: 736–739.

123 Balasubramanyam, K., Altaf, M., Varier, R.A. et al. (2004). Polyisoprenylated benzophenone, garcinol, a natural histone acetyltransferase inhibitor, represses chromatin transcription and alters global gene expression. *J. Biol. Chem.* 279: 33716–33726.

124 Arif, M., Pradhan, S.K., Vedamurthy, B.M. et al. (2009). Mechanism of p300 specific histone acetyltransferase inhibition by small molecules. *J. Med. Chem.* 52: 267–277.

125 Singh, J., Salcius, M., Liu, S.W. et al. (2008). DcpS as a therapeutic target for spinal muscular atrophy. *ACS Chem. Biol.* 3: 711–722.

126 Gogliotti, R.G., Cardona, H., Singh, J. et al. (2013). The DcpS inhibitor RG3039 improves survival, function and motor unit pathologies in two SMA mouse models. *Hum. Mol. Genet.* 22: 4084–4101.

127 Deng, X., Shao, G., Zhang, H.T. et al. (2017). Protein arginine methyltransferase 5 functions as an epigenetic activator of the androgen receptor to promote prostate cancer cell growth. *Onco Ther.* 36: 1223–1231.

128 Chung, J.I.H., Sloan, S., Scherle, P. et al. (2019). PRMT5 is a key epigenetic regulator that promotes transcriptional activation in mantle cell lymphoma by regulating the lysine methyltransferase SETD7 and MLL1 activity. *Blood* 134: 2777.

129 Bezzi, M., Teo, S.X., Muller, J. et al. (2013). Regulation of constitutive and alternative splicing by PRMT5 reveals a role for Mdm4 pre-mRNA in sensing defects in the spliceosomal machinery. *Genes Dev.* 27: 1903–1916.

130 Radzisheuskaya, A., Shliaha, P.V., Grinev, V. et al. (2019). PRMT5 methylome profiling uncovers a direct link to splicing regulation in acute myeloid leukemia. *Nat. Struct. Mol. Biol.* 26: 999–1012.

131 Meister, G. and Fischer, U. (2002). Assisted RNP assembly: SMN and PRMT5 complexes cooperate in the formation of spliceosomal UsnRNPs. *EMBO J.* 21: 5853–5863.

132 Brehmer, D., Beke, L., Wu, T. et al. (2021). Discovery and pharmacological characterization of JNJ-64619178, a novel small-molecule inhibitor of PRMT5 with potent antitumor activity. *Mol. Cancer Ther.* 20: 2317–2328.

133 Antonysamy, S., Bonday, Z., Campbell, R.M. et al. (2012). Crystal structure of the human PRMT5:MEP50 complex. *PNAS* 109: 17960–17965.

134 Pande, V., Sun, W., Beke, L. et al. (2020). A chemical probe for the methyl transferase PRMT5 with a novel binding mode. *ACS Med. Chem. Lett.* 11: 2227–2231.

135 Haque, T., Cadenas, F.L., Xicoy, B. et al. (2021). Phase 1 Study of JNJ-64619178, a protein arginine methyltransferase 5 inhibitor, in patients with lower-risk myelodysplastic syndromes. *Blood* 138: 2606–2606.

136 Liu, Y.-C. and Cheng, S.-C. (2015). Functional roles of DExD/H-box RNA helicases in Pre-mRNA splicing. *J. Biomed. Sci.* 22: 54.

137 Hönig, A., Auboeuf, D., Parker, M.M. et al. (2002). Regulation of alternative splicing by the ATP-dependent DEAD-box RNA helicase p72. *Mol. Cell. Biol.* 22: 5698–5707.

138 Absmeier, E., Santos, K.F., and Wahl, M.C. (2016). Functions and regulation of the Brr2 RNA helicase during splicing. *Cell Cycle* 15: 3362–3377.

139 Naineni, S.K., Robert, F., Nagar, B., and Pelletier, J. (2022). Targeting DEAD-box RNA helicases: the emergence of molecular staples, *WIREs. RNA* e1738.

140 Iwatani-Yoshihara, M., Ito, M., Klein, M.G. et al. (2017). Discovery of allosteric inhibitors targeting the spliceosomal RNA helicase Brr2. *J. Med. Chem.* 60: 5759–5771.

141 Ito, M., Iwatani, M., Yamamoto, T. et al. (2017). Discovery of spiro[indole-3,2'-pyrrolidin]-2(1H)-one based inhibitors targeting Brr2, a core component of the U5 snRNP. *Bioorg. Med. Chem.* 25: 4753–4767.

142 Shadrick, W.R., Ndjomou, J., Kolli, R. et al. (2013). Discovering new medicines targeting helicases: challenges and recent progress. *SLAS Discovery* 18: 761–781.

143 Aukema, K.G., Chohan, K.K., Plourde, G.L. et al. (2009). Small molecule inhibitors of yeast pre-mRNA splicing. *ACS Chem. Biol.* 4: 759–768.

144 Pawellek, A., McElroy, S., Samatov, T. et al. (2014). Identification of small molecule inhibitors of pre-mRNA splicing. *J. Biol. Chem.* 289: 34683–34698.

145 O'Brien, K., Matlin, A.J., Lowell, A.M., and Moore, M.J. (2008). The biflavonoid isoginkgetin is a general inhibitor of Pre-mRNA splicing. *J. Biol. Chem.* 283: 33147–33154.

146 Effenberger, K.A., Perriman, R.J., Bray, W.M. et al. (2013). A high-throughput splicing assay identifies new classes of inhibitors of human and yeast spliceosomes. *J. Biomol. Screening* 18: 1110–1120.

147 You, Y.J., Zheng, X.G., Yong, K., and Ahn, B.Z. (1998). Naphthazarin derivatives: synthesis, cytotoxic mechanism and evaluation of antitumor activity. *Arch. Pharmacal Res.* 21: 595–598.

148 Wan, L., Ottinger, E., Cho, S., and Dreyfuss, G. (2008). Inactivation of the SMN complex by oxidative stress. *Mol. Cell* 31: 244–254.

149 Nakajima, H., Hori, Y., Terano, H. et al. (1996). New antitumor substances, FR901463, FR901464 and FR901465. II. Activities against experimental tumors in mice and mechanism of action. *J. Antibiot. (Tokyo)* 49: 1204–1211.

150 Sakai, Y., Yoshida, T., Ochiai, K. et al. (2002). GEX1 compounds, novel antitumor antibiotics related to herboxidiene, produced by Streptomyces sp. I. Taxonomy, production, isolation, physicochemical properties and biological activities. *J. Antibiot. (Tokyo)* 55: 855–862.

151 Kaida, D., Motoyoshi, H., Tashiro, E. et al. (2007). Spliceostatin A targets SF3b and inhibits both splicing and nuclear retention of pre-mRNA. *Nat. Chem. Biol.* 3: 576–583.

152 Fan, L., Lagisetti, C., Edwards, C.C. et al. (2011). Sudemycins, novel small molecule analogues of FR901464, induce alternative gene splicing. *ACS Chem. Biol.* 6: 582–589.

153 Albert, B.J., McPherson, P.A., O'Brien, K. et al. (2009). Meayamycin inhibits pre-messenger RNA splicing and exhibits picomolar activity against multidrug-resistant cells. *Mol. Cancer Ther.* 8: 2308–2318.

154 Liu, X., Biswas, S., Berg, M.G. et al. (2013). Genomics-guided discovery of thailanstatins A, B, and C As pre-mRNA splicing inhibitors and antiproliferative agents from *Burkholderia thailandensis* MSMB43. *J. Nat. Prod.* 76: 685–693.

155 Teng, T., Tsai, J.H., Puyang, X. et al. (2017). Splicing modulators act at the branch point adenosine binding pocket defined by the PHF5A-SF3b complex. *Nat. Commun.* 8: 15522.

156 Corrionero, A., Miñana, B., and Valcárcel, J. (2011). Reduced fidelity of branch point recognition and alternative splicing induced by the anti-tumor drug spliceostatin A. *Genes Dev.* 25: 445–459.

157 Roybal, G.A. and Jurica, M.S. (2010). Spliceostatin A inhibits spliceosome assembly subsequent to prespliceosome formation. *Nucleic Acids Res.* 38: 6664–6672.

158 Folco, E.G., Coil, K.E., and Reed, R. (2011). The anti-tumor drug E7107 reveals an essential role for SF3b in remodeling U2 snRNP to expose the branch point-binding region. *Genes Dev.* 25: 440–444.

159 Mizui, Y., Sakai, T., Iwata, M. et al. (2004). Pladienolides, new substances from culture of *Streptomyces platensis* Mer-11107. III. In vitro and in vivo antitumor activities. *J. Antibiot. (Tokyo)* 57: 188–196.

160 Sakai, T., Sameshima, T., Matsufuji, M. et al. (2004). Pladienolides, new substances from culture of *Streptomyces platensis* Mer-11107. I. Taxonomy, fermentation, isolation and screening. *J. Antibiot. (Tokyo)* 57: 173–179.

161 Kotake, Y., Sagane, K., Owa, T. et al. (2007). Splicing factor SF3b as a target of the antitumor natural product pladienolide. *Nat. Chem. Biol.* 3: 570–575.

162 Iwata, M., Ozawa, Y., Uenaka, T. et al. (2004). E7107, a new 7-urethane derivative of pladienolide D, displays curative effect against several human tumor xenografts. *Cancer Res.* 64: 691–691.

163 Hsu, T.Y.T., Simon, L.M., Neill, N.J. et al. (2015). The spliceosome is a therapeutic vulnerability in MYC-driven cancer. *Nature* 525: 384–388.

164 Webb, T.R., Joyner, A.S., and Potter, P.M. (2013). The development and application of small molecule modulators of SF3b as therapeutic agents for cancer. *Drug Discovery Today* 18: 43–49.

165 Lu, S.X., De Neef, E., Thomas, J.D. et al. (2021). Pharmacologic modulation of RNA splicing enhances anti-tumor immunity. *Cell* 184: 4032–4047.e31.

166 Bowling, E.A., Wang, J.H., Gong, F. et al. (2021). Spliceosome-targeted therapies trigger an antiviral immune response in triple-negative breast cancer. *Cell* 184: 384–403.e21.

167 Hong, D.S., Kurzrock, R., Naing, A. et al. (2014). A phase I, open-label, single-arm, dose-escalation study of E7107, a precursor messenger ribonucleic acid (pre-mRNA) splicesome inhibitor administered intravenously on days 1 and 8 every 21 days to patients with solid tumors. *Invest. New Drugs* 32: 436–444.

168 Osman, S., Albert, B.J., Wang, Y. et al. (2011). Structural requirements for the antiproliferative activity of pre-mRNA splicing inhibitor FR901464. *Chemistry (Easton)* 17: 895–904.

169 Makowski, K., Vigevani, L., Albericio, F. et al. (2017). Sudemycin K: a synthetic antitumor splicing inhibitor variant with improved activity and versatile chemistry. *ACS Chem. Biol.* 12: 163–173.

170 Effenberger, K.A., Anderson, D.D., Bray, W.M. et al. (2014). Coherence between cellular responses and in vitro splicing inhibition for the anti-tumor drug pladienolide B and its analogs. *J. Biol. Chem.* 289: 1938–1947.

171 Villa, R., Kashyap, M.K., Kumar, D. et al. (2013). Stabilized cyclopropane analogs of the splicing inhibitor FD-895. *J. Med. Chem.* 56: 6576–6582.

172 Seiler, M., Yoshimi, A., Darman, R. et al. (2018). H3B-8800, an orally available small-molecule splicing modulator, induces lethality in spliceosome-mutant cancers. *Nat. Med.* 24: 497–504.

173 Amit, M., Donyo, M., Hollander, D. et al. (2012). Differential GC content between exons and introns establishes distinct strategies of splice-site recognition. *Cell Rep.* 1: 543–556.

174 Cheung, A.K., Hurley, B., Kerrigan, R. et al. (2018). Discovery of small molecule splicing modulators of survival motor neuron-2 (SMN2) for the treatment of spinal muscular atrophy (SMA). *J. Med. Chem.* 61: 11021–11036.

175 Woll, M.G., Qi, H., Turpoff, A. et al. (2016). Discovery and optimization of small molecule splicing modifiers of survival motor neuron 2 as a treatment for spinal muscular atrophy. *J. Med. Chem.* 59: 6070–6085.

176 Palacino, J., Swalley, S.E., Song, C. et al. (2015). SMN2 splice modulators enhance U1–pre-mRNA association and rescue SMA mice. *Nat. Chem. Biol.* 11: 511–517.

177 Campagne, S., Boigner, S., Rüdisser, S. et al. (2019). Structural basis of a small molecule targeting RNA for a specific splicing correction. *Nat. Chem. Biol.* 15: 1191–1198.

178 Sivaramakrishnan, M., McCarthy, K.D., Campagne, S. et al. (2017). Binding to SMN2 pre-mRNA-protein complex elicits specificity for small molecule splicing modifiers. *Nat. Commun.* 8: 1476.

179 Bhattacharyya, A., Trotta, C.R., Narasimhan, J. et al. (2021). Small molecule splicing modifiers with systemic HTT-lowering activity. *Nat. Commun.* 12: 7299.

180 Lally, C., Jones, C., Farwell, W. et al. (2017). Indirect estimation of the prevalence of spinal muscular atrophy Type I, II, and III in the United States. *Orphanet J. Rare Dis.* 12: 175.

181 Kolb, S.J., Battle, D.J., and Dreyfuss, G. (2007). Molecular functions of the SMN complex. *J. Child Neurol.* 22: 990–994.

182 Paushkin, S., Gubitz, A.K., Massenet, S., and Dreyfuss, G. (2002). The SMN complex, an assemblyosome of ribonucleoproteins. *Curr. Opin. Cell Biol.* 14: 305–312.

183 Oskoui, M., Levy, G., Garland, C.J. et al. (2007). The changing natural history of spinal muscular atrophy type 1. *Neurology* 69: 1931–1936.

184 Cho, S. and Dreyfuss, G. (2010). A degron created by SMN2 exon 7 skipping is a principal contributor to spinal muscular atrophy severity. *Genes Dev.* 24: 438–442.

185 Gendron, N.H. and MacKenzie, A.E. (1999). Spinal muscular atrophy: molecular pathophysiology. *Curr. Opin. Neurol.* 12.

186 Avila, A.M., Burnett, B.G., Taye, A.A. et al. (2007). Trichostatin A increases SMN expression and survival in a mouse model of spinal muscular atrophy. *J. Clin. Invest.* 117: 659–671.

187 Brichta, L., Hofmann, Y., Hahnen, E. et al. (2003). Valproic acid increases the SMN2 protein level: a well-known drug as a potential therapy for spinal muscular atrophy. *Hum. Mol. Genet.* 12: 2481–2489.

188 Andreassi, C., Angelozzi, C., Tiziano, F.D. et al. (2004). Phenylbutyrate increases SMN expression in vitro: relevance for treatment of spinal muscular atrophy. *Eur. J. Hum. Genet.* 12: 59–65.

189 Chang, J.G., Hsieh-Li, H.M., Jong, Y.J. et al. (2001). Treatment of spinal muscular atrophy by sodium butyrate. *PNAS* 98: 9808–9813.

190 Hastings, M.L., Berniac, J., Liu, Y.H. et al. (2009). Tetracyclines that promote SMN2 exon 7 splicing as therapeutics for spinal muscular atrophy. *Sci. Transl. Med.* 1: 5ra12.

191 Angelozzi, C., Borgo, F., Tiziano, F.D. et al. (2008). Salbutamol increases SMN mRNA and protein levels in spinal muscular atrophy cells. *J. Med. Genet.* 45: 29–31.

192 Grzeschik, S.M., Ganta, M., Prior, T.W. et al. (2005). Hydroxyurea enhances SMN2 gene expression in spinal muscular atrophy cells. *Ann. Neurol.* 58: 194–202.

193 Passini, M.A., Bu, J., Richards, A.M. et al. (2011). Antisense oligonucleotides delivered to the mouse CNS ameliorate symptoms of severe spinal muscular atrophy. *Sci. Transl. Med.* 3: 72ra18.

194 Lim, S.R. and Hertel, K.J. (2001). Modulation of survival motor neuron pre-mRNA splicing by inhibition of alternative 3' splice site pairing. *J. Biol. Chem.* 276: 45476–45483.

195 Porensky, P.N., Mitrpant, C., McGovern, V.L. et al. (2012). A single administration of morpholino antisense oligomer rescues spinal muscular atrophy in mouse. *Hum. Mol. Genet.* 21: 1625–1638.

196 Hua, Y., Vickers, T.A., Okunola, H.L. et al. (2008). Antisense masking of an hnRNP A1/A2 intronic splicing silencer corrects SMN2 splicing in transgenic mice. *Am. J. Hum. Genet.* 82: 834–848.

197 Wurster, C.D. and Ludolph, A.C. (2018). Nusinersen for spinal muscular atrophy. *Ther. Adv. Neurol. Disord.* 11: 1756285618754459.

198 Shadid, M., Badawi, M., and Abulrob, A. (2021). Antisense oligonucleotides: absorption, distribution, metabolism, and excretion. *Expert Opin. Drug Metab. Toxicol.* 17: 1281–1292.

199 Ratni, H., Mueller, L., and Ebeling, M. (2019). Chapter 3 – rewriting the (tran)script: application to spinal muscular atrophy. In: *Prog. Med. Chem.* (ed. D.R. Witty and B. Cox), 119–156. Elsevier.

200 Thorne, N., Shen, M., Lea, W.A. et al. (2012). Firefly luciferase in chemical biology: a compendium of inhibitors, mechanistic evaluation of chemotypes, and suggested use as a reporter. *Chem. Biol.* 19: 1060–1072.

201 Naryshkin, N.A., Weetall, M., Dakka, A. et al. (2014). SMN2 splicing modifiers improve motor function and longevity in mice with spinal muscular atrophy. *Science* 345: 688–693.

202 Kletzl, H., Marquet, A., Günther, A. et al. (2019). The oral splicing modifier RG7800 increases full length survival of motor neuron 2 mRNA and survival of motor neuron protein: results from trials in healthy adults and patients with spinal muscular atrophy. *Neuromuscul. Disord.* 29: 21–29.

203 Pinard, E., Green, L., Reutlinger, M. et al. (2017). Discovery of a novel class of survival motor neuron 2 splicing modifiers for the treatment of spinal muscular atrophy. *J. Med. Chem.* 60: 4444–4457.

204 Giovanni, B., Enrico, B., Claudia, C. et al. (2020). Pooled safety data from the risdiplam (RG7916) clinical trial development program (1267). *Neurology* 94: 1267.

205 Basil, T.D., Ricardo, M., Maria, M.-B. et al. (2021). FIREFISH Part 2: 24-month efficacy and safety of risdiplam in infants with type 1 spinal muscular atrophy (SMA) (4126). *Neurology* 96: 4126.

206 Oskoui, M., Day, J.W., Deconinck, N. et al. (2023). Two-year efficacy and safety of risdiplam in patients with type 2 or non-ambulant type 3 spinal muscular atrophy (SMA). *J. Neurol.* 270: 2531–2546.

207 Ratni, H., Ebeling, M., Baird, J. et al. (2018). Discovery of risdiplam, a selective survival of motor neuron-2 (SMN2) gene splicing modifier for the treatment of spinal muscular atrophy (SMA). *J. Med. Chem.* 61: 6501–6517.

208 Woll, M.G., Naryshkin, N.A., and Karp, G.M. (2018). Drugging pre-mRNA splicing. In: *RNA Therapeutics* (ed. A.L. Garner), 135–176. Cham: Springer International Publishing.

209 Hug, N., Longman, D., and Cáceres, J.F. (2016). Mechanism and regulation of the nonsense-mediated decay pathway. *Nucleic Acids Res.* 44: 1483–1495.

210 Baker, K.E. and Parker, R. (2004). Nonsense-mediated mRNA decay: terminating erroneous gene expression. *Curr. Opin. Cell Biol.* 16: 293–299.

211 Finkbeiner, S. (2011). Huntington's disease. *Cold Spring Harbor Perspect. Biol.* 3.

212 Bates, G.P., Dorsey, R., Gusella, J.F. et al. (2015). Huntington disease. *Nat. Rev. Dis. Primers* 1: 15005.

213 Garber, K. (2023). Drugging RNA. *Nat. Biotechnol.* 41: 745–749.

214 Krach, F., Stemick, J., Boerstler, T. et al. (2022). An alternative splicing modulator decreases mutant HTT and improves the molecular fingerprint in Huntington's disease patient neurons. *Nat. Commun.* 13: 6797.

215 Keller, C.G., Shin, Y., Monteys, A.M. et al. (2022). An orally available, brain penetrant, small molecule lowers huntingtin levels by enhancing pseudoexon inclusion. *Nat. Commun.* 13: 1150.

216 Zafferani, M., Martyr, J.G., Muralidharan, D. et al. (2022). Multiassay profiling of a focused small molecule library reveals predictive bidirectional modulation of the lncRNA MALAT1 triplex stability in vitro. *ACS Chem. Biol.* 17: 2437–2447.

217 Furuzono, T., Murata, A., Okuda, S. et al. (2021). Speeding drug discovery targeting RNAs: an iterative "RNA selection-compounds screening cycle" for exploring RNA-small molecule pairs. *Biorg. Med. Chem.* 36: 116070.

218 Hermann, T. and Westhof, E. (2000). Rational drug design and high-throughput techniques for RNA targets. *Comb. Chem. High Throughput Screening* 3: 219–234.

219 Chappie, T.A., Abdelmessih, M., Ambroise, C.W. et al. (2022). Discovery of small-molecule CD33 pre-mRNA splicing modulators. *ACS Med. Chem. Lett.* 13: 55–62.

220 Londregan, A.T., Wei, L., Xiao, J. et al. (2018). Small molecule proprotein convertase subtilisin/kexin type 9 (PCSK9) inhibitors: hit to lead optimization of systemic agents. *J. Med. Chem.* 61: 5704–5718.

221 Londregan, A.T., Aspnes, G., Limberakis, C. et al. (2018). Discovery of N-(piperidin-3-yl)-N-(pyridin-2-yl)piperidine/piperazine-1-carboxamides as small molecule inhibitors of PCSK9. *Bioorg. Med. Chem. Lett.* 28: 3685–3688.

222 Li, W., Ward, F.R., McClure, K.F. et al. (2019). Structural basis for selective stalling of human ribosome nascent chain complexes by a drug-like molecule. *Nat. Struct. Mol. Biol.* 26: 501–509.

223 Petersen, D.N., Hawkins, J., Ruangsiriluk, W. et al. (2016). A small-molecule anti-secretagogue of PCSK9 targets the 80S ribosome to inhibit PCSK9 protein translation. *Cell Chem. Biol.* 23: 1362–1371.

224 Li, H., Qiu, J., and Fu, X.D. (2012). RASL-seq for massively parallel and quantitative analysis of gene expression. *Curr. Protoc. Mol. Biol.*; Chapter 4: Unit 4.13.1-9.

225 Simon, J.M., Paranjape, S.R., Wolter, J.M. et al. (2019). High-throughput screening and classification of chemicals and their effects on neuronal gene expression using RASL-seq. *Sci. Rep.* 9: 4529.

226 Alpern, D., Gardeux, V., Russeil, J. et al. (2019). BRB-seq: ultra-affordable high-throughput transcriptomics enabled by bulk RNA barcoding and sequencing. *Genome Biol.* 20: 71.

227 Li, J., Ho, D.J., Henault, M. et al. (2022). DRUG-seq provides unbiased biological activity readouts for neuroscience drug discovery. *ACS Chem. Biol.* 17: 1401–1414.

228 Ye, C., Ho, D.J., Neri, M. et al. (2018). DRUG-seq for miniaturized high-throughput transcriptome profiling in drug discovery. *Nat. Commun.* 9: 4307.

8

Prospects for Riboswitches in Drug Development

Michael G. Mohsen[1,2] *and Ronald R. Breaker*[1,2,3]

[1] *Department of Molecular, Cellular and Developmental Biology, Yale University, New Haven, CT 06511, USA*
[2] *Howard Hughes Medical Institute, Yale University, New Haven, CT 06511, USA*
[3] *Department of Molecular Biophysics and Biochemistry, Yale University, New Haven, CT 06511, USA*

8.1 Introduction

8.1.1 The Known Landscape of Riboswitches

Riboswitches are gene regulatory elements commonly located in the 5′ untranslated regions (UTRs) of bacterial messenger RNAs (mRNAs) [1–4]. A riboswitch typically comprises an aptamer domain that, upon binding its target ligand, alters the folding of an adjoining expression platform [5–7]. Each expression platform exploits one of several possible gene regulatory mechanisms, for example by exerting control over transcription, translation, or RNA processing (Figure 8.1) [8–12]. Numerous examples of genetic "ON" switches, wherein increasing concentration of the target ligand increases expression of the downstream gene, and "OFF" switches have been found in nature (Figure 8.2).

In addition various tandem riboswitch arrangements that sense multiple input ligands have been identified [13], which adds to the diversity of riboswitch functions. Over 55 distinct classes of riboswitches have been experimentally validated to date, which sense diverse ligands such as nucleotide derivatives, elemental ions, amino acids, and signaling molecules [12, 14]. Though most prevalent in bacteria, riboswitches have been discovered in organisms spanning all three domains of life [14]. The natural diversity of riboswitch classes, their mechanisms for gene control, and their phylogenetic distributions suggest that these RNAs could be exploited as tools and as targets by drug developers.

8.1.2 Riboswitches in Drug Development

The ability of riboswitches to sense a target ligand and modulate expression of a downstream gene has interested researchers from diverse disciplines, including those in drug development [15–18]. Perhaps the most apparent connection to drug development is the consideration of riboswitches as possible drug targets

RNA as a Drug Target: The Next Frontier for Medicinal Chemistry, First Edition.
Edited by John Schneekloth and Martin Pettersson.

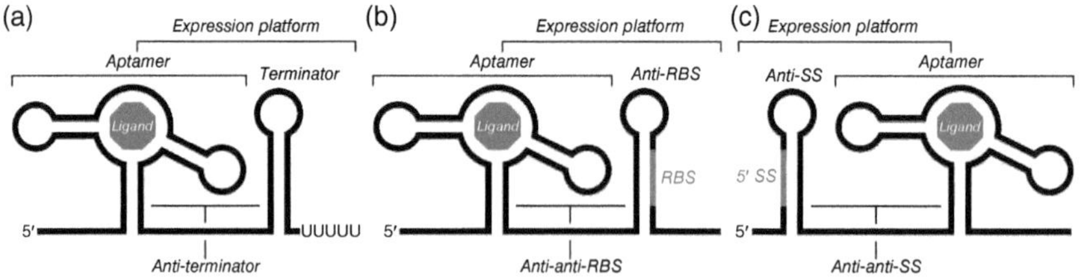

Figure 8.1 Natural riboswitches employ various expression platforms to regulate gene expression. (a) Ligand binding by the aptamer domain regulates the formation of a transcription terminator stem, which attenuates transcription of the full-length mRNA. (b) A ribosome-binding site (RBS) is occluded by an anti-RBS stem, the formation of which is regulated by ligand binding by the adjoining aptamer domain. (c) Some riboswitches in eukaryotes regulate splicing by hiding or revealing a 5′ splice site.

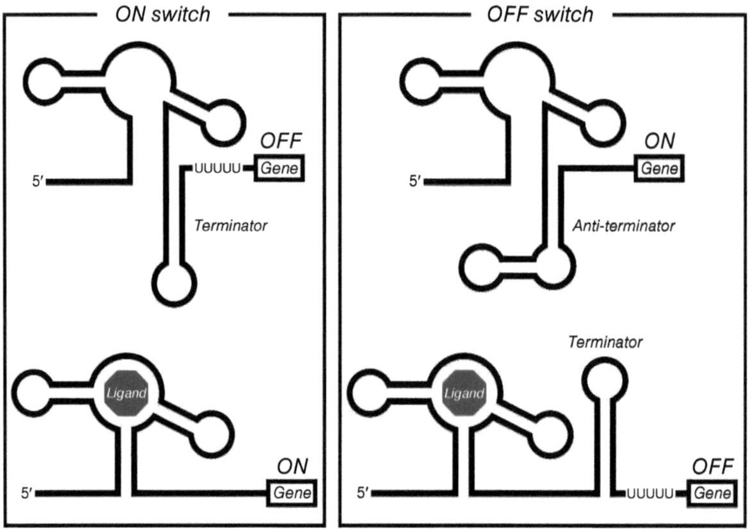

Figure 8.2 Riboswitches can occur as ON or OFF switches. Left: an example of a transcriptional ON switch. In the ligand-free state, a terminator attenuates transcription of downstream genes. When sufficient concentrations of ligand are present in the cell, part of the aptamer structure may act as an anti-terminator. Gene expression is thus turned ON. Right: an example of a transcriptional OFF switch. In the ligand-free state, an anti-terminator structure prevents formation of the competing terminator stem. When ligand accumulates in the cell, the aptamer binds, and the terminator stem is presented. Gene expression is thus turned OFF.

[19–21]. One application is to identify small molecules that simulate binding of the natural ligand to the riboswitch aptamer to turn off the expression of an essential gene (Figure 8.3a). Because riboswitches are mostly found in bacteria, this approach lends itself to the development of novel RNA-targeting antibiotics where there is a lower risk of unwanted interactions with an equivalent RNA in eukaryotes. A second application involves using riboswitch-based biosensors to report on the disruption of an essential physiological process or metabolic pathway. Paired with a high-throughput screening (HTS) approach, riboswitch sensors

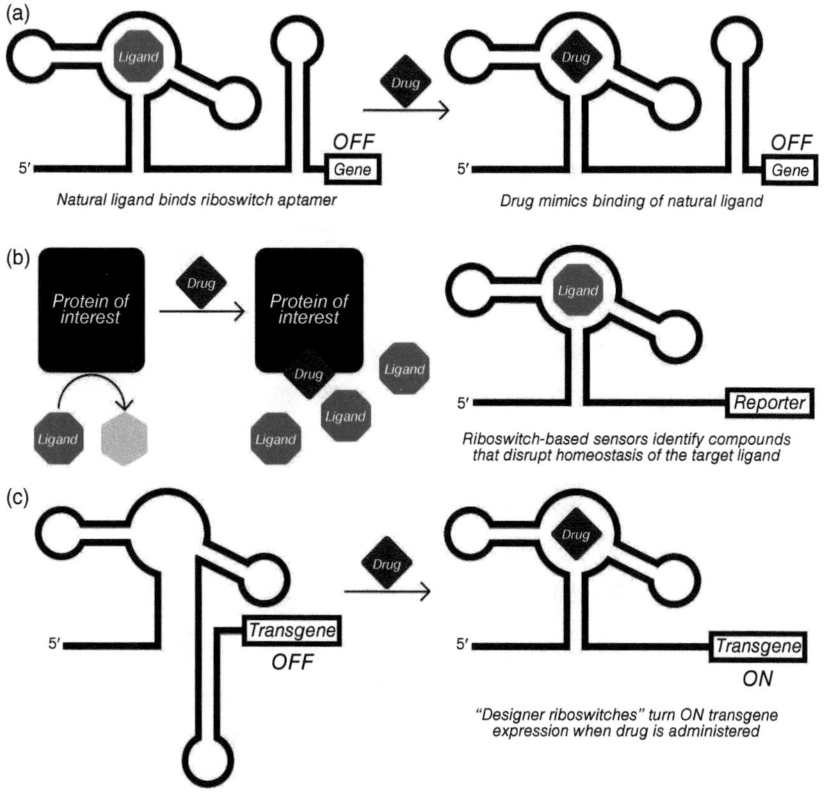

Figure 8.3 Riboswitches as targets and tools in drug development. (a) Riboswitch aptamers are targeted by small molecule drugs that, for example, can mimic the binding of the native ligand. (b) Riboswitches used as sensors for their native ligand can be employed to screen for small molecule inhibitors of a protein of interest that processes the ligand. (c) "Designer riboswitches" that sense drug or drug-like compounds can be used to turn on expression of a therapeutic transgene in response to the drug.

provide information about how small-molecule compounds in the screen may cause a buildup or depletion of the ligand, presumably by disrupting the function of a metabolic enzyme or a protein involved in a key aspect of bacterial physiology [22–24] (Figure 8.3b). The goal of this approach is to produce novel antibiotic compounds that disrupt new targets and pathways. A third application entails engineering riboswitches that regulate gene expression in response to drug-like compounds [25] (Figure 8.3c). Such a device could be employed in human gene therapy applications to precisely regulate the expression of a therapeutic transgene.

8.1.3 The Need for Novel Antibiotics

The development of antibiotics was one of the defining medical breakthroughs of the twentieth century [26]. The common use (and misuse) of antibiotics combined with the ability of bacterial pathogens to rapidly evolve has led to the development and spread of antimicrobial resistance [27]. Following the current trend,

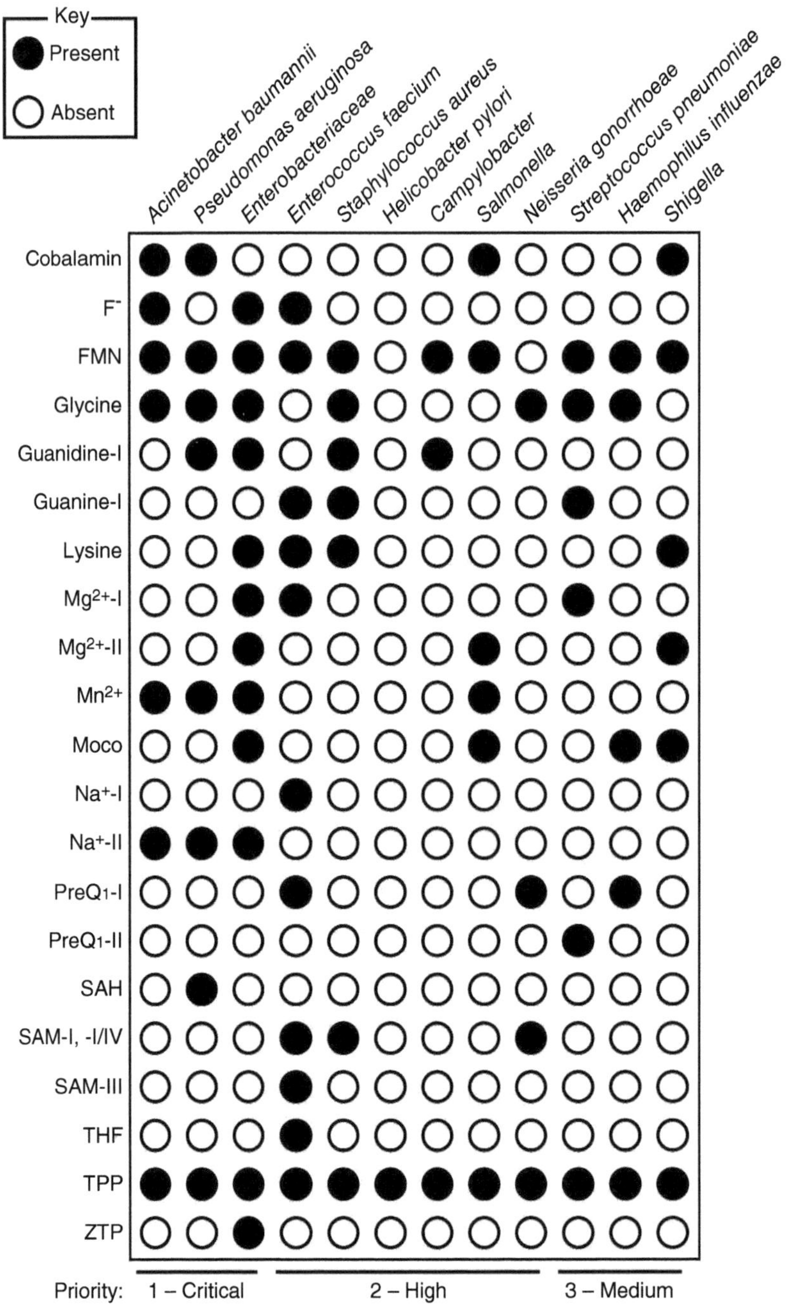
Key
Present
Absent
Acinetobacter baumannii
Pseudomonas aeruginosa
Enterobacteriaceae
Enterococcus faecium
Staphylococcus aureus
Helicobacter pylori
Campylobacter
Salmonella
Neisseria gonorrhoeae
Streptococcus pneumoniae
Haemophilus influenzae
Shigella
Cobalamin
F⁻
FMN
Glycine
Guanidine-I
Guanine-I
Lysine
Mg2+-I
Mg2+-II
Mn2+
Moco
Na+-I
Na+-II
PreQ1-I
PreQ1-II
SAH
SAM-I, -I/IV
SAM-III
THF
TPP
ZTP
Priority:
1 – Critical
2 – High
3 – Medium

antimicrobial resistance is predicted to lead to 10 million deaths per year by 2050 [26]. To address this urgent threat, new classes of chemical compounds that target novel targets or pathways are needed [23, 28]. Two of the three drug development modalities introduced above are related to the development of novel antibiotic compounds.

8.2 Riboswitches as Drug Targets

8.2.1 Why Target Riboswitches?

RNA is widely recognized as a clinically useful target in bacterial pathogens and humans [29, 30]. RNA molecules, like proteins, possess dynamic structures that undergo conformation changes, which can be influenced by small molecules [20]. For example, most antibiotics in clinical use target bacterial ribosomes, and nearly all of these compounds have been shown to bind ribosomal RNAs rather than ribosomal proteins [31].

Among the diverse types of RNAs present in cells, riboswitches are especially attractive as drug targets [32]. Whereas the interaction between other RNA targets and small molecules is mostly fortuitous, riboswitch aptamers often form structurally sophisticated binding pockets that specifically bind small-molecule ligands even in the presence of highly similar compounds that exist within cells [19]. Thus, compounds that target RNA ligand-binding pockets might be identified in a manner analogously to that for pockets made by proteins. Bacterial pathogens might also have greater difficulty developing resistance to a drug that targets a riboswitch aptamer because a mutation to a conserved nucleotide in the aptamer that avoids drug binding might also confer loss of binding to the native ligand. Because riboswitches often control the expression of genes important to bacterial survival, it is likely that disrupting riboswitch function would affect bacterial viability or virulence [20].

Additionally, various riboswitch classes are predicted to be present in bacterial pathogens identified by the World Health Organization's global priority pathogens list [19, 21] (Figure 8.4), which includes 12 species of bacteria that exhibit medium,

Figure 8.4 Riboswitch classes predicted to be present in the 12 members of the World Health Organization global priority pathogens list. These riboswitch classes include Cobalamin [33], Fluoride (F^-) [34], FMN (flavin mononucleotide) [35], Glycine [36], Guanidine-I [37], Guanine-I [38], Lysine [39], Mg^{2+}-I [40], Mg^{2+}-II [41], Mn^{2+} [42], molybdenum cofactor (Moco) [43], Na^+-I [44], Na^+-II [45], $PreQ_1$-I (pre-queuosine$_1$) [46], $PreQ_1$-II [47], SAH (*S*-adenosylhomocysteine) [48], SAM-I (*S*-adenosylmethionine) [49], SAM-I/IV [50], SAM-III [51], THF (tetrahydrofolate) [52], TPP (thiamin pyrophosphate) [53], and ZTP (5-aminoimidazole-4-carboxamide riboside 5′-triphosphate) [54]. Though many classes are represented, not all are likely to make useful targets (see Section 8.2.2). Riboswitches for the same ligand that employ different binding pockets are separated into different rows, whereas those that are known to employ highly similar binding pockets (e.g. SAM-I and SAM-I/IV [55]) are grouped. The data summarized in this graphic was collected from Rfam 14.9 [56].

high, or critical antimicrobial resistance [57]. None of these riboswitches have been discovered to occur naturally in humans. It is thus possible that drugs targeted to one of these riboswitches may have a low chance of interfering with human physiology.

8.2.2 Features of a Druggable Riboswitch

Riboswitches that control essential genes and function as OFF switches are perhaps more pharmacologically relevant [21]. A drug compound that binds such a riboswitch with affinity comparable to or greater than that of the native ligand would force the riboswitch to be in the OFF state regardless of the concentration of the native ligand inside the cell. Thus, the riboswitch will be unable to regulate essential downstream genes in response to fluctuating concentrations of the native ligand. Specifically, the riboswitch is tricked into acting as if there is an abundance of an essential ligand when in fact the cell is being starved of the molecule. However, some riboswitches might not fully suppress gene expression [58] and permit a level of gene expression that is sufficient for bacterial survival even when there is a high concentration of a ligand analog.

Features of the aptamer-binding pocket can also affect the suitability of a riboswitch as a drug target. Many existing drug compounds have complex, hydrophobic chemical structures. Thus, aptamer-binding pockets that are small, polar, or solvent-exposed might be unable to bind molecules with drug-like properties [59, 60]. The challenge for medicinal chemists is to identify compounds with the appropriate mix of drug-like properties and the characteristics needed to be recognized by natural aptamers.

Finally, riboswitch classes that are widespread over many genera would make ideal target candidates for development of broad-spectrum antibiotics. The common riboswitch classes that sense FMN, TPP, SAM, or AdoCbl appear to be the best-suited targets to achieve broad-spectrum efficacy. Other riboswitch classes that are more narrowly distributed could be targets for developing narrow-spectrum antibiotics. Historically, broad-spectrum antibiotic agents have been preferred, but narrow-spectrum compounds could help to avoid damaging the human microbiome and present a lower risk for developing antimicrobial resistance in the environment [61].

8.2.3 Riboswitch-Targeted Drugs

8.2.3.1 Small Molecules Targeting FMN Riboswitches

FMN (flavin mononucleotide, Figure 8.5) riboswitches exhibit many of the druggable features discussed above [35, 65, 66]. FMN riboswitches from *Bacillus subtilis* turn off expression of essential genes in response to increased FMN levels in the cell [35]. Subsequently, it was discovered that the natural antibacterial agent roseoflavin targets FMN riboswitches, mimicking the binding of the native ligand [58]. The synthetic compound 5FDQD (Figure 8.5), developed as an FMN mimic using medicinal chemistry principles, also targets FMN riboswitches [62]. 5FDQD

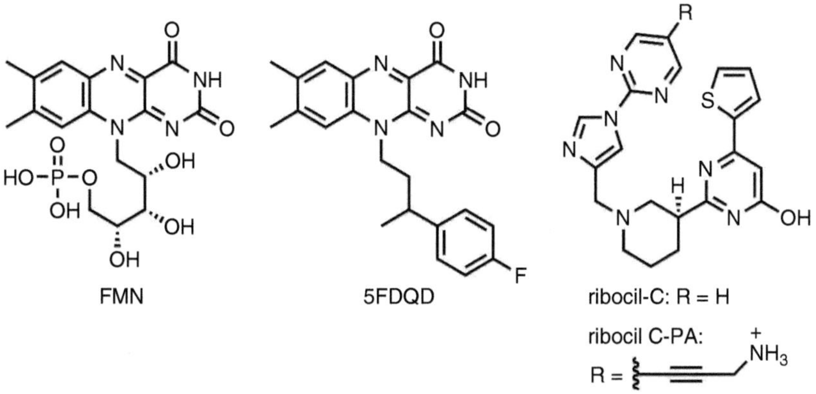

Figure 8.5 Chemical structures of flavin mononucleotide (FMN) (the native ligand of FMN riboswitches [35]) and FMN riboswitch-targeting compounds 5FDQD [62], ribocil-C [63], and ribocil C-PA [64].

was found to be nearly as effective as broad-spectrum antibacterial compounds vancomycin and metronidazole at curing mice infected with *Clostridioides difficile* [62]. Notably, 5FDQD showed markedly less alteration in culturable cecal flora relative to vancomycin and metronidazole [62]. Compounds that bind FMN riboswitches with even greater affinity have also been reported [67], suggesting that medicinal chemistry approaches can be used to make additional improvements to this class of compounds.

Another example of a synthetic compound that targets FMN riboswitches is ribocil, which was discovered through a phenotypic screen [63]. Ribocil is a racemic mixture of ribocil-A (*R* enantiomer) and ribocil-B (*S* enantiomer), the latter of which was determined to be the active compound [63]. Ribocil-B was further improved by medicinal chemistry approaches, which led to the development of ribocil-C [63]. Moreover, the chemical scaffold of ribocil differs substantially from that of FMN and other compounds that target FMN riboswitches (Figure 8.5). Whereas FMN binds the *E. coli* FMN riboswitch with a K_D of <10 nM [35], ribocil binds the same riboswitch with a K_D of 13 nM [68] and ribocil-C binds with a K_D of <1 nM [63]. Ribocil-C was found to be effective at treating Gram-positive bacteria in infectious settings, but less so with Gram-negative bacteria, which are known to exclude or eject many compounds [21, 69]. Recently, an improved ribocil C-PA was developed that was 16-fold more potent against Gram-negative bacteria *E. coli* and *K. pneumoniae* [64]. Using rational design principles, a quaternary amine was installed at a solvent-exposed site, which had the desired effects of increased entry and accumulation in Gram-negative bacteria [64].

8.2.3.2 Other Riboswitches Targeted in Proof-of-Principle Demonstrations

There are numerous proof-of-principle reports describing novel ligand development for various riboswitches [70–81]. Much work has been performed in developing synthetic ligands that target *glmS* ribozymes, riboswitches that use glucosamine-6-phosphate as a cofactor for self-cleavage [70–72]. Several reports describe synthetic ligand mimics of guanine that bind Guanine-I riboswitches with high affinity [73–75]. Synthetic ligands and probes have been developed using a combination of HTS and structure–activity relationship (SAR) approaches that target $PreQ_1$ riboswitches [76, 77]. ZTP riboswitches were targeted with synthetic ZMP analogs in which the sugar-phosphate moiety is replaced with various functional groups, including simple heterocycles [78]. Fragment-based approaches have led to the development of compounds that bind TPP riboswitches [79–81]. The antibacterial and antifungal compound pyrithiamine is converted to pyrithiamine pyrophosphate inside cells, which also binds and disrupts TPP riboswitches [82, 83]. Moreover, its discovery predates that of TPP riboswitches by more than half a century [53, 65]. Though many of the compounds described in these reports are not as advanced as the FMN-targeting compounds, the diversity of riboswitches that have been targeted is indicative of the potential of this technology.

8.2.4 Barriers and Future Developments

A potential pitfall is that ligands developed in vitro, either through rational design or by screening compound libraries, that tightly bind a riboswitch aptamer target in a test tube may fail to cause antibacterial effects in vivo. High-throughput screening approaches sometimes use in vivo assays, which can circumvent this problem, but access to sufficiently diverse chemical libraries remains a substantial barrier that must be addressed [21]. Another related possibility is that antibacterial compounds that are intended to disrupt riboswitch function might instead target other aspects of bacterial physiology. For example, synthetic lysine analogs that bind Lysine riboswitches in vitro also display antibacterial activity, but the mechanism of antibacterial activity is likely via lysyl-tRNA synthetases [84, 85].

In addition to continuing to develop ligands that bind known riboswitches, additional riboswitch targets are likely to emerge as orphan riboswitches (ligand unknown) [86] and yet-undiscovered riboswitches are likely to continue to be experimentally validated. It is hypothesized that most – if not all – of the widely distributed riboswitch classes have already been discovered [12]. Undiscovered riboswitch classes are therefore likely to be rare and narrowly distributed. Some of these latter classes likely will present intriguing candidates for narrow-spectrum antibiotic development.

8.3 Riboswitches as Tools for Antibiotic Drug Development

8.3.1 Riboswitches as Biosensors

Riboswitches can be used as tools to identify compounds that disrupt key aspects of bacterial metabolism or physiology. Riboswitches or riboswitch aptamers can be exploited in the construction of biosensors that report to researchers the relative concentrations of their target ligands [87, 88]. This is achieved by installing a riboswitch upstream of a reporter gene such as *lacZ* (β-galactosidase) [22–24], or by producing an allosteric device in which the riboswitch regulates a fluorogenic aptamer [89–91]. Bacterial cells that express this biosensor are then subjected to a high-throughput screen to identify small molecules that alter the intracellular concentration of the target ligand. A plausible cause for changes in ligand concentration could be that the small molecule disrupts the activity of a protein that is important for ligand homeostasis. This can subsequently be confirmed by performing the requisite assays with the protein of interest. Hit compounds identified through this approach could be further improved through medicinal chemistry approaches to enhance their disruptive effects, leading to the development of new antibacterial compounds.

8.3.2 A Riboswitch-Based Fluoride Sensor Illuminates Agonists of Fluoride Toxicity

In a prior report [22], the fluoride riboswitch was exploited using this approach to identify agonists of fluoride toxicity. Fluoride possesses substantial antibacterial effects [92, 93] and is generally toxic to organisms in all three domains of life [22]. Thus, compounds that specifically increase fluoride toxicity in bacteria could exploit the antibacterial action of this anion, and these could be valuable to combating antimicrobial resistance, particularly for topical or surface treatments. Researchers constructed a fluoride sensor by inserting a Fluoride riboswitch upstream of a *lacZ* reporter gene. The model gram-positive bacterial organism *Escherichia coli* expressing this reporter was subjected to a high-throughput screen in the presence of fluoride. Several hit compounds associated with increased reporter signals were identified. The most active hit compound was further improved by structure–activity relationship analysis to yield a series of diaryl urea and diaryl thiourea compounds that were confirmed experimentally as potent agonists of fluoride toxicity (Figure 8.6a). Various types of fluoride agonists presumably could be made to shuttle fluoride into cells, block its export, or act by inhibiting cell wall or lipid biosynthesis, thus increasing fluoride transport into the cell [22, 94–96]. Although the reported compounds do not appear potent enough to gain widespread use as antibiotics in combination with fluoride, the results showcased the utility of riboswitches as tools for developing drugs for other bacterial targets.

8.3.3 A Riboswitch-Based ZTP Sensor Identifies Inhibitors of Folate Biosynthesis

In a subsequent report [23], researchers employed another riboswitch to search for inhibitors of folate biosynthesis in *E. coli*. The folate metabolic pathway is essential in all species and therefore is an attractive target for antibiotic drug development [97]. Dihydropteroate synthase is a folate biosynthesis enzyme that is not found in humans, and therefore can be targeted without concern for disrupting folate metabolism in patients [98]. A class of antibacterial agents known as sulfonamides, which contain a characteristic sulfonamide linkage, was developed long ago that specifically target this enzyme [99].

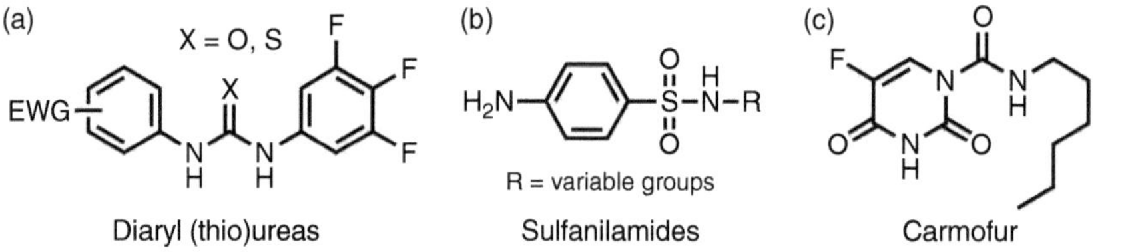

Figure 8.6 Chemical scaffolds of compounds identified in HTS campaigns that employed a riboswitch-based sensor. (a) Agonists of fluoride toxicity in *E. coli* and *S. mutans* discovered through a HTS effort that employed an F^- riboswitch reporter. The best-performing compounds employed a diaryl urea or diaryl thiourea scaffold in which one aryl moiety contained electron withdrawing groups at the meta and/or para positions. (b) Inhibitors of folate biosynthesis in *E. coli* discovered through a HTS effort that employed a ZTP riboswitch reporter. The best-performing compounds employed a sulfanilamide scaffold. (c) Inhibitors of SAH nucleosidase in *E. coli* discovered through a HTS effort that employed a SAH riboswitch-based sensor. A confirmed active compound identified is carmofur (1-hexylcarbamoyl-5-fluorouracil).

To search for inhibitors of folate biosynthesis with different chemical structures or novel biochemical mechanisms of action, researchers exploited a riboswitch that senses ZTP (5-aminoimidazole-4-carboxamide riboside 5′-triphosphate) [23, 54]. ZTP is proposed to function as an alarmone that produces a stress response when the cell is starved of essential folate derivatives, particularly 10-formyl-tetrahydrofolate [100]. Grafting a ZTP riboswitch upstream of the open reading frame (ORF) of a *lacZ* mRNA allowed for monitoring of intracellular ZTP levels. Numerous hit compounds were identified in a high-throughput screen that produced an increase in ZTP concentration. Most of the hits carry a sulfanilamide scaffold containing the characteristic sulfonamide linkage (Figure 8.6b). Based on this chemical similarity, these compounds presumably employ a similar mechanism of action to previously reported sulfonamide antimicrobials. It is likely that this screening campaign mostly yielded sulfonamide-containing compounds and few other types of folate inhibitor classes at least in part due to the relative low chemical diversity of compounds in the library.

8.3.4 A Riboswitch-Based SAH Sensor Reveals an Inhibitor of SAH Nucleosidase

S-adenosylhomocysteine (SAH) is a by-product of cellular transmethylation biochemistry involving *S*-adenosylmethionine (SAM) [101]. SAH buildup can cause inhibition of cellular transmethylation reactions, rendering its detoxification essential [101]. SAH nucleosidase is the enzyme responsible for recycling SAH in bacteria [102], identifying it as a critical target for antibiotic drug development [103]. Immucillin-based compounds have been developed to target SAH nucleosidase, but unfortunately there is reported cross-reactivity with human methylthioadenosine phosphorylase as well as poor cellular permeability [103–105].

To develop screening methods that address these issues, researchers recently exploited a SAH riboswitch as an in vivo sensor for this by-product of SAM-dependent methylation reactions. A riboswitch-reporter fusion construct was used to search for new compounds that disrupt SAH nucleosidase activity in *E. coli* [24]. An active compound, carmofur (1-hexylcarbamoyl-5-fluorouracil), was identified (Figure 8.6c) and validated using genetic (riboswitch mutant) and biochemical (enzyme kinetics) assays [24]. Carmofur is approved for use as an antineoplastic drug for cancer treatment [106], making its immediate implementation as an antibacterial agent unlikely. However, it presents a novel chemical scaffold that could presumably be further improved by medicinal chemistry techniques.

8.3.5 Barriers and Future Developments

A major barrier to any high-throughput screening effort is access to a large and diverse chemical library. Additionally, because the reporters often rely on fluorescence signal to detect changes in ligand concentration, many autofluorescent compounds are typically discounted as false positives. In principle, active compounds could also be autofluorescent, but they are not suitable for the assay in its current format. For future screening efforts, multiple reporters with distinct emission wavelengths could be used to accommodate fluorescent compounds whose emissions overlap with that of one of the reporters. Also, bactericidal compounds may be so potent that they cause bacterial cell death at the concentrations used in the screening assay. In this case, the reporter activity would be low, despite the possibility that the compound has the desired effect. While it is difficult to avoid this problem, one method might be to screen certain compounds at reduced concentrations.

Future efforts will likely target pathways that are unique to bacteria, to avoid off-target effects in humans. Pathways widespread in pathogenic bacteria, but less common in bacteria that compose the human gut microbiome, are of particular interest. Prime candidates for future endeavors include TPP riboswitches, which represent the most widespread class and thus might be well suited for the development of broad-spectrum antibiotics [14, 21].

8.4 Application of Riboswitches in Gene Therapy

8.4.1 Considerations for Designer Riboswitches

Genetically encodable synthetic devices that allow for conditional regulation of gene expression are proving to be increasingly useful in a host of applications including synthetic biology, functional genomics, biosensing, and therapeutics [107, 108]. Such genetic switches would be ideally suited for regulating the expression of a transgene in human gene therapy applications, in which transgene expression is chemically induced by a drug. Genetic switches could be employed as important components of gene therapy systems to treat a wide array of human health issues including pathological diseases, genetic disorders, and cancer.

Protein-based genetic switches, such as the tetracycline-responsive Tet-ON/Tet-OFF systems, have achieved success in preclinical gene therapy applications [109–111]. However, these switches are immunogenic and prohibitively large (>1 kb), producing a substantial genetic footprint and hindering delivery [112, 113]. Riboswitches offer tremendous potential for overcoming these challenges. However, natural examples respond to fundamental metabolites such as nucleic acid derivatives, ions, or amino acids [14]. The concentrations of these ligands cannot be safely manipulated in humans, precluding the use of most known natural riboswitches for human gene therapy applications. Recently, riboswitches with alternative aptamer and expression platform domains have been engineered to regulate gene expression in response to other ligands [114]. Relative to protein switches, these "designer riboswitches" are notably smaller (<200 bases), nonimmunogenic [112], and modular in design [115]. The relatively compact size makes it easier to include RNA-based switches in a delivery vector alongside a therapeutic protein of interest. Additionally, while it is a considerable challenge to modify a protein switch to respond to a different drug, it is comparatively straightforward to evolve aptamers for new compounds.

The first consideration in developing a designer riboswitch is the target ligand. In principle, an RNA aptamer can be generated as a receptor for almost any target using in vitro selection [116, 117]. Drug-like compounds that exhibit excellent bioavailability, safety, pharmacodynamics, and pharmacokinetics are ideal candidates for this effort. Recently, researchers have exploited natural riboswitch scaffolds to generate aptamers for new compounds that maintain the natural scaffold [118–120]. This strategy appears to increase the likelihood that RNA aptamers will fold reliably (and function) inside cells. Aptamers can then be grafted onto expression platforms to produce engineered riboswitches [120]. In some reports, aptamer and expression platform domains are evolved together [121], or a communication module that enables allostery is developed [115, 122–124].

An important consideration is that designer riboswitches should be implemented as ON switches, so that the drug is only administered while treatment is required. Ideally, there would be zero gene expression in the absence of the drug. Administering the drug at carefully measured doses would enable exploring the dynamic range of the switch, a valuable feature of this type of personalized medicine. If the aptamer and drug exhibit 1 : 1 binding, it should theoretically be possible to explore intermediate gene expression levels between fully OFF and ON states over two orders of magnitude of drug concentrations. Furthermore, developing an aptamer with high affinity for the drug is imperative, as low concentrations of the drug will minimize off-target effects.

8.4.2 Eukaryotic Expression Platforms

With most bacterial riboswitches, the aptamer domain regulates a transcription terminator stem or an anti-Shine-Dalgarno sequence [8, 9]. These expression platforms do not readily conform to the mechanisms used for gene expression and regulation in humans. Thus, different expression platforms must be developed to control the expression of genes in patients using synthetic riboswitches. Self-cleaving ribozymes are a common expression platform employed by researchers when engineering a riboswitch intended for human applications [112, 125–130]. These ribozymes function naturally as *cis*-acting RNAs that improve the rate constant of RNA strand scission by internal phosphoester transfer (often by 6 orders of magnitude or greater) [131–139]. Self-cleaving ribozymes can be fused with aptamers to generate allosteric ribozymes in which self-cleaving activity is conditional on the presence or absence of the target ligand [122–124, 140].

Allostery can occur in two distinct ways: (i) an inactive ribozyme is turned on by the presence of the target ligand or (ii) an active ribozyme is inhibited by the presence of the target ligand. The latter model is well suited for gene therapy applications and could be used to control gene expression by inserting such a switch in the 3′ UTR of an mRNA [141]. When the drug is absent, the ribozyme rapidly cleaves off the 3′ poly-A tail from the precursor mRNA. The cleaved precursor mRNA is degraded by the exosome [142, 143], keeping background gene expression levels very low. When the drug is administered, the ribozyme is disabled, and gene expression is turned on. These features were showcased in a recent report describing the regulation of a rapid self-cleaving ribozyme with antisense morpholino oligonucleotides [112]. One drawback of this approach is that it would require injections of morpholino oligonucleotides. The ability to externally control the switch with an oral inducer that is less invasive would be a preferred treatment option.

Curiously, allosteric self-cleaving ribozymes have not been found to control gene expression in nature [144]. Though it could simply be the case that these examples are yet to be discovered, it merits exploring other possible expression platforms that more directly interface with mammalian gene regulatory machinery. For example, a recent report describes an engineered riboswitch that uses the initial or "P1" stem of a guanine aptamer to hide or reveal a polyadenylation sequence [145]. This approach is attractive because of the simplicity of the design. However, a second engineered riboswitch that incorporated a self-cleaving ribozyme was required in tandem to sufficiently improve the dynamic range. Similarly, researchers have developed riboswitches that control alternative splicing by hiding or revealing a 5′ splice site within the P1 stem of a tetracycline aptamer [113, 146]. Another report describes an engineered riboswitch that regulates an internal ribosome entry site (IRES) in response to theophylline [147]. One drawback of this approach is that the IRES itself is quite large and would consume valuable vector space. Additionally, it is unlikely to be a generalizable approach to engineering riboswitches without much trial-and-error experimentation during the design process.

In another example, researchers used tetracycline to hide or reveal a microRNA (miRNA) binding site [148]. A disadvantage noted by the authors is that this approach might disrupt the natural miRNA system within the cell and produce unwanted off-target effects. Recently, an aptamer that binds a tetracycline repressor (TetR) protein was exploited to regulate alternative splicing [149]. This involves expressing a foreign protein, which could present issues with both immunogenicity and vector space limitations. Another example involved a theophylline aptamer that regulated a -1 ribosomal frameshifting element [150].

This approach produces nonsense protein products which could also pose issues with immunogenicity.

8.4.3 Barriers and Future Developments

Many proof-of-principle studies have been published using ribozyme-based expression platforms, among other mechanisms for gene control. There are various aspects to consider when selecting an expression platform, including the length of the construct (including aptamer and expression platform) in nucleotides, the relative ease with which allostery is expected to be achieved with an aptamer domain (design difficulty), whether the design is reasonably expected to modular, expected off-target effects from the nature of the expression platform itself, and the expected dynamic range. We have evaluated these features for several eukaryotic expression platforms (Figure 8.7). Some devices, such as allosteric ribozymes, could be implemented with various placements within an mRNA, whereas others must be positioned precisely to exhibit gene control.

We considered expression platforms that can simply be contained within the P1 stem of an aptamer (such as hiding or revealing a polyadenylation signal, miRNA-binding site, or Kozak sequence) as favorable. Constructs that involve another relatively small domain (such as a self-cleaving ribozyme or a short intron sequence) were considered intermediate and those that involved a large domain (IRES, frameshifting element) were considered unfavorable.

For design difficulty, some constructs are relatively straightforward to design (those that involve hiding or revealing a sequence via ligand-mediated formation

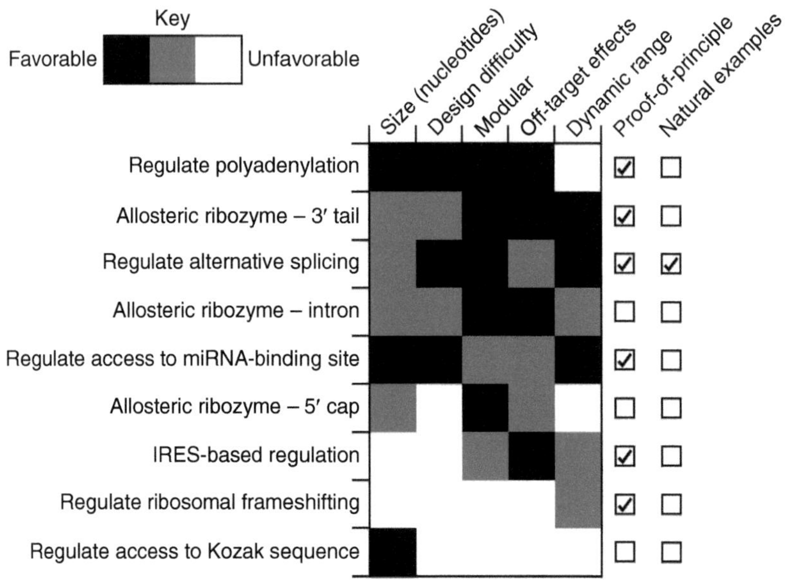

Figure 8.7 Evaluation of mammalian expression platforms that could be applied to regulate gene expression in eukaryotes.

of a P1 stem). Development of constructs considered intermediate in this category might involve screening many constructs, but numerous literature precedents exist to guide researchers (e.g. allosteric ribozymes). Constructs considered unfavorably might require substantial trial and error to develop (e.g. regulating a large domain such as an IRES or frameshifting element). Devices inserted in the 5′ UTR (e.g. for regulating access to a Kozak sequence) are likely to be incredibly challenging to implement as ON switches. This is likely true because highly structured RNAs such as aptamers that occur between the 5′ cap and start codon have been shown to reduce translation of the associated ORF [151], thereby potentially reducing overall gene expression even when the riboswitch would be in the ON state.

Some engineered RNA switches are expected to be (or have been reported to be) modular in architecture, wherein the aptamer domain can be swapped out for another with different ligand specificity and the device still functions reasonably well. This characteristic is desirable because it reduces the time required to develop a device that responds to a different compound and still maintains robust switch function. Lastly, we considered the expected or reported ranges for potential ON-switch devices that could be (or have been) developed. For devices such as allosteric ribozymes, which are expected to have extremely low expression in the OFF state, a large dynamic range may not be required as even low gene expression levels might be sufficient to provide the therapeutic effect.

A common theme among reported examples is that the compounds used to control the riboswitch are often repeated from the same group of classic aptamers (guanine, tetracycline, and theophylline). There is a pressing need for aptamers that respond to drug-like compounds like those described earlier (see Section 8.4.1).

8.5 Concluding Remarks

Numerous bacterial discoveries have led to fundamental molecular biology tools, such as polymerase chain reaction (PCR) [152], restriction enzyme technology [153], and novel therapeutic technologies (e.g. clustered regularly interspaced short palindromic repeats [CRISPR] [154]). Since the first experimentally validated bacterial riboswitch was reported just over 20 years ago [33], riboswitch-based technologies have seen substantial progress in preclinical drug development. Despite this, many exciting challenges remain. Known bacterial riboswitches present a valuable and still largely untapped collection of targets for the development of new antibacterial agents. Furthermore, the discovery and validation of new riboswitch classes is a driving force for identifying new biological targets for antibiotic development. In addition to presenting novel riboswitch classes themselves, new proteins have been discovered by pathways that are elucidated by riboswitch discovery – such as guanidine hydrolases [155, 156]. The prospect of discovering hypothesized riboswitches that naturally occur in humans would present tantalizing opportunities for drug development researchers, especially with the increase in interest in RNA drug development resulting from the advent of mRNA vaccines [157]. Meanwhile, synthetic biologists seek to advance riboswitch technology ever closer to human gene therapy applications.

Acknowledgment

We thank members of the Breaker laboratory for helpful comments and discussions. RNA research in the Breaker laboratory is supported by the Howard Hughes Medical Institute and grants from the NIH. M.G.M. is a Howard Hughes Medical Institute Awardee of the Life Sciences Research Foundation.

References

1 Mandal, M. and Breaker, R.R. (2004). Gene regulation by riboswitches. *Nat. Rev. Mol. Cell Biol.* 5: 451–463.
2 Winkler, W.C. and Breaker, R.R. (2005). Regulation of bacterial gene expression by riboswitches. *Annu. Rev. Microbiol.* 59: 487–517.
3 Serganov, A. and Nudler, E. (2013). A decade of riboswitches. *Cell* 152: 17–24.
4 Sherwood, A.V. and Henkin, T.M. (2016). Riboswitch-mediated gene regulation: novel RNA architectures dictate gene expression responses. *Annu. Rev. Microbiol.* 70: 361–374.
5 Henkin, T.M. (2008). Riboswitch RNAs: using RNA to sense cellular metabolism. *Genes Dev.* 22: 3383–3390.
6 Lotz, T.S. and Suess, B. (2018). Small-molecule-binding riboswitches. *Microbiol. Spectrum* 6.
7 Bédard, A.S.V., Hien, E.D.M., and Lafontaine, D.A. (2020). Riboswitch regulation mechanisms: RNA, metabolites and regulatory proteins. *Biochim. Biophys. Acta, Gene Regul. Mech.* 194501.
8 Breaker, R.R. (2018). Riboswitches and translation control. *Cold Spring Harbor Perspect. Biol.* 10.
9 Turnbough, C.L. (2019). Regulation of bacterial gene expression by transcription attenuation. *Microbiol. Mol. Biol. Rev.* 83.
10 Ariza-Mateos, A., Nuthanakanti, A., and Serganov, A. (2021). Riboswitch mechanisms: new tricks for an old dog. *Biochem.* 86: 962–975.
11 Scull, C.E., Dandpat, S.S., Romero, R.A., and Walter, N.G. (2021). Transcriptional riboswitches integrate timescales for bacterial gene expression control. *Front. Mol. Biosci.* 7.
12 Kavita, K. and Breaker, R.R. (2023). Discovering riboswitches: the past and the future. *Trends Biochem. Sci.* 48: 119–141.
13 Sherlock, M.E., Higgs, G., Yu, D. et al. (2022). Architectures and complex functions of tandem riboswitches. *RNA Biol.* 19: 1059–1076.
14 McCown, P.J., Corbino, K.A., Stav, S. et al. (2017). Riboswitch diversity and distribution. *RNA* 23: 995–1011.
15 Breaker, R.R. (2009). Riboswitches: from ancient gene-control systems to modern drug targets. *Future Microbiol.* 4: 771–773.

16 Topp, S. and Gallivan, J.P. (2010). Emerging applications of riboswitches in chemical biology. *ACS Chem. Biol.* 5: 139–148.

17 Machtel, P., Bąkowska-Żywicka, K., and Żywicki, M. (2016). Emerging applications of riboswitches – from antibacterial targets to molecular tools. *J. Appl. Genet.* 57: 531–541.

18 Hallberg, Z.F., Su, Y., Kitto, R.Z., and Hammond, M.C. (2017). Engineering and in vivo applications of riboswitches. *Annu. Rev. Biochem.* 86: 515–539.

19 Blount, K.F. and Breaker, R.R. (2006). Riboswitches as antibacterial drug targets. *Nat. Biotechnol.* 24: 1558–1564.

20 Deigan, K.E. and Ferré-D'Amaré, A.R. (2011). Riboswitches: discovery of drugs that target bacterial gene-regulatory RNAs. *Acc. Chem. Res.* 44: 1329–1338.

21 Panchal, V. and Brenk, R. (2021). Riboswitches as drug targets for antibiotics. *Antibiotics* 10 (1): 1–22.

22 Nelson, J.W., Plummer, M.S., Blount, K.F. et al. (2015). Small molecule fluoride toxicity agonists. *Chem. Biol.* 22: 527–534.

23 Perkins, K.R., Atilho, R.M., Moon, M.H., and Breaker, R.R. (2019). Employing a ZTP riboswitch to detect bacterial folate biosynthesis inhibitors in a small molecule high-throughput screen. *ACS Chem. Biol.* 14: 2841–2850.

24 Sadeeshkumar, H., Balaji, A., Sutherland, A. et al. (2023). Employing an SAH riboswitch to detect the effects of SAH nucleosidase inhibitors in a small molecule high-throughput screen. *Anal. Biochem.* 666: 115047.

25 Link, K.H. and Breaker, R.R. (2009). Engineering ligand-responsive gene-control elements: lessons learned from natural riboswitches. *Gene Ther.* 16: 1189–1201.

26 Hutchings, M., Truman, A., and Wilkinson, B. (2019). Antibiotics: past, present and future. *Curr. Opin. Microbiol.* 51: 72–80.

27 Prescott, J.F. (2014). The resistance tsunami, antimicrobial stewardship, and the golden age of microbiology. *Vet. Microbiol.* 171: 273–278.

28 Terreni, M., Taccani, M., and Pregnolato, M. (2021). New antibiotics for multidrug-resistant bacterial strains: Latest research developments and future perspectives. *Mol. Ther.* 26.

29 Hong, W., Zeng, J., and Xie, J. (2014). Antibiotic drugs targeting bacterial RNAs. *Acta Pharm. Sin. B* 4: 258–265.

30 Childs-Disney, J.L., Yang, X., Gibaut, Q.M.R. et al. (2022). Targeting RNA structures with small molecules. *Nat. Rev. Drug Discovery* 21: 736–762.

31 Sutcliffe, J.A. (2005). Improving on nature: antibiotics that target the ribosome. *Curr. Opin. Microbiol.* 8: 534–542.

32 Matzner, D. and Mayer, G. (2015). (Dis)similar analogues of riboswitch metabolites as antibacterial lead compounds. *J. Med. Chem.* 58: 3275–3286.

33 Nahvi, A., Sudarsan, N., Ebert, M.S. et al. (2002). Genetic control by a metabolite binding mRNA. *Chem. Biol.* 9: 1043–1049.

34 Baker, J.L., Sudarsan, N., Weinberg, Z. et al. (2012). Widespread genetic switches and toxicity resistance proteins for fluoride. *Science* 335: 233–235.

35 Winkler, W.C., Cohen-Chalamish, S., and Breaker, R.R. (2002). An mRNA structure that controls gene expression by binding FMN. *Proc. Natl. Acad. Sci. U. S. A.* 99: 15908–15913.

36 Mandal, M., Lee, M., Barrick, J.E. et al. (2004). A glycine-dependent riboswitch that uses cooperative binding to control gene expression. *Science* 306: 275–279.

37 Nelson, J.W., Atilho, R.M., Sherlock, M.E. et al. (2017). Metabolism of free guanidine in bacteria is regulated by a widespread riboswitch class. *Mol. Cell* 65: 220–230.

38 Mandal, M., Boese, B., Barrick, J.E. et al. (2003). Riboswitches control fundamental biochemical pathways in *Bacillus subtilis* and other bacteria. *Cell* 113: 577–586.

39 Sudarsan, N., Wickiser, J.K., Nakamura, S. et al. (2003). An mRNA structure in bacteria that controls gene expression by binding lysine. *Genes Dev.* 17: 2688–2697.

40 Dann, C.E., Wakeman, C.A., Sieling, C.L. et al. (2007). Structure and mechanism of a metal-sensing regulatory RNA. *Cell* 130: 878–892.

41 Park, S.Y., Cromie, M.J., Lee, E.J., and Groisman, E.A. (2010). A bacterial mRNA leader that employs different mechanisms to sense disparate intracellular signals. *Cell* 142: 737–748.

42 Price, I.R., Gaballa, A., Ding, F. et al. (2015). Mn^{2+}-sensing mechanisms of *yybP-ykoY* orphan riboswitches. *Mol. Cell* 57: 1110–1123.

43 Regulski, E.E., Moy, R.H., Weinberg, Z. et al. (2008). A widespread riboswitch candidate that controls bacterial genes involved in molybdenum cofactor and tungsten cofactor metabolism. *Mol. Microbiol.* 68: 918–932.

44 White, N., Sadeeshkumar, H., Sun, A. et al. (2022). Na^+ riboswitches regulate genes for diverse physiological processes in bacteria. *Nat. Chem. Biol.* 18: 878–885.

45 White, N., Sadeeshkumar, H., Sun, A. et al. (2022). Lithium-sensing riboswitch classes regulate expression of bacterial cation transporter genes. *Sci. Rep.* 12.

46 Roth, A., Winkler, W.C., Regulski, E.E. et al. (2007). A riboswitch selective for the queuosine precursor $preQ_1$ contains an unusually small aptamer domain. *Nat. Struct. Mol. Biol.* 14: 308–317.

47 Meyer, M.M., Roth, A., Chervin, S.M. et al. (2008). Confirmation of a second natural $preQ_1$ aptamer class in *Streptococcaceae* bacteria. *RNA* 14: 685–695.

48 Wang, J.X., Lee, E.R., Morales, D.R. et al. (2008). Riboswitches that sense *S*-adenosylhomocysteine and activate genes involved in coenzyme recycling. *Mol. Cell* 29: 691–702.

49 Winkler, W.C., Nahvi, A., Sudarsan, N. et al. (2003). An mRNA structure that controls gene expression by binding *S*-adenosylmethionine. *Nat. Struct. Biol.* 10: 701–707.

50 Weinberg, Z., Wang, J.X., Bogue, J. et al. (2010). Comparative genomics reveals 104 candidate structured RNAs from bacteria, archaea, and their metagenomes. *Genome Biol.* 11: 1–17.

51 Fuchs, R.T., Grundy, F.J., and Henkin, T.M. (2006). The SMK box is a new SAM-binding RNA for translational regulation of SAM synthetase. *Nat. Struct. Mol. Biol.* 13: 226–233.

52 Ames, T.D., Rodionov, D.A., Weinberg, Z., and Breaker, R.R. (2010). A eubacterial riboswitch class that senses the coenzyme tetrahydrofolate. *Chem. Biol.* 17: 681–685.

53 Winkler, W., Nahvi, A., and Breaker, R.R. (2002). Thiamine derivatives bind messenger RNAs directly to regulate bacterial gene expression. *Nature* 419: 952–956.

54 Kim, P.B., Nelson, J.W., and Breaker, R.R. (2015). An ancient riboswitch class in bacteria regulates purine biosynthesis and one-carbon metabolism. *Mol. Cell* 57: 317–328.

55 Trausch, J.J., Xu, Z., Edwards, A.L. et al. (2014). Structural basis for diversity in the SAM clan of riboswitches. *Proc. Natl. Acad. Sci. U. S. A.* 111: 6624–6629.

56 Kalvari, I., Nawrocki, E.P., Ontiveros-Palacios, N. et al. (2021). Rfam 14: expanded coverage of metagenomic, viral and microRNA families. *Nucleic Acids Res.* 49: D192–D200.

57 Asokan, G.V., Ramadhan, T., Ahmed, E., and Sanad, H. (2019). WHO global priority pathogens list: A bibliometric analysis of medline-pubmed for knowledge mobilization to infection prevention and control practices in Bahrain. *Oman Med. J.* 34: 184–193.

58 Lee, E.R., Blount, K.F., and Breaker, R.R. (2009). Roseoflavin is a natural antibacterial compound that binds to FMN riboswitches and regulates gene expression. *RNA Biol.* 6: 187–194.

59 Warner, K.D., Hajdin, C.E., and Weeks, K.M. (2018). Principles for targeting RNA with drug-like small molecules. *Nat. Rev. Drug Discovery* 178 (17): 547–558.

60 Hewitt, W.M., Calabrese, D.R., and Schneekloth, J.S. (2019). Evidence for ligandable sites in structured RNA throughout the Protein Data Bank. *Bioorg. Med. Chem.* 27: 2253–2260.

61 Melander, R.J., Zurawski, D.V., and Melander, C. (2018). Narrow-spectrum antibacterial agents. *Medchemcomm* 9: 12–21.

62 Blount, K.F., Megyola, C., Plummer, M. et al. (2015). Novel riboswitch-binding flavin analog that protects mice against *Clostridium difficile* infection without inhibiting cecal flora. *Antimicrob. Agents Chemother.* 59: 5736–5746.

63 Howe, J.A., Wang, H., Fischmann, T.O. et al. (2015). Selective small-molecule inhibition of an RNA structural element. *Nature* 526: 672–677.

64 Motika, S.E., Ulrich, R.J., Geddes, E.J. et al. (2020). Gram-negative antibiotic active through inhibition of an essential riboswitch. *J. Am. Chem. Soc.* 142: 10856–10862.

65 Mironov, A.S., Gusarov, I., Rafikov, R. et al. (2002). Sensing small molecules by nascent RNA: a mechanism to control transcription in bacteria. *Cell* 111: 747–756.

66 Serganov, A., Huang, L., and Patel, D.J. (2009). Coenzyme recognition and gene regulation by a flavin mononucleotide riboswitch. *Nature* 458: 233–237.

67 Vicens, Q., Mondragón, E., Reyes, F.E. et al. (2018). Structure-activity relationship of flavin analogues that target the flavin mononucleotide riboswitch. *ACS Chem. Biol.* 13: 2908–2919.

68 Howe, J.A., Xiao, L., Fischmann, T.O. et al. (2016). Atomic resolution mechanistic studies of ribocil: a highly selective unnatural ligand mimic of the *E. coli* FMN riboswitch. *RNA Biol.* 13: 946–954.

69 Wang, H., Mann, P.A., Xiao, L. et al. (2017). Dual-targeting small-molecule inhibitors of the *Staphylococcus aureus* FMN riboswitch disrupt riboflavin homeostasis in an infectious setting. *Cell Chem. Biol.* 24: 576–588.e6.

70 Mayer, G. and Famulok, M. (2006). High-throughput-compatible assay for *glmS* riboswitch metabolite dependence. *ChemBioChem* 7: 602–604.

71 Fei, X., Holmes, T., Diddle, J. et al. (2014). Phosphatase-inert glucosamine 6-phosphate mimics serve as actuators of the *glmS* riboswitch. *ACS Chem. Biol.* 9: 2875–2882.

72 Matzner, D., Schüller, A., Seitz, T. et al. (2017). Fluoro-carba-sugars are glycomimetic activators of the *glmS* ribozyme. *Chem. A Eur. J.* 23: 12604–12612.

73 Kim, J.N., Blount, K.F., Puskarz, I. et al. (2009). Design and antimicrobial action of purine analogues that bind guanine riboswitches. *ACS Chem. Biol.* 4: 915–927.

74 Mulhbacher, J., Brouillette, E., Allard, M. et al. (2010). Novel riboswitch ligand analogs as selective inhibitors of guanine-related metabolic pathways. *PLoS Pathog.* 6: 1–11.

75 Matyjasik, M.M., Hall, S.D., and Batey, R.T. (2020). High affinity binding of N_2-modified guanine derivatives significantly disrupts the ligand binding pocket of the guanine riboswitch. *Mol. Ther.* 25: 2295.

76 Connelly, C.M., Numata, T., Boer, R.E. et al. (2019). Synthetic ligands for $PreQ_1$ riboswitches provide structural and mechanistic insights into targeting RNA tertiary structure. *Nat. Commun.* 10: 1–12.

77 Balaratnam, S., Rhodes, C., Bume, D.D. et al. (2021). A chemical probe based on the $PreQ_1$ metabolite enables transcriptome-wide mapping of binding sites. *Nat. Commun.* 12: 1–15.

78 Tran, B., Pichling, P., Tenney, L. et al. (2020). Parallel discovery strategies provide a basis for riboswitch ligand design. *Cell Chem. Biol.* 27: 1241–1249.e4.

79 Chen, L., Cressina, E., Leeper, F.J. et al. (2010). A fragment-based approach to identifying ligands for riboswitches. *ACS Chem. Biol.* 5: 355–358.

80 Cressina, E., Chen, L., Abell, C. et al. (2011). Fragment screening against the thiamine pyrophosphate riboswitch *thiM*. *Chem. Sci.* 2: 157–165.

81 Warner, K.D., Homan, P., Weeks, K.M. et al. (2014). Validating fragment-based drug discovery for biological RNAs: lead fragments bind and remodel the TPP riboswitch specifically. *Chem. Biol.* 21: 591–595.

82 Tracy, A.H. and Elderfield, R.C. (1941). Studies in the pyridine series. II. Synthesis of 2-methyl-3-(β-hydroxyethyl)pyridine and of the pyridine analog of thiamine (vitamin b1). *J. Organomet. Chem.* 6: 54–62.

83 Sudarsan, N., Cohen-Chalamish, S., Nakamura, S. et al. (2005). Thiamine pyrophosphate riboswitches are targets for the antimicrobial compound pyrithiamine. *Chem. Biol.* 12: 1325–1335.

84 Blount, K.F., Wang, J.X., Lim, J. et al. (2007). Antibacterial lysine analogs that target lysine riboswitches. *Nat. Chem. Biol.* 3: 44–49.

85 Ataide, S.F., Wilson, S.N., Dang, S. et al. (2007). Mechanisms of resistance to an amino acid antibiotic that targets translation. *ACS Chem. Biol.* 2: 819–827.

86 Greenlee, E.B., Stav, S., Atilho, R.M. et al. (2018). Challenges of ligand identification for the second wave of orphan riboswitch candidates. *RNA Biol.* 15: 377–390.

87 Jaffrey, S.R. (2018). RNA-based fluorescent biosensors for detecting metabolites in vitro and in living cells. *Adv. Pharmacol.* 82: 187–203.

88 Su, Y. and Hammond, M.C. (2020). RNA-based fluorescent biosensors for live cell imaging of small molecules and RNAs. *Curr. Opin. Biotechnol.* 63: 157–166.

89 Paige, J.S., Nguyen-Duc, T., Song, W., and Jaffrey, S.R. (2012). Fluorescence imaging of cellular metabolites with RNA. *Science* 335: 1194.

90 Su, Y., Hickey, S.F., Keyser, S.G.L., and Hammond, M.C. (2016). In vitro and in vivo enzyme activity screening via RNA-based fluorescent biosensors for *S*-adenosyl-l-homocysteine (SAH). *J. Am. Chem. Soc.* 138: 7040–7047.

91 Manna, S., Truong, J., and Hammond, M.C. (2021). Guanidine biosensors enable comparison of cellular turn-on kinetics of riboswitch-based biosensor and reporter. *ACS Synth. Biol.* 10: 566–578.

92 Li, L. (2003). The biochemistry and physiology of metallic fluoride: action, mechanism, and implications. *Crit. Rev. Oral Biol. Med.* 14: 100–114.

93 Barbier, O., Arreola-Mendoza, L., and Del Razo, L.M. (2010). Molecular mechanisms of fluoride toxicity. *Chem. Biol. Interact.* 188: 319–333.

94 Francisco, G.D., Li, Z., Albright, J.D. et al. (2004). Phenyl thiazolyl urea and carbamate derivatives as new inhibitors of bacterial cell-wall biosynthesis. *Bioorg. Med. Chem. Lett.* 14: 235–238.

95 Li, Z., Francisco, G.D., Hu, W. et al. (2003). 2-Phenyl-5,6-dihydro-2H-thieno[3,2-c]pyrazol-3-ol derivatives as new inhibitors of bacterial cell wall biosynthesis. *Bioorg. Med. Chem. Lett.* 13: 2591–2594.

96 Russell, A.D. (2004). Whither triclosan? *J. Antimicrob. Chemother.* 53: 693–695.

97 Bourne, C.R. (2014). Utility of the biosynthetic folate pathway for targets in antimicrobial discovery. *Antibiotics* 3: 1–28.

98 Bermingham, A. and Derrick, J.P. (2002). The folic acid biosynthesis pathway in bacteria: evaluation of potential for antibacterial drug discovery. *BioEssays* 24: 637–648.

99 Roland, S., Ferone, R., Harvey, R.J. et al. (1979). The characteristics and significance of sulfonamides as substrates for *Escherichia coli* dihydropteroate synthase. *J. Biol. Chem.* 254: 10337–10345.

100 Bochner, B.R. and Ames, B.N. (1982). ZTP (5-amino 4-imidazole carboxamide riboside 5′-triphosphate): A proposed alarmone for 10-formyl-tetrahydrofolate deficiency. *Cell* 29: 929–937.

101 Lu, S.C. (2000). *S*-Adenosylmethionine. *Int. J. Biochem. Cell Biol.* 32: 391–395.

102 Parveen, N. and Cornell, K.A. (2011). Methylthioadenosine/*S*-adenosylhomocysteine nucleosidase, a critical enzyme for bacterial metabolism. *Mol. Microbiol.* 79: 7–20.

103 Gutierrez, J.A., Crowder, T., Rinaldo-Matthis, A. et al. (2009). Transition state analogs of 5′-methylthioadenosine nucleosidase disrupt quorum sensing. *Nat. Chem. Biol.* 5: 251–257.

104 Singh, V., Shi, W., Evans, G.B. et al. (2004). Picomolar transition state analogue inhibitors of human 5′-methylthioadenosine phosphorylase and X-ray structure with MT-immucillin-A. *Biochemistry* 43: 9–18.

105 Singh, V., Evans, G.B., Lenz, D.H. et al. (2005). Femtomolar transition state analogue inhibitors of 5′-methylthioadenosine/*S*-adenosylhomocysteine nucleosidase from *Escherichia coli*. *J. Biol. Chem.* 280: 18265–18273.

106 Wu, K., Xiu, Y., Zhou, P. et al. (2019). A new use for an old drug: carmofur attenuates lipopolysaccharide (LPS)-induced acute lung injury via inhibition of FAAH and NAAA activities. *Front. Pharmacol.* 10: 818.

107 Yokobayashi, Y. (2019). Aptamer-based and aptazyme-based riboswitches in mammalian cells. *Curr. Opin. Chem. Biol.* 52: 72–78.

108 Nomura, Y. and Yokobayashi, Y. (2015). Aptazyme-based riboswitches and logic gates in mammalian cells. *Methods Mol. Biol.* 1316: 141–148.

109 Gossen, M., Freundlieb, S., Bender, G. et al. (1995). Transcriptional activation by tetracyclines in mammalian cells. *Science* 268: 1766–1769.

110 Guilbaud, M., Devaux, M., Couzinié, C. et al. (2019). Five years of successful inducible transgene expression following locoregional adeno-associated virus delivery in nonhuman primates with no detectable immunity. *Hum. Gene Ther.* 30: 802–813.

111 Das, T., Tenenbaum, L., and Berkhout, B. (2016). Tet-on systems for doxycycline-inducible gene expression. *Curr. Gene Ther.* 16: 156–167.

112 Zhong, G., Wang, H., He, W. et al. (2020). A reversible RNA on-switch that controls gene expression of AAV-delivered therapeutics in vivo. *Nat. Biotechnol.* 38: 169–175.

113 Finke, M., Brecht, D., Stifel, J. et al. (2021). Efficient splicing-based RNA regulators for tetracycline-inducible gene expression in human cell culture and *C. elegans*. *Nucleic Acids Res.* 49: E71.

114 Tickner, Z.J. and Farzan, M. (2021). Riboswitches for controlled expression of therapeutic transgenes delivered by adeno-associated viral vectors. *Pharmaceuticals* 14.

115 Felletti, M., Stifel, J., Wurmthaler, L.A. et al. (2016). Twister ribozymes as highly versatile expression platforms for artificial riboswitches. *Nat. Commun.* 7: 2–9.

116 Ellington, A.D. and Szostak, J.W. (1990). In vitro selection of RNA molecules that bind specific ligands. *Nature* 346: 818–822.

117 Tuerk, C. and Gold, L. (1990). Systematic evolution of ligands by exponential enrichment: RNA ligands to bacteriophage T4 DNA polymerase. *Science* 249: 505–510.

118 Porter, E.B., Polaski, J.T., Morck, M.M., and Batey, R.T. (2017). Recurrent RNA motifs as scaffolds for genetically encodable small-molecule biosensors. *Nat. Chem. Biol.* 13: 295–301.

119 Dey, S.K., Filonov, G.S., Olarerin-George, A.O. et al. (2022). Repurposing an adenine riboswitch into a fluorogenic imaging and sensing tag. *Nat. Chem. Biol.* 18: 180–190.

120 Mohsen, M.G., Midy, M.K., Balaji, A., and Breaker, R.R. (2023). Exploiting natural riboswitches for aptamer engineering and validation. *Nucleic Acids Res.* 51: 966–981.

121 Boussebayle, A., Torka, D., Ollivaud, S. et al. (2019). Next-level riboswitch development-implementation of Capture-SELEX facilitates identification of a new synthetic riboswitch. *Nucleic Acids Res.* 47: 4883–4895.

122 Tang, J. and Breaker, R.R. (1997). Rational design of allosteric ribozymes. *Chem. Biol.* 4: 453–459.

123 Soukup, G.A. and Breaker, R.R. (1999). Engineering precision RNA molecular switches. *Proc. Natl. Acad. Sci. U. S. A.* 96: 3584–3589.

124 Koizumi, M., Soukup, G.A., Kerr, J.N.Q., and Breaker, R.R. (1999). Allosteric selection of ribozymes that respond to the second messengers cGMP and cAMP. *Nat. Struct. Biol.* 6: 1062–1071.

125 Zhong, G., Wang, H., Bailey, C.C. et al. (2016). Rational design of aptazyme riboswitches for efficient control of gene expression in mammalian cells. *Elife* 5.

126 Rehm, C., Klauser, B., Finke, M., and Hartig, J.S. (2021). Engineering aptazyme switches for conditional gene expression in mammalian cells utilizing an in vivo screening approach. *Methods Mol. Biol.* 2323: 199–212.

127 Mustafina, K., Fukunaga, K., and Yokobayashi, Y. (2020). Design of mammalian ON-riboswitches based on tandemly fused aptamer and ribozyme. *ACS Synth. Biol.* 9: 19–25.

128 Mustafina, K., Nomura, Y., Rotrattanadumrong, R., and Yokobayashi, Y. (2021). Circularly-permuted pistol ribozyme: a synthetic ribozyme scaffold for mammalian riboswitches. *ACS Synth. Biol.* 10: 2040–2048.

129 Stifel, J. and Hartig, J.S. (2021). Ribozymes for regulation of gene expression. *Ribozymes* 505–518.

130 Felletti, M. and Hartig, J.S. (2017). Ligand-dependent ribozymes. *Wiley Interdiscip. Rev.: RNA* 8.

131 Tang, J. and Breaker, R.R. (2000). Structural diversity of self-cleaving ribozymes. *Proc. Natl. Acad. Sci. U. S. A.* 97: 5784–5789.

132 Scott, W.G. (2007). Ribozymes. *Curr. Opin. Struct. Biol.* 17: 280–286.

133 Doherty, E.A. and Doudna, J.A. (2001). Ribozyme structures and mechanisms. *Annu. Rev. Biophys. Biomol. Struct.* 30: 457–475.

134 Rossi, J.J. (1992). Ribozymes. *Curr. Opin. Biotechnol.* 3: 3–7.

135 Peng, H., Latifi, B., Müller, S. et al. (2021). Self-cleaving ribozymes: Substrate specificity and synthetic biology applications. *RSC Chem. Biol.* 2: 1370–1383.

136 Weinberg, C.E., Weinberg, Z., and Hammann, C. (2019). Novel ribozymes: discovery, catalytic mechanisms, and the quest to understand biological function. *Nucleic Acids Res.* 47: 9480–9494.

137 Lee, K.Y. and Lee, B.J. (2017). Structural and biochemical properties of novel self-cleaving ribozymes. *Mol. Ther.* 22.

138 Jimenez, R.M., Polanco, J.A., and Lupták, A. (2015). Chemistry and biology of self-cleaving ribozymes. *Trends Biochem. Sci* 40: 648–661.

139 Roth, A. and Breaker, R. (2021). Ribozyme discovery in bacteria. *Ribozymes* 281–302.

140 Soukup, G.A. and Breaker, R.R. (1999). Nucleic acid molecular switches. *Trends Biotechnol.* 17: 469–476.

141 Wieland, M. and Hartig, J.S. (2008). Artificial riboswitches: synthetic mRNA-based regulators of gene expression. *ChemBioChem* 9: 1873–1878.

142 Houseley, J., LaCava, J., and Tollervey, D. (2006). RNA-quality control by the exosome. *Nat. Rev. Mol. Cell Biol.* 7: 529–539.

143 West, S., Gromak, N., Norbury, C.J., and Proudfoot, N.J. (2006). Adenylation and exosome-mediated degradation of cotranscriptionally cleaved pre-messenger RNA in human cells. *Mol. Cell* 21: 437–443.

144 Panchapakesan, S.S.S. and Breaker, R.R. (2021). The case of the missing allosteric ribozymes. *Nat. Chem. Biol.* 17: 375–382.

145 Spöring, M., Boneberg, R., and Hartig, J.S. (2020). Aptamer-mediated control of polyadenylation for gene expression regulation in mammalian cells. *ACS Synth. Biol.* 9: 3008–3018.

146 Weigand, J.E. and Suess, B. (2007). Tetracycline aptamer-controlled regulation of pre-mRNA splicing in yeast. *Nucleic Acids Res.* 35: 4179.

147 Ogawa, A. (2011). Rational design of artificial riboswitches based on ligand-dependent modulation of internal ribosome entry in wheat germ extract and their applications as label-free biosensors. *RNA* 17: 478–488.

148 Mou, H., Zhong, G., Gardner, M.R. et al. (2018). Conditional regulation of gene expression by ligand-induced occlusion of a microRNA target sequence. *Mol. Ther.* 26: 1277–1286.

149 Mol, A.A., Groher, F., Schreiber, B. et al. (2019). Robust gene expression control in human cells with a novel universal TetR aptamer splicing module. *Nucleic Acids Res.* 47: e132–e132.

150 Lin, Y.H. and Chang, K.Y. (2016). Rational design of a synthetic mammalian riboswitch as a ligand-responsive -1 ribosomal frame-shifting stimulator. *Nucleic Acids Res.* 44: 9005–9015.

151 Werstuck, G. and Green, M.R. (1998). Controlling gene expression in living cells through small molecule-RNA interactions. *Science* 282: 296–298.

152 Saiki, R.K., Scharf, S., Faloona, F. et al. (1985). Enzymatic amplification of β-globin genomic sequences and restriction site analysis for diagnosis of sickle cell anemia. *Science* 230: 1350–1354.

153 Roberts, R.J. (2005). How restriction enzymes became the workhorses of molecular biology. *Proc. Natl. Acad. Sci. U. S. A.* 102: 5905–5908.

154 Jinek, M., Chylinski, K., Fonfara, I. et al. (2012). A programmable dual-RNA-guided DNA endonuclease in adaptive bacterial immunity. *Science* 337: 816–821.

155 Wang, B., Xu, Y., Wang, X. et al. (2021). A guanidine-degrading enzyme controls genomic stability of ethylene-producing cyanobacteria. *Nat. Commun.* 121 (12): 1–13.

156 Funck, D., Sinn, M., Fleming, J.R. et al. (2022). Discovery of a Ni2+-dependent guanidine hydrolase in bacteria. *Nature* 603: 515–521.

157 Pardi, N., Hogan, M.J., Porter, F.W., and Weissman, D. (2018). mRNA vaccines-a new era in vaccinology. *Nat. Rev. Drug Discovery* 17: 261–279.

9

Small Molecules That Degrade RNA

Noah A. Springer[1,2], Samantha M. Meyer[1,2], Amirhossein Taghavi[1], Jessica L. Childs-Disney[1], and Matthew D. Disney[1,2]

[1] *Department of Chemistry, The Herbert Wertheim UF Scripps Institute for Biomedical Innovation & Technology, Jupiter, FL 33458, USA*
[2] *The Scripps Research Institute, Jupiter, FL 33458, USA*

9.1 Antisense Oligonucleotide Degraders

The most common method to degrade a cellular RNA is by inducing ribonuclease (RNase H) cleavage upon binding of an antisense oligonucleotide (ASO). ASOs are modified oligonucleotides that base pair to target RNAs and either facilitate degradation, [1] act as steric blockers to alter splicing, [2] and/or inhibit translation [3]. For ASOs that degrade their target, the DNA/RNA heteroduplex is recognized by endogenous RNase H1 that cleaves the RNA strand of these hybrids, leading to specific degradation of target RNAs within cells [1, 4]. After cleavage via RNase H1, the target RNA is then fully degraded by exoribonucleases XRN1 (5′-3′ exoribonuclease 1), XRN2 (5′-3′ exoribonuclease 2), and the exosome complex [5]. Because only the RNA strand of the ASO/RNA duplex is cleaved, the ASO can be recycled and therefore acts sub-stoichiometrically. This process enables potent knockdown of a gene product in cells.

ASOs have been useful as chemical tools for knocking down targets in cell culture but are increasingly becoming viable drugs for some targets. The first ASO with an RNase H1-mediated mechanism of action, Fomiversen, was originally approved by the United States Food and Drug Administration (FDA) in 1998 to treat cytomegalovirus (CMV) retinitis [6], though it was later taken off the market. More recently, Inotersen was approved by the FDA in 2018 to treat hereditary transthyretin amyloidosis (hATTR) [7], competing with the small interfering RNA (siRNA) drug patisiran [8]. Additionally, although it functions via splicing modulation rather than RNase H1-mediated degradation, the success of nusinersen [9] demonstrates that ASOs can become blockbuster drugs. The design of potent ASOs is relatively straightforward when compared to other technologies since Watson-Crick base-pairing rules allow for rapid ASO design against any known RNA sequence. Key to the selectivity of an ASO is selection of unique sequences

RNA as a Drug Target: The Next Frontier for Medicinal Chemistry, First Edition.
Edited by John Schneekloth and Martin Pettersson.

in the RNA target. However, hybridization-free energy, cellular abundance, and the energetics of on- and off-targets can also affect selectivity; such complexities should be carefully considered [10, 11]. Nonetheless, various modifications to the nucleotide bases, ribose, and phosphodiester backbone have been identified that enhance the metabolic stability of ASOs, as well as influence tissue uptake and the thermodynamic stability of its interaction with the target RNA [12, 13]. The success of nusinersen demonstrates the potential of ASOs in the clinic, despite the challenges associated with the modality in general, centered on its lack of oral bioavailability and tissue distribution largely limited to the liver and kidney [13]. As exemplified by nusinersen, treatment directly into the cerebrospinal fluid can allow for distribution throughout the central nervous system [9]. Although ASOs are a promising technology with the potential to transform therapeutics targeting RNAs, the remainder of this chapter will focus on small molecules that have similar targeted RNA degradation capabilities.

9.2 Small-Molecule Direct Degraders

Many routes have been explored to identify small molecules capable of inducing degradation of nucleic acids. These generally fall into three categories: natural products, metal ion-dependent molecules, and metal ion-independent molecules.

Complex natural products that induce nucleic acid degradation include bleomycin and the enediynes. Bleomycin (described further in Section 9.2.2) induces degradation of DNA and RNA via oxygen activation and hydrogen abstraction [14–16]. The enediyne natural products were initially discovered due to their antibiotic and antitumor effects [17]. These small molecules undergo a Bergman cyclization upon binding to DNA [18], resulting in a diradical formation, leading to hydrogen atom abstraction and DNA double-strand cleavage [19, 20].

Metals and metal complexes have long been used to facilitate DNA degradation, commonly in DNA fingerprinting analyses. Some of these molecules, including iron (II) ethylenediaminetetraacetic acid (EDTA) [21] and 1,10-phenanthroline-copper complexes [22], function by producing hydroxyl radicals, which degrade DNA by hydrogen atom abstraction. Other examples include photoactivatable compounds such as rhodium (II) 9,10-phenanthrenequinonediimine complexes [23], among many others, as reviewed previously [24]. Many metal ions and metal ion complexes, such as tris(1,10- phenanthroline) ruthenium(II) complexes [25, 26], also show the ability to cleave RNA, as reviewed previously [27, 28]. These complexes often contain Zn^{2+}, Cu^{2+}, or a lanthanide ion to catalyze the reaction [27, 28]. One application of these metal ion complexes is for "artificial ribonucleases," where the metal ion complexes are appended to an oligonucleotide that directs selective cleavage [29]. Additionally, some metal ion complexes alone can show modest RNA sequence preference, even in unstructured RNAs [30].

Nonmetal-based small molecules also facilitate cleavage of nucleic acids. These include photoactivatable DNA cleavers such as anthraquinones, acridine-linked nitrobenzamides, porphyrins, riboflavin, napthalimides, and more, and have been previously reviewed [24]. Some of these, such as riboflavins [31], can also lead to RNA degradation. Hydroxyl radical-generating molecules such as *N*-hydroxypyridinethiones [32] can also induce both DNA and RNA degradation via hydrogen abstraction [33]. Most of these approaches, however, have not been used in cells or preclinical animal models of disease.

9.2.1 *N*-Hydroxypyridine-2(1*H*)-thione (*N*-HPT) Conjugates

Early work toward the deliberate design of small molecule RNA-targeted degraders with activity in cells involved directly appending degrading moieties onto small molecule RNA binders. The first example of such a molecule utilized a derivative of *N*-hydroxypyridine-2(1*H*)-thione (*N*-HPT) [34]. Upon ultraviolet light irradiation, *N*-HPT produces hydroxyl radicals that initiate a radical cascade culminating in cleavage of the phosphodiester bonds of RNA [33]. An *N*-HPT derivative (1-hydroxy-6-thioxo-1,6-dihydropyridine-2-carboxylic acid) was coupled to a previously validated dimeric compound (2H-4) that binds the RNA repeat expansion causative of myotonic dystrophy type 1 (DM1) [34, 35].

DM1 is caused by a trinucleotide repeat expansion in the 3' untranslated region (UTR) of the dystrophia myotonica protein kinase (*DMPK*) gene [36]. The repeat expansion ranges anywhere from 100 to several thousand r(CUG) repeats [dubbed $r(CUG)^{exp}$]. This $r(CUG)^{exp}$ forms a stable secondary structure comprising 1×1 nucleotide UU internal loops. The loops are high affinity binding sites for various RNA-binding proteins such as the muscleblind-like 1 (MBNL1) splicing factor. The repeats sequester MBNL1 in the nucleus, preventing it from performing its canonical role as a splicing modulator, thereby leading to deregulation of alternative pre-mRNA splicing [37–39]. Early studies showed displacing these protein–RNA interactions with ASOs reversed disease phenotypes, demonstrating that the $r(CUG)^{exp}$ is the toxic entity operating in DM1 [40–42].

The heterobifunctional direct degrader (2H-4-*N*-HPT) reduced the target RNA levels in transfected HeLa cells by ~50% at a dose of 5 μM after 12–16 h, with degradation plateauing around 5 h post-photolysis [34]. Additionally, 2H-4-*N*-HPT, as well as the irradiation, did not affect the viability of cells, suggesting the compound did not result in widespread cell toxicity. While this study served as a proof of principle that small molecules could induce degradation of RNAs in cells, the obvious limitation of this approach was the requirement of irradiation to induce hydroxyl radical formation and thus its intractability *in vivo*. Nonetheless, this study was an important proof of concept that small molecules can be programmed to degrade an RNA target in cells selectively.

9.2.2 Bleomycin

Bleomycins are a group of natural products from *Streptomyces verticillus* that were discovered in 1966 and soon thereafter were shown to have anticancer properties [43, 44]. Bleomycin has been used in combination with other drugs to treat a variety of cancers, including testicular cancer [45], squamous cell carcinoma [46],

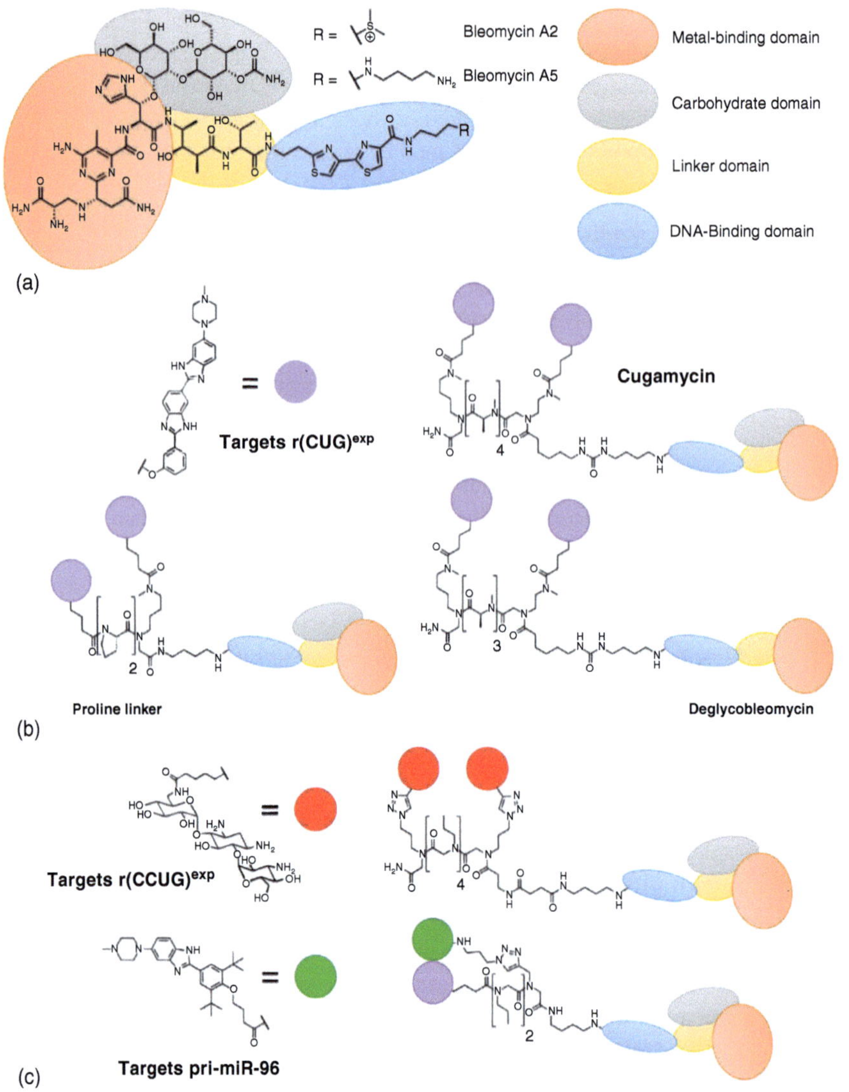

Figure 9.1 Bleomycin degraders. (a) The natural product bleomycin, with each functional domain highlighted. (b) Cugamycin, a r(CUG)^{exp}-targeting bleomycin conjugate (top right) with two functional derivatives (bottom left and bottom right). (c) Two other bleomycin conjugates targeting r(CCUG)^{exp} (top) and pri-miR-96 (bottom).

and Hodgkin's [47] and non-Hodgkin's [48] lymphoma. Its anticancer properties are believed to be primarily derived from its ability to induce double-strand breaks in DNA. Bleomycin is composed of four domains: a metal-binding domain, a carbohydrate domain, a linker domain, and a DNA-binding domain (Figure 9.1a). The metal-binding domain is responsible for forming a metal ion complex, which can activate oxygen to extract a hydrogen from the nucleic acid backbone [14, 49–51]. The carbohydrate domain appears to be important for cell recognition and uptake as well as DNA binding and cleavage efficiency [52–54]. The linker domain length and composition are both critical for efficient cleavage of DNA [52, 55, 56]. Finally, the bithiazole and adjacent cation comprise the DNA-binding domain, which facilitates bleomycin's affinity toward DNA, as well as contributes to its specificity [57, 58]. These four domains function together to facilitate nucleic acid cleavage.

Moreover, bleomycin also cleaves RNA [15, 16, 59, 60]. After it was initially demonstrated that high concentrations of activated bleomycin could weakly cleave $tRNA^{Phe}$ [16], work by the Hecht group showed that bleomycin cleavage of RNA was site selective [15]. Bleomycin efficiently and selectively degraded $tRNA^{His}$ precursor without any degradation of $tRNA^{Tyr}$ precursor RNA [15]. Later, using a series of designed RNA constructs, bleomycin A5 was demonstrated to preferentially cleave hairpin RNAs with longer AU-rich sequences, particularly those rich in purines [60].

To examine whether RNA in cells could be degraded by bleomycin, the microRNA (miRNA) genome was mined for sequences with the potential to be degraded. One potential target of bleomycin A5 is the primary transcript of miRNA (pri-miR)-10b, which contains an AU-rich sequence (AUAUAU). Treatment of both HeLa cells transfected with pri-miR-10b, as well as a triple-negative breast cancer cell line that overexpresses miR-10b, with nanomolar concentrations of bleomycin A5, reduced the abundance of both pri- and mature miR-10b [60]. These studies support that bleomycin A5 could be useful as part of a heterobifunctional small molecule aimed at targeted RNA degradation.

9.2.3 Bleomycin Conjugates

To overcome the promiscuous nature of bleomycin to cleave both DNA and RNA sequences, bleomycin conjugates have been developed to impart selectivity. These include sequence-selective oligonucleotide-bleomycin conjugates targeting DNA [61, 62], some of which show RNA degradation capabilities as well [63]. However, this section will primarily focus on RNA-targeted small-molecule-bleomycin conjugates that have been recently developed. In these molecules, an RNA-binding module drives the selective recognition of the target RNA, bringing the bleomycin proximal to induce direct cleavage. Off-target cleavage of DNA is further reduced if the small molecule is coupled to the free amine in the DNA-binding domain, removing the positive charge and weakening interactions with DNA [52, 64]. To date, bleomycin-based direct degraders have been developed to target the RNA repeat expansions that cause DM1 and myotonic dystrophy type 2 (DM2), as well as oncogenic pri-microRNAs (Figure 9.1b).

9.2.3.1 Bleomycin Degraders Targeting the r(CUG) Repeat Expansion That Causes DM1

Since the RNA repeat expansion in *DMPK* mRNA is the toxic, disease-causing entity, direct degradation of the RNA is an attractive therapeutic strategy. Coupling the terminal primary amine of bleomycin A5 to a previously validated $r(CUG)^{exp}$-binding small molecule yielded Cugamycin, a direct degrader of the RNA repeat expansion [65, 66]. Cugamycin degraded 30–40% of *DMPK* mRNA in patient-derived fibroblasts and myoblasts (noting that the mutant r(CUG)^{exp} allele accounts for 50–70% of total *DMPK* in human DM1 skeletal muscle [67]) and ~40% of the r(CUG)^{exp}-containing mRNA in a DM1 mouse model [65, 66]). In addition to degrading the disease-causing RNA, Cugamycin rescued mis-splicing events associated with MBNL1 sequestration and decreased myotonia, a hallmark of DM1, in an *in vivo* mouse model [66]. Impressively, Cugamycin rescued 97% of splicing defects in a DM1 mouse model, shifting them toward the splicing pattern observed in wild-type mice [66]. These promising results demonstrated the potential and feasibility of bleomycin-conjugated degraders as therapeutics against disease-associated RNAs.

Two interesting findings resulted from these studies. First, while acylation of the DNA-binding domain did not eliminate bleomycin-induced DNA damage, attaching the RNA-binding moieties reduced DNA-double strand breaks (as measured by γ-H2AX staining) to the level of untreated cells at the effective dose of 1 μM [66]. This supported the hypothesis that converting bleomycin to an RNA degrader by coupling to its DNA-binding site would enhance the selectivity of bleomycin for RNA. Second, when treated at doses that nearly equivalently degraded *DMPK* RNA, Cugamycin showed increased specificity relative to a locked nucleic acid (LNA) gap-mer complementary to the repeat expansion. Additionally, the LNA degraded all mRNAs with short r(CUG) repeats that were examined, as well as *DMPK* mRNA, whereas Cugamycin specifically degraded the *DMPK* mRNA. Notably, the short r(CUG) repeats in various transcripts do not adopt a periodic array of UU internal loops formed by r(CUG)^{exp}, the source of Cugamycin specificity for *DMPK* [66].

Later studies improved upon Cugamycin by separately optimizing the RNA-binding and bleomycin moieties. First, bleomycin was exchanged for deglycobleomycin, where the carbohydrate domain of bleomycin was removed [68] (Figure 9.1b). As mentioned in Section 9.2.2, the carbohydrate domain contributes to cleavage efficiency, cell permeability, and DNA-binding affinity via hydrogen bonding to the DNA backbone [52–54]. While Cugamycin cleaved DNA *in vitro* at concentrations above 500 nM, its deglycobleomycin derivative showed no DNA-cleaving ability up to 2 μM [68]. In DM1 myotubes, Cugamycin-induced DNA damage only at the highest concentration tested, 25 μM, whereas the deglycobleomycin derivative showed no DNA damage at any concentration tested (up to 25 μM) [68]. Further, this difference in DNA cleavage activity was not due to variations in cellular uptake, as Cugamycin showed similar cell permeability to its deglycobleomycin derivative [68].

In a subsequent study, the dimeric RNA-binding moiety of Cugamycin was optimized by varying the linker composition and length [69]. Changing the linker of the dimeric RNA-binding moiety from four *N*-methyl alanine residues in Cugamycin to two proline residues increased the affinity to RNA approximately threefold *in vitro* [69]. However, this change in linker composition and length changed the subcellular localization of the r(CUG)^{exp}-binder from primarily nuclear (where the toxic RNA resides) to both nuclear and cytoplasmic [69]. The resultant bleomycin conjugate with the short proline linker was approximately fivefold more potent than Cugamycin in DM1 patient-derived myotubes, as measured by the decrease in *DMPK* mRNA abundance and the rescue of the *MBNL1* splicing defect [69]. Together, these studies demonstrate that bleomycin-based direct degraders can be optimized via medicinal chemistry approaches. To date, only the bleomycin sugar composition and linker length of Cugamycin have been explored. Future medicinal chemistry investigations around Cugamycin could reveal other modifications that improve potency, cellular uptake, and cleavage efficiency.

9.2.3.2 Bleomycin Degraders Targeting r(CCUG) Repeat Expansion that Causes DM2

DM2 is caused by a tetranucleotide RNA repeat expansion [r(CCUG)^{exp}] in intron 1 of CHC-type zinc finger nucleic acid binding protein (*CNBP*) pre-mRNA [70]. Like the pathology of DM1, the repeat expansion sequesters RNA-binding proteins such as MBNL1 [71], resulting in nuclear foci and pre-mRNA splicing defects, specifically exclusion of exon 11 in the insulin receptor (*IR*) pre-mRNA, rendering cells resistant to insulin [72]. In addition, r(CCUG)^{exp} also causes retention of the intron in which it is harbored [73]. A previously identified dimeric small molecule that binds r(CCUG)^{exp} was coupled to bleomycin A5 in a similar manner as Cugamycin [74, 75] (Figure 9.1c). The bleomycin conjugate cleaved a r(CCUG) repeat *in vitro* and in the *CNBP* mRNA in DM2 fibroblasts, without significantly increasing DNA damage compared to untreated cells [75]. The bleomycin conjugate was more potent than its parent compound, decreasing *CNBP* mRNA abundance, improving mis-splicing of insulin receptor exon 11, and reducing nuclear foci, all by approximately 50%; the binder alone at the same dose only improved splicing and reduced foci by ~20% [75]. Importantly, this r(CCUG)^{exp}-targeting bleomycin conjugate was more selective than an ASO targeting the same sequence, as the ASO exacerbated DM2 splicing defects via off-target degradation of *MBNL1* mRNA, which also contains a short r(CCUG) repeat. However, the short repeat does not form the hairpin structure recognized by the bleomycin conjugate and is thus unaffected by the direct degrader compound [75]. This study demonstrated that bleomycin conjugates can be utilized against at least two repeat expansion disorders and that bleomycin-conjugated direct degraders show greater specificity than ASOs targeting the same repeat expansion. It also highlights more broadly that structure-specific RNA-targeted small molecules could have advantages over sequence-specific targeting in some cases.

9.2.3.3 Bleomycin Degraders Targeting Oncogenic Precursor microRNAs

MiRNAs are a class of small noncoding (nc)RNAs that modulate the translation of many genes via base pairing to the 3′ UTR of target mRNAs. This base pairing can lead to either translational repression or directed degradation of the bound mRNA. Previous work has shown that small-molecule RNA binders can inhibit miRNA processing by the enzymes Dicer and Drosha, affecting the levels of specific mature miRNAs (see Chapter 6 for more details).

The first miRNA targeted via bleomycin-based direct degraders was pri-miR-96 [76]. Mature miR-96 inhibits apoptosis in cancer cells by repressing the translation of pro-apoptotic transcription factor Forkhead box protein O1 (FOXO1) [77].

Previous studies had identified a compound, Targaprimir-96 (TGP-96), that inhibits biogenesis of pri-miRNA-96 by binding to the Drosha processing site [78]. Inhibition of miRNA processing by Drosha resulted in a de-repression of the miR-96 target FOXO1, thus triggering apoptosis of cancer cells [78]. TGP-96 was converted into a bleomycin degrader (TGP-96-bleo) via amide coupling to the bleomycin A5 free amine [76] (Figure 9.1c). Similar to the results seen for Cugamycin, attaching the RNA binder to the acylated bleomycin conjugate reduced DNA cleavage *in vitro* and decreased DNA damage in cells when compared to free bleomycin [76].

Moreover, since TGP-96 inhibits processing of pri-miR-96 by binding to the Drosha processing site, its mode of action increases pri-miR-96 levels while decreasing mature miR-96 levels. However, because TGP-96-bleo functions via direct degradation of the RNA, a reduction in both mature and pri-miR-96 levels was observed upon treatment with 500 nM of TGP-96-bleo [76]. Additionally, miRNA sequencing revealed that upon TGP-96-bleo treatment, miR-96 was downregulated to a greater and more statistically significant extent than the rest of the miRNAs detected [76].

Importantly, this study developed a method to identify the precise small-molecule binding sites within RNA targets in cells, dubbed Ribo-SNAP-Map [76]. To do so, cells were treated with TGP-96-bleo, TGP-96, or an acylated bleomycin compound alone. RNA was extracted from the cells and subjected to reverse transcription quantitative polymerase chain reaction (RT-qPCR) using a gene-specific forward primer for pri-miR-96 and a universal reverse primer. The resulting cDNA was then subjected to Sanger sequencing. Because TGP-96-bleo functions by cleaving the pri-miR-96 RNA target, one would expect to identify an increase in cleaved RNA fragments. Indeed, cDNA corresponding to cleaved RNA fragments was identified uniquely in TGP-96-bleo-treated samples, corresponding to a cleavage site 5–7 nucleotides away from the predicted and *in vitro*-validated binding site for TGP-96 [76]. These studies both confirmed target engagement and mapped the binding site of TGP-96-bleo to pri-miR-96 in cells.

9.2.3.4 Conclusions and Outlook for Bleomycin-Based Direct Degraders

To date, bleomycin conjugates have shown promise as chemical biology tools both in cells and *in vivo* [66, 76]. By directly appending RNA-binding moieties to the DNA-binding domain of bleomycin A5, the nuclease-like ability of bleomycin to cleave nucleotides can be co-opted to target RNA specifically. This has resulted in the design of heterobifunctional small molecules capable of inducing degradation of target RNAs in cells, with the most promising degrader, Cugamycin, showing activity in a DM1 transgenic mouse model. Additionally, as a natural product, bleomycin has been optimized by nature to both enter cells and cleave nucleotides.

However, optimization of bleomycin conjugates by medicinal chemistry is limited. While studies with deglycobleomycin conjugates showed less off-target DNA cleavage while retaining RNA cleavage, more significant chemical optimization of bleomycin is synthetically difficult. While total synthesis of bleomycin, allowing for alteration of the various domains, is possible, it is realistically impractical for use in development of mass-produced drugs. For this reason, future endeavors to optimize bleomycin conjugates may be more fruitful through optimization of linker length, rigidity, orientation, and composition, allowing for improved RNA cleavage.

9.3 Ribonuclease Targeting Chimeras (RiboTACs)

Over the past two decades, significant research effort has been expended to develop proteolysis-targeting chimeras (PROTACs). PROTACs, first reported in 2001, are heterobifunctional small molecules containing an E3 ubiquitin ligase-recruiting moiety connected via a linker to a protein target-binding moiety [79]. These molecules recruit target proteins to an E3 ubiquitin ligase, facilitating the transfer of ubiquitin to the target protein. Polyubiquitination marks the target protein for degradation via the proteasome, leading to specific, quick, and oftentimes dramatic degradation of target proteins in cells. Due to extensive optimization by medicinal chemistry, there are orally bioavailable PROTACs in clinical trials targeting a variety of protein targets in cancer with promising safety and efficacy data [80].

Like PROTACs, ribonuclease-targeting chimeras (RiboTACs) are heterobifunctional molecules that induce degradation of a target. RiboTACs are composed of a ribonuclease-recruiting moiety attached to an RNA-binding moiety via a linker. These molecules allow a ribonuclease to be activated in local proximity to a target RNA, facilitating the target RNA's subsequent enzymatic degradation (Figure 9.2). Although still in its infancy, RiboTACs have been developed to degrade target RNAs in cells and in *in vivo* models of disease [81–83].

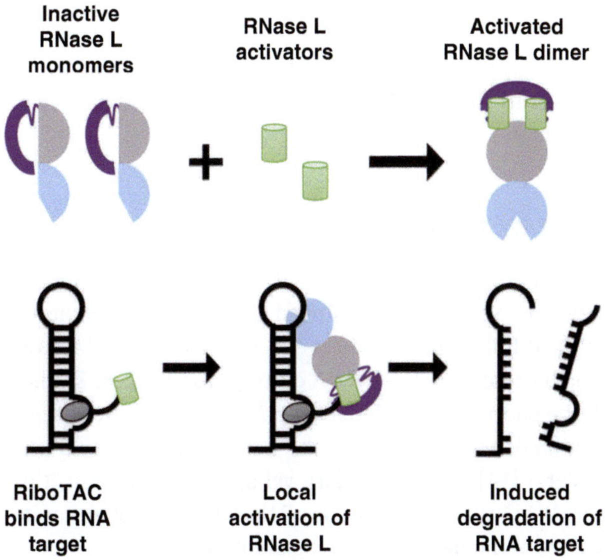

Figure 9.2 RNase L activation and proposed mechanism of action. RNase L is endogenously activated upon induced dimerization from 2′-5′ oligoadenylates (top). RiboTACs are heterobifunctional ligands that locally activate RNase L in proximity to a target RNA, stimulating the degradation of the RNA (bottom).

9.3.1 RNase L is an Endogenous Endoribonuclease That Functions as Part of the Innate Immune Response

As aforementioned, RiboTACs recruit an endogenous nuclease to induce degradation of the RNA target. While many ribonucleases are excreted from the cell into the extracellular space and thus are not suitable for targeted RNA degradation within cells [84], Ribonuclease L (RNase L) is present in the cytoplasm of most cell types [85, 86] and therefore amenable for use as proof of concept.

RNase L functions as part of the innate viral immune response. In the absence of viral infection, RNase L is present as an inactive monomer. The presence of viral double-stranded RNA and interferon signaling activates 2′,5′-oligoadenylate synthetase (OAS), initiating the synthesis of 2′-5′-oligoadenylates (2′-5′poly(A)) [87–89]. The 2′-5′A oligonucleotides activate RNase L by binding to the monomeric protein and inducing a conformational change that results in the formation of an active homodimer [90]. Activated RNase L then rapidly degrades most cellular and viral RNAs, showing sequence specificity for cleavage between the +1 and +2 nucleotides after an unpaired uridine [91–93]. This rapid RNA degradation halts viral replication and ultimately kills the infected cell [91].

Several attributes make RNase L an attractive ribonuclease to utilize for targeted degradation of RNAs. First, RNase L is an endonuclease, cleaving the RNA internally, rather than from the 5′ or 3′ ends, allowing degradation of the RNA at sites adjacent to the small-molecule binding site. Second, RNase L has inherent sequence preferences, contributing to the overall observed selectivity of the chimera. Third, RNase L is present in the cytoplasm of most cell types [85, 86], so targets in a variety of tissues could be cleaved by this enzyme.

As detailed later, it is important to note that RiboTACs provoke degradation without affecting levels of RNAs or proteins upstream of RNase L [81, 82]. That is, they induce degradation of a specific RNA target locally without causing widespread degradation of RNA observed upon viral infection.

9.3.2 First-Generation RiboTACs Targeting Oncogenic miRNAs

The first RiboTAC consisted of a previously designed and validated small molecule that binds pri-miR-96 (TGP-96; see Section 9.2.3.3) linked to 2′-5′A_4 as the RNase L recruiter (Figure 9.3a). The ideal linker distance between TGP-96 and 2′-5′A_4 was investigated using an *in vitro*, fluorescence-based RNA cleavage assay. These studies revealed the RiboTAC with the shortest linker length (no *N*-propyl glycine spacer) induced RNA cleavage marginally better relative to the longer linkers ($n = 3$ and $n = 9$ *N*-propyl glycine spacers) [94]. In a secondary validation experiment, this RiboTAC, TGP-96-RL (Figure 9.3a), was able to induce RNase L oligomerization to approximately 50% of the extent of the native 2′-5′A_4 ligand [94].

In cells, TGP-96-RL decreased mature miR-96 levels to approximately the same extent as the parent ligand, TGP-96 [94]. However, these two molecules have different mechanisms of action. TGP-96 inhibits Drosha processing of pri-miR-96, leading to a dose-dependent increase in pri-miR-96 abundance and a subsequent

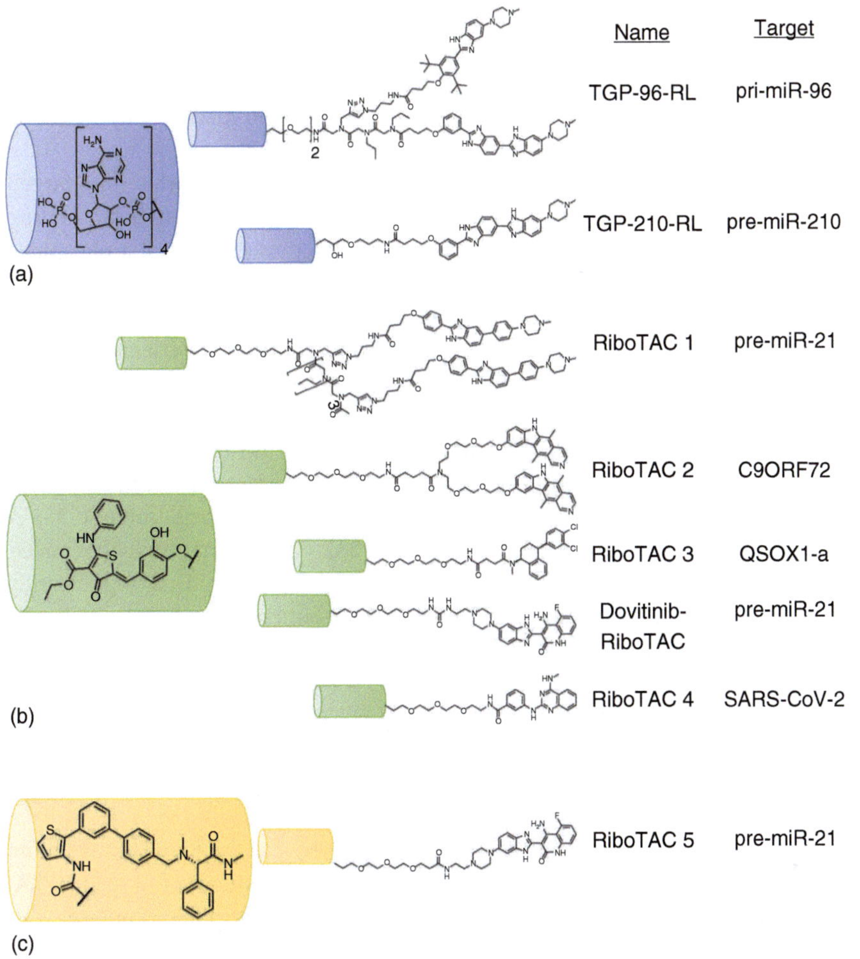

Figure 9.3 RiboTAC degraders. (a) 2′-5′ oligoadenylate (2′-5′A)-based RiboTACs. Early RiboTACs utilized the native ligand for RNase L, 2′-5′A, to recruit RNase L to target RNAs. (b) Later RiboTACs replaced 2′-5′A with the small molecule C1-3 to activate RNase L. (c) Further RiboTACs replaced C1-3 with WuXi DEL as the RNase L activator. The name and primary target for each RiboTAC is listed to the right.

decrease in mature miR-96 abundance [78, 94]. In contrast, TGP-96-RL recruits RNase L to cleave the target RNA, resulting in dose-dependent decreases in both pri-miR-96 and mature miR-96 abundances [94]. To confirm this RiboTAC functions via an RNase L-mediated mechanism of action, knockdown and knock-in validation experiments were completed via small interfering (si)RNAs targeted to RNase L and forced expression of RNase L, respectively. Supporting the proposed mechanism of action, knockdown of RNase L eliminated the observed decrease in pri-miR-96 levels upon treatment with TGP-96-RL. Conversely, forced overexpression of RNase L led to an increase in degradation of pri-miR-96. In addition, TGP-96-RL de-repressed FOXO1, a regulator of apoptosis in cancer cells and a miR-96 target, while having no effect in a healthy control cell line [94]. Thus, although the potency of TGP-96 was not dramatically improved, converting the molecule to a RiboTAC changed the mechanism of action of the molecule from inhibiting Drosha processing to degradation of pri-miR-96 mediated by RNase L, and thus provided data to support RiboTAC proof of concept.

Building upon the success of TGP-96-RL, a second RiboTAC, this time targeting the precursor to miR-210 (pre-miR-210), was developed (Figure 9.3a). Mature miR-210 is upregulated in hypoxic cancers where it represses glycerol-3-phosphate dehydrogenase 1-like (GPD1L) translation. Repression of GPD1L inhibits degradation of hypoxia-inducible factor 1-alpha (HIF1α), resulting in the transcription of hypoxia-associated genes [95, 96]. Thus, degradation of miR-210 presents a possible therapeutic avenue for hypoxic cancers.

A previously validated molecule, TGP-210, had been shown to bind the Dicer processing site of pre-miR-210, thus inhibiting its biogenesis [97]. Three RiboTACs varying in their RNase L activating moiety ($2'$-$5'A_{2\text{-}4}$) were synthesized and tested in an RNase L-dependent *in vitro* RNA cleavage assay. Only the tetrameric 2′-5′A ligand induced degradation of pre-miR-210 [98]. Moreover, although conversion of TGP-210 to the RiboTAC TGP-210-RL (Figure 9.3a) did not significantly affect RNA-binding affinity, it did decrease DNA-binding affinity of the ligand approximately 2-fold, increasing the selectivity window of the ligand. Further, preincubation of TGP-210-RL with RNase L only modestly reduced binding affinity to RNA while ablating binding to DNA. Cellular uptake and localization experiments revealed that although TGP-210-RL showed a ~40% reduction in cell permeability relative to TGP-210, the RiboTAC was preferentially localized in the cytoplasm where RNase L is also present, whereas the parent compound localized to the nucleus [98]. Collectively, these results suggested that the RiboTAC was more selective in cells than the parent compound, owing to its reduced affinity for DNA, its localization outside of the nucleus, and its co-localization in the cytoplasm with RNase L.

In cells, TGP-210-RL reduced the abundances of both pre- and mature miR-210, whereas the parent compound TGP-210 only decreased the mature miR-210 abundance. This decrease in pre-miR-210 was RNase L-dependent, as demonstrated by siRNA knockdown and overexpression knock-in experiments. MiRNA sequencing also showed the target (miR-210) was the most downregulated miRNA of the miRNAs detected. RT-qPCR analysis confirmed the downstream target (GPDL1) was de-repressed at the mRNA level with a concomitant decrease in *HIF-1α* transcript abundance [98]. TGP-210-RL at a dose of 500 nM induced cellular apoptosis in a caspase assay to a similar extent as a miR-210-targeting LNA. This effect was diminished upon overexpression of miR-210, suggesting the induction of apoptosis was mediated by miR-210 degradation [98].

In all, these first-generation RiboTACs demonstrated the feasibility of locally recruiting an endogenous ribonuclease to degrade target RNAs. They were successful in leading to significant degradation of their targets at sub-micromolar doses in cellular models of disease. However, these molecules are not drug-like. The 2′-5′ oligoadenylate used to activate and recruit RNase L is large and negatively charged.

Thus, subsequent efforts were focused on finding drug-like small-molecule RNase L recruiters.

9.3.3 Small-Molecule-Based RiboTACs

In 2007, the Silverman lab identified two small molecules (a 2-aminothiophene and a thienopyrimidinone) from a library of 32,000 compounds that dimerize and activate RNase L *in vitro* with mid-micromolar potency [99] (C1 and C2, Figure 9.4a). These molecules compete with the endogenous 2′-5′A ligand for binding to the RNase, indicating that they bind the same site within the protein [99]. Finally, both molecules were able to suppress viral replication in cells and did so in an RNase L-dependent fashion [99]. These studies demonstrate that small molecules can indeed dimerize and activate RNase L, albeit at higher concentrations than the native 2′-5′A ligand [99].

Medicinal chemistry was employed to define the structure–activity relationships (SAR) surrounding the two RNase L-activating small molecules, with the goals of discovering more potent derivatives and identifying a position to tether to an RNA-binding module (Figure 9.4a). For the 2-aminothiophene compound (Figure 9.4a, C1), several potential points of linker attachment were probed via addition of methoxy groups [81]. These analogs were then compared to the parent

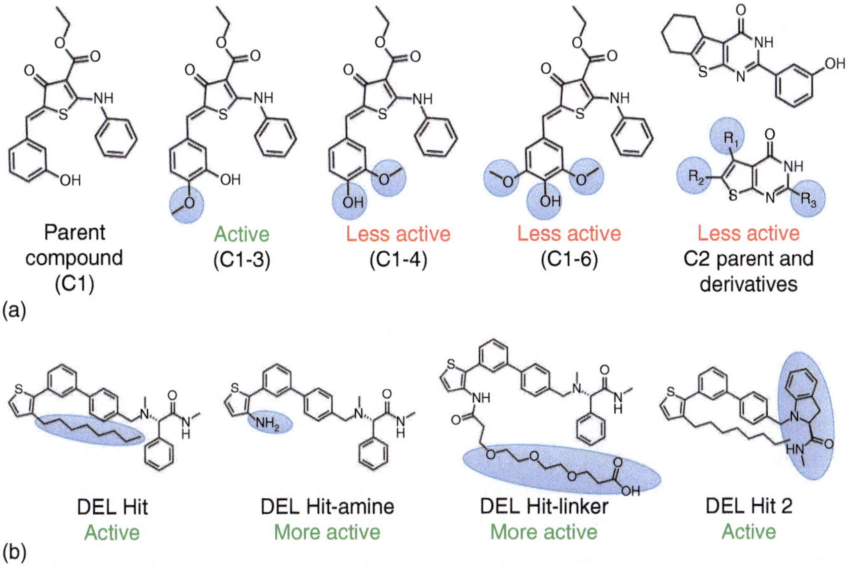

Figure 9.4 Structure-activity relationships of RNase L activators. The hit compounds and derivatives thereof were assessed for activity in a fluorescence-based *in vitro* cleavage assay. (a) One of the high-throughput screening hits from the Silverman laboratory, C1 [99], can tolerate para-methoxy substitutions, but not other methoxy substitution patterns. The other screening hit (C2) and its derivatives were all less active than C1-3. (b) The primary DEL Hit activated RNase L. Substitution of the octyl chain for a primary amine or polyethylene glycol linker increased activation. Additionally, a DEL hit that replaced the phenylalanine scaffold with an indoline retained RNase L-activating activity.

compound in the previously described *in vitro* RNA cleavage assay using an RNA sensor with preferred RNase L cleavage sites (Section 9.3.2). One analog, C1-3, showed increased activity relative to the parent, while structurally similar analogs, such as C1-4, showed minimal RNase L activation [81]. For the thienopyrimidinone (Figure 9.4a, C2), many derivatives were synthesized and tested for RNase L activation, but none showed higher activation of RNase L than C1-3 [81]. For these reasons, C1-3 was chosen as the RNase L small-molecule recruiter for second-generation RiboTACs.

As a proof-of-concept study for small-molecule-based RiboTACs, C1-3 was conjugated to a dimeric RNA binder of pre-miR-21 dubbed TGP-21, yielding RiboTAC 1 (Figure 9.3b). MiR-21 is an oncogenic miRNA that plays an important role in triple-negative breast cancer [100]. TGP-21 binds pre-miR-21's Dicer processing site, thus inhibiting its processing into the mature miRNA [81]. Converting the pre-miR-21 binder to RiboTAC 1 significantly enhanced potency and specificity of the molecule. RiboTAC 1 decreased the IC_{50} for reduction in miR-21 levels from approximately 1 μM to 50 nM, a 20-fold improvement [81]. Additionally, reduction in pre-miR-21 levels was RNase L-dependent, as the reduction was fully ablated in RNase L knockdown cells. Furthermore, RiboTAC 1 reduced miR-21 levels to a statistically significant extent after 12 h, with the reduction persisting for up to 4 days after treatment; the parent compound acted less quickly and sustained the effect for a shorter period of time [81]. RiboTAC 1 showed a more specific miRNA inhibition profile relative to the binder alone, and no changes in abundance of highly abundant RNA transcripts (such as ribosomal and transfer RNAs) were found upon treatment with the RiboTAC [81]. These results suggested that a small-molecule-based RiboTAC can dramatically improve potency and specificity of a miRNA-binding molecule.

One potential issue that could arise with ligand-induced activation of RNase L could be activation of the RNase L-mediated innate immune response. If RiboTACs broadly activate RNase L throughout the cell, then RNase L could degrade many cellular RNAs. However, if RiboTACs function via local activation of RNase L in proximity to the RNA target, then one would not expect the immune response to be activated. To test this hypothesis, the expression levels of several markers of the innate immune response were examined by RT-qPCR and enzyme-linked immunosorbent assay (ELISA) upon RiboTAC treatment [81]. While transfection of the native RNase L ligand ($2'$-$5'A_4$) resulted in an increase in expression of innate immune response biomarkers, treatment with RiboTAC 1 did not affect the biomarkers relative to a DMSO control [81]. These results support the mechanism of local, transient activation of RNase L rather than a cell-wide innate immune response.

In addition to showing selective degradation of the target miRNA-21 in cells, RiboTAC 1 de-repressed miR-21's downstream protein targets (PDCD4 and PTEN) and inhibited cellular proliferation. In pharmacokinetics studies, the pre-miR-21 RiboTAC was able to sustain low nanomolar concentrations in the plasma for at least 24 h after intraperitoneal injection at 10 mg/kg. Additionally, in a mouse model of breast cancer, the RiboTAC reduced tumor colonization in the lung as well as reduced both pre- and mature miR-21 abundances [81]. In all, this study demonstrated for the first time that a RiboTAC with a small-molecule-based activator of RNase L could significantly improve potency and selectivity of RNA-binding small molecules with *in vivo* efficacy.

Since this inaugural work, the small-molecule-based RiboTAC strategy has been applied to various targets with similar success (Figure 9.3). C1-3-based RiboTACs have been utilized to degrade $r(G_4C_2)^{exp}$ [83], which causes C9orf72-associated amyotrophic lateral sclerosis and frontotemporal dementia (collectively c9ALS/FTD), an RNA structure present in the SARS-CoV-2 genome [101], and a specific isoform of quiescin sulfhydryl oxidase 1 (*QSOX1*) mRNA that facilitates invasion and proliferation of breast cancer cells [102] (Figure 9.3b). The c9ALS/FTD-targeting RiboTAC (RiboTAC 2, Figure 9.3b) demonstrated increased potency relative to the RNA binder and reduced cellular phenotypes in c9ALS/FTD in a mouse model [83]. The *QSOX1* RiboTAC (RiboTAC 3, Figure 9.3b) was derived from a fragment that bound *QSOX1* mRNA in cells, where it targeted a structure found in the *QSOX1a* isoform that is absent in the 1b isoform. The fragment had a very modest effect (~15% reduction) on *QSOX1a* protein expression, with no effect on mRNA abundance. Upon its conversion to a RiboTAC (Figure 9.3b), levels of *QSXO1a* mRNA were reduced while *QSXO1b* abundance was not. The same trend was observed at the protein level, thus demonstrating the degrader was isoform-specific. Further, RiboTAC 3 was more potent than the parent fragment, as the RiboTAC doubled the effect on QSOX1a protein expression (35% decrease for the RiboTAC vs. 15% decrease for the parent) at half the concentration (10 μM for the RiboTAC vs. 20 μM for the parent) [102].

Another interesting case study showed that known drugs with canonical activity against a protein target can be reprogrammed to affect an RNA selectively by conversion to a RiboTAC. Dovitinib is a receptor tyrosine kinase (RTK) inhibitor that has shown similar efficacy against renal cell carcinoma (RCC) in a Phase III clinical trial as an approved RCC therapeutic (sorafenib) [103]. Dovitinib also binds pre-miR-21's Dicer processing site [82], albeit with much lower affinity than RTKs (~3 μM vs. low nM, respectively [104]), and inhibits the miRNA's biogenesis. To assess whether selectivity could be improved for the RNA target, C1-3 was conjugated to Dovitinib to create Dovitinib-RiboTAC (Figure 9.3b). Dovitinib-RiboTAC decreased mature miR-21 levels approximately 25 times more potently than Dovitinib itself while inhibiting RTK signaling less potently by approximately 100-fold, resulting in a 2500-fold increase in selectivity for the RNA target. Additionally, Dovitinib-RiboTAC was more selective than Dovitinib across both the proteome and transcriptome [82].

Dovitinib-RiboTAC was subsequently tested in two mouse models of miR-21-regulated disease. First, the RiboTAC inhibited colonization of breast cancer cells to the lung in a xenograft mouse model studying miR-21 associated metastasis of a triple-negative breast cancer cell line (MDA-MB-231) [82]. Additionally, Dovitinib-RiboTAC rescued hallmarks of Alport Syndrome, a genetic kidney disease where miR-21 inhibition has shown therapeutic potential [105], in a mouse model [82, 106]. In both mouse models, pre- and mature miR-21 levels were decreased, and peroxisome proliferator-activated receptor alpha (PPARα) protein, a direct target of miR-21, was de-repressed upon addition of the Dovitinib-RiboTAC

[82]. This case study demonstrates the advantage of RiboTACs in not only increasing potency via degradation of the target but also to reprogram activity away from a canonical protein target towards an RNA target.

9.3.4 Comparison of Bleomycin-Based Direct Degraders and RiboTACs

As outlined thus far, bleomycin and RiboTAC degraders are both capable of degrading specific targeted RNAs in cells and *in vivo*. While bleomycin degrades RNA directly by hydrogen extraction, RiboTACs function indirectly by recruiting an endogenous ribonuclease. To assess the degradation capabilities of these in parallel, the miRNA 17–92 cluster was chosen as a test case. The miRNA 17–92 cluster encodes six miRNAs and is transcriptionally regulated by the oncogene *c-myc* [107]. To assess the differences between bleomycin-mediated direct cleavage and RiboTAC-mediated enzymatic cleavage, a bleomycin conjugate and RiboTAC were created from a small molecule that binds the Dicer processing sites of three of the miRNAs in the cluster, thereby inhibiting their biogenesis [108]. When converted to a bleomycin conjugate, the abundance of pri-miR-17-92 was reduced by approximately 30% at a dose of 100 nM, causing a concomitant change in all six mature miRNAs encoded by the cluster. In contrast, due to the subcellular localization of RNase L in the cytoplasm, the RiboTAC did not degrade the nuclear pri-miRNA. Rather, treatment with 500 nM of the RiboTAC led to specific degradation of the three pre-miRNAs and reduction of levels of the mature miRNAs thereof that are bound by the parent molecule, without affecting the levels of the other three miRNAs in the cluster (pre- or mature) [108]. This analysis showed that the co-localization of the target and the degrader can affect whether cleavage is observed, or upon which form of the transcript its effect is exerted. It is also possible that differences in cleaved targets could be due to the different sequence specificity of the two modalities. RNase L's preference for unpaired uridines and bleomycin's preference for AU-rich and purine-rich sequences could further allow rational design of more specific degraders.

9.3.5 Discovery of Additional Small-Molecule RNase L Activators

The initial small-molecule RNase L activators were discovered using a high-throughput screen, as described in Section 9.3.3. This high-throughput screen of over 30,000 compounds afforded two molecules capable of activating RNase L [99], one of which was optimized and successfully utilized in RiboTACs [81] (Figure 9.4a). To identify new RNase L activators with different chemotypes and improved properties, a 2.8 billion compound 2nd-Generation DELopen library (where DEL is DNA-encoded library) from WuXi AppTech was screened for binding to recombinant RNase L protein [109]. Of the ~1600 compounds that specifically bound to RNase L, the four most enriched and redundant hits were examined for RNase L-activating activity. Two of the four compounds showed dose-dependent activation of RNase L in the *in vitro* fluorescence-based RNA cleavage assay. These hit molecules from the DEL screen contained a long alkyl chain as their terminal building block (Figure 9.4b). When this alkyl chain was removed from the molecule and replaced with a primary amine to enhance solubility, enhanced

RNase L activation was observed. Amide coupling of a polyethylene glycol (PEG) linker to this amine further enhanced solubility and increased the activation of RNase L induced by the compound even more than the amine derivative [109] (Figure 9.4b).

Because this DEL hit activated RNase L and tolerated linker attachment, it was utilized as the RNase L-recruiting moiety of a RiboTAC. As a test case, Dovitinib, the RTK inhibitor that also binds the Dicer processing site of pre-miR-21 [82] (described in Section 9.3.3), was attached to the RNase L DEL hit, yielding the molecule RiboTAC 5 (Figure 9.3c). RiboTAC 5 decreased the levels of pre-miR-21 by ~30% at a dose of 5 μM in MDA-MB-231 cells, comparable to the 40% decrease at the same dose of Dovitinib-RiboTAC (with the C1-3 RNase L recruiter) [82, 109]. This decrease was RNase L-dependent, as a CRISPR knockout of RNase L abolished all activity of RiboTAC 5 against pre-miR-21 [109]. Additionally, treatment with 5 μM of RiboTAC 5 decreased the miR-21-associated invasive phenotype of MDA-MB-231 cells [109].

The success of this DEL screen demonstrates that different chemotypes can activate RNase L for use in RiboTACs. The DELopen RNase L recruiter and C1-3 are rather structurally dissimilar but are both capable of activating RNase L at mid-micromolar doses. RiboTACs have progressed from utilizing the endogenous oligonucleotide activator of RNase L to two different small-molecule activators for RNase L recruitment (C1-3 and the DELopen recruiter). Further identification of functional chemotypes and medicinal chemistry optimization of these RNase L activators could enable more drug-like RiboTACs with improved solubility and reduced molecular weight without compromising efficacy.

Additionally, DEL screening can be used to identify chemotypes that bind to other RNA effector proteins, widening the scope of enzymes recruited by RiboTACs. This will allow RiboTACs to be fine-tuned based on substrate specificity and effector protein subcellular localization. As seen with the miR-17-92 example (in Section 9.3.4), RNase L is less efficient at cleaving nuclear RNAs, likely due to its predominant localization in the cytoplasm [86]. However, if ligands were identified that bind to and recruit nuclear ribonucleases, RiboTACs could be developed to specifically degrade nuclear RNAs, expanding the scope of targetable RNAs and potentially increasing target specificity. DEL technology provides a facile way to quickly screen and identify these chemical binders.

9.3.6 Conclusions and Outlook for RiboTACs

As described in Section 9.3.3, early RiboTACs have shown promising results inducing the degradation of disease-associated RNAs, both noncoding and coding (Figure 9.3). Additionally, three RiboTACs (two targeting pre-miR-21 that operates in many cancers and Alport Syndrome [81, 82] and one targeting $r(G_4C_2)^{exp}$ in ALS/FTD [83]) have shown efficacy in mouse models of disease, suggesting they could be further optimized into therapeutics. One key to developing RiboTACs with activity in mouse models of disease without noticeable toxicity was the identification of a small molecule (rather than the 2′-5′-oligoadenylate) that was capable of locally activating RNase L to degrade the target RNAs without activating the RNase L-mediated innate immune response [81, 82]. This allowed specific, targeted degradation without the potentially harmful side effects of immune system stimulation.

While the development of small-molecule-based RiboTACs has improved drug-likeness and cellular permeability by replacing the large, negatively charged, 2′-5′A RNase L recruiter with the smaller heterocyclic molecules, there is still much room for optimization. Further, significant work remains to be done with regard to medicinal chemistry optimization of the linker connecting the RNA-binding domain to the RNase L recruiting domain. Currently, all C1-3-based RiboTACs utilize a four-unit PEG linker to connect the RNase L-recruiter to the RNA-binding module. Related studies in the PROTAC field have shown that linker length and composition can be crucially important for effective degradation and influence physicochemical properties of the chimera [110]. Studies are needed to assess whether linkers need to be optimized for each RNA target, as is the case for PROTACs, and if drug-likeness can be improved through these modifications [110].

Despite efficacy in mouse models of disease [81–83] and several lines of data supporting RNase L-dependency (such as RNase L knockdown and overexpression experiments [94, 98]), the precise mechanism of action of RiboTACs has yet to be elucidated. Like PROTACs, RiboTACs may require a stable and productive ternary complex for efficient degradation. However, one can also envision a mechanism wherein the RiboTAC dissociates from the target RNA, enabling it to then activate RNase L in local proximity of the RNA. The ternary complex model has some support from previous studies: when RNase L was immunoprecipitated from cells, pri-miR-96 levels were selectively enriched from cells treated with the pri-miR-96 RiboTAC, while an off-target pri-miRNA was not enriched [94]. Further studies will be required to fully understand this mechanism and thus inform the design of RiboTACs with improved degradation efficiency.

Thus far, RiboTACs have used the induced proximity of RNase L to degrade target RNAs. Its nearly ubiquitous tissue expression [85] and endoribonuclease activity have allowed RNase L to successfully induce degradation of a variety of RNAs in various cell lines and animal models. The sequence specificity of RNase L [91–93] has enabled RiboTACs to have fewer off-targets than their parent compounds [81]. However, its low expression levels and localization to the cytoplasm may limit the amount of observed degradation. Additionally, RiboTACs that recruit RNase L must not only bind RNase L but also activate the enzyme. To further improve selectivity and potency of RiboTACs, one can envision recruiting other cellular ribonucleases to degrade target RNA transcripts. Future work may explore which other nucleases are capable of being recruited to RNAs by small-molecule ligands.

9.4 Summary and Outlook for Small-Molecule RNA Degraders

This chapter has explored the recent advances in RNA-targeted small-molecule degraders, focusing primarily on two types of molecules: bleomycin direct degraders and RiboTACs. While both modalities are in their infancy, these molecules have shown that RNA can be degraded selectively by small molecules in cells and *in vivo*, rescuing disease phenotypes. Bleomycin degraders directly cleave RNA by metal activation of oxygen, leading to hydrogen abstraction and RNA backbone cleavage. By appending the bleomycin A5 moiety to selective RNA binders, degradation can be specifically targeted to RNAs of interest, showing efficacy in degrading an RNA repeat expansion and pri-miRNAs. Indeed, bleomycin conjugates are likely better suited for nuclear RNA targets than a RiboTAC, as RNase L is primarily located in the cytoplasm [86]. RiboTACs, on the other hand, function by activating an endogenous endoribonuclease (RNase L) in local proximity to an RNA of interest. Both the native 2′-5′poly(A) and two heterocyclic small molecules can induce activation of RNase L, resulting in selective degradation of target RNAs when a component of a chimera. RiboTACs induce the cleavage of their cognate RNAs in cells and *in vivo* including noncoding pri- and pre-miRNAs and mRNAs harboring repeat expansions.

While results from these bleomycin degraders and RiboTACs have been encouraging thus far, work remains to optimize these small molecules for therapeutic potential. For bleomycin conjugates, deglycobleomycin appears to have fewer off-target DNA cleavage effects. Additionally, improving RNA-binding affinity via linker optimization increases the extent of cleavage. However, no work has been completed to optimize the linker between bleomycin A5 and the RNA-binding moieties, which could increase RNA cleavage efficiency and/or alter selectivity. For RiboTACs, improvement from the oligonucleotide natural ligand to a small-molecule RNase L activator improved drug-likeness tremendously; however, the molecules still fall outside of the typical Rule of 5 parameters for drug-likeness [111]. While much work still remains, RiboTACs have the advantage of being amenable to medicinal chemistry optimization, which could one day yield an orally bioavailable drug, whereas the alternative approach to therapeutically cleaving RNAs, ASOs, must be delivered via injection. Additionally, as with bleomycin conjugates, no work has been done to optimize the chemical properties of the linkers to increase cleavage efficiency. Future work in the field of RNA small-molecule degraders should continue to optimize these molecules to improve efficiency of RNA cleavage, drug-likeness, and pharmacokinetic parameters.

RNA small-molecule degraders have the potential to combine the benefits of ASO degraders and those of small molecules, with the goal of obtaining an orally bioavailable therapeutic. An advantage of this approach is that target validation can be completed in the same way for ASOs and small-molecule degraders – by depletion of the target as assessed by RNA-seq analysis or RT-qPCR. Further, the capability to sub-stoichiometrically degrade RNA by ASOs, RiboTACs, and bleomycin conjugates allows for potent activity, particularly for the latter when compared to RNA binders alone. Small-molecule binders and RiboTACs can rely on traditional medicinal chemistry strategies to optimize affinity, selectivity, potency, and physicochemical properties. Both bleomycin conjugates and RiboTACs have bright futures for the development of RNA-targeted therapeutics that will only improve with further optimization.

References

1 Wu, H., Lima, W.F., Zhang, H. et al. (2004). Determination of the role of the human RNase H1 in the pharmacology of DNA-like antisense drugs. *J. Biol. Chem.* 279 (17): 17181–17189.

2 Scharner, J., Ma, W.K., Zhang, Q. et al. (2020). Hybridization-mediated off-target effects of splice-switching antisense oligonucleotides. *Nucleic Acids Res.* 48 (2): 802–816.

3 Melton, D.A. (1985). Injected anti-sense RNAs specifically block messenger RNA translation in vivo. *Proc. Natl. Acad. Sci. U. S. A.* 82 (1): 144–148.

4 Stein, H. and Hausen, P. (1969). Enzyme from calf thymus degrading the RNA moiety of DNA-RNA hybrids: effect on DNA-dependent RNA polymerase. *Science* 166 (3903): 393–395.

5 Lima, W. F., C. L. De Hoyos, X.-h. Liang and S. T. Crooke (2016) RNA cleavage products generated by antisense oligonucleotides and siRNAs are processed by the RNA surveillance machinery. *Nucleic Acids Res.,* 44(7), 3351-3363.

6 Roehr, B. (1998). Fomivirsen approved for CMV retinitis. *J. Int. Assoc. Phys. AIDS Care* 4 (10): 14–16.

7 Keam, S.J. (2018). Inotersen: first global approval. *Drugs* 78 (13): 1371–1376.

8 Hoy, S.M. (2018). Patisiran: first global approval. *Drugs* 78 (15): 1625–1631.

9 Hoy, S.M. (2017). Nusinersen: first global approval. *Drugs* 77 (4): 473–479.

10 Herschlag, D. (1991). Implications of ribozyme kinetics for targeting the cleavage of specific RNA molecules in vivo: more isn't always better. *Proc. Natl. Acad. Sci. U. S. A.* 88 (16): 6921–6925.

11 Watt, A.T., Swayze, G., Swayze, E.E., and Freier, S.M. (2020). Likelihood of nonspecific activity of gapmer antisense oligonucleotides is associated with relative hybridization free energy. *Nucleic Acid Ther.* 30 (4): 215–228.

12 Crooke, S.T., Baker, B.F., Crooke, R.M., and Liang, X.-H. (2021). Antisense technology: an overview and prospectus. *Nat. Rev. Drug Discovery* 20 (6): 427–453.

13 Geary, R.S., Norris, D., Yu, R., and Bennett, C.F. (2015). Pharmacokinetics, biodistribution and cell uptake of antisense oligonucleotides. *Adv. Drug Delivery Rev.* 87: 46–51.

14 Stubbe, J. and Kozarich, J.W. (1987). Mechanisms of bleomycin-induced DNA degradation. *Chem. Rev.* 87 (5): 1107–1136.

15 Carter, B.J., de Vroom, E., Long, E.C. et al. (1990). Site-specific cleavage of RNA by Fe(ii)· Bleomycin. *Proc. Natl. Acad. Sci. U. S. A.* 87 (23): 9373–9377.

16 Magliozzo, R.S., Peisach, J., and Ciriolo, M.R. (1989). Transfer RNA is cleaved by activated bleomycin. *Mol. Pharmacol.* 35 (4): 428–432.

17 Ishida, N., Miyazaki, K., Kumagai, K., and Rikimaru, M. (1965). Neocarzinostatin, an antitumor antibiotic of high molecular weight isolation, physicochemical properties and biological activities. *J. Antibiot. Series A* 18 (2): 68–76.

18 Bergman, R.G. (1973). Reactive 1, 4-dehydroaromatics. *Acc. Chem. Res.* 6 (1): 25–31.

19 Joshi, M.C. and Rawat, D.S. (2012). Recent developments in enediyne chemistry. *Chem. Biodivers.* 9 (3): 459–498.

20 Smith, A.L. and Nicolaou, K.C. (1996). The enediyne antibiotics. *J. Med. Chem.* 39 (11): 2103–2117.

21 Dixon, W.J., Hayes, J.J., Levin, J.R. et al. (1991). Hydroxyl radical footprinting. In: *Methods in Enzymology*, vol. 208, 1991, 380–413. Academic Press.

22 Sigman, D.S., Kuwabara, M.D., Chen, C.-H.B., and Bruice, T.W. (1991, 1991). Nuclease activity of 1,10-phenanthroline-copper in study of protein—DNA interactions. In: *Methods in Enzymology*, vol. 208, 414–433. Academic Press.

23 Chow, C.S. and Barton, J.K. (1992). Transition metal complexes as probes of nucleic acids. In: *Methods in Enzymology*, vol. 212, 1992, 219–242. Academic Press.

24 Armitage, B. (1998). Photocleavage of nucleic acids. *Chem. Rev.* 98 (3): 1171–1200.

25 Chow, C.S. and Barton, J.K. (1990). Shape-selective cleavage of trnaphe by transition metal complexes. *J. Am. Chem. Soc.* 112 (7): 2839–2841.

26 Chow, C.S., Behlen, L.S., Uhlenbeck, O.C., and Barton, J.K. (1992). Recognition of tertiary structure in tRNAs by $Rh(phen)_2phi^{3+}$, a new reagent for RNA structure-function mapping. *Biochemistry* 31 (4): 972–982.

27 Lönnberg, H. (2011). Cleavage of RNA phosphodiester bonds by small molecular entities: a mechanistic insight. *Org. Biomol. Chem.* 9 (6): 1687–1703.

28 Morrow, J.R. and Iranzo, O. (2004). Synthetic metallonucleases for RNA cleavage. *Curr. Opin. Chem. Biol.* 8 (2): 192–200.

29 Niittymäki, T. and Lönnberg, H. (2006). Artificial ribonucleases. *Org. Biomol. Chem.* 4 (1): 15–25.

30 Cacciapaglia, R., Casnati, A., Mandolini, L. et al. (2007). Efficient and selective cleavage of RNA oligonucleotides by calix[4]arene-based synthetic metallonucleases. *J. Am. Chem. Soc.* 129 (41): 12512–12520.

31 Burgstaller, P. and Famulok, M. (1997). Flavin-dependent photocleavage of RNA at G•U base pairs. *J. Am. Chem. Soc.* 119 (5): 1137–1138.

32 Adam, W., Ballmaier, D., Epe, B. et al. (1995). *N*-hydroxypyridinethiones as photochemical hydroxyl radical sources for oxidative DNA damage. *Angew. Chem. Int. Ed. Engl.* 34 (19): 2156–2158.

33 Chaulk, S.G., Pezacki, J.P., and MacMillan, A.M. (2000). Studies of RNA cleavage by photolysis of *N*-hydroxypyridine-2(1h)-thione. A new photochemical footprinting method. *Biochemistry* 39 (34): 10448–10453.

34 Guan, L. and Disney, M.D. (2013). Small-molecule-mediated cleavage of RNA in living cells. *Angew. Chem. Int. Ed. Engl.* 52 (5): 1462–1465.

35 Childs-Disney, J., Hoskins, J., Rzuczek, S.G. et al. (2012). Rationally designed small molecules targeting the RNA that causes myotonic dystrophy type 1 are potently bioactive. *ACS Chem. Biol.* 7 (5): 856–862.

36 Brook, J.D., McCurrach, M.E., Harley, H.G. et al. (1992). Molecular basis of myotonic dystrophy: expansion of a trinucleotide (CTG) repeat at the 3′ end of a transcript encoding a protein kinase family member. *Cell* 68 (4): 799–808.

37 Taneja, K.L., McCurrach, M., Schalling, M. et al. (1995). Foci of trinucleotide repeat transcripts in nuclei of myotonic dystrophy cells and tissues. *J. Cell Biol.* 128 (6): 995–1002.

38 Jiang, H., Mankodi, A., Swanson, M.S. et al. (2004). Myotonic dystrophy type 1 is associated with nuclear foci of mutant RNA, sequestration of muscleblind proteins and deregulated alternative splicing in neurons. *Hum. Mol. Genet.* 13 (24): 3079–3088.

39 Nakamori, M., Sobczak, K., Puwanant, A. et al. (2013). Splicing biomarkers of disease severity in myotonic dystrophy. *Ann. Neurol.* 74 (6): 862–872.

40 Wheeler, T.M., Sobczak, K., Lueck, J.D. et al. (2009). Reversal of rna dominance by displacement of protein sequestered on triplet repeat RNA. *Science* 325 (5938): 336–339.

41 Wheeler, T.M., Leger, A.J., Pandey, S.K. et al. (2012). Targeting nuclear RNA for in vivo correction of myotonic dystrophy. *Nature* 488 (7409): 111–115.

42 Jauvin, D., Chrétien, J., Pandey, S.K. et al. (2017). Targeting DMPK with antisense oligonucleotide improves muscle strength in myotonic dystrophy type 1 mice. *Mol. Ther. Nucleic Acids* 7: 465–474.

43 Umezawa, H., Ishizaka, M., Kimura, K. et al. (1968). Biological studies on individual bleomycins. *J. Antibiot.* 21 (10): 592–602.

44 Umezawa, H., Maeda, K., Takeuchi, T., and Okami, Y. (1966). New antibiotics, bleomycin A and B. *J. Antibiot.* 19 (5): 200–209.

45 de Wit, R., Stoter, G., Kaye, S.B. et al. (1997). Importance of bleomycin in combination chemotherapy for good-prognosis testicular nonseminoma: a randomized study of the European organization for research and treatment of cancer genitourinary tract cancer cooperative group. *J. Clin. Oncol.* 15 (5): 1837–1843.

46 Sadek, H., Azli, N., Wendling, J.L. et al. (1990). Treatment of advanced squamous cell carcinoma of the skin with cisplatin, 5-fluorouracil, and bleomycin. *Cancer* 66 (8): 1692–1696.

47 Yagoda, A., Mukherji, B., Young, C. et al. (1972). Bleomycin, an antitumor antibiotic. clinical experience in 274 patients. *Ann. Intern. Med.* 77 (6): 861–870.

48 Skarin, A.T., Rosenthal, D.S., Moloney, W.C., and Iii, E.F. (1977). Combination chemotherapy of advanced non-hodgkin lymphoma with bleomycin, adriamycin, cyclophosphamide, vincristine, and prednisone (bacop). *Blood* 49 (5): 759–770.

49 Burger, R.M. (1998). Cleavage of nucleic acids by bleomycin. *Chem. Rev.* 98 (3): 1153–1170.

50 Hecht, S.M. (1986). The chemistry of activated bleomycin. *Acc. Chem. Res.* 19 (12): 383–391.

51 Kane, S.A. and Hecht, S.M. (1994). Polynucleotide recognition and degradation by bleomycin. *Prog. Nucleic Acid Res. Mol. Biol.* 49: 313–352.

52 Boger, D.L. and Cai, H. (1999). Bleomycin: synthetic and mechanistic studies. *Angew. Chem. Int. Ed. Engl.* 38 (4): 448–476.

53 Goodwin, K.D., Lewis, M.A., Long, E.C., and Georgiadis, M.M. (2008). Crystal structure of DNA-bound Co (iii)· bleomycin B2: insights on intercalation and minor groove binding. *Proc. Natl. Acad. Sci. U. S. A.* 105 (13): 5052–5056.

54 Schroeder, B.R., Ghare, M.I., Bhattacharya, C. et al. (2014). The disaccharide moiety of bleomycin facilitates uptake by cancer cells. *J. Am. Chem. Soc.* 136 (39): 13641–13656.

55 Boger, D.L., Colletti, S.L., Honda, T., and Menezes, R.F. (1994). Total synthesis of bleomycin A2 and related agents. 1. Synthesis and DNA binding properties of the extended C-terminus: Tripeptide S, tetrapeptide S, pentapeptide S, and related agents. *J. Am. Chem. Soc.* 116 (13): 5607–5618.

56 Boger, D.L., Colletti, S.L., Teramoto, S. et al. (1995). Synthesis of key analogs of bleomycin A2 that permit a systematic evaluation of the linker region: Identification of an exceptionally prominent role for the l-threonine substituent. *Bioorg. Med. Chem.* 3 (9): 1281–1295.

57 Chien, M., Grollman, A.P., and Horwitz, S.B. (1977). Bleomycin-DNA interactions: fluorescence and proton magnetic resonance studies. *Biochemistry* 16 (16): 2641–2647.

58 Kilkuskie, R.E., Suguna, H., Yellin, B. et al. (1985). Oxygen transfer by bleomycin analogs dysfunctional in DNA cleavage. *J. Am. Chem. Soc.* 107 (1): 260–261.

59 Abraham, A.T., Lin, J.-J., Newton, D.L. et al. (2003). RNA cleavage and inhibition of protein synthesis by bleomycin. *Chem. Biol.* 10 (1): 45–52.

60 Angelbello, A.J. and Disney, M.D. (2018). Bleomycin can cleave an oncogenic noncoding RNA. *ChemBioChem* 19 (1): 43–47.

61 Sergeev, D.S., Zarytova, V.F., Mamaev, S.V. et al. (1992). Sequence-specific cleavage of single-stranded DNA by oligonucleotides conjugated to bleomycin. *Antisense Res. Dev.* 2 (3): 235–241.

62 Sergeyev, D.S. and Zarytova, V.F. (1996). Interaction of bleomycin and its oligonucleotide derivatives with nucleic acids. *Russ. Chem. Rev.* 65 (4): 355.

63 Vorobjev, P.E., Smith, J.B., Pyshnaya, I.A. et al. (2003). Site-specific cleavage of RNA and DNA by complementary DNA–bleomycin A5 conjugates. *Bioconjugate Chem.* 14 (6): 1307–1313.

64 Wu, W., Vanderwall, D.E., Turner, C.J. et al. (1996). Solution structure of Co•bleomycin A2 green complexed with d(CCAGGCCTGG). *J. Am. Chem. Soc.* 118 (6): 1281–1294.

65 Rzuczek, S.G., Colgan, L.A., Nakai, Y. et al. (2017). Precise small-molecule recognition of a toxic CUG RNA repeat expansion. *Nat. Chem. Biol.* 13 (2): 188–193.

66 Angelbello, A.J., Rzuczek, S.G., McKee, K.K. et al. (2019). Precise small-molecule cleavage of an r(CUG) repeat expansion in a myotonic dystrophy mouse model. *Proc. Natl. Acad. Sci. U. S. A.* 116 (16): 7799–7804.

67 Wojciechowska, M., Sobczak, K., Kozlowski, P. et al. (2018). Quantitative methods to monitor RNA biomarkers in myotonic dystrophy. *Sci. Rep.* 8 (1): 5885.

68 Angelbello, A.J., DeFeo, M.E., Glinkerman, C.M. et al. (2020). Precise targeted cleavage of a r(CUG) repeat expansion in cells by using a small-molecule–deglycobleomycin conjugate. *ACS Chem. Biol.* 15 (4): 849–855.

69 Benhamou, R.I., Abe, M., Choudhary, S. et al. (2020). Optimization of the linker domain in a dimeric compound that degrades an r(CUG) repeat expansion in cells. *J. Med. Chem.* 63 (14): 7827–7839.

70 Liquori, C.L., Ricker, K., Moseley, M.L. et al. (2001). Myotonic dystrophy type 2 caused by a CCTG expansion in intron 1 of ZNF9. *Science* 293 (5531): 864–867.

71 Perdoni, F., Malatesta, M., Cardani, R. et al. (2009). RNA/MBNL1-containing foci in myoblast nuclei from patients affected by myotonic dystrophy type 2: an immunocytochemical study. *Eur. J. Histochem.* 53 (3): e18.

72 Savkur, R.S., Philips, A.V., and Cooper, T.A. (2001). Aberrant regulation of insulin receptor alternative splicing is associated with insulin resistance in myotonic dystrophy. *Nat. Genet.* 29 (1): 40–47.

73 Sznajder, Ł.J., Thomas, J.D., Carrell, E.M. et al. (2018). Intron retention induced by microsatellite expansions as a disease biomarker. *Proc. Natl. Acad. Sci. U. S. A.* 115 (16): 4234–4239.

74 Lee, M.M., Pushechnikov, A., and Disney, M.D. (2009). Rational and modular design of potent ligands targeting the RNA that causes myotonic dystrophy 2. *ACS Chem. Biol.* 4 (5): 345–355.

75 Benhamou, R.I., Angelbello, A.J., Andrews, R.J. et al. (2020). Structure-specific cleavage of an RNA repeat expansion with a dimeric small molecule is advantageous over sequence-specific recognition by an oligonucleotide. *ACS Chem. Biol.* 15 (2): 485–493.

76 Li, Y. and Disney, M.D. (2018). Precise small molecule degradation of a noncoding RNA identifies cellular binding sites and modulates an oncogenic phenotype. *ACS Chem. Biol.* 13 (11): 3065–3071.

77 Guttilla, I.K. and White, B.A. (2009). Coordinate regulation of foxo1 by miR-27a, miR-96, and miR-182 in breast cancer cells. *J. Biol. Chem.* 284 (35): 23204–23216.

78 Velagapudi, S.P., Cameron, M.D., Haga, C.L. et al. (2016). Design of a small molecule against an oncogenic noncoding RNA. *Proc. Natl. Acad. Sci. U. S. A.* 113 (21): 5898–5903.

79 Sakamoto, K.M., Kim, K.B., Kumagai, A. et al. (2001). Protacs: chimeric molecules that target proteins to the Skp1-Cullin-F box complex for ubiquitination and degradation. *Proc. Natl. Acad. Sci. U. S. A.* 98 (15): 8554–8559.

80 Gao, X., Burris Iii, H.A., Vuky, J. et al. (2022). Phase 1/2 study of ARV-110, an androgen receptor (AR) protac degrader, in metastatic castration-resistant prostate cancer (mCRPC). *J. Clin. Oncol.* 40 (6): 17.

81 Costales, M.G., Aikawa, H., Li, Y. et al. (2020). Small-molecule targeted recruitment of a nuclease to cleave an oncogenic RNA in a mouse model of metastatic cancer. *Proc. Natl. Acad. Sci. U. S. A.* 117 (5): 2406–2411.

82 Zhang, P., Liu, X., Abegg, D. et al. (2021). Reprogramming of protein-targeted small-molecule medicines to RNA by ribonuclease recruitment. *J. Am. Chem. Soc.* 143 (33): 13044–13055.

83 Bush, J.A., Aikawa, H., Fuerst, R. et al. (2021). Ribonuclease recruitment using a small molecule reduced c9ALS/FTD r(G_4C_2) repeat expansion in vitro and in vivo ALS models. *Sci. Transl. Med.* 13 (617): eabd5991.

84 Åsa, S., Fagerberg, L., Schwenk, J.M. et al. (2019). The human secretome. *Sci. Signaling* 12 (609): eaaz0274.

85 Fredrik, P., Nielsen, J., Alm, T. et al. (2015). Tissue-based map of the human proteome. *Science* 347 (6220): 1260419.

86 Thul, P.J., Lovisa, Å., Wiking, M. et al. (2017). A subcellular map of the human proteome. *Science* 356 (6340): eaal3321.

87 Kerr, I.M. and Brown, R.E. (1978). pppA2'p5'A2'p5'A: an inhibitor of protein synthesis synthesized with an enzyme fraction from interferon-treated cells. *Proc. Natl. Acad. Sci. U. S. A.* 75 (1): 256–260.

88 Donovan, J., Dufner, M., and Korennykh, A. (2013). Structural basis for cytosolic double-stranded RNA surveillance by human oligoadenylate synthetase 1. *Proc. Natl. Acad. Sci. U. S. A.* 110 (5): 1652–1657.

89 Lin, R.-J., Yu, H.-P., Chang, B.-L. et al. (2009). Distinct antiviral roles for human 2′, 5′-oligoadenylate synthetase family members against dengue virus infection. *J. Immunol.* 183 (12): 8035–8043.

90 Dong, B. and Silverman, R.H. (1995). 2-5A-dependent RNase molecules dimerize during activation by 2-5A. *J Biol Chem* 270 (8): 4133–4137.

91 Wreschner, D.H., McCauley, J.W., Skehel, J.J., and Kerr, I.M. (1981). Interferon action—sequence specificity of the ppp $(A2'p)_n$A-dependent ribonuclease. *Nature* 289 (5796): 414–417.

92 Floyd-Smith, G., Slattery, E., and Lengyel, P. (1981). Interferon action: RNA cleavage pattern of a (2′-5′) oligoadenylate—dependent endonuclease. *Science* 212 (4498): 1030–1032.

93 Han, Y., Donovan, J., Rath, S. et al. (2014). Structure of human RNase L reveals the basis for regulated RNA decay in the IFN response. *Science* 343 (6176): 1244–1248.

94 Costales, M.G., Matsumoto, Y., Velagapudi, S.P., and Disney, M.D. (2018). Small molecule targeted recruitment of a nuclease to RNA. *J. Am. Chem. Soc.* 140 (22): 6741–6744.

95 Mathew, L.K. and Simon, M.C. (2009). miR-210: A sensor for hypoxic stress during tumorigenesis. *Mol. Cell* 35 (6): 737–738.

96 Huang, X., Ding, L., Bennewith, K.L. et al. (2009). Hypoxia-inducible miR-210 regulates normoxic gene expression involved in tumor initiation. *Mol. Cell* 35 (6): 856–867.

97 Costales, M.G., Haga, C.L., Velagapudi, S.P. et al. (2017). Small molecule inhibition of microRNA-210 reprograms an oncogenic hypoxic circuit. *J. Am. Chem. Soc.* 139 (9): 3446–3455.

98 Costales, M.G., Suresh, B., Vishnu, K., and Disney, M.D. (2019). Targeted degradation of a hypoxia-associated non-coding RNA enhances the selectivity of a small molecule interacting with RNA. *Cell Chem. Biol.* 26 (8): 1180–1186.e1185.

99 Thakur, C.S., Jha, B.K., Dong, B. et al. (2007). Small-molecule activators of RNase L with broad-spectrum antiviral activity. *Proc. Natl. Acad. Sci. U. S. A.* 104 (23): 9585–9590.

100 Krichevsky, A.M. and Gabriely, G. (2009). miR-21: A small multi-faceted RNA. *J. Cell. Mol. Med.* 13 (1): 39–53.

101 Haniff, H.S., Tong, Y., Liu, X. et al. (2020). Targeting the SARS-CoV-2 RNA genome with small molecule binders and ribonuclease targeting chimera (RIBOTAC) degraders. *ACS Cent. Sci.* 6 (10): 1713–1721.

102 Tong, Y., Gibaut, Q.M.R., Rouse, W. et al. (2022). Transcriptome-wide mapping of small-molecule RNA-binding sites in cells informs an isoform-specific degrader of QSOX1 mRNA. *J. Am. Chem. Soc.* 144 (26): 11620–11625.

103 Motzer, R.J., Porta, C., Vogelzang, N.J. et al. (2014). Dovitinib versus sorafenib for third-line targeted treatment of patients with metastatic renal cell carcinoma: an open-label, randomised phase 3 trial. *Lancet Oncol.* 15 (3): 286–296.

104 Trudel, S., Li, Z.H., Wei, E. et al. (2005). Chir-258, a novel, multitargeted tyrosine kinase inhibitor for the potential treatment of t(4;14) multiple myeloma. *Blood* 105 (7): 2941–2948.

105 Gomez, I.G., MacKenna, D.A., Johnson, B.G. et al. (2015). Anti–microRNA-21 oligonucleotides prevent Alport nephropathy progression by stimulating metabolic pathways. *J. Clin. Investig.* 125 (1): 141–156.

106 Cosgrove, D., Meehan, D.T., Grunkemeyer, J.A. et al. (1996). Collagen col4a3 knockout: a mouse model for autosomal Alport syndrome. *Genes Dev.* 10 (23): 2981–2992.

107 Mu, P., Han, Y.-C., Betel, D. et al. (2009). Genetic dissection of the mir-17~92 cluster of micrornas in myc-induced b-cell lymphomas. *Genes Dev.* 23 (24): 2806–2811.

108 Liu, X., Haniff, H.S., Childs-Disney, J. et al. (2020). Targeted degradation of the oncogenic microRNA 17-92 cluster by structure-targeting ligands. *J. Am. Chem. Soc.* 142 (15): 6970–6982.

109 Meyer, S.M., Tanaka, T., Zanon, P.R.A. et al. (2022). DNA-encoded library screening to inform design of a ribonuclease targeting chimera (RiboTAC). *J. Am. Chem. Soc.* 144 (46): 21096–21102.

110 Troup, R.I., Fallan, C., and Baud, M.G.J. (2020). Current strategies for the design of protac linkers: a critical review. *Explor. Targeted Antitumor Ther.* 1 (5): 273–312.

111 Lipinski, C.A., Lombardo, F., Dominy, B.W., and Feeney, P.J. (2001). Experimental and computational approaches to estimate solubility and permeability in drug discovery and development settings. *Adv. Drug Delivery Rev.* 46 (1): 3–26.

10

Approaches to the Identification of Molecules Altering Programmed Ribosomal Frameshifting in Viruses

Elinore A. VanGraafeiland[1], Diego M. Arévalo[2], and Benjamin L. Miller[1,2,3]

[1] *University of Rochester, Department of Biochemistry and Biophysics, 601 Elmwood Ave, Rochester, NY 14642, USA*
[2] *University of Rochester, Department of Chemistry, 252 Elmwood Ave, Rochester, NY 14611, USA*
[3] *University of Rochester, Department of Dermatology, 601 Elmwood Ave, Rochester, NY 14642, USA*

10.1 Introduction

The diverse roles of RNA in normal and aberrant human biology, more of which are discovered on a near-daily basis, have driven an increasing interest in RNA as a therapeutic target since pioneering studies by Czarnik [1], Wong [2], and others in the 1990s. In eukaryotic cells, RNA is responsible for the maintenance, regulation, and processing of genetic information. As such, RNAs are often implicated in cancers, viral infections, and other diseases [3]. Currently, the vast majority of therapeutics focus on protein targets, accounting for approximately only 0.05% of the human genome [4]. RNAs are an attractive alternative, as they may circumvent some challenges often experienced with more traditional drug targets. For example, difficult-to-drug or "undruggable" proteins can be targeted by modulating the translation efficiency, mRNA abundance, or stability of the corresponding protein RNA [4, 5]. Many RNAs important to pathogenic organisms do not have close orthologs in humans, making them ideal targets for selective compounds [5]. In one important example of this, pathogenic viruses, including human immunodeficiency virus type 1 (HIV-1), coronaviruses including severe acute respiratory syndrome coronavirus 2 (SARS-CoV-2), influenza virus, and respiratory syncytial virus, have life cycles that are absolutely dependent on an RNA-specific process known as Programmed Ribosomal Frameshifting (PRF). RNAs involved in PRF are therefore particularly intriguing candidates for drug discovery. This review will discuss the history and current state of the art of efforts to target viral RNAs involved in PRF as a method for interfering with the viral life cycle.

One of the first examples discovered of frameshifting in eukaryotic systems was the Rous sarcoma virus (RSV), in 1985 [6]. Initial work showed that the Gag and Gag-pol poly proteins were produced in a roughly 20 : 1 ratio, that Gag and Pol were in different reading frames, and that frameshifting was sequence specific [6]. Later work in 1988 showed frameshifting was stimulated by a combination of a heptameric

RNA as a Drug Target: The Next Frontier for Medicinal Chemistry, First Edition.
Edited by John Schneekloth and Martin Pettersson.

A/U rich sequence that permitted "slippage" of the ribosome into the −1 frame and a downstream structured RNA (described as a "stem-loop" but subsequently determined to form a pseudoknot) capable of causing ribosomal pausing [7]. Further, the stimulatory pseudoknot of RSV was sensitive to changes to its structure [7], and frameshifting efficiency could be modulated by changing that RNA's secondary structure or by mutations to the upstream "slippery" sequence [8].

Frameshifting activity has also been observed in viruses that cause a greater impact on public health. Both the influenza virus and the respiratory syncytial virus have overlapping reads in their genomes that require frameshifting events for translation of important viral proteins. Influenza requires a +1 frameshift to translate the polypeptide PA-X: the PA protein is involved in viral polymerase activity, while the *N*-terminal domain of PA-X has been reported to have activity repressing the host cell immune systems [9]. Respiratory syncytial virus, on the other hand, has overlapping reading frames in the gene for an internal virion matrix protein, M2. The upstream ORF M2-1 is involved in viral RNA replication, while the downstream out-of-frame ORF M2-2 has activity regulating transcription and replication [10]. For both viruses, frameshifting plays an important role for the viral life cycle [9, 10].

While other forms of PRF have been discovered, the most common in viruses is a shift in the −1 direction, leading to the production of a new protein product [11]. Viruses use −1 PRF, shown in Figure 10.1,[1] to maintain optimal ratios of proteins and enzymes, and disrupting the efficiency of frameshifting can impact viral viability and viral replication (RSV [8], SARS-CoV [13–15], HIV [16, 17], SARS-CoV-2 [18, 19]).

The mechanism of −1 programmed ribosomal frameshifting (PRF) is the subject of ongoing research, but three mechanisms have been proposed. These are (1) the docking of a frameshift-stimulating stem loop in the A-site of the ribosome during translation resulting in the slippage of the single P-site tRNA when the A-site is vacant during translation (Figure 10.2a, below), (2) the frameshift-stimulating sequence interacts with the mRNA entry channel or exterior of the ribosome resulting in both the A- and P-site tRNAs to slip while the aa-tRNA accommodates the A-site (Figure 10.2b, below), and (3) both the A- and P-site tRNAs experience slippage during translocation [21, 22]. Recent studies by the Ermolenko Lab found that frameshift-causing hairpins (also called stemloops) such as those used by HIV, discussed further below, inhibit A-site tRNA binding and mRNA translocation in manners similar to mechanisms (1) and (3) [21]. It was assumed that the mRNA stemloop and pseudoknots (used as frameshift signals by some other viruses) facilitate ribosome pausing due to high thermodynamic stability throughout the entire RNA structure [20]. However, the translating ribosome is only capable of unwinding three base pairs at a time, and hence the overall thermodynamic stability of stemloops and pseudoknots should not have an impact on frameshifting [20].

1 Reprinted (adapted) with permission from Anokhina, V.S. and Miller, B.L. (2021). Targeting ribosomal frameshifting as an antiviral strategy: from HIV-1 to SARS-CoV-2. *Acc. Chem. Res.* 54 (17): 3349–3361. https://doi.org/10.1021/acs.accounts.1c00316. Copyright 2021 American Chemical Society.

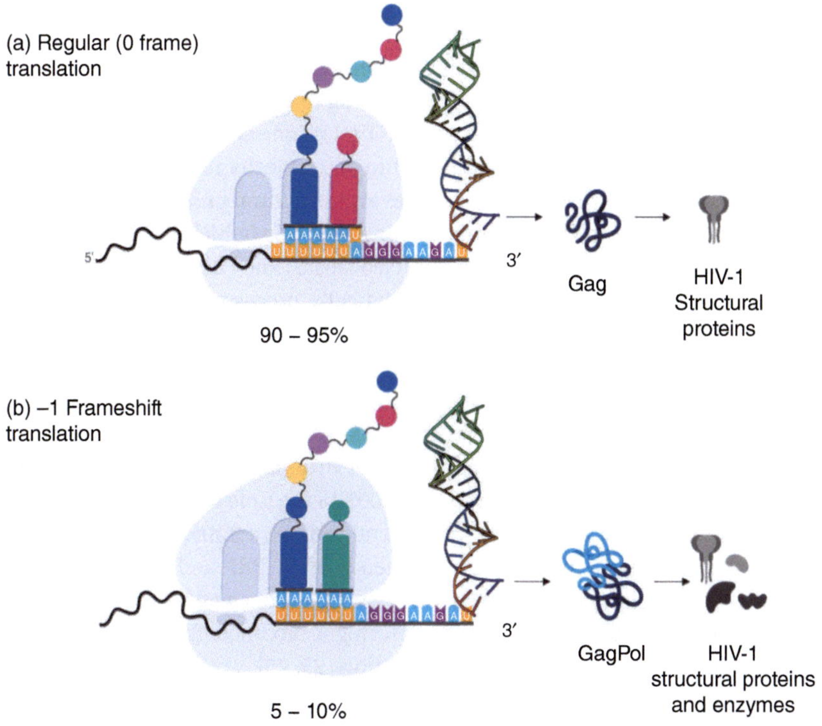

Figure 10.1 During translation of an mRNA containing a frameshift-stimulating element (FSE), the ribosome translates the transcript, reaches the FSE, overcomes its hindrance to translation and unwinds it, and terminates translation when it reaches the stop codon within the FSE (a, top). However, some of the time the ribosome is unable to easily overcome the hindrance to translation presented by the FSE, resulting in a shifting of the ribosome into the −1 open reading frame (b, bottom). Source: Anokhina and Miller [12]/with permission of Springer Nature. For HIV, a −1 frameshifting event is required for the production of viral enzymes (Gag and GagPol) essential for viral replication.

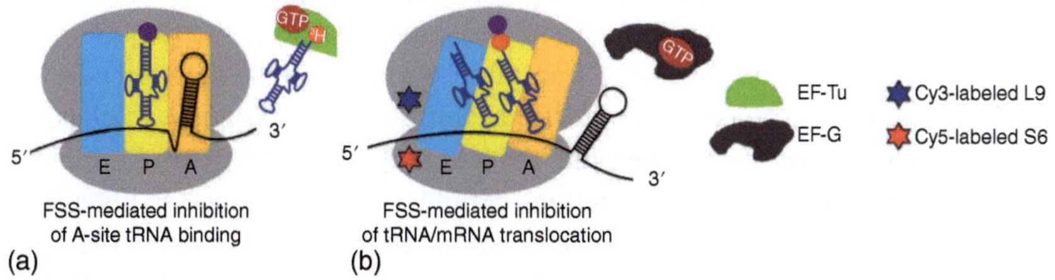

Figure 10.2 Mechanisms of frameshifting, as described by Bao et al. [20] (a, left, Mechanism 1) Frameshift-stimulating stem loops can dock in the A-site of the ribosome, preventing the incoming tRNA from docking, resulting in the slippage of the tRNA in the P-site. (b, right, Mechanism 2) Alternatively, frameshift-stimulating elements can interact with the exterior of the ribosome, including the mRNA entry channel, preventing translocation of the ribosome and inducing frameshifting of the tRNAs in the P- and A-sites. In both cases, the ribosome must unfold the hindering RNA structure to continue translation. Source: Bao et al. [20]/Springer Nature/CC BY 4.0.

Instead, it has been posited that a frameshift signal inhibits tRNA binding by interacting with the A-site. This was demonstrated using a construct that expanded the length of a hairpin frameshift-stimulating element (FSE) by six base pairs; this failed to inhibit tRNA binding to the A-site, pointing to the first mechanism [20].

The human immunodeficiency virus type 1 (HIV-1) is one of the more well-known examples of retroviruses employing frameshifting as a mechanism to produce and regulate the relative quantities of viral enzymes and structural proteins. The *gag-pol* HIV-1 mRNA codes for translation of two polyproteins: Gag (which is proteolytically processed to yield HIV matrix, capsid, and nucleocapsid) and Pol, which only forms as a Gag-Pol fusion polyprotein. Pol is proteolytically processed to yield protease, reverse transcriptase, and integrase enzymes. Gag-Pol forms when -1 PRF causes the ribosome to move in to a new reading frame, skipping the stop codon on the gag gene during translation [21, 23]. The frameshift efficiency, resulting in the formation of the Gag-Pol polyprotein, is approximately 5–10%, and this stoichiometry has been shown to be necessary for proper packaging of virus particles [21]. For example, mutants that result in Gag-Pol being produced 100% of the time were unable to make viral particles [23]. As discussed above in a general context, a frameshift stimulatory element (FSE, Figure 10.3) regulates the frequency of −1 PRF and hence the ratio of Gag and Gag-Pol. Therefore, we and others hypothesized several years ago that a compound that could bind to the FSE mRNA might modulate frameshifting, and consequently inhibit viral assembly and replication [23, 25].

10.2 Mechanisms of Frameshifting

To begin to understand how to target the FSE RNA, it is useful to understand what is necessary to facilitate a frameshifting event. Frameshifting can only occur when two elements are present: a highly conserved UUUUUUA sequence, known as the slippery sequence (Figure 10.3, boxed in blue), and a downstream frameshift stimulatory stem–loop (Figure 10.3, upper stem) [23, 24]. The slippery sequence is where the shift of one nucleotide causes a change in reading frame during translation, while the stimulatory stem has been posited to pause the ribosome [24]. Studies elucidating the structure of the HIV-1 frameshift element mRNA determined that the slippery sequence is proceeded by the frameshift stimulatory signal, which is an irregular helix made up of an upper and lower stem [24, 25]. Of note, shortening or removing the stem–loop, along variations of the HIV FSE sequence do not affect tRNA binding to the A-site [20]. It has been posited that the interaction of the FSE stem–loop is not sequence-specific, most likely involving recognition of the RNA's sugar-phosphate backbone [20].

A common method for investigating frameshifting that can also be employed to test the influence of compounds is through use of a dual reporter assay. In the assay, the slippery sequence and FSE are sandwiched between two different reporters, typically *Renilla* luciferase (Rluc) and firefly luciferase (Fluc) or other reporter genes. Rluc and Fluc yield enzymes acting on substrates to produce luminescence at different wavelengths (colors) [26]. In cellular systems (or sometimes

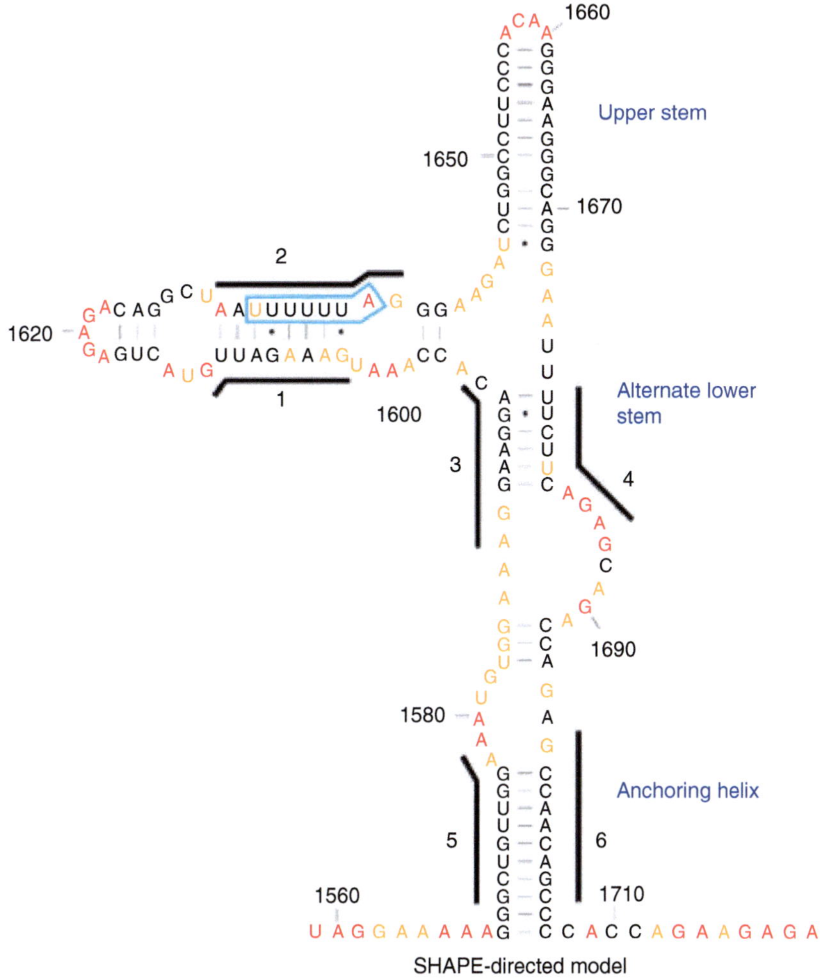

Figure 10.3 The SHAPE-determined model of the HIV gag-pol frameshift sequence RNA. Source: Low et al. [24]/with permission of American Chemical Society.

in a cellular lysate such as rabbit reticulocyte lysate), the downstream reporter is only expressed when frameshifting occurs while the upstream reporter is always expressed, allowing for an assay capable of measuring frameshifting efficiency for a given FSE [26].

10.3 Targeting Frameshifting in HIV

Dual-reporter assays were employed extensively in analyzing one of the more prominent classes of compounds that bind the FSE mRNA: aminoglycosides. Guanidinoneomycin B, an exhaustively guanidine-derivatized analog of neomycin B, is an example of this, and was studied extensively by Butcher and Tor [27]. However, aminoglycosides are generally regarded as binding to RNA targets in a non-selective manner [28]. The nature of aminoglycosides to bind indiscriminately to RNA has been attributed to their conformational flexibility, which allows aminoglycosides to conform to varied RNA targets [28, 29]. Recently, nucleic acid dye tags were used to study the frameshifting event for HIV-1 [30]. Peptide-based and peptidomimetic compounds have been used with considerable success for targeting the HIV-1 FSE. These compounds were studied over a period of several years by the Miller group. Initial hit compounds were identified using a resin-bound variant of a library generation method called dynamic combinatorial chemistry. This uses reversible reactions to create dynamic combinatorial libraries, which can undergo evolution based on the selection pressure of library members binding preferentially to a nucleic acid (or other) target [31]. While many exchange chemistries are possible, here the reversible exchange was facilitated by the presence of cysteine residues present in each library member, allowing for the formation of resin-bound disulfides and subsequent reversible disulfide exchange between resin-bound materials and solution-phase compounds [31]. In the screen targeting the HIV-1 FSE RNA, an 11,325 member Resin Bound Dynamic Combinatorial Library (RBDCL) was prepared. The equilibrium of the reversible exchange between the solid-phase and solution-phase monomers was altered when fluorescently tagged RNA was introduced, allowing for the identification of an initial hit compound (Figure 10.4, **1**)[2] via

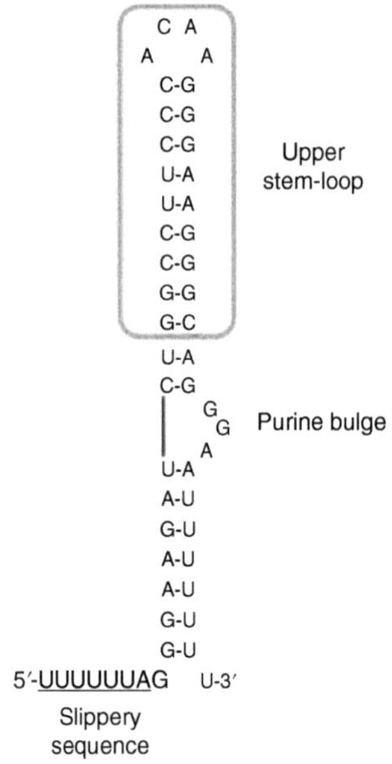

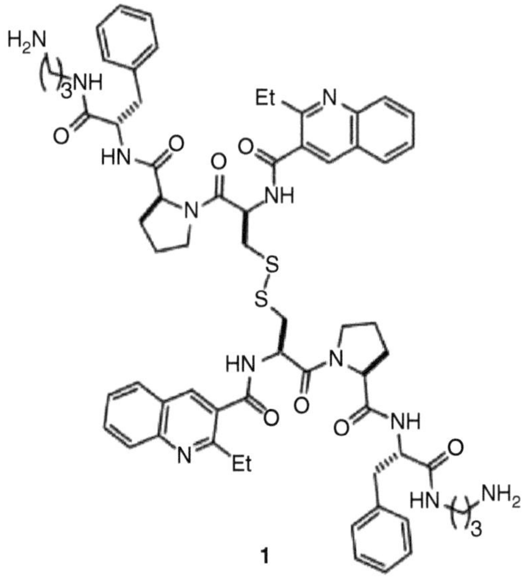

1

Figure 10.4 The initial lead compound (right) determined via the RBDCL [32] for the HIV gag-pol FSE RNA (left) [33]. Source: (a) Palde et al. [33]/with permission of American Chemical Society; (b) McNaughton et al. [32]/with permission of American Chemical Society.

2 Reprinted (adapted) with permission from Palde, P.B., Ofori, L.O., Gareiss, P.C. et al. (2010). Strategies for recognition of stem-loop RNA structures by synthetic ligands: application to the HIV-1 frameshift stimulatory sequence. *J. Med. Chem.* 53 (16): 6018–6027. https://doi.org/10.1021/jm100231t. Copyright 2010 American Chemical Society.

fluorescence microscopy, followed by mass spectrometry [32]. The library members incorporated heterocyclic moieties to facilitate binding to the HIV-1 FSE RNA; the primary compound identified from the screen was symmetrical, with quinoline groups as the heterocycle [32, 33]. Post identification validation involved testing for affinity and specificity via surface plasmon resonance (SPR). This yielded a K_D of $4.1 \pm 2.4\,\mu M$ and showed that the compound displayed no apparent affinity to related RNA sequences [32].

Based on this initial hit, several structural hypotheses were tested to yield compounds with higher affinity and selectivity for the FSE mRNA. One set of initial experiments focused on structure activity relationships of the 2-ethylquinoline 3-carboxamide moiety. Modifying the 2-ethyl to methyl or proton yielded insignificant decreases in affinity of the compound for the FSE RNA [33]. However, reducing the π-surface by replacing 2-ethylquinoline with 2-methyl-3-carboxypyridine resulted in ablation of binding to the FSE RNA [33]. Another point of modification on the lead compound was to test a suitable bioisostere for the disulfide bridge of the compound, due to susceptibility of disulfides to reduction or exchange in a cellular environment [16, 33]. While disulfides have served a structural role in bioactive peptides, thioesters and carbon linkers have been demonstrated to enhance biostability without affecting function of the compound [33]. To that end, the Miller lab synthesized and tested the activity of olefin and hydrocarbon analogs of the lead compound (Figure 10.5). It was found that the Z-isomer of the olefin displayed greater affinity for the FSE RNA over the E-isomer [33]. The Z-isomer olefin analog displayed over fourfold increase of affinity relative to the hydrocarbon analog; it was reasoned that this was due to the increased flexibility and hydrophobicity of the fully saturated analog [33]. Further experiments demonstrated that analogs were selective for binding the stem–loop RNA. Interestingly, the monomeric compound, while able to bind to the FSE RNA, had binding ablated in the presence of yeast tRNA, showing that its binding to the FSE RNA was nonspecific [33]. Similar binding behavior was observed with 2-ethylquinoline 3-carboxylic acid, which binds to RNA non-specifically, suggesting that the entire peptide and quinoline is necessary for selective binding to the FSE RNA [33].

Increasing the pi-surface area available for binding by replacing the 2-ethylquinoline with a benzo[g]quinoline enhanced affinity (Figure 10.5, **2–8**). These analogs were tested to determine binding kinetics, as the equilibrium dissociation constant K_D on its own does not provide the full picture of the binding event. The dissociation rate, k_d, is regarded as an important determinant of selectivity for protein binders, and this represented an opportunity to test the idea in the context of RNA [34]. Slower dissociation rates indicate longer residence times and greater target selectivity [35]. With that in mind, binding experiments using SPR were carried out with immobilized biotinylated FSE RNA on the surface. The determined off-rates for compound **1**, along with the analogs, were 10^{-2} to $10^{-3}\,s^{-1}$, which is a stark contrast to the fast on- and off-rate of a tested aminoglycoside, Neomycin [33]. With promising results, these analogs were tested in cells via a MTT assay, serving

Figure 10.5 The N-methylation and triazole analogs of the olefin FSE RNA-binding compound. Source: Hilimire et al. [16]/with permission of American Chemical Society.

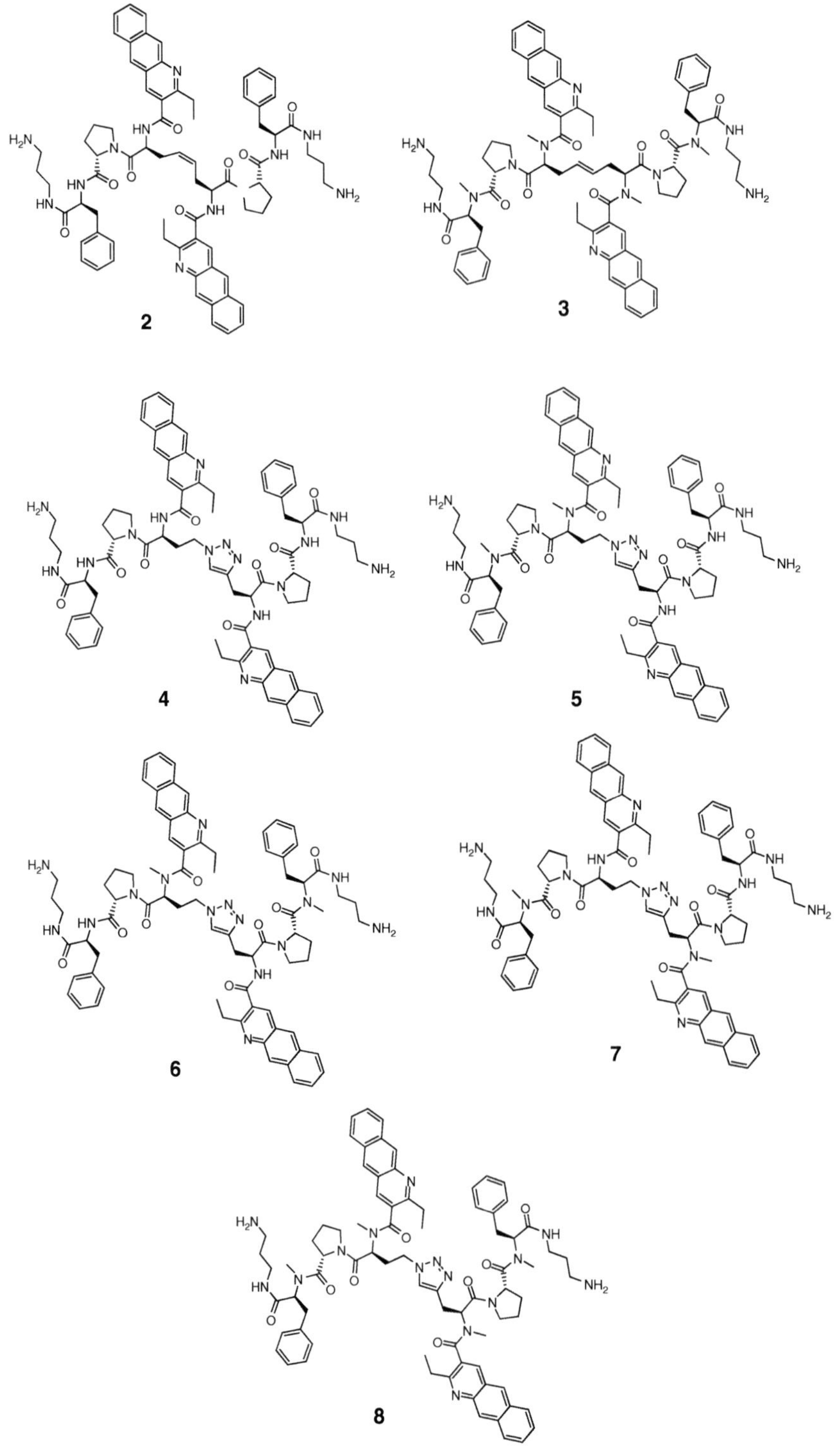

as a reporter for mitochondrial activity, and found no statistically significant cell toxicity with cells treated with compounds up to 1 mM [33].

Two further modifications introduced were N-methylation and 1,4-triazole as an alternative disulfide bioisotere to the olefin. N-methylation was used to further enhance binding selectivity of the olefin analog (Figure 10.5, **3**), as this modification often improves affinity, selectivity, and activity of peptides [36, 37]. Triazole was chosen as a bioisotere (Figure 10.5, **4–8**) due to the robust metal-catalyzed Huisgen cycloaddition chemistry that was readily available, and that despite the precedent for triazole to be used in other targets, including RNA, they have not been used as a bioisostere for disulfides [16]. The structural similarities between disulfides, olefins, and triazoles were clear, based on density functional theory (DFT) calculations, though the disulfide torsional bond rotation is distinct from that of olefins and triazoles [16]. What was found from these experiments is that inclusion of a triazole in the structure had no effect on affinity, while N-methylation had a modest effect [16]. It was observed that N-methyl analog **3** had a dissociation constant (K_D) for the FSE RNA of 13.0 ± 5.0 nM, a five-fold increase in affinity over the olefin-containing compound [16]. Cell permeability and toxicity experiments revealed that compound **6** was non-toxic up to 110 µM, and compound **8** was the most cell permeable as determined via flow cytometry [16]. These N-methyl analogs were also studied for frameshift modulating and anti-HIV activity using pseudotyped HIV, and were found to enhance frameshifting at levels consistent with their relative potencies, and likewise to interfere with the infectivity of pseudotyped HIV. Finally, compounds were found to be active against both laboratory HIV-1 strains (HIV_{IIIB}) and a multi-drug-resistant patient isolate of HIV-1 [16, 36].

Success with replacing portions of the peptide with non-peptidic bioisosteres led to the question: could one incorporate other bioisosteric peptide mimics to further evolve these HIV-1 FSE binders to something entirely non-peptidic? To address that question, we hypothesized that the 2,5-diketopiperazine (DKP) could be integrated into FSE-binding molecules, and perhaps serve more broadly as desirable scaffold for RNA-binding compounds. DKP is a considered a "privileged structure," defined as a substructure exhibiting good drug-like properties and often molecules able to specifically bind a broad range of biological targets [39]. DKPs are known to offer bioavailability and biostability advantages relative to simple peptides, due to improved stability, protease resistance, and conformational rigidity [40, 41]. The DKP has at least four points of functionality, making it a particularly diversifiable scaffold that can cover a great deal of chemical space. However, prior to our work, it had yet to be used as part of an RNA-binding compound. Thus a DKP-containing compound (**10**) was designed, synthesized, and tested alongside a non-DKP-containing compound (**9**) to determine the effects this new scaffold has on binding to the FSE RNA (Figure 10.6). Initial DFT simulations suggested that the DKP and non-DKP analogs adopted similar orientations and distances, having only a 1 Å RMS difference between the two [38]. Affinity and selectivity experiments for both analogs determined that the incorporation of the DKP scaffold did not impair binding, and competition with five-fold excess yeast tRNA did not yield notable changes in binding constants [38]. In contrast, a DKP containing

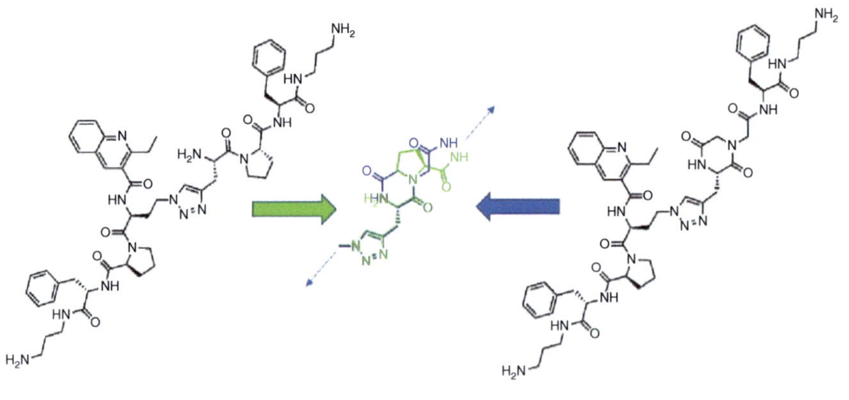

9 **10**

Figure 10.6 The DKP (**10**) and non-DKP (**9**) containing analogs. They both adopt similar structural and 3D space. Source: Arévalo et al. [38]/with permission of Royal Society of Chemistry.

half-compound displayed no binding to the RNA, demonstrating the necessity of the entire compound [38].

To determine where the DKP-containing compound was binding onto the FSE RNA, a series of surface plasmon resonance (SPR) competition experiments were performed by co-injecting the DKP compound with five-fold excess of stem and loop swapped FSE RNA mutants, along with FSE RNA (Figure 10.7). The competition experiment revealed that WT HIV-1 FSE RNA had ablated approximately 40% of total binding based on R_{max} value, suggesting that the affinity of the DKP-containing compound is impacted by whether the RNA is immobilized or in solution [38]. Of

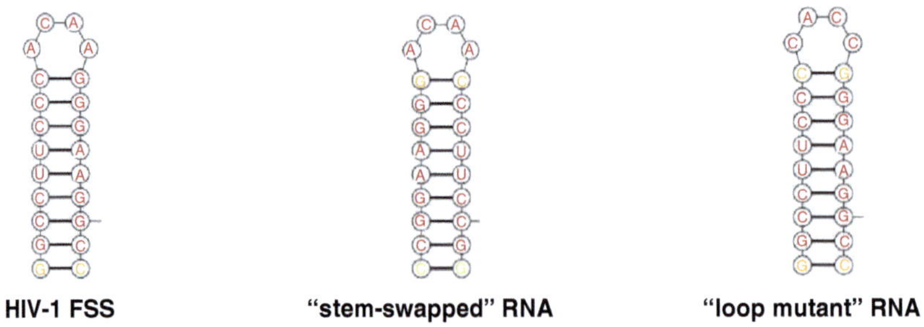

Conditions	K_D	*R*(max)	Δ[*R*(max)], %
5 μM **10**	5.04×e^{-7}	15.9	0
5 μM **10** + 25 μM HIV – 1 FSS	6.5×e^{-7}	9.6	40
5 μM **10** + 25 μM "stem-swapped" RNA	6.4×e^{-7}	13	18
5 μM **10** + 25 μM "loop mutant"	6.3×e^{-7}	15.2	4

Figure 10.7 DKP containing compound co-inject competition experiments with WT HIV-1 FSE RNA, "stem-swapped" and "loop" mutant RNAs via SPR. Source: Arévalo et al. [38]/with permission of Royal Society of Chemistry.

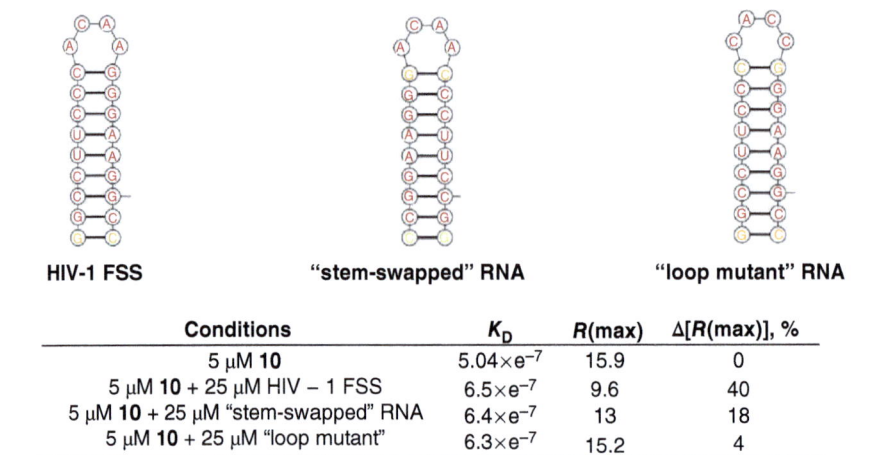

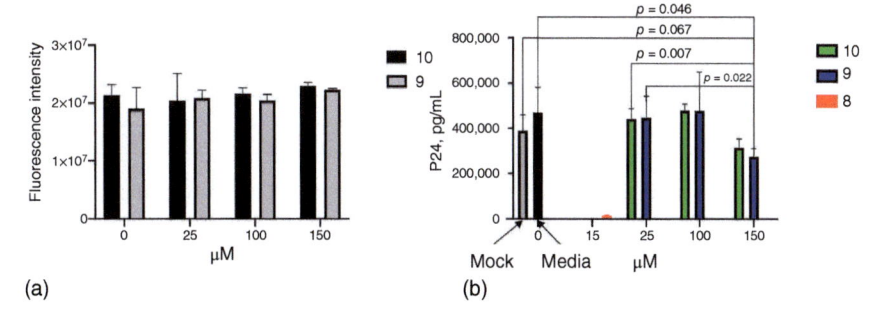

Figure 10.8 The toxicity and anti-HIV activity assays, from left to right. Both analogs are non-toxic up to 150 μM in MT-2 cells and display modest anti-HIV activity. Source: Arévalo et al. [38]/with permission of Royal Society of Chemistry.

the two mutant RNA that were co-injected, the stem-swapped RNA sequence caused an 18% decrease in R_{max}, while the loop-swapped mutant only competed off 4% (Figure 10.7). This finding suggests that most of the interactions of DKP analog to the FSE RNA is at the loop region [38]. Toxicity assays performed with MT-2 cells treated with both analogs have shown that they both do not show any notable toxicity up to 150 μM (Figure 10.8). The anti-HIV activity was not impacted with the inclusion of the DKP scaffold, though there was a loss of activity compared to the control [38].

10.4 Targeting Frameshifting in SARS-CoV-1 and SARS-CoV-2

Much like HIV-1, frameshifting in coronaviruses such as SARS-Cov-1 and -Cov-2 acts as a regulatory mechanism that controls the ratio of the production of non-structural proteins and enzymes. Specifically, genes *orf1a* and *orf1b* have an overlap in reading frames in the genome, requiring a frameshifting event during translation to produce the out-of-frame downstream polyprotein pp1ab in addition to the in-frame upstream polyprotein pp1a [42]. These polyproteins are further processed into nonstructural viral proteins such as proteases for viral protein processing (part of pp1a) and replication enzymes, including the RNA-dependent RNA polymerase (in pp1ab) [42].

While disrupting frameshifting of the HIV gag-pol polyprotein can abolish viral reproduction, changing the frameshift efficiency of beta coronaviruses such as SARS-CoV-1 and 2 impacts early viral growth kinetics, viral infectivity, and viral replication (Figure 10.9) [13, 14].

As previously stated, frameshifting requires an upstream slippery sequence and downstream frameshift-stimulating structure. In the case of beta coronaviruses, the canonical FSE is a three-stem, three-loop H-type pseudoknot [43, 44] capable of forming upstream and downstream interactions with neighboring RNA [45, 46] and dimerizing with another FSE [47]. This structure is conserved in coronaviruses, and

Slippery site sequence	% −1 PRF	Standard deviation	Plaque size	TCID$_{50}$
U UUA AAC (WT)	14.4	2.35	+ + +	4.53
U UUU UUU	4.88	1.31	+ +	<1
A AAA AAU	2.33	0.55	+	<1
U UUG AAC	0.15	0.03	−	ND

Figure 10.9 Mutating the SARS-CoV-1 slippery sequence reduces frameshift efficiency, which negatively impacts viral plaque size and infectivity. Source: Plant et al. [13]/with permission of American Society for Microbiology. Frameshift efficiency was measured in Vero E6 cells by incorporating either a wild-type or mutant slippery sequence and the FSE into a dual luciferase reporter plasmid. Clones of the SARS-CoV-1 genome were transfected into Vero E6 cells to measure infectivity of transcripts.

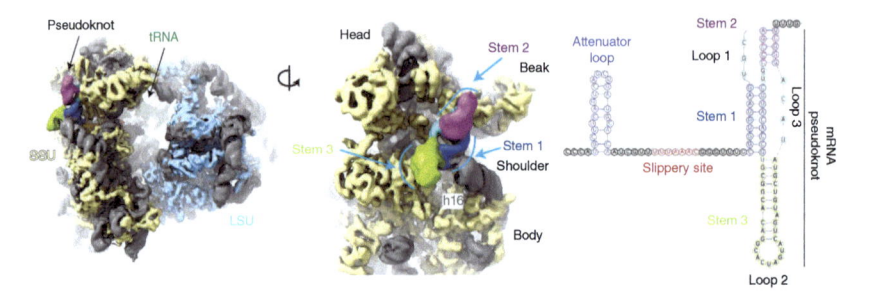

Figure 10.10 SARS-CoV-2 orf1ab FSE (green, purple, and blue) and ribosome (large subunit, light blue; small subunit, light green) captured together prior to a frameshifting event. The viral RNA is in the 0 frame, with a stop codon incorporated in the upstream slippery sequence. The presence of a mutant eRF1 prevents the release of the nascent polypeptide. The experiment was performed in rabbit reticulocyte lysate. Cryo-EM resolution ranged from 2.2 to 7.4 Å. Source: Bhatt et al. [18]/American Association for the Advancement of Science/CC BY 4.0.

changing the structure results in a corresponding change in frameshift efficiency [13]. An upstream hairpin stem loop, known as the attenuator stem loop, adds additional regulation to frameshift efficiency [44, 48].

The mechanism of frameshifting in coronaviruses is still under investigation, but cryo-EM and crystallography data from the Ban Lab shows the FSE wedged into the mRNA entry channel during translation (Figure 10.10) [18], providing evidence of a mechanism for inhibiting ribosomal translocation and causing ribosomal stalling required for a frameshifting event to occur.

One of the challenges of targeting frameshifting in SARS-CoV-2 is the complexity of the frameshift-stimulating element (FSE). Originally believed to be a three-stemmed, three-looped H-type pseudoknot, research by the Woodside group and others have shown that while this conformation occurs in isolation (Figure 10.11), the RNA element is context-dependent and can assume multiple conformations and associations with upstream and downstream RNA sequences, especially in a cellular environment (Figures 10.12 and 10.13) [18, 45, 49].

Initial structural data was obtained based on the canonical pseudoknot structure located at the 3′ end of orf1a. Composed of three stems and three loops, this

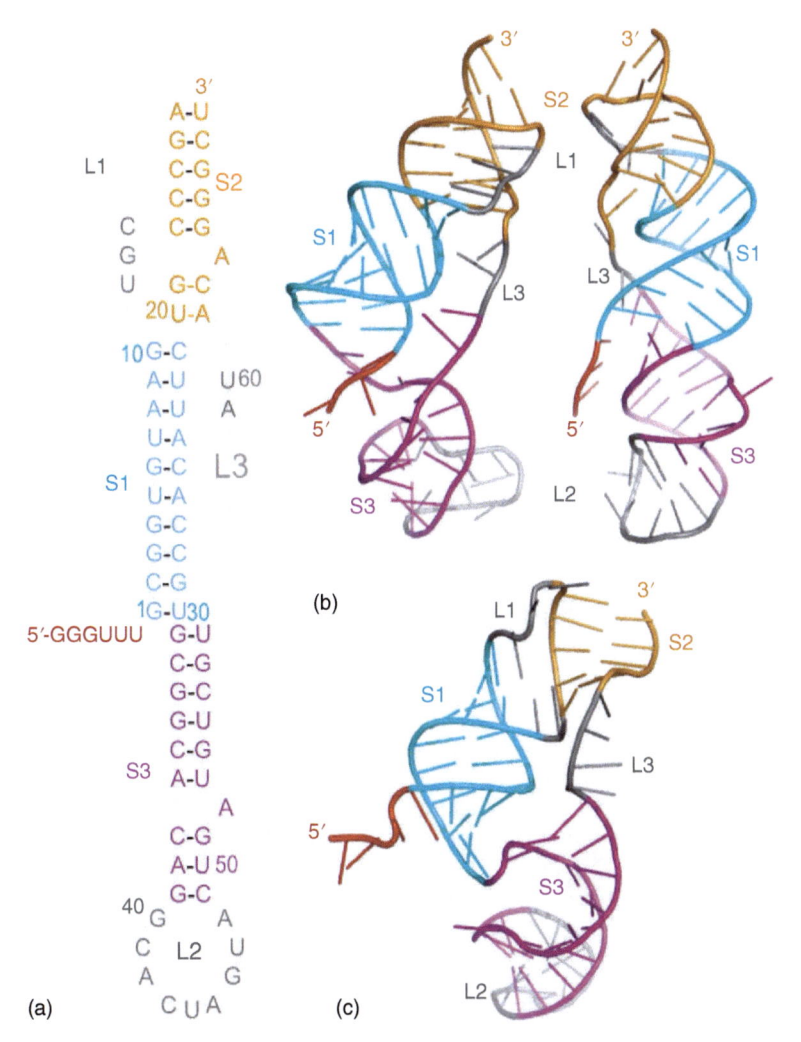

Figure 10.11 (a) SARS-CoV-2 FSE. Slippery sequence (red), stem 1 (blue), stem 2 (yellow), stem 3 (purple), loops (gray). (b) 5′ end of the FSE threaded (left) and unthreaded (right) through the middle of the structure, modeled with molecular dynamics simulations. Source: [49, 50]/PLOS, CC BY 4.0; /Springer Nature/CC-BY 4.0. (c) Cryo-EM structure from Bhatt et al. Source: Adapted from Bhatt et al. [18].

structure harbors the stop codon for orf1a within stem 1 (Figure 10.11, blue), and was generated based on molecular dynamics simulations by the Woodside lab and cryo-EM data from the Ban lab. Interestingly, the predicted structures included a conformer with the 5′ end (Figure 10.11, red) threaded through loop 3 and also a conformer with the 5′ end remaining on the exterior of the construct. It was also posited that it was likely that this element may be likely to fold into multiple conformations as the RNA undergoes multiple cycles of unfolding and refolding [49, 50].

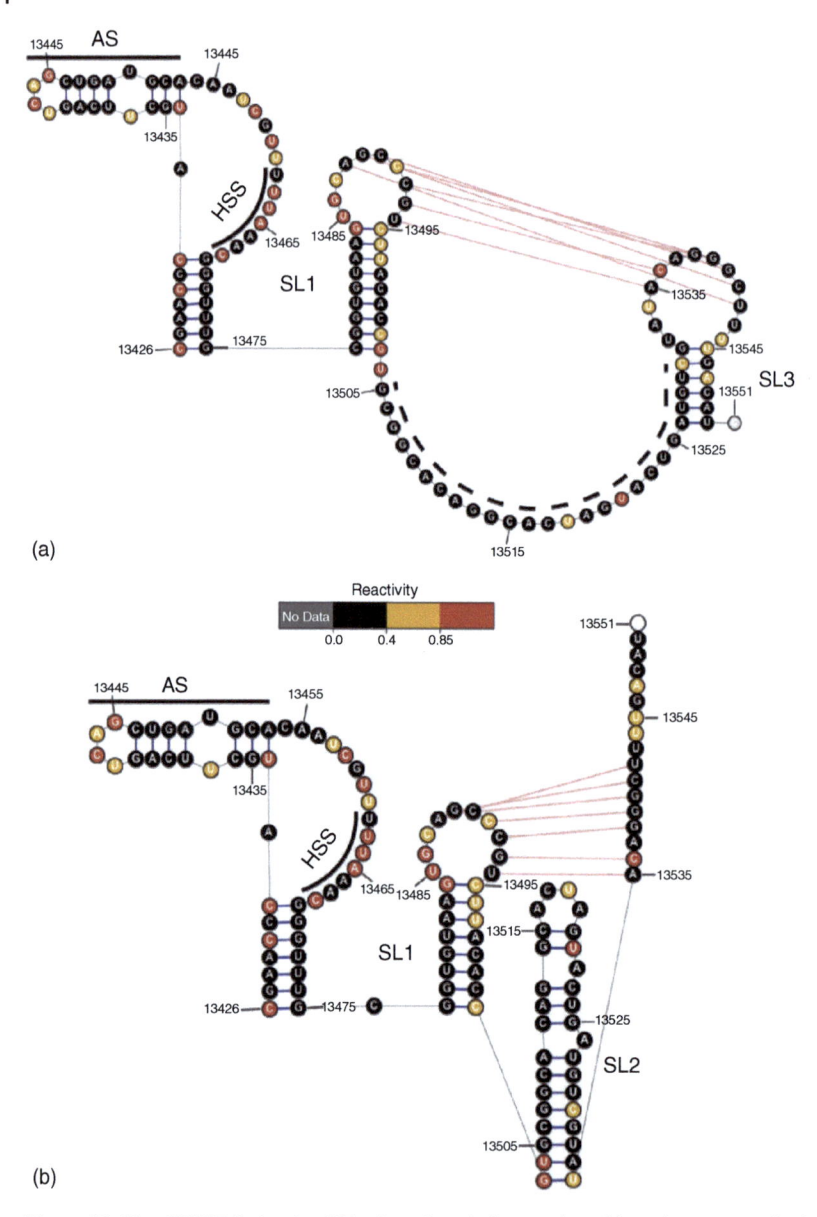

Figure 10.12 SHAPE (selective 2′ hydroxyl acylation analyzed by primer extension) data from Vero E6 cells infected with SARS-CoV-2 identified two possible conformations, (a) and (b). (a) had a higher probability of formation than (b). Source: Huston et al. [45]/with permission of Elsevier.

Later structural analyses by the Pyle lab indicated that the canonical pseudoknot could, in fact, form multiple conformations in a cellular environment [45]. While SHAPE-MaP data from multiple reads encompassing the FSE and surrounding RNA indicated that the canonical three stem-three loop H-type pseudoknot could form (Figure 10.12b), a second conformer was also likely to form that, rather than

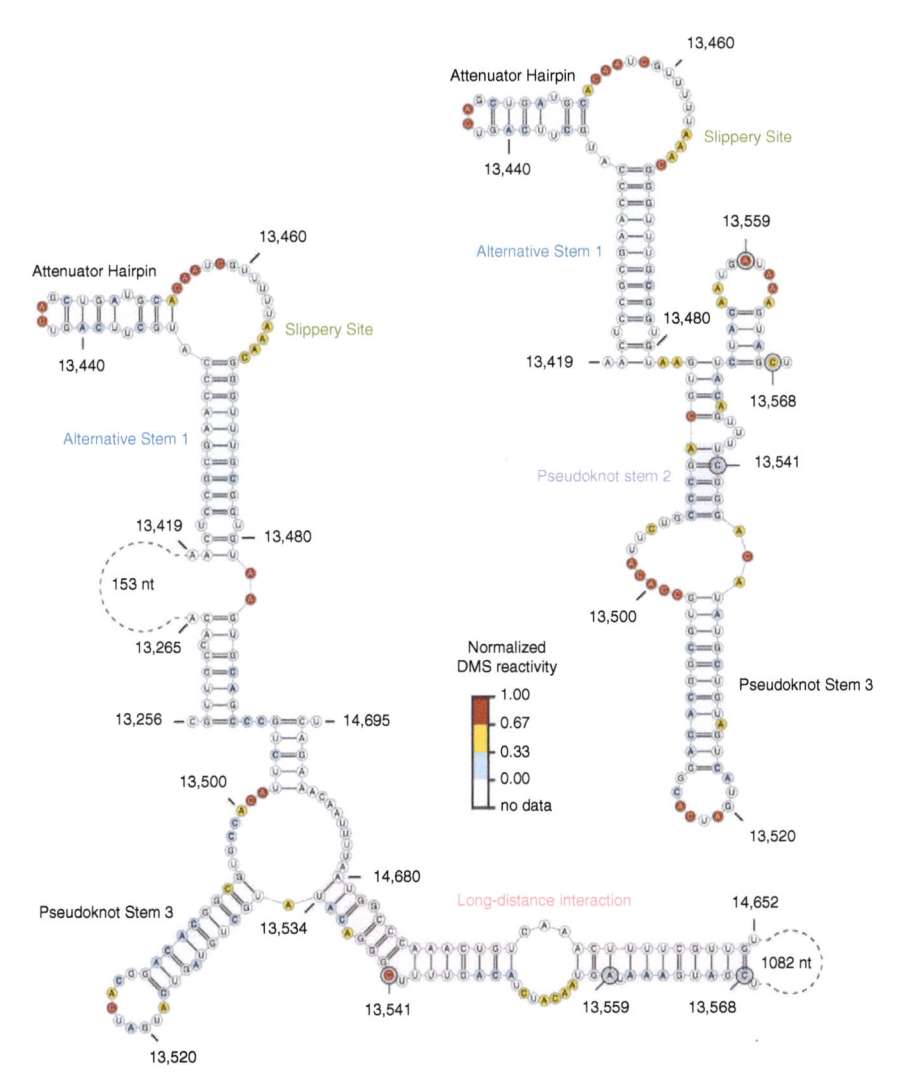

Figure 10.13 DMS reactivities of the SARS-CoV-2 FSE analyzed by full-genome RT-PCR in Huh7 cells. Abundance of each cluster: 45% (left), 55% (right). The FSE is shown with extensive interactions with upstream and downstream nucleotides. Source: Lan et al. [46]/Springer Nature/CC BY 4.0.

a tightly structured pseudoknot, formed two distinct stem loops connected by an unstructured region that was capable of interacting with other regions of RNA (Figure 10.12a). In fact, when they expanded the length of RNA studied to a 749 nucleotide surrounding the FSE, they observed that the FSE formed interactions with RNA located 260 or 470 nucleotides upstream of the FSE [45].

This finding that the SARS-CoV-2 orf1ab FSE is capable of extended interactions in a cellular environment was corroborated by the Rouskin Lab, who used DMS-MaPSeq with the DREEM clustering algorithm to show that the canonical pseudoknot, while capable for forming the 3 stem/3 loop structure in isolation, had extensive upstream and downstream interactions with other regions of the viral RNA in infected Vero and Huh7 cells (Figure 10.13) [46].

Early research on targeting the SARS-CoV-2 FSE relied on previous research on the SARS-CoV-1 FSE. The two RNA elements have nearly identical sequences, differing by only two nucleotides in the loop 3 region. In 2011, the small-molecule 2-{[4-(2-methylthiazol-4-ylmethyl)-[1,4]diazepane-1-carbonyl]amino}benzoic acid ethyl ester (MTDB (**11**), Figure 10.14) was reported as a frameshifting modulator for the SARS-CoV-1 FSE after it was identified as binding to the FSE via a virtual docking screen. Though its binding affinity was quite low ($K_d = 210 \pm 20\,\mu M$), cell-free and *in cellulo* studies confirmed that it was effective at inhibiting frameshift efficiency for SARS-CoV-1 (Figure 10.14) [53]. With the emergence of SARS-CoV-2, MTDB showed similar activity with the SARS-CoV-2 FSE (Figure 10.14)[3]; this finding along with the sequence similarity between the two viruses [44] allowed researchers to gain valuable early insights into the novel virus' frameshifting behavior and its impact on viral replication.

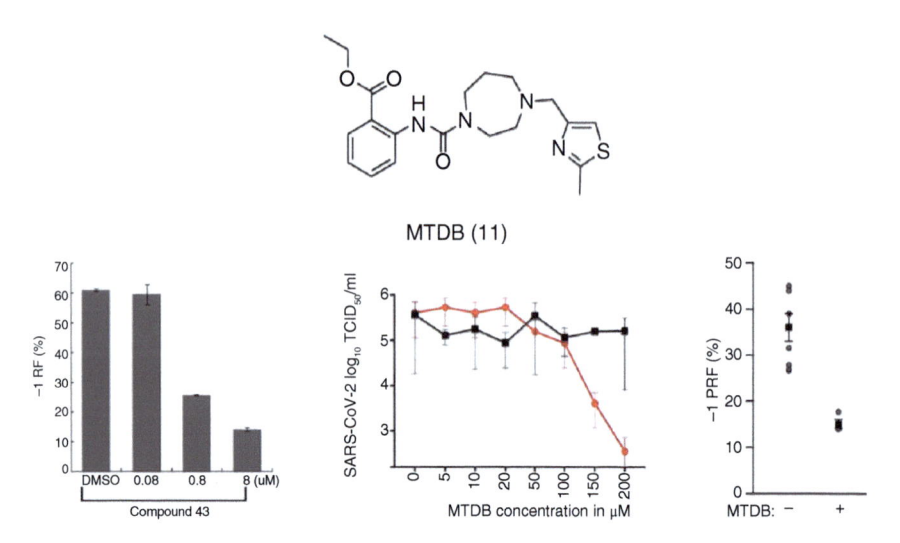

Figure 10.14 MTDB (**11**, also labeled compound 43, top). (Left) Concentration-dependent inhibition of frameshift efficiency in HEK293T cells containing the SARS-CoV-1 FSE sandwiched between an upstream renilla luciferase and a downstream firefly-renilla luciferase fusion protein in the −1 reading frame, treated with MTDB. Source: Adapted from Park et al. [51]. Though MTDB inhibits frameshifting at sub-micromolar concentrations (left) and viral infectivity at micromolar concentrations (middle). Source: [18, 52], it is unlikely that it does so by binding to the FSE, to which it binds only weakly [53]. MTDB (5 µM) also reduces frameshifting of the SARS-CoV-2 ORF1ab FSE in a dual luciferase assay in rabbit reticulocyte lysate (right). Source: Kelly et al. [44]/with permission of Elsevier.

---

3 Reprinted (adapted) with permission from Park, S.J., Kim, Y.G., Park, H.J. (2011). Identification of RNA pseudoknot-binding ligand that inhibits the −1 ribosomal frameshifting of SARS-coronavirus by structure-based virtual screening. *J. Am. Chem. Soc.* 133 (26): 10094–10100. https://doi.org/10.1021/ja1098325. Copyright 2011 American Chemical Society.

Merafloxacin (**12**) was identified as an inhibitor of SARS-CoV-2 −1 PRF via a dual reporter assay combined with a high-throughput screen of 4434 compounds from collections of FDA-approved drugs, the Pharmakon 1600 collection, and the Tested-In-Human collection [19]. Merafloxacin is a member of the fluoroquinolone class of antibacterial agents, and the only fluoroquinolone of 40 tested in the screen to have a significant impact on frameshifting [19].

Merafloxacin (**12**)[18]

Merafloxacin (**12**). Source: Borthwick [40]/with permission of American Society for Microbiology.

While the mechanism of inhibition has yet to be elucidated, shortening the distal sidechain merafloxacin and adding a terminal alcohol group partially restored frameshifting activity and viral titer, and frameshifting activity and viral titer were completely restored by replacing the pyrrolidine moiety with a piperidine moiety (Figure 10.15) [19]. These results suggest that frameshifting activity of merafloxacin is tied to the specific structure of the compound rather than the underlying fluoroquinolone backbone.

Merafloxacin does appear to specifically affect the frameshifting of betacoronaviruses, with some impact on frameshifting of alphacoronaviruses, as observed in HEK293T cells transfected with a dual reporter plasmid containing the FSE of various viruses and subsequently treated with merafloxacin [19].

Rather than target the FSE itself, the Disney Lab turned its focus to the upstream attenuator hairpin, shown to assist in regulation of frameshifting (Figure 10.16) [54]. Using an RNA-focused compound library, they identified a small molecule (C5 (**15**), Figure 10.17) capable of binding to the 1x1 UU internal loop in the attenuator

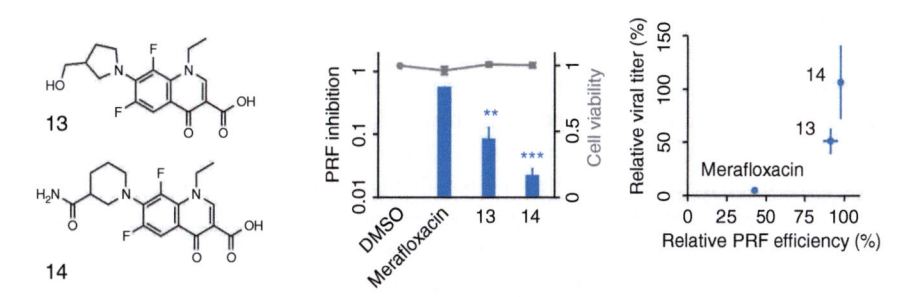

Figure 10.15 Analogs of merafloxacin partially (**13**, 20 μM) and mostly (**14**, 20 μM) restore frameshift efficiency (middle) and viral titer (right) in Vero E6 cells infected with SARS-CoV-2. Source: Sun et al. [19]/National Academy of Sciences/CC BY 4.0.

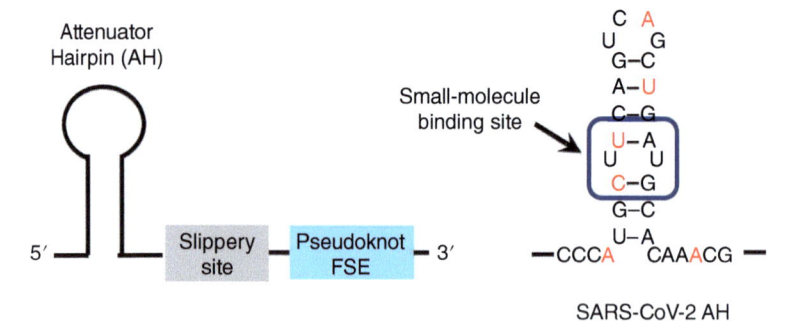

Figure 10.16 (left) Diagram of the location of the attenuator hairpin in relation to the slippery site and FSE in SARS-CoV-1 and SARS-CoV-2. (right) The SARS-CoV-2 attenuator hairpin contains a small-molecule-binding site in a 1 × 1 U-U internal loop that is not present in the SARS-CoV-1 attenuator hairpin. Differences between the SARS-CoV-1 and -2 attenuator hairpins are shown by the nucleotides in red. Source: Haniff et al. [48]/with permission of American Chemical Society.

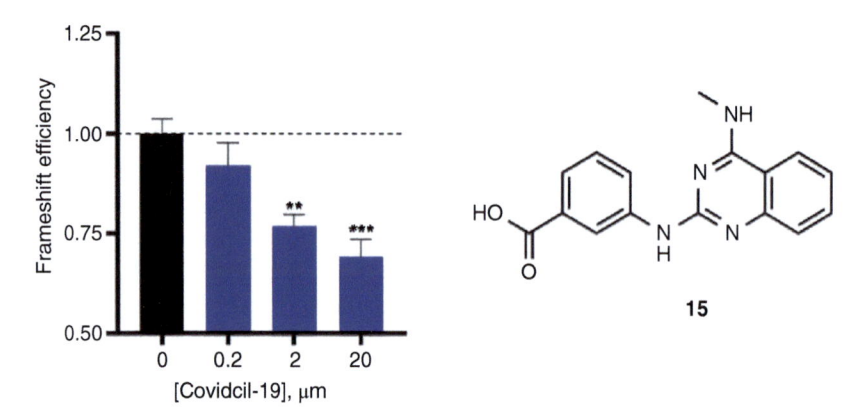

Figure 10.17 Compound C5 (Covidcil-19 (**15**), right) reduced frameshift efficiency in a concentration-dependent manner when a dual luciferase reporter plasmid containing the slippery sequence and FSE between in-frame Renilla luciferase and firefly luciferase in the −1 frame is transfected in HEK293T cells (top). At 2 μM, frameshift efficiency was reduced to roughly 50% in the presence of C5 versus vehicle alone. Source: Haniff et al. [48]/with permission of American Chemical Society.

hairpin [48], which is absent in the attenuator hairpin of SARS-CoV-1 [48, 54]. They then used Chem-CLIP (chemical cross-linking and isolation by pull-down) to selectively target and isolate the SARS-CoV-2 RNA in a cellular environment, then built onto that design with an RNA-degrading chimera—linking a RNase L-recruiter molecule to C5 to selectively target and cleave the attenuator hairpin (Figure 10.18). The effect on frameshifting was measured with a dual luciferase reporter system in HEK293T cells. Not only did C5 inhibit frameshifting by binding to the attenuator hairpin, the C5-Chem-CLIP construct allowed the SARS-CoV-2 RNA to be isolated without pulling down cellular RNA, and the C5-RIBOTAC construct recruited RNase L for the selective degradation of the entire SARS-CoV-2 RNA while having no effect on SARS-CoV-1 RNA counts [48].

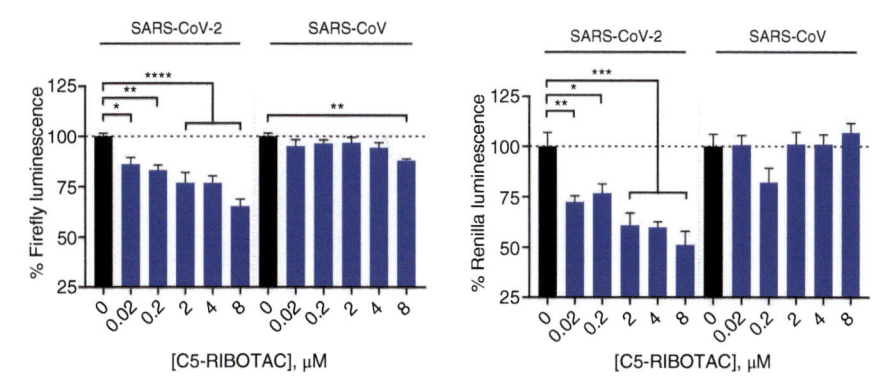

Figure 10.18 The C5-RIBOTAC (ribonuclease targeting chimera) recruits Rnase L for degradation of SARS-CoV-2 RNA in HEK293T cells. A dual luciferase reporter system shows a decrease in both Renilla (upstream of attenuator hairpin and FSE) and firefly (downstream of FSE) luciferases, as the ribonuclease does not differentiate between different sections of the reporter system when it is recruited by C5-RIBOTAC binding to the attenuator hairpin. Source: Haniff et al. [48]/with permission of American Chemical Society.

	Structure	EC_{50} (µM)
16		13.0
17		25.2
18		12.0

Geneticin (19)

Figure 10.19 Analogs (**16–18**) of geneticin (**19**) have improved antiviral activity and inhibition of frameshift efficiency over geneticin, an aminoglycoside capable of reducing frameshift efficiency. Source: Varricchio et al. [55]/with permission of Elsevier. Frameshift efficiency was measured with a dual luciferase assay in Vero E6 cells.

Nafamostat (**20**)

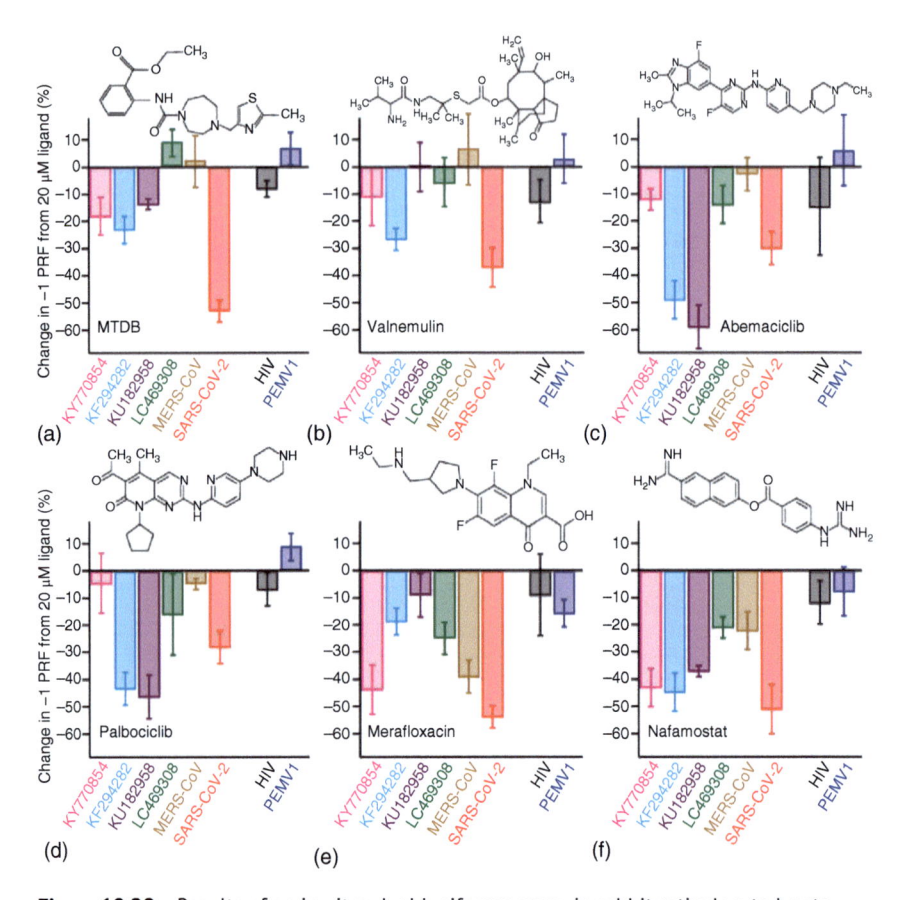

Figure 10.20 Results of an in vitro dual luciferase assay in rabbit reticulocyte lysate observing the effects of six compounds, including MTDB (a), merafloxacin (e), and nafamostat (f) on frameshift efficiency for FSEs from different coronaviruses, as well as HIV and PEMV1 as controls. Source: Munshi et al. [57]/MDPI/CC BY 4.0. Valnemulin (b) is an antibiotic approved for veterinary use, Abemaciclib (c) and Palbociclib (d) are CDK4/6 kinase inhibitors approved for breast cancer treatment. Viruses KY770854 and KF294282 are alpha coronaviruses isolated from bats, and KU182958 and LC469308 are beta coronaviruses also isolated from bats. PEMV1 is the pea enation mosaic virus, which has a 2 stem H-type pseudoknot FSE.

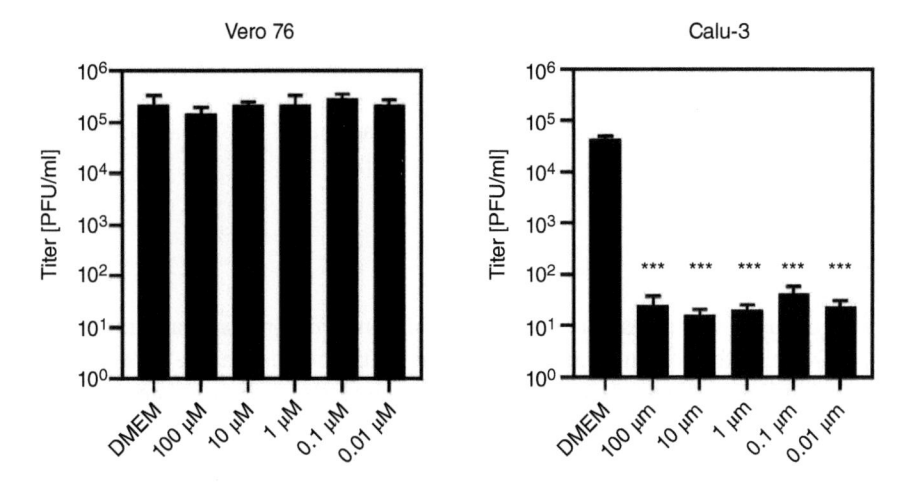

Figure 10.21 Nafamostat does not reduce viral titer at 100 µM in Vero E6 cells but does reduce viral titer at all concentrations in Calu-3 cells. Cells were treated with nafamostat for one hour, then infected with SARS-CoV-2 before being washed and treated with nafamostat again for another 24 hours. Source: Jäger et al. [58]/MDPI/CC BY 4.0.

As mentioned above, aminoglycosides are a class of compounds known to bind to RNA secondary structures. One aminoglycoside, geneticin (**19**), shows antiviral activity against multiple viruses. Geneticin is also capable of reducing frameshift efficiency for SARS-CoV-2 at high concentration (600 µM) in Vero E6 cells, as shown with a dual reporter assay [55]. Further analysis with *in silico* docking experiments with geneticin and the SARS-CoV-2 FSE suggested 3 potential docking sites on the FSE, one of which was confirmed *in vitro* by mutating the residues involved and observing a corresponding decrease in frameshift inhibition in the presence of geneticin and merafloxacin (as a control) [55]. These docking experiments were followed up by virtually screening the RNA against a library of RNA binders; the most potent of these compounds had $EC_{50} = 12\,\mu M$ and reduced frameshift efficiency in a dual luciferase assay to ~65% versus untreated Vero E6 cells (500 µM compound) (Figure 10.19) [55]. The authors of this study hypothesized that the compounds shown in the table have a similar binding mode to geneticin based on the docking studies, but further experiments are needed to support this hypothesis.

Nafamostat (**20**) was in clinical trials as a protease inhibitor for SARS-CoV-2 during the COVID-19 pandemic [56]. However, it also showed inhibition of frameshifting for a spectrum of betacoronaviruses, including SARS-CoV-2, while only slightly modulating frameshifting for two other frameshifting viruses not belonging to the coronavirus family [57]. Nafamostat was identified by Munshi et al. as an inhibitor of frameshifting through a screen of 1814 FDA-approved drugs combined with a cell-free dual reporter assay, along with valnemulin (antibiotic), palbociclib, and abemaciclib (kinase inhibitors). Out of those four, nafamostat, despite its broader effect, consistently strongly inhibited frameshifting (<40% inhibition) across most of the coronavirus strains tested (Figure 10.20) [57].

Nafamostat reduces viral titer in Calu-3 cells, which express the protease TMPRSS2, but not Vero 76 cells, which do not express TMPRSS2 (Figure 10.21) [58]. It can be inferred, therefore, that while nafamostat is a frameshifting inhibitor, its effects on viral infection in cells are likely to be a result of its protease inhibition activity rather than its frameshifting inhibition [58].

10.5 Conclusions

The RNAs used by viruses to regulate essential frameshift processes are intriguing drug targets, as they circumvent many of the potential pitfalls that are encountered in more traditional drug targets such as proteins and DNA. Efforts to date targeting these RNAs also highlight the need for greater chemical diversity in RNA-targeted compounds, especially for small-molecule binders with lower weight and higher specificity. Of the viruses discussed herein, the Miller group at Rochester has identified compounds that bind to the HIV-1 FSE RNA, building from initial identification via a Resin-Bound Dynamic Combinatorial Library (RBDCL) to afford compounds with exceptionally high affinity and selectivity. These compounds have been demonstrated to alter frameshift efficiency, and interfere with replication of HIV-1, including a multidrug-resistant patient isolate, in human cells [16]. Frameshifting of the SARS-CoV-2 orf1ab FSE has been targeted by a variety of small molecules [19, 48, 51, 55, 57]. Many of these are capable of binding to the SARS-CoV-2 orf1ab FSE and decreasing frameshift efficiency, which is disruptive to viral replication, though more work is needed in this area to develop a more robust and non-toxic small-molecule binder.

As it stands, there is a tremendous amount of potential in targeting RNA that extends beyond the work presented here for HIV-1 and SARS-CoV-2 RNA. 90% of the human genome consists of non-coding RNAs, which have important and varied roles in most aspects of gene expression, ranging from transcription, translation and serving as scaffolds for membrane-less organelles [59]. With advances in structural biology, these RNAs and others that were historically difficult to characterize will benefit from adaptation and further development of technologies that have been previously used for protein targets, including mass spectrometry screening and DNA-encoded libraries [59]. These advancements are welcome, as commonly used methods for targeting RNA rely on the use of single-stranded antisense oligonucleotides (ASO) and double-stranded small interfering RNAs (siRNA) [60]. While exciting research tools, both ASOs and siRNAs have proven challenging in clinical application. For example, siRNAs often cause allergic reactions, display poor cell permeability, and have limited ability to cross the brain–blood barrier [60]. Currently, there are precious few therapeutically relevant compounds that target RNA [60], underscoring the unmet need for a greater understanding of the chemical space of RNA binders.

References

1 Mei, H.-Y., Mack, D.P., Galan, A.A. et al. (1997). Discovery of selective, small-molecule inhibitors of RNA complexes—1. The tat protein/TAR RNA

complexes required for HIV-1 transcription. *Bioorg. Med. Chem.* 5 (6): 1173–1184. https://doi.org/10.1016/S0968-0896(97)00064-3.

2 Hendrix, M., Priestley, E.S., Joyce, G.F., and Wong, C.-H. (1997). Direct observation of aminoglycoside–RNA interactions by surface plasmon resonance. *JACS* 119 (16): 3641–3648. https://doi.org/10.1021/ja964290o.

3 Šponer, J., Bussi, G., Krepl, M. et al. (2018). RNA structural dynamics As captured by molecular simulations: a comprehensive overview. *Chem. Rev.* 118 (8): 4177–4338. https://doi.org/10.1021/acs.chemrev.7b00427.

4 Warner, K.D., Hajdin, C.E., and Weeks, K.M. (2018). Principles for targeting RNA with drug-like small molecules. *Nat. Rev. Drug Discovery* 17 (8): 547–558. https://doi.org/10.1038/nrd.2018.93.

5 Juru, A.U. and Hargrove, A.E. (2021). Frameworks for targeting RNA with small molecules. *J. Biol. Chem.* 296: https://doi.org/10.1074/jbc.REV120.015203.

6 Jacks, T. and Varmus, H.E. (1985). Expression of the rous sarcoma virus *Pol* gene by ribosomal frameshifting. *Science* 230 (4731): 1237–1242. https://doi.org/10.1126/science.2416054.

7 Jacks, T., Madhani, H., Masiarz, F., and Varmus, H.E. Signals for ribosomal frameshift in the Rous sarcoma virus gag-pol region. *Cell* https://doi.org/10.1016/0092-8674(88)90031-1.

8 Nikolić, E.I.C., King, L.M., Vidakovic, M. et al. (2012). Modulation of ribosomal frameshifting frequency and its effect on the replication of Rous sarcoma virus. *J. Virol.* 86 (21): 11581–11594. https://doi.org/10.1128/JVI.01846-12.

9 Firth, A.E., Jagger, B.W., Wise, H.M. et al. (2012). Ribosomal frameshifting used in influenza A virus expression occurs within the sequence UCC_UUU_CGU and is in the +1 direction. *Open Biol.* 2 (10): 120109. https://doi.org/10.1098/rsob.120109.

10 Bermingham, A. and Collins, P.L. (1999). The M2–2 protein of human respiratory syncytial virus is a regulatory factor involved in the balance between RNA replication and transcription. *Proc. Natl. Acad. Sci. U.S.A.* 96 (20): 11259–11264. https://doi.org/10.1073/pnas.96.20.11259.

11 Atkins, J.F., Loughran, G., Bhatt, P.R. et al. (2016). Ribosomal frameshifting and transcriptional slippage: from genetic steganography and cryptography to adventitious use. *Nucleic Acids Res.* 44 (15): 7007–7078. https://doi.org/10.1093/nar/gkw530.

12 Anokhina, V.S. and Miller, B.L. (2021). Targeting ribosomal frameshifting as an antiviral strategy: from HIV-1 to SARS-CoV-2. *Acc. Chem. Res.* 54 (17): 3349–3361. https://doi.org/10.1021/acs.accounts.1c00316.

13 Plant, E.P., Rakauskaitė, R., Taylor, D.R., and Dinman, J.D. (2010). Achieving a golden mean: mechanisms by which coronaviruses ensure synthesis of the correct stoichiometric ratios of viral proteins. *J. Virol.* 84 (9): 4330–4340. https://doi.org/10.1128/jvi.02480-09.

14 Plant, E.P., Sims, A.C., Baric, R.S. et al. (2013). Altering SARS coronavirus frameshift efficiency affects genomic and subgenomic RNA production. *Viruses* 5 (1): 279–294. https://doi.org/10.3390/v5010279.

15 Ahn, D.G., Lee, W., Choi, J.K. et al. (2011). Interference of ribosomal frameshifting by antisense peptide nucleic acids suppresses SARS coronavirus replication. *Antiviral Res.* 91 (1): 1–10. https://doi.org/10.1016/j.antiviral.2011.04.009.

16 Hilimire, T.A., Chamberlain, J.M., Anokhina, V. et al. (2017). HIV-1 frameshift RNA-targeted triazoles inhibit propagation of replication-competent and multi-drug-resistant HIV in human cells. *ACS Chem. Biol.* 12 (6): 1674–1682. https://doi.org/10.1021/acschembio.7b00052.

17 Shehu-Xhilaga, M., Crowe, S.M., and Mak, J. (2001). Maintenance of the gag/gag-pol ratio is important for human immunodeficiency virus type 1 RNA dimerization and viral infectivity. *J. Virol.* 75 (4): 1834–1841. https://doi.org/10.1128/JVI.75.4.1834-1841.2001.

18 Bhatt, P.R., Scaiola, A., Loughran, G. et al. (2021). Structural basis of ribosomal frameshifting during translation of the SARS-CoV-2 RNA genome. *Science* 372 (6548): 1306–1313. https://doi.org/10.1126/science.abf3546.

19 Sun, Y., Abriola, L., Niederer, R.O. et al. (2021). Restriction of SARS-CoV-2 replication by targeting programmed −1 ribosomal frameshifting. *Proc. Natl. Acad. Sci. U.S.A.* 118 (26): e2023051118. https://doi.org/10.1073/pnas.2023051118.

20 Bao, C., Zhu, M., Nykonchuk, I. et al. (2022). Specific length and structure rather than high thermodynamic stability enable regulatory MRNA stem-loops to pause translation. *Nat. Commun.* 13 (1): 988. https://doi.org/10.1038/s41467-022-28600-5.

21 Bao, C., Loerch, S., Ling, C. et al. (2020). MRNA stem-loops can pause the ribosome by hindering A-site TRNA binding. *eLife* 9: e55799. https://doi.org/10.7554/eLife.55799.

22 Dinman, J.D. (2012). Mechanisms and implications of programmed translational frameshifting. *WIREs RNA* 3 (5): 661–673. https://doi.org/10.1002/wrna.1126.

23 Hung, M., Patel, P., Davis, S., and Green, S.R. (1998). Importance of ribosomal frameshifting for human immunodeficiency virus type 1 particle assembly and replication. *J. Virol.* 72 (6): 4819–4824.

24 Low, J.T., Garcia-Miranda, P., Mouzakis, K.D. et al. (2014). Structure and dynamics of the HIV-1 frameshift element RNA. *Biochemistry* 53 (26): 4282–4291. https://doi.org/10.1021/bi5004926.

25 Brakier-Gingras, L., Charbonneau, J., and Butcher, S.E. (2012). Targeting frameshifting in the human immunodeficiency virus. *Expert Opin. Ther. Targets* 16 (3): 249–258. https://doi.org/10.1517/14728222.2012.665879.

26 Grentzmann, G., Ingram, J.A., Kelly, P.J. et al. (1998). A dual-luciferase reporter system for studying recoding signals. *RNA* 4 (4): 479–486.

27 Staple, D.W., Venditti, V., Niccolai, N. et al. (2008). Guanidinoneomycin B recognition of an HIV-1 RNA helix. *ChemBioChem* 9 (1): 93–102. https://doi.org/10.1002/cbic.200700251.

28 Chittapragada, M., Roberts, S., and Ham, Y.W. (2009). Aminoglycosides: molecular insights on the recognition of RNA and aminoglycoside mimics. *Perspect. Med. Chem.* 3: 21–37.

29 Blount, K.F., Zhao, F., Hermann, T., and Tor, Y. (2005). Conformational constraint as a means for understanding RNA-aminoglycoside specificity. *JACS* 127 (27): 9818–9829. https://doi.org/10.1021/ja050918w.

30 Lyon, K., Aguilera, L.U., Morisaki, T. et al. (2019). Live-cell single RNA imaging reveals bursts of translational frameshifting. *Mol. Cell* 75 (1): 172–183.e9. https://doi.org/10.1016/j.molcel.2019.05.002.

31 McNaughton, B.R. and Miller, B.L. (2006). Resin-bound dynamic combinatorial chemistry. *Org. Lett.* 8 (9): 1803–1806. https://doi.org/10.1021/ol060330+.

32 McNaughton, B.R., Gareiss, P.C., and Miller, B.L. (2007). Identification of a selective small-molecule ligand for HIV-1 frameshift-inducing stem-loop RNA from an 11,325 member resin bound dynamic combinatorial library. *JACS* 129 (37): 11306–11307. https://doi.org/10.1021/ja072114h.

33 Palde, P.B., Ofori, L.O., Gareiss, P.C. et al. (2010). Strategies for recognition of stem-loop RNA structures by synthetic ligands: application to the HIV-1 frameshift stimulatory sequence. *J. Med. Chem.* 53 (16): 6018–6027. https://doi.org/10.1021/jm100231t.

34 Copeland, R.A., Pompliano, D.L., and Meek, T.D. (2006). Drug–target residence time and its implications for lead optimization. *Nat. Rev. Drug Discovery* 5 (9): 730–739. https://doi.org/10.1038/nrd2082.

35 Swinney, D.C. (2004). Biochemical mechanisms of drug action: what does it take for success? *Nat. Rev. Drug Discovery* 3 (9): 801–808. https://doi.org/10.1038/nrd1500.

36 Hilimire, T.A., Bennett, R.P., Stewart, R.A. et al. (2016). *N*-Methylation as a strategy for enhancing the affinity and selectivity of RNA-binding peptides: application to the HIV-1 frameshift-stimulating RNA. *ACS Chem. Biol.* 11 (1): 88–94. https://doi.org/10.1021/acschembio.5b00682.

37 Chatterjee, J., Rechenmacher, F., and Kessler, H. (2013). *N*-Methylation of peptides and proteins: an important element for modulating biological functions. *Angew. Chem. Int. Ed.* 52 (1): 254–269. https://doi.org/10.1002/anie.201205674.

38 Arévalo, D.M., Anokhina, V.S., Swart, O.L.R., and Miller, B.L. (2022). Expanding the known structure space for RNA binding: a test of 2,5-diketopiperazine. *Org. Biomol. Chem.* 20 (3): 606–612. https://doi.org/10.1039/D1OB01976G.

39 DeSimone, R.W., Currie, K.S., Mitchell, S.A. et al. (2004). Privileged structures: applications in drug discovery. *Comb. Chem. High Throughput Screening* 7 (5): 473–494. https://doi.org/10.2174/1386207043328544.

40 Borthwick, A.D. (2012). 2,5-Diketopiperazines: synthesis, reactions, medicinal chemistry, and bioactive natural products. *Chem. Rev.* https://pubs.acs.org/doi/full/10.1021/cr200398y.

41 Giessen, T.W. and Marahiel, M.A. (2015). Rational and combinatorial tailoring of bioactive cyclic dipeptides. *Front. Microbiol.* 6: 785. https://doi.org/10.3389/fmicb.2015.00785.

42 Malone, B., Urakova, N., Snijder, E.J., and Campbell, E.A. (2022). Structures and functions of coronavirus replication–transcription complexes and their relevance for SARS-CoV-2 drug design. *Nat. Rev. Mol. Cell Biol.* 23 (1): 21–39. https://doi.org/10.1038/s41580-021-00432-z.

43 Plant, E.P., Pérez-Alvarado, G.C., Jacobs, J.L. et al. (2005). A three-stemmed MRNA pseudoknot in the SARS coronavirus frameshift signal. *PLoS Biol.* 3 (6): 1012–1023. https://doi.org/10.1371/journal.pbio.0030172.

44 Kelly, J.A., Olson, A.N., Neupane, K. et al. (2020). Structural and functional conservation of the programmed −1 ribosomal frameshift signal of SARS coronavirus 2 (SARS-CoV-2). *J. Biol. Chem.* 295 (31): 10741–10748. https://doi.org/10.1074/jbc.AC120.013449.

45 Huston, N.C., Wan, H., Strine, M.S. et al. (2021). Comprehensive in vivo secondary structure of the SARS-CoV-2 genome reveals novel regulatory motifs and mechanisms. *Mol. Cell* 81 (3): 584–598.e5. https://doi.org/10.1016/j.molcel.2020.12.041.

46 Lan, T.C.T., Allan, M.F., Malsick, L.E. et al. (2022). Secondary structural ensembles of the SARS-CoV-2 RNA genome in infected cells. *Nat. Commun.* 13 (1): 1128. https://doi.org/10.1038/s41467-022-28603-2.

47 Ishimaru, D., Plant, E.P., Sims, A.C. et al. (2013). RNA dimerization plays a role in ribosomal frameshifting of the SARS coronavirus. *Nucleic Acids Res.* 41 (4): 2594–2608. https://doi.org/10.1093/nar/gks1361.

48 Haniff, H.S., Tong, Y., Liu, X. et al. (2020). Targeting the SARS-CoV-2 RNA genome with small molecule binders and ribonuclease targeting chimera (RIBOTAC) degraders. *ACS Cent. Sci.* 6 (10): 1713–1721. https://doi.org/10.1021/acscentsci.0c00984.

49 Omar, S.I., Zhao, M., Sekar, R.V. et al. (2021). Modeling the structure of the frameshift-stimulatory pseudoknot in SARS-CoV-2 reveals multiple possible conformers. *PLoS Comput. Biol.* 17 (1): https://doi.org/10.1371/journal.pcbi.1008603.

50 Neupane, K., Zhao, M., Lyons, A. et al. (2021). Structural dynamics of single SARS-CoV-2 pseudoknot molecules reveal topologically distinct conformers. *Nat. Commun.* 12 (1): 4749. https://doi.org/10.1038/s41467-021-25085-6.

51 Park, S.J., Kim, Y.G., and Park, H.J. (2011). Identification of RNA pseudoknot-binding ligand that inhibits the −1 ribosomal frameshifting of SARS-coronavirus by structure-based virtual screening. *JACS* 133 (26): 10094–10100. https://doi.org/10.1021/ja1098325.

52 Bhatt, P.R., Scaiola, A., Loughran, G. et al. Structural basis of ribosomal frameshifting during translation of the SARS-CoV-2 RNA genome. *Science* 372: *bioRxiv* 2020, 2020.10.26.355099.

53 Ritchie, D.B., Soong, J., Sikkema, W.K.A., and Woodside, M.T. (2014). Anti-frameshifting ligand reduces the conformational plasticity of the SARS virus pseudoknot. *JACS* 136 (6): 2196–2199. https://doi.org/10.1021/ja410344b.

54 Cho, C.-P., Lin, S.-C., Chou, M.-Y. et al. (2013). Regulation of programmed ribosomal frameshifting by co-translational refolding RNA hairpins. *PLoS One* 8 (4): e62283. https://doi.org/10.1371/journal.pone.0062283.

55 Varricchio, C., Mathez, G., Pillonel, T. et al. (2022). Geneticin shows selective antiviral activity against SARS-CoV-2 by interfering with programmed −1 ribosomal frameshifting. *Antiviral Res.* 208: 105452. https://doi.org/10.1016/j.antiviral.2022.105452.

56 Zhuravel, S.V., Khmelnitskiy, O.K., Burlaka, O.O. et al. (2021). Nafamostat in hospitalized patients with moderate to severe COVID-19 pneumonia: a randomised phase II clinical trial. *eClinicalMedicine* 41: 101169. https://doi.org/10.1016/j.eclinm.2021.101169.

57 Munshi, S., Neupane, K., Ileperuma, S.M. et al. (2022). Identifying inhibitors of −1 programmed ribosomal frameshifting in a broad spectrum of coronaviruses. *Viruses* 14 (2): 177. https://doi.org/10.3390/v14020177.

58 Jäger, N., Hoffmann, M., Pöhlmann, S., and Krüger, N. (2022). Nafamostat-mediated inhibition of SARS-CoV-2 ribosomal frameshifting is insufficient to impair viral replication in vero cells. comment on Munshi et al. identifying inhibitors of −1 programmed ribosomal frameshifting in a broad spectrum of coronaviruses. *Viruses* 2022, 14, 177. *Viruses* 14 (7): 1526. https://doi.org/10.3390/v14071526.

59 Garner, A.L. (2023). Contemporary progress and opportunities in RNA-targeted drug discovery. *ACS Med. Chem. Lett.* 14 (3): 251–259. https://doi.org/10.1021/acsmedchemlett.3c00020.

60 Shao, Y. and Zhang, Q.C. (2020). Targeting RNA Structures in diseases with small molecules. *Essays Biochem.* 64 (6): 955–966. https://doi.org/10.1042/EBC20200011.

11

RNA–Protein Interactions: A New Approach for Drugging RNA Biology

Dalia M. Soueid and Amanda L. Garner

Department of Medicinal Chemistry, College of Pharmacy, University of Michigan, Ann Arbor, Michigan 48109, USA

One of the many mechanisms by which RNAs are regulated in the cell is through interactions with RNA-binding proteins (RBPs). Indeed, the extent to which the cell utilizes RBP-mediated RNA regulation is astonishing. RBPs have classically been defined by the presence of one or more RNA-binding domain (RBD), which are capable of recognizing specific sequences and/or structural motifs on an RNA [1–6]. Preliminary analyses using sequence alignment of known RBPs and computational prediction to map various RBDs across organisms led to the uncovering of ~500 RBPs in mice and ~700 in humans [7–9]. With the advent of large-scale sequencing technologies, these lists continue to grow. It is now estimated that there are over 2000 RBPs in humans, many of which do not contain canonical RBDs, redefining our perception of RBPs and their roles in regulating cellular RNA biology [10]. These discoveries were catalyzed by an explosion in the development of new methods, providing novel insights into the regulation of RNA biology, including RNA-centric and protein-centric approaches which enable mapping RNA–protein interactions (RPIs) across the transcriptome [11, 12]. As numerous RBP-recognition motifs can exist within a single RNA molecule, RNAs are often invariably bound and regulated by multiple RBPs, resulting in the formation of complex and dynamic ribonucleoprotein complexes (RNPs). These complexes play fundamental roles in controlling nearly all aspects of gene expression from splicing to translation, modulating RNAs throughout their entire lifecycle from birth (i.e. transcription) to death (i.e. degradation) [13]. Accordingly, dysregulation of the networking between RNAs and RBPs has been shown to lead to a number of human diseases, including neurodegenerative disorders and cancers. This connection between RBP biology and disease, in turn, has catalyzed an interest in drugging RPIs. Herein, we will discuss the molecular basis for RPIs and highlight the significance of RPIs including several well-validated examples in which dysregulation of these interactions could be the basis for disease. We will then summarize experimental methods developed to detect these interactions with the purpose of promoting drug discovery efforts.

RNA as a Drug Target: The Next Frontier for Medicinal Chemistry, First Edition.
Edited by John Schneekloth and Martin Pettersson.

11.1 Molecular Basis of RNA–Protein Interactions

RBPs have traditionally been defined by the presence of one or more canonical RBDs [1], such as RNA recognition motifs (RRMs) [14], double-stranded RBDs [15], zinc fingers [16], and K homology domains among others [17]. While RBPs often contain multiple copies of the same type of RBD, they can also contain a combination of distinct RBDs that direct their binding to diverse RNA motifs. RBDs are typically <100 amino acids, and only a small portion of the domain is responsible for interacting with an RNA [18]. As such, the binding footprint for an RBD on an RNA is only 6–8 nucleotides in length [19]. RBPs gain specificity by binding to multiple RNA motifs within a single substrate. Intrinsically disordered regions and linkers are also characteristic of many RBPs, which enable these proteins to engage in multivalent binding to an RNA [20]. Other levels of RBP regulation include posttranslational modifications and protein–protein interactions (PPIs) [21, 22]. The combination of all these elements in the protein, in addition to abundance, localization, and RNA-binding site arrangement within the secondary structure of an RNA substrate, contributes to the specificity observed for select RPIs. Later, we will highlight key RBDs and discuss their modes of molecular recognition of an RNA. A summary of examples of RBPs that utilize these domains, as well as their biological functions, can be found in Table 11.1.

11.1.1 RNA Recognition Motifs (RRMs)

RRMs, also referred to as RNP domains, are not only the most abundant protein domains found in RBPs but they are also one of the most abundant protein domains found in eukaryotes [41, 42]. RRM-containing proteins play a functional role in a majority of posttranscriptional gene regulation including mRNA and rRNA processing, RNA nuclear export, and RNA stability [13]. In addition to interacting with RNAs, RRMs also interact with DNA and facilitate PPIs [14]. This commonly occurring protein domain consists of roughly 90 amino acids with two conserved central sequences termed RNP1 (8 bases) and RNP2 (6 bases), which are responsible for RNA binding [43]. These conserved sequences contain primarily aromatic and positively charged amino acids and are defined by the following sequences: **RNP1** – [RK]-G-[*FY]-[GA]-[*FY]-[ILV]-X-[FY] and **RNP2** – [ILV]-[*FY]-[ILV]-X-N-L, where "X" is any amino acid and "*" denotes the aromatic residue which interacts directly with RNA [44, 45].

While RRMs have been shown to bind to virtually all single-stranded RNA sequences *in vitro* [14], structural studies have demonstrated how different RRMs achieve binding specificity for unique RNA sequences. Despite having similar folds, each RRM-containing RBP or individual RRMs within a protein containing multiple RRMs, exhibit varied specificities and binding affinities for certain RNA sequences [46, 47]. The typical fold of an RRM consists of four β-sheets packed against two α-helices in the arrangement $\beta_1\alpha_1\beta_2\beta_3\alpha_2\beta_4$ (Figure 11.1) [41]. The β_1 and β_3 strands make up the primary RNA binding surface, driven primarily by three aromatic residues in RNP1 and RNP2 where two of the residues stack with

Table 11.1 Representative examples of RBPs and RBP families harboring various RBDs and their broad cellular functions.

RBDs	RBPs/Families	Main function
RRM	Musashi	Regulate mRNA translation in neural development and maintenance of adult neural stem cells [23]
	hnRNPs	Broadly involved in nucleic acid metabolism: splicing, mRNA stabilization, transcriptional/translational regulation [24]
	SR Proteins (contain RG domains)	Splice site recognition and major players in recruitment and stabilization of components of the core spliceosome [25]
	Hu Antigen Proteins	HuB, HuC, and HuD function in neuronal differentiation and plasticity; HuR mostly functions in cellular stress response [26]
dsRBD	Staufen	Mainly important for RNA localization, also play conserved roles in early differentiation of neurons and plasticity of mature neurons [27]
	Dicer	Riboendonuclease that functions as a critical regulator of the biogenesis of small RNAs, including microRNAs, small interfering RNAs, and small nucleolar RNAs [28, 29]
	TARBP	Various roles in innate immune response and cellular stress response; integral part of the RNA-induced silencing complex with Dicer and Argonaute proteins [30]
ZnF	Mbnl	Important regulators of tissue-specific alternative splicing that have a key role in terminal muscle differentiation; transcript-dependent activators or repressors of splicing [31]
	TTP	Regulates translation (via degradation or repression) of proinflammatory cytokines by binding to mRNA [32]
	Roquin & Regnase	Important roles in the prevention of inflammatory and autoimmune diseases through inducing degradation/translational repression of target mRNAs relevant to T cell differentiation [33]

(Continued)

Table 11.1 (Continued)

RBDs	RBPs/Families	Main function
KH	STAR	Signal transducer and activator of RNA which binds to mRNA targets and regulates processes such as cell cycle and tissue development [34]
	FUBP	Broad functions in RNA processing including mRNA splicing, stability, export, and translation and also exhibit transcriptional control through binding to ssDNA sequences [35]
	Vigilin	Evolutionarily conserved family of proteins containing tandem KH domains, which perform numerous cellular functions including mRNA stabilization, translational regulation, stress granule component, tRNA shuttling, P-body regulation, and heterochromatin regulation [36]
	NusA, NusB, NusE, NusG	Regulate different phases of initiation, elongation, and termination of bacterial transcription through interactions with bacterial RNA polymerase and RNA [37]
CSD	Lin28	Protein, which is expressed at different developmental stages of various tissues and organs, plays important functions as a cell division activator and inhibitor of differentiation, and interacts with both pre-miRNAs and mRNAs [38]
YTH	YTHDF & YTHDC family	Function as essential readers of m^6A modifications, playing important regulatory roles in almost all stages of methylated RNA metabolism and are involved in the development and progression of many tumors [39]
PUF	Pumilio and FBF (PUF) Family	Highly conserved eukaryotic RBPs which interact with regulatory elements in the 3′ UTR of mRNA targets to promote RNA decay and translational repression and also promote ribosome stalling, recruitment of miRNAs, and chromosomal instability [40]

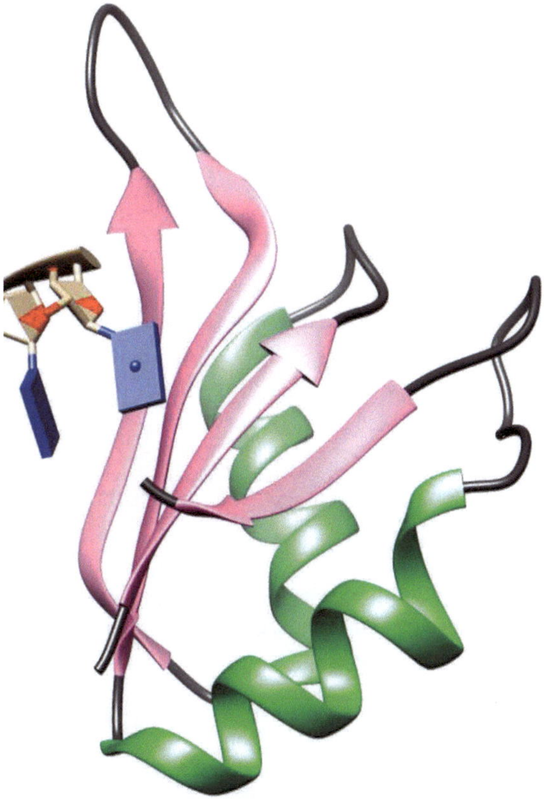

Figure 11.1 HuD RRM interacting with c-fos RNA. Pink: β-sheet, green: α-helix, gray: loop, and tan: RNA (PDB: 1FXL).

the bases of the nucleotides and a third aromatic residue is often inserted between two sugar rings of the dinucleotide (Figure 11.2) [41]. This β-sheet surface of the RRM shows intrinsic preference for a particular RNA sequence. Structures of RRMs bound to various RNAs have revealed a more complex mode of binding involving interactions in the protein loops (as little as 1 or as many as 3) connecting the β-sheets and α-helices. The loops primarily on the bottom end of the RRM structure (loops 1, 3, and 5) have been shown to engage in RNA interactions in many proteins (Figure 11.3), although exceptions have also been reported (e.g. NELF E) [48–50]. Interestingly, some loops have been shown to recognize a certain shape in an RNA as opposed to sequence by binding to the phosphodiester backbone of the major groove [48]. In some cases, when an aromatic residue is missing from the RNP consensus sequence, interactions which utilize the loop portions become the predominant mode of binding [51]. This loop-mediated binding mode was hypothesized to have evolved later to expand the RNA recognition landscape of RRMs [14]. As such, RRMs are often considered "plastic," owing to their ability to bind to a wide range of RNA targets, driven by their many modes of binding and flexible linker regions separating the domains, leading to their wide range of functional activities [41].

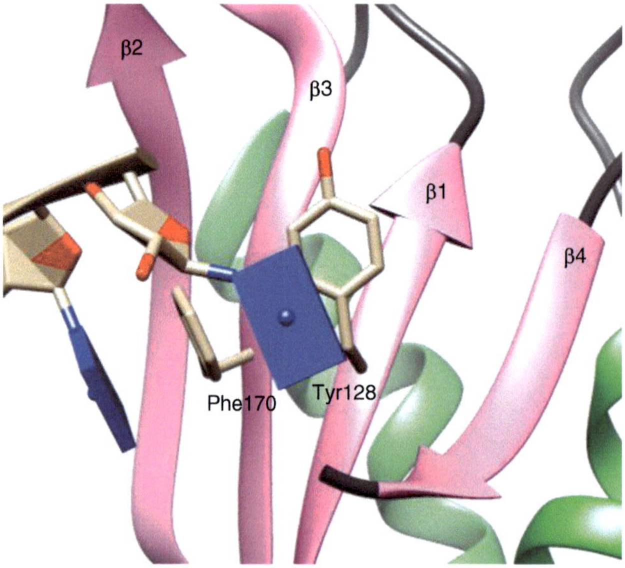

Figure 11.2 HuD RRM β1 and β3 aromatic residue stacking interaction with dinucleotide. Pink: β-sheet, green: α-helix, gray: loop, and tan: RNA (PDB: 1FXL).

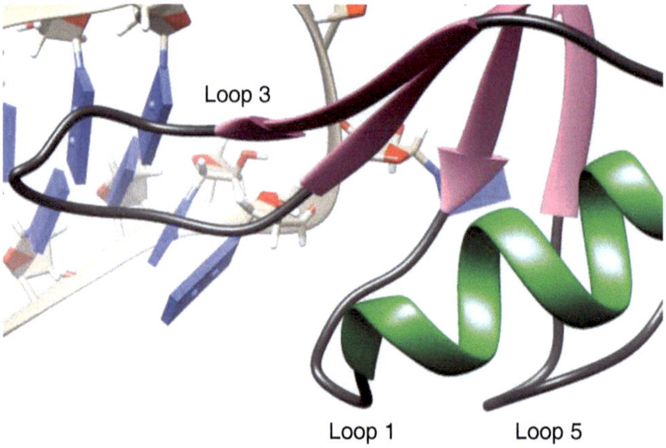

Figure 11.3 RRM-containing RBMY loop interaction with hairpin RNA. Pink: β-sheet, green: α-helix, gray: loop, and tan: RNA. (PDB: 2FY1).

11.1.2 Double-Stranded RNA-Binding Domains (dsRBD)

Double-stranded RNA-binding domains (dsRBD), which are the second most abundant RBD, represent a small protein domain (70 amino acids) that interacts with double-stranded regions of RNA and contain a conserved $\alpha_1\beta_1\beta_2\beta_3\alpha_2$ topology (Figure 11.4) [18]. Unlike other RBDs, dsRBDs typically recognize RNA secondary structure rather than sequence [52]. dsRBDs primarily recognize A-form helices of RNA, but can also bind to RNA hairpin structures [53, 54]. These proteins interact with the RNA in both the minor and major grooves using three distinct regions

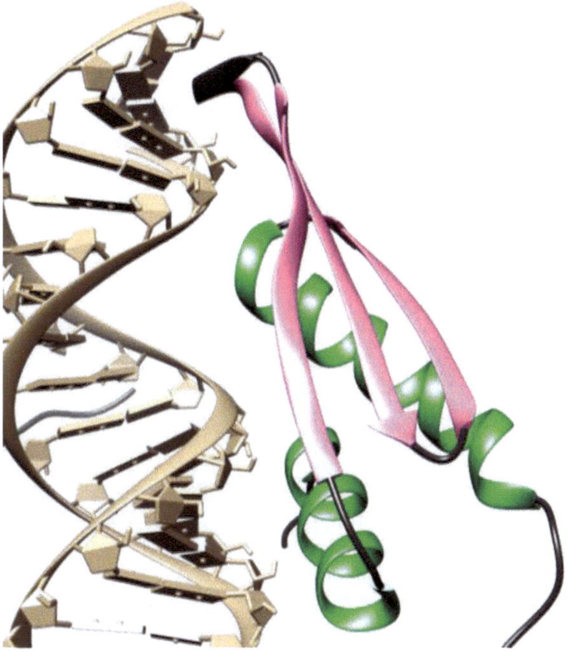

Figure 11.4 Stau1 dsRBD in complex with dsRNA. Interaction through 2 minor grooves and 1 major groove. Pink: β-sheet, green: α-helix, gray: loop, and tan: RNA. (PDB: 6HTU).

from the protein to interact with three distinct regions on the RNA (Figure 11.4) [54, 55]. Like many RBDs, dsRBDs are often found in multiple copies in an RBP. A widespread auxiliary function of these domains is their role in regulating nucleocytoplasmic transport of an RNA; however, they also function in RNA interference, RNA processing, RNP and RNA localization, as well as RNA editing and translational control [15, 56, 57].

11.1.3 Zinc Finger (ZnF) Domains

Zinc finger (ZnF) domains, more commonly thought of as DNA-binding transcription factors, also are involved in many RNA-binding events [16]. ZnFs can be found alone in an RBP as tandem repeats or in combination with other RBDs [18]. These domains are among the smallest of RBDs at 30 amino acids in length displaying a conserved $\beta_1\beta_2\alpha_1$ fold held together through coordination of a Zn^{2+} ion (Figure 11.5) [18]. There are many types of ZnFs including CCHH, CCCH, and CCCC, where C represents cysteine and H is histidine, describing the amino acids in the ZnF domain which coordinate to the Zn^{2+} ion [18]. CCHH is the most common domain capable of binding both DNA and RNA [58, 59]. Further evidence of RNA binding by ZnFs came from structures of CCCH, CCHC, and CCCC ZnFs solved in complex with single-stranded RNAs [31, 60–62]. ZnF recognition of an RNA sequence is based on the type of ZnF domain present. For example, CCCH ZnF proteins typically bind to AU-rich elements (AREs) located in the 3′ untranslated region (3′ UTR) of mRNAs [63]. The primary mode of interaction between the protein and RNA is mediated through hydrogen bonding of the protein backbone atoms with Watson–Crick edges of the bases (Figure 11.5) [61]. This binding mode, however, is not standard for all ZnF domains. A unique binding mechanism is observed, for example, with MBNL1 whose crystal structure demonstrated that it binds to 5′ GCU 3′ sequences with its ZnF3 and ZnF4 domains [31]. In addition to hydrogen bonding interactions with the protein backbone, this RPI is mediated by stacking interactions and hydrogen bonds involving main chain atoms of the protein (Figure 11.6). Much of the structural data available for ZnF domains has provided insights into the possible functions of these

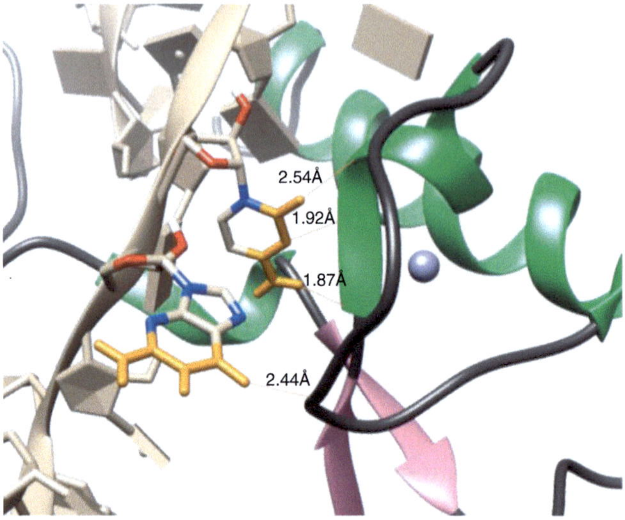

Figure 11.5 Mbnl1 ZnF 1 and 2 in complex with cardiac troponin T mRNA. Pink: β-sheet, green: α-helix, orange: Watson–Crick edges of base and hydrogen bonds (with distance) gray: loop, and tan: RNA. (PDB: 5U9B).

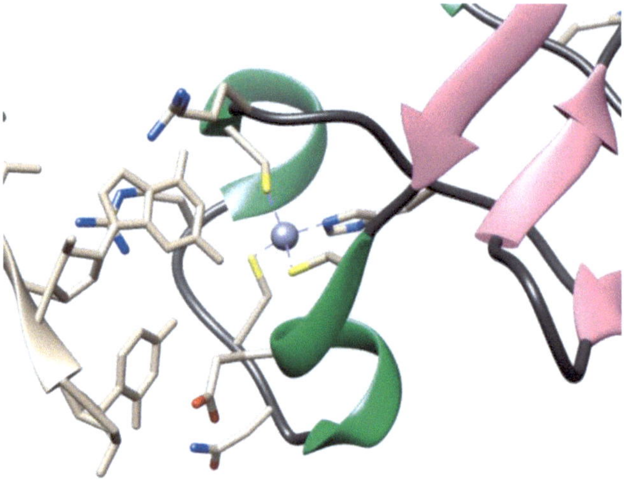

Figure 11.6 Mbnl1 ZnF 4 stacking with RNA. Pink: β-sheet, green: α-helix, gray: loop, and tan: RNA. (PDB: 3D2S).

protein as alternative splicing regulators [31, 64]. However, due to the wide variety of interactions possible through ZnF domains binding, more structural information is needed to fully understand their diverse binding modes, and ultimately the specific function(s) of these small RBDs [18].

11.1.4 K Homology (KH) Domains

K Homology (KH) domains are ~70 amino acids in length and separated into two categories: type I in eukaryotes and type II in prokaryotes, each of which exhibits different folds. The topology of the type I KH domain is described as $\beta_1\alpha_1\alpha_2\beta_2\beta_3\alpha_3$, while the reverse is true of the type II fold that contains an $\alpha_1\beta_1\beta_2\alpha_2\alpha_3\beta_3$ topology (Figure 11.7a) [17, 65]. The binding surface of a KH domain forms a small crevice through the α1 and α2 helices on one side and the β1 sheet on the other. This

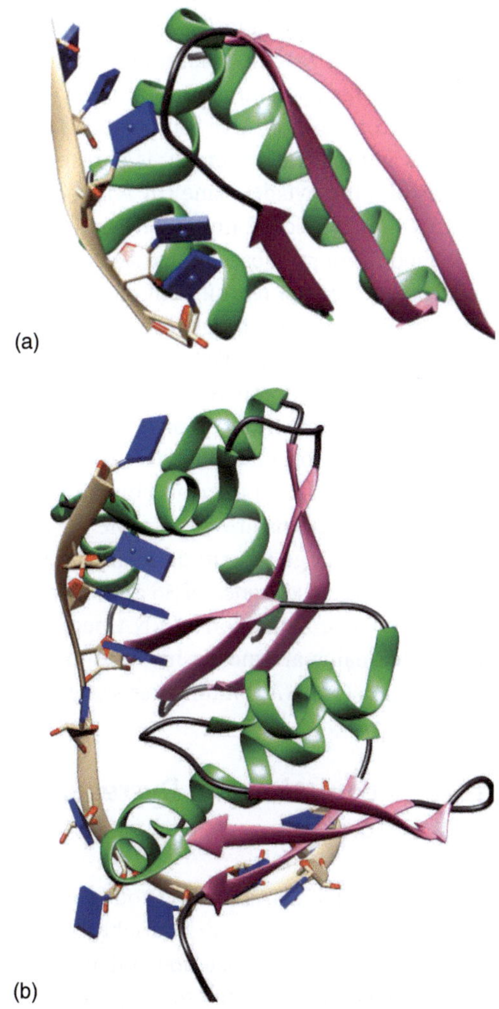

Figure 11.7 (a) Poly(c) binding protein KH interaction with 4 nucleotide region of RNA. (PDB: 2PY9) (b) NusA tandem KH interacting with 11 nucleotide region of RNA. Pink: β-sheet, green: α-helix, grey: loop, and tan: RNA. (PDB: 2ATW).

small pocket cannot accommodate a large structure; thus, RNA recognition by a KH domain is accomplished through only four residues [17]. Nonetheless, KH domains can still interact with many different combinations of four nucleobases (Figure 11.7a) [18]. Binding to a particular four-base sequence on its own yields relatively low micromolar affinity; however [18], when multiple KH domains are present, as seen with the other RBDs, there is a cooperative effect resulting in higher binding affinities. Using NusA as an example, this protein contains two KH domains separated by a short linker allowing for numerous contacts between the domains and forms a larger plane of interaction on the RNA resulting in nanomolar binding affinity (Figure 11.7b) [66].

11.1.5 Other RBDs

The other RBDs include cold shock domains (CSD), YT521-B homology domains (YTH), RGG/RG domains, DEAD/DEAH box helicase domains, Pumilio (PUF) domains, Piwi/Argonaute/Zwille (PAZ) domains, and Sm domains. CSDs are comprised of ~70 amino acids and, similar to RRMs, contains an RNP1 and RNP2 motif [67]. This domain, more commonly found in eukaryotes, contains a β-barrel structure composed of five antiparallel β-sheets [67]. The YTH domain, roughly 100–150 amino acids in length, is part of a family of proteins, which function as readers of 6-methyladenosine (m^6A) modifications, which are the most common internal modification found on RNAs [68]. Binding of YTH-containing RBPs to m^6A modifications subsequently results in either a decrease in RNA stability and degradation through recruitment of the CCR4-NOT complex [69] or regulation of translation efficiency through interactions with the translation initiation machinery and the ribosome [70]. RGG/RG motifs are defined by sequences rich in arginine residues, which are positively charged and capable of mediating hydrogen bonding and amino-aromatic interactions [71]. This motif is found in more than 1000 proteins and has important functions in transcription, splicing, DNA damage signaling, and mRNA translation through binding to RNA and DNA [72–77]. DEAD/DEAH box helicase domains are responsible for unwinding DNA and dsRNA [78]. PUF domains are a large protein domain consisting of eight α-helices, which repeat a highly conserved sequence of 36 amino acids [79, 80]. Some functions of the PUF proteins include regulation of RNA decay and translational repression [81]. PAZ and Sm domains are mostly involved in microRNA (miRNA) binding and small nuclear RNA (snRNA) binding, respectively [10].

11.2 Regulation and Dysregulation of RNA–Protein Interactions

RBP regulation of RNAs is carried out at every step in the lifecycle of an RNA, and as highlighted above, RNAs are invariably bound by both specific and nonspecific RBPs from transcription to translation as depicted in Figure 11.8 [82]. As a model type of RNA by which to exemplify the impact of RBPs on an RNA's lifespan, we will use

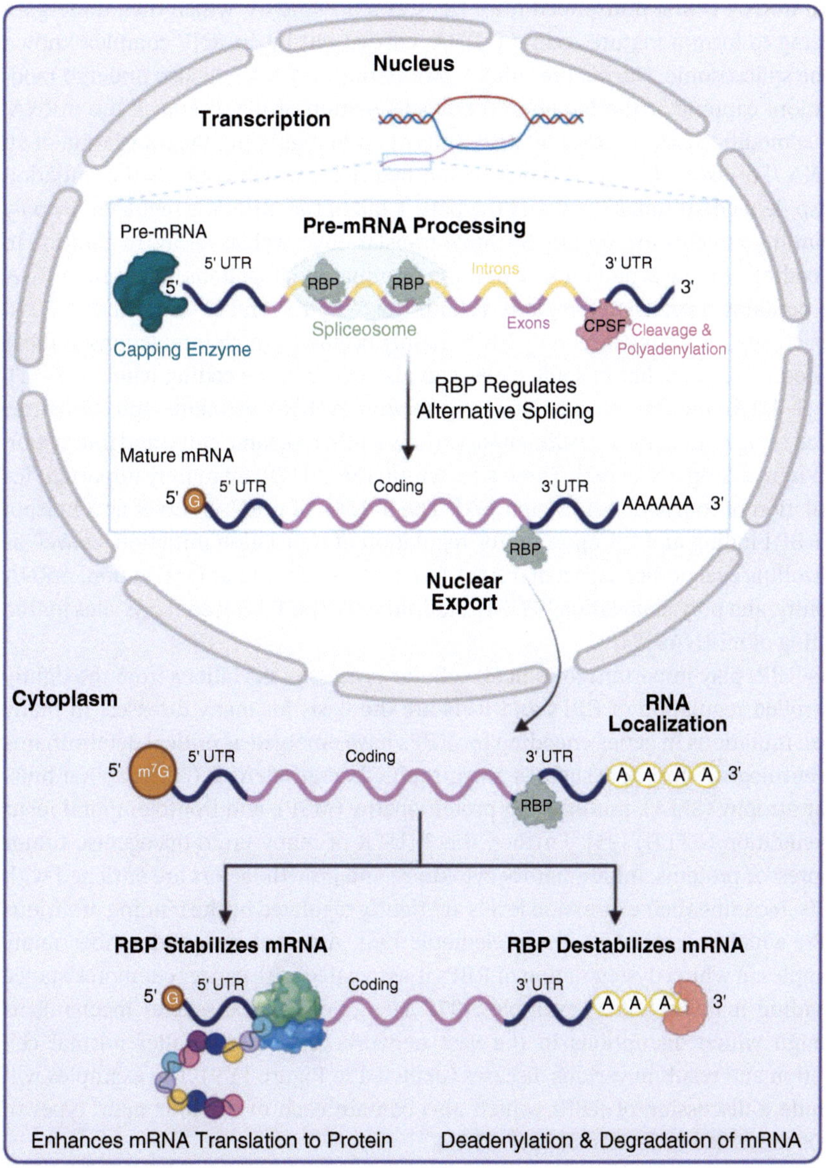

Figure 11.8 Representation of cellular functions of RBPs acting on mRNA targets from transcription through pre-mRNA processing to translation. Figure created in BioRender.

mRNAs, which not only contain the code or "message" to make a protein but also contain sites which provide information for regulation of its nuclear export, subcellular localization, translation, and stability by RBPs [13, 82]. We encourage readers to consults previous reviews to learn more about RBP regulation of non-coding RNAs [83–85], as well as RNA-modifying enzymes [86, 87].

An mRNA is first transcribed from DNA as a pre-mRNA, which then undergoes splicing to form a mature coding mRNA, carried out by an RNP complex known as the spliceosome. During pre-mRNA processing, an RNA will also undergo modification: capping at the 5′ end and polyadenylation of the 3′ end of the mRNA. These modifications are read by RBPs important in regulating the translation of an mRNA. For example, the 5′ cap is bound by eIF4E, which controls the initiation of cap-dependent translation, and the poly A tail of the mRNA is regulated by poly A binding proteins to similarly facilitate translation as well as decay. In addition to the coding sequence, and outside of these terminal modifications, a mature mRNA also contains untranslated regions at both the 5′ and 3′ end (5′ UTR and 3′ UTR, respectively). RNA regulation by RBPs mainly occurs through interactions at these noncoding regions, but in some cases, can also occur in the coding region [88–91]. The 5′ UTR contains various *cis*-acting regulatory RNA elements and structures which serve roles in the recruitment of various RBPs, ribosome entry, and interaction with non-coding RNAs [92]. These sites within the 5′ UTR are mainly important for regulation of translation initiation [93]. The 3′ UTR of mRNAs serves as a hotspot for RBP binding and is important for regulation of translation initiation, as well as controlling every other aspect of mRNA fate such as subcellular localization, mRNA stability, and polyadenylation [93, 94]. Additionally, the 3′ UTR contains sites for the binding of miRNAs [94].

As RBPs play important roles in all cellular processes, deviations from the tightly controlled regulation of RBPs and RPIs are the basis for many diseases. In many cases, mutations in genes encoding for RBPs have emerged as critical determinants of neurological disorders such as amyotrophic lateral sclerosis (ALS), spinal muscular atrophy (SMA), multisystem proteinopathy (MSP), and frontotemporal lobar degeneration (FTLD) [95]. Further, the 3′ UTR of many proto-oncogenes, tumor suppressor proteins, inflammatory cytokines, and growth factors are enriched with AREs, meaning their expression levels are tightly regulated by the binding of various RBPs, which interact with those elements [96]. A recent review describes many examples in which dysregulation of RBPs is associated with cancer chemoresistance providing many excellent examples [97]. Here we describe several mechanisms through which disruptions in the vast network of RPIs may alter normal cell function and result in various diseases (depicted in Figure 11.9). The examples will include a discussion of RBPs, which also contain each of the four main types of RBDs presented in Sections 11.1.1–11.1.4.

11.2.1 Poor Quality Control Leads to Over- and Underproduction of RBPs

Aberrant expression of RBPs causing upregulation or downregulation of an individual protein contributes to disease onset. This is the case for the RRM-containing proteins heterogenous ribonucleoprotein A/B (hnRNP A/B) and Musashi 1/2 (Msi1/2). Depleted levels of the alternative splicing regulators hnRNP A/B, suppressed directly by impaired cholinergic signaling, cause key disease hallmarks in Alzheimer's disease [98]. At the same time, hnRNP A1 overexpression has also been

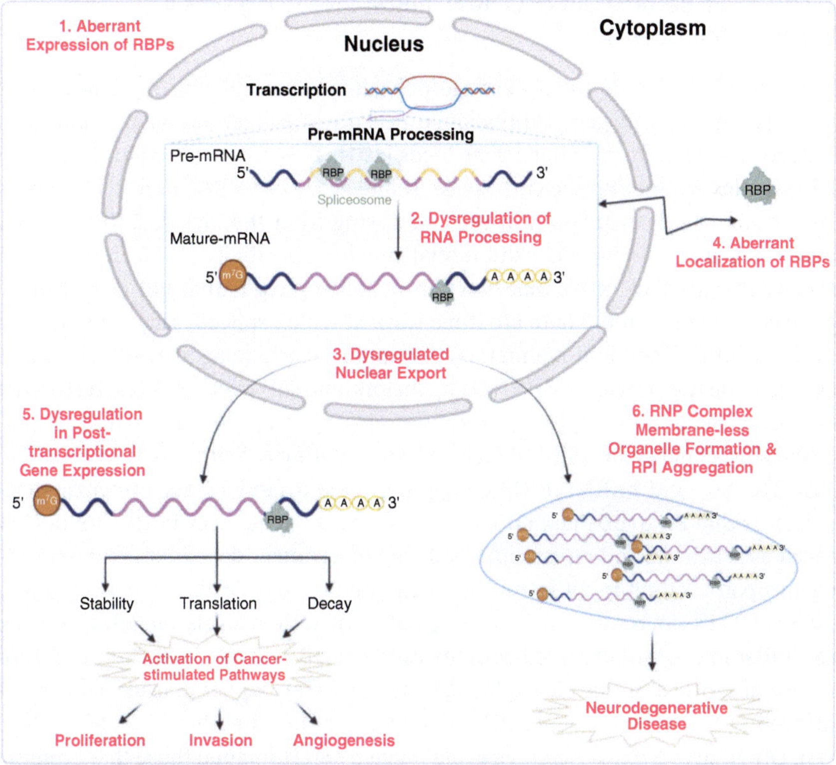

Figure 11.9 Representation of several ways in which RBPs and RPIs can be dysregulated in cells contributing to two main disease areas: cancer and neurodegeneration. Figure created in BioRender.

linked to induced alternative splicing of the amyloid precursor protein mRNA and reduced Aβ levels, further suggesting that hnRNP A/B reduction could contribute to Alzheimer's Disease onset [99]. Msi1/2 overexpression, on the other hand, is found to contribute to almost all hematological malignancies and is correlative with poor clinical prognosis in these malignancies [100]. Msi1/2 play distinct roles in the development and maintenance of neural cells with high levels of transcripts present in the brain during postnatal development, low expression persisting into adulthood, and a resurgence of expression in various malignancies [101]. This family of proteins contains tandem RRM domains and bind the sequence motif 5′ UAGUAG 3′ in the 3′ UTR of target RNAs [102]. Msi1/2 have emerged as biomarkers and therapeutic targets. One interaction with which Msi1/2 are hypothesized to contribute to disease pathogenesis is by binding to and repressing the translation of the *Numb1* mRNA, resulting in increased NOTCH1 signaling in cancer and leukemia patients [23]. This mRNA encodes for the Numb1 protein, which is involved in controlling cell fate decisions in the central and peripheral nervous system through inhibition of NOTCH1 [103].

11.2.2 RBPs Become Out of Control, mRNA Processing Gets a Makeover (and Hates It)

In addition to 5′ capping and 3′ cleavage/polyadenylation, splicing of pre-mRNAs is a vital step in dictating gene expression, especially in eukaryotes where many proteins are produced from a single gene locus [104]. This process is controlled by an RNP complex containing the core spliceosome, accessory RBPs, and RNA. This is a major point of dysregulation in the cell arising from the fact that RBP–mRNA interactions are transient and exhibit relatively low specificity [105]. Here we will focus on the auxiliary RBPs that function in splicing regulation but do not make up the core spliceosome. There are three ways in which spliceopathy is induced in cells in an RBP-dependent manner: (i) disruption of a splicing element, (ii) mutations affecting the activity of RBP splicing factors, and (iii) toxic RNA (example to be discussed in Section 11.2.3) [105]. Disruptions in a splicing element refer to a mutation causing a change in splice site recognition affecting recognition by *trans*-acting RBPs. The SR- and hnRNP RRM-containing protein families are principle splicing factors that bind auxiliary enhancer and silencer sequences in the pre-mRNA and act as activators and repressors of splicing in a context-dependent manner contingent upon binding to an intron or an exon [106, 107]. Mutations affecting the activity of RBPs can result in up/downregulation of protein levels and affect splicing in a similar manner as observed with the hnRNP A/B example in Section 11.2.1. In the case of serine arginine-rich splicing factor 1 (Srsf1), depletion leads to aberrant expression of its primary target BIN1, leading to reduced ability to repress c-Myc [108]. Other targets whose splicing is regulated by Srsf1 include those that promote proto-oncogenic transformation [109]. Major splicing regulators are essential to normal cellular function due to the significance of the mRNAs they produce, as well as the fact that many of these regulators are responsible for the alternative splicing of hundreds of transcripts, demonstrating the multitude of processes affected by a single RBP [110–112]. Further information about the effects of splicing dysregulation in cancer can be found in a recent review [113].

11.2.3 RBP Shuttling of mRNA Becomes Askew

Mature mRNAs are immediately exported from the nucleus to the cytoplasm after processing is complete. Many proteins are involved in making sure RNAs are exported properly from the nucleus to the cytoplasm and further to the site of translation including the nuclear pore complex and other RBPs. This is a vital step in the regulation of gene expression in which aberrantly transcribed or processed mRNAs are not shuttled from the nucleus, as well as the fact that this step is highly controlled by extracellular signaling and stress responses [114]. At the same time, however, nuclear retention of RNA may also contribute to dysregulation and is the basis for several diseases [115]. One of the most well-characterized examples of this is the mutation causing the multisystemic disorder, myotonic dystrophy (DM1), and other repeat disorders [116, 117]. DM1 is caused by a CTG expanded repeat in the *Dystrophia Myotonica Protein Kinase* (*DMPK*) gene resulting in mutant mRNA transcripts harboring a $(CUG)_n$ (n = fifty to a few thousand) expanded repeat in the 3′ UTR [118–122]. In normal cells, DMPK mRNA is transcribed, transported to nuclear speckles, and then exported from the nucleus. The $(CUG)_{exp}$ repeats prevent its entry into nuclear speckles, and instead causes the RNA to accumulate in separate and distinct nuclear foci, and in the process, sequester the ZnF-containing RBP Muscleblind-like protein 1 (Mbnl1) to those foci. Subsequently, Mbnl1 is prohibited from carrying out its role as an essential regulator of alternative splicing, resulting in many mis-spliced RNAs in DM1. The $(CUG)_{exp}$ nuclear foci are suggested to be the source of pathology in DM1 with an increased number of repeats correlative with disease severity due to enhanced ability to accumulate and recruit more Mbnl1 proteins [123]. This is also a case to exemplify a disease in which the driver of the disease is a toxic gain of function in the RNA, which causes an RBPs' functions to lead to symptoms rather than the RBP being the main pathological driver.

11.2.4 The RBP is Lost and Wreaks Havoc on the Cell

As mentioned in Section 11.1, localization of an RBP plays a large role in dictating which RNAs it may interact with where mis-localization of the RBP will cause adverse effects through binding to off-target RNAs. Various mutations in RRM-containing protein TDP-43 promote mislocalization to subcellular locations in the cytoplasm, while others can cause retention in the nucleus [110, 124, 125]. Previous reports have shown that mutant forms of TDP-43 increased mislocalization to the mitochondria, thereby leading to the repression of the expression of mitochondrial RNAs [126]. Similarly, the KH domain-containing RBP Src associated in mitosis of 68 kDa (Sam68) undergoes various posttranslational modifications, which greatly influence its biochemical properties, fine tuning its subcellular localization, and ability to interact with signaling proteins and target RNAs. Sam68, an almost exclusively nuclear protein containing a nuclear localization signal, is localized to the cytoplasm in some cells and plays a role in translational regulation of target mRNAs [127, 128]. However, various cancer types show that higher Sam68 expression in the cytoplasm contributes to tumor progression and metastasis [129]. Upregulation and increased cytoplasmic localization of Sam68 significantly correlate with pathological grade in patients with renal cell carcinoma [130], tumor-nodule metastasis and other outcomes in breast cancer patients [131], and lymph node metastasis in patients with early-stage cervical cancer [131].

11.2.5 RBPs Dictate Which mRNAs are Translated, Favoring their Toxic Friends

One of the most direct impacts RBPs have on regulating gene expression is through interacting with transcripts in the cytoplasm, where they influence stability and translational efficiency of target RNAs. The dsRBD-containing RBP Staufen1 (Stau1) is a multifunctional protein that regulates all aspects of RNA metabolism; here, we will discuss its role in translation and decay and its contribution to cancer [132]. Stau1 binds to the 5′ UTR of target RNAs, simultaneously with the ribosome, and transports an mRNA to the site of translation in the rough endoplasmic reticulum to promote protein synthesis [133]. Staul can also bind to regulatory motifs in the 3′ UTR of transcripts to promote mRNA stabilization, enhancing translation [134]. In undifferentiated C2C12 myoblasts, for example, Staul directly binds to and stabilizes the 3′ UTR of Dvl2 mRNA, promoting cell proliferation. During myogenesis, Staul levels become reduced, and along with it the half-life of Dvl2 mRNA, prompting the induction of myogenic differentiation [135]. Staul can also bind to double-stranded regions downstream of the stop codon in the 3′ UTR of transcripts, and through direct interaction with the ATP-dependent helicase UPF1 to enhance its activity, promote Staul-mediated decay [136]. Through these various functions, Staul can support cellular proliferation, tumor growth, and metastasis in cancer through stabilization of transcripts promoting those functions such as SIRT1 mRNA [137]. Staul-mediated decay may also contribute to increased growth of cancer cells through targeting proteins, which act as transcription and tumor suppressors such as ZNF331 [138]. Alternatively, Staul has the capacity to be able to inhibit cancer growth by promoting the decay of transcription factors such as RAX2 [139]. Like the previous examples highlighted, the role of Staul in disease progression is context dependent, stressing the importance of maintaining proper regulation of the broader network of interactions between RNA and RBPs.

11.2.6 RBPs and RNA Become Very Clique-y, Form Their Own Complex and Cause Stress to the Rest of the Cell

The RBP fused in sarcoma (FUS), containing both an RRM and ZnF, is highly mutated in ALS patients, where mutations largely occur in prion-like domains of the protein priming it for aggregation [140]. Furthermore, previous studies have found that while nuclear FUS does not incorporate into stress granules, mutant FUS can bind and sequester nuclear localized FUS to cytoplasmic stress granules [141]. More broadly, many RBPs display a propensity to assemble in membrane-less compartments through the process of liquid–liquid phase separation (LLPS) [142]. These compartments, composed primarily of RBPs and RNAs, are dynamic and reversible and allow for the exchange of macromolecules with their surrounding environment [143]. LLPS particles are often held together by the accumulation of multiple weak interactions between RNAs and RBPs [143–145]. These interactions generally engage the low complexity intrinsically disordered regions that are characteristic of many RBPs. Various RNP complexes, such as the nucleolus, stress granules, P-bodies, paraspeckles, Cajal bodies, and others, are proposed to form following the principles of phase separation [146–149]. In the case of some disease states, LLPS condensates can transition to more viscous states with reduced fluidity and even further to more dense pathological aggregates [150, 151]. This is the case for many degenerative brain diseases which are characterized by plaque-like aggregates composed of RBPs. Additionally, many disease-associated RBPs contain disordered prion-like domains, facilitating PPIs and accelerating liquid to solid-phase transitions.

11.3 Experimental Methods to Detect and Screen for Small Molecules that Modulate RNA–Protein Interactions

Due to the increasing evidence of RPI dysregulation in diseases, targeting RBPs and RPIs has surfaced as a new subject in RNA-targeted drug discovery [152]. The last two decades have uncovered many networks of RPIs and resulted in the application of existing methods and development of new technologies for detecting and validating RPIs *in vitro* and *in cellulo*. Here, we will highlight methods that can be used to detect and validate RPIs, as well as discover small-molecule modulators of RPIs. Examples of hits identified using these approaches will also be discussed and can be found in Table 11.2.

11.3.1 *In vitro* Fluorescence-Based Assays

Fluorescence-based assays, including fluorescence polarization (FP)- and fluorescence resonance energy transfer (FRET)-based methods (Figure 11.10), provide quantitative measures of an RPI resulting in an ability to measure accurate binding affinities and determine IC_{50} values for inhibitors. SPR and ITC are also powerful tools for the quantitative characterization of RPIs [153–157]; however, these techniques require specialized instrumentation and are not considered high-throughput for inhibitor discovery. FP utilizes a fluorophore-labeled biomolecule, in this case a fluorescently labeled RNA probe, which tumbles in solution at a rate dependent upon the size of the molecule [157–162]. An RPI is detectable when there are changes in polarization caused by protein binding to the fluorescently labeled RNA, slowing the rotation and emitting an FP signal. FRET, on the other hand, utilizes donor and acceptor fluorophore pairs where excitation of the donor fluorophore results in the transfer of energy to the acceptor fluorophore when in close proximity [163–165]. In the case of an RPI, the donor and acceptor fluorophores are conjugated to the RNA and protein. Both FP and FRET are compatible with high-throughput small-molecule screening and accordingly have been used to identify inhibitors of RPIs. Select examples of RBP-binding compounds discovered using these approaches include multiple inhibitors of Lin28 [164, 166] binding to pre-let-7 substrates and disrupters of the binding of Msi1/2 [167] and eIF4E [168] to RNAs comprising consensus binding sequences (Table 11.2).

11.3.2 *In vitro* Chemiluminescence-Based Assays

Although robust and high-throughput, fluorescence-based assays are prone to compound interference by autofluorescent molecules or compounds that can function as fluorescence quenchers [169]. To overcome these limitations, chemiluminescence-based detection assays for RPIs have been developed, including catalytic enzyme-linked click chemistry assay (cat-ELCCA) and split enzyme assay (SEA) technology (Figure 11.11) [170, 171]. Both of these methods are plate

Table 11.2 Select examples of RBP-binding compounds discovered using assays mentioned in Sections 11.3.1–11.3.2.

Compound	Structure	Target	Activity	Assay
PH-43	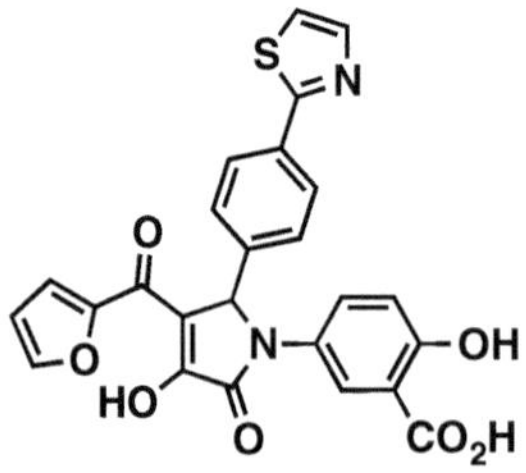	Lin28	IC_{50} : 5 μM K_d : 16 μM	FP
Ro 08-2750	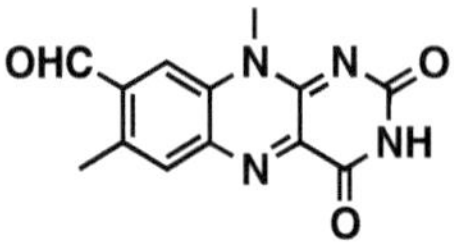	Msi2	IC_{50} : 2.7 μM K_d : 11 μM	FP
eFFECTOR 634	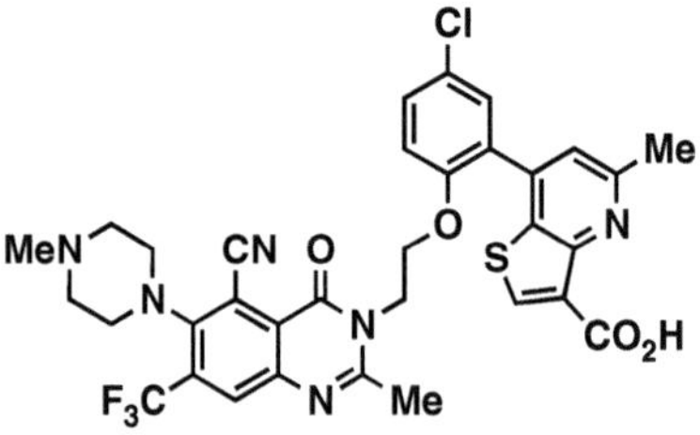	eIF4E	5.6 μM	FP
compound 1	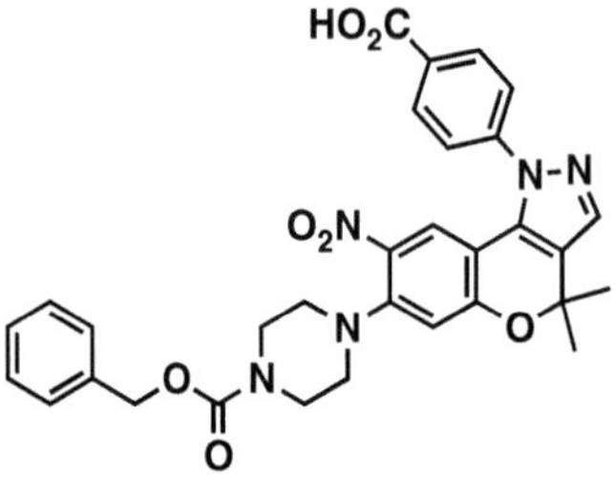	Lin28	IC_{50} : 4 μM K_d : 3.5 μM	FRET
CCG-233094	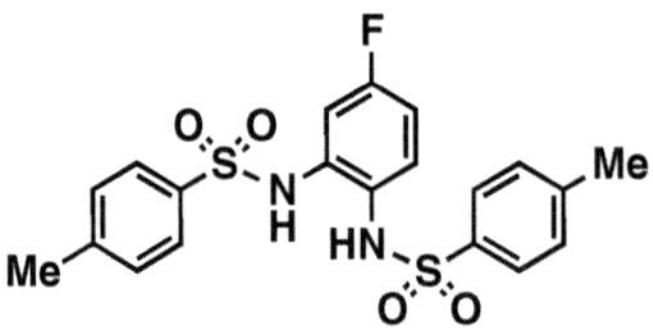	Lin28	IC_{50} : 8.3 μM K_d : 300 nM	cat-ELCCA

based, amenable for high-throughput screening, and rely on click chemistry-based detection strategies.

Cat-ELCCA has been applied to multiple biochemical systems, including monitoring the enzymatic activities of ghrelin *O*-acyltransferase (GOAT) [172] and Dicer [173–175], and biomolecular interactions including RPIs (e.g. Lin28-pre-let-7 interaction [176]) and PPIs (e.g. eIF4E-4E-BP1 PPI [177]). For RPIs, a biotinylated-RBP

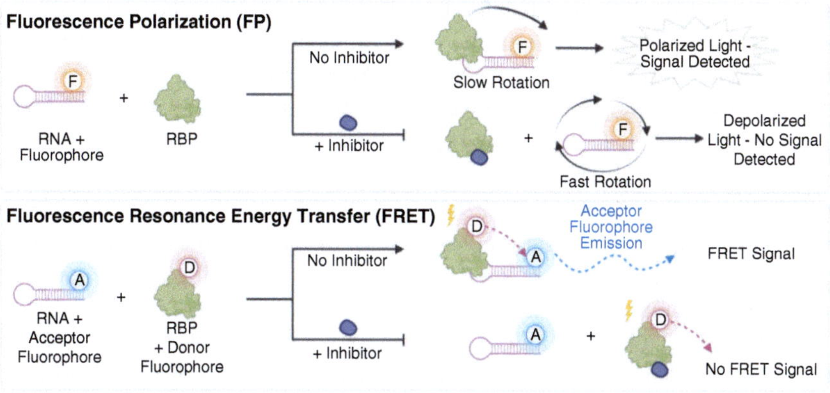

Figure 11.10 Schematic representation of fluorescence polarization and fluorescence resonance energy transfer assays to detect RPIs and their inhibition. Figure created in BioRender.

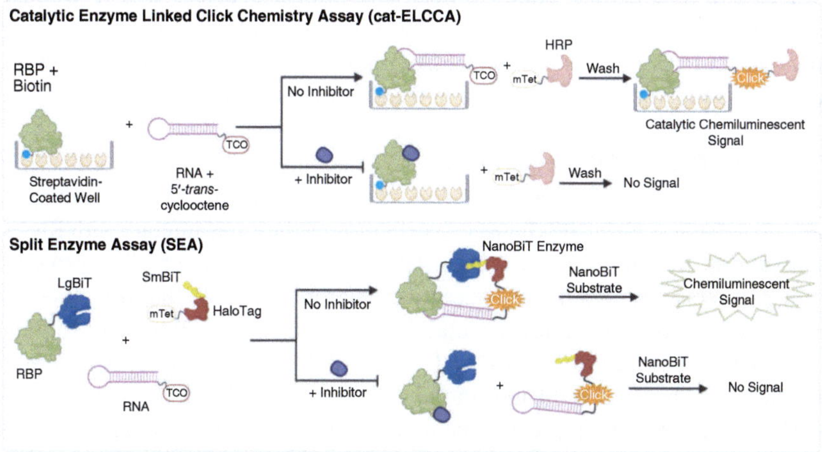

Figure 11.11 Schematic representation of catalytic enzyme linked click chemistry assay and split enzyme assay to detect RPIs and their inhibition. Figure created in BioRender.

is immobilized onto a streptavidin-coated well plate and treated with an RNA substrate harboring a *trans*-cyclooctene (TCO) click chemistry handle. Signal is generated in this assay when the TCO-labeled RNA becomes covalently conjugated to a methyltetrazine (mTet)-functionalized horseradish peroxidase (HRP) via inverse-electron demand Diels–Alder-based click chemistry. Chemiluminescence results after the addition of an HRP substrate. Key advantages of cat-ELCCA are enhanced sensitivity due to catalytic signal amplification and minimal compound interference compared to fluorescence-based detection assays. Using this strategy, a high-throughput screen was conducted against the pre-let-7-Lin28 RPI resulting in the discovery of a novel Lin28 inhibitory scaffold (Table 11.2) [176]. There are, however, a couple of limitations to this approach including the use of costly streptavidin-coated plates needed for protein immobilization and the multiple washing steps required throughout the assay protocol. This ultimately led to the development of a second click chemistry-based biorthogonal assay.

SEA is a protein complementation-based assay that utilizes a split luciferase that is able to produce catalytic signal amplification following interaction between a target RNA and RBP [171]. The split NanoLuc Binary Technology (NanoBiT) system from Promega is comprised of an 18 kDa larger subunit as well as an 11 amino acid peptide making up the small subunit (SmBiT) [178]. These two components were intentionally engineered to have low affinity for each other with a K_d of 190 μM, allowing for the components conjugated to these two subunits to be the main driver of interaction [178]. Like cat-ELCCA, SEA also uses a TCO-labeled RNA. LgBiT is fused to the RBP of interest, while SmBiT contains the mTet modification, which is appended via conjugation to HaloTag [179]. Signal results when the RBP binds to the target RNA following a covalent click chemistry reaction between the TCO and mTet components, placing SmBiT and LgBiT in close enough proximity to assemble the active NanoBiT enzyme which produces a chemiluminescent signal following treatment with NanoLuc substrate. SEA has been utilized to detect RPIs in 384-well plate format with robust assay statistics and was further able to detect inhibition by a small molecule (CCG-233094 in Table 11.2) without the need to wash away unbound species due to the low inherent affinity of the NanoBiT subunits [171].

11.3.2.1 Cell-Based RPI Detection Assays

While enabling assay technologies, *in vitro* methods come with a major drawback as they do not assess how RBPs behave in cells or how they may interact with RNAs in cells due to the absence of post-translational modifications or other protein-binding partners present in the native cellular environment [169, 180, 181]. Indeed, many RBPs function in complexes containing multiple RPIs or PPIs that facilitate the interaction between the RNA and RBP [180]. This biological complexity necessitates the need for cell-based methods to detect specific RPIs that are also amenable to high-throughput experimentation and are reversible to allow for the identification of inhibitors of the interaction. Cell-based platforms for detecting and screening RPIs also come with an additional advantage in that they also allow for simultaneous assessment of cellular permeability, activity, and cytotoxicity.

Cell-based FRET and fluorescence *in situ* hybridization (FISH) coupled with immunofluorescence have broad applications and can be used to demonstrate interaction and co-localization of an RNA and RBP [182–184]. However, FRET, in addition to the limitations in fluorescence-based methods already discussed, is also highly dependent upon the ratios of the interacting partners to produce a signal. Additionally, for these imaging-based methods to be made high-throughput, highly specialized and expensive high-content imaging equipment is necessary. With FISH coupled with immunofluorescence specifically, there is no evidence of a direct interaction between an RNA and protein, just co-localization of the components [185]. These methods also typically require cell fixation and permeabilization to be used with antibodies, making them not suitable for high-throughput experimentation. Furthermore, only a fraction of RBPs have validated antibodies for use, making

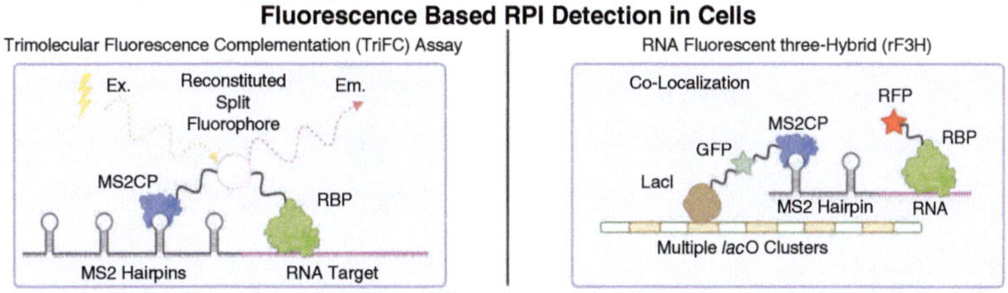

Figure 11.12 Schematic representation of trimolecular fluorescence complementation assay and RNA fluorescent three-hybrid assay to detect RPIs in a cell-based setting. Figure created in BioRender.

these approaches not ideal or maybe even not an option for the detection of poorly characterized RPIs [186].

Additional methods include the trimolecular fluorescence complementation (TriFC) assay and RNA fluorescent three-hybrid (rF3H) assay (Figure 11.12). TriFC, originally established for the visualization of cellular PPIs, utilizes a split fluorophore as the detection method, brought together by other interacting units [187–190]. In this case, an RNA target sequence is appended to the sequence coding for the MS2 hairpin RNA. The RNA bacteriophage MS2 coat protein (MS2CP), which binds to the MS2 hairpin RNA, is fused to a portion of a split fluorophore [191]. The RBP-of-interest is fused to the second half of the split fluorophore. When the RBP binds to the RNA target adjacent to the MS2 hairpin RNA, the fluorophore is reconstituted and will exhibit a fluorescence signal at its specific excitation and emission wavelength, driven by the RPI. This assay has not been used for screening inhibitors likely due to the irreversibility of the complementation between the fluorophore protein fragments leading to high background and resulting in an inability of this method to measure RPI dynamics [192]. In rF3H, an MS2 stem-loop-labeled RNA (similar to that used in TriFC) is anchored to a specific locus by a fusion protein containing the MS2CP, a GFP, and an anchoring protein. Specific anchor proteins may direct the locus of the trap, with LacI binding to an integrated lab operon shown as an example in Figure 11.12. Other loci include the Lamin B1 anchor localizing to the nuclear lamina or the Coilin protein localizing to Cajal bodies [193]. Interaction of the RBP fused to another fluorescent protein (RFP) with the RNA target will give insight into co-localization of the protein to that specific cellular compartment. This method, while not advantageous for screening, could be useful for signal detection for certain disease contexts by enrichment of signal at a specific locus.

11.3.3 Cell-Based RNA–Protein Interaction Screening

The limitations observed with *in vitro* small molecule screening, coupled with the absence of cell-based screening methods for RPIs, led to the development of additional cell-based RPI assays. RNA interaction with protein-mediated complementation assay (RiPCA; Figure 11.13), in similar manner to cat-ELCCA and SEA, leverages biorthogonal chemistry strategies for the detection of specific interactions

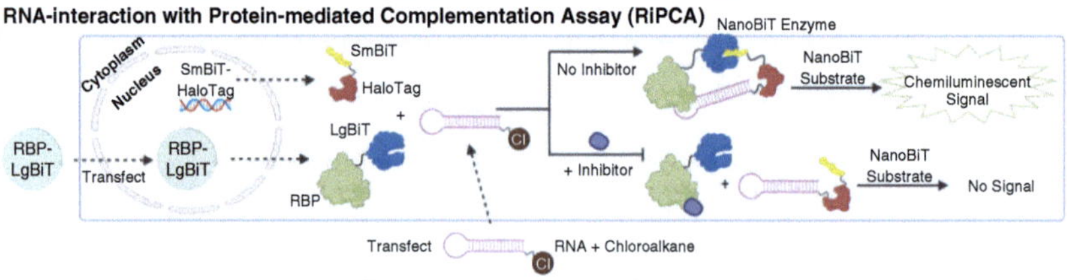

Figure 11.13 Schematic representation of RNA interaction with protein-mediated complementation assay to detect RPIs in the presence of an inhibitor and without in a cell-based setting. Figure created in BioRender.

[194–196]. The RBP-of-interest is fused to the LgBiT subunit, while the SmBiT is fused to HaloTag (HT). Flp-In HEK293T cells are engineered to stably express the SmBiT-HT fusion protein, which are subsequently transiently transfected with a plasmid encoding the RBP fused to LgBiT. The RNA, functionalized with a PEGylated chloroalkane substrate for conjugation to HT, is co-transfected alongside the RBP-LgBiT. Signal is detected following HT covalently modifying the RNA target and the RBP binding to the RNA, bringing LgBiT and SmBiT in proximity to interact and form the catalytically active NanoLuc enzyme, which results in the production of chemiluminescent signal following treatment with NanoLuc substrate. Carried out in this way, a new cell line does not need to be generated for each RBP- or RPI-of-interest, rather, a different RBP would just need to be cloned into the plasmid-containing LgBiT. RiPCA is suitable for screening to identify inhibitors of an RPI, is amenable to high-throughput experimentation, and results in sensitive signal generated by the complex that is stabilized by the covalent bond between HT and the RNA. Additionally, the cells are not lysed or permeabilized to allow for signal detection because RiPCA uses Promega's Live-Cell NanoBiT detection reagent. Some limitations to this approach include potential issues with overexpression of the RBP because it is transiently transfected through the plasmid on top of endogenous expression. Moreover, the RNA must be generated through chemical synthesis due to requirement of a site-specific nucleobase modification for coupling to the chloroalkane handle for HT conjugation, limiting the length of RNA that can be used due to limitations of RNA chemical synthesis.

11.4 Closing Remarks

Sequencing of the human genome catalyzed expanded exploration of RNA biology. From these investigations, we have come to appreciate not only the complexity and significance of cellular RNAs but also how entangled the cellular lifecycle of an RNA is with a cadre of regulatory proteins. As we continue to push the boundaries of drug discovery toward the targeting of historically difficult-to-drug areas of biology, RNAs and RPIs have emerged as exciting challenges for the field of medicinal chemistry. In learning more about RBPs and RPIs, we hope that new insights will be gleaned with respect to molecular recognition principles for binding to RNAs that can be applied toward our pursuit of developing small molecule-based, RNA-targeted therapeutics, as well as reveal new mechanisms for impacting RNA biology in disease states for the development of next-generation medicines.

References

1 Lunde, B.M., Moore, C., and Varani, G. (2007). RNA-binding proteins: modular design for efficient function. *Nat Rev Mol Cell Biol.* 8 (6): 479–490. https://doi.org/10.1038/nrm2178. PubMed PMID: 17473849; PMCID: PMC5507177.

2 Murzin, A.G., Brenner, S.E., Hubbard, T., and Chothia, C. (1995). SCOP: a structural classification of proteins database for the investigation of sequences and structures. *J Mol Biol.* 247 (4): 536–540. https://doi.org/10.1006/jmbi.1995.0159. PubMed PMID: 7723011.

3 Letunic, I., Doerks, T., and Bork, P. (2009). SMART 6: recent updates and new developments. *Nucleic Acids Res.* 37 (Database issue): D229–D232. Epub 20081031. https://doi.org/10.1093/nar/gkn808. PubMed PMID: 18978020; PMCID: PMC2686533.

4 Finn, R.D., Mistry, J., Tate, J. et al. (2010). The Pfam protein families database. *Nucleic Acids Res.* 38 (Database issue): D211–D222. Epub 20091117. https://doi.org/10.1093/nar/gkp985. PubMed PMID: 19920124; PMCID: PMC2808889.

5 Wilson, D., Pethica, R., Zhou, Y. et al. (2009). SUPERFAMILY--sophisticated comparative genomics, data mining, visualization and phylogeny. *Nucleic Acids Res.* 37 (Database issue): D380–D386. Epub 20081126. https://doi.org/10.1093/nar/gkn762. PubMed PMID: 19036790; PMCID: PMC2686452.

6 Marchler-Bauer, A., Zheng, C., Chitsaz, F. et al. (2013). CDD: conserved domains and protein three-dimensional structure. *Nucleic Acids Res.* 41 (Database issue): D348–D352. Epub 20121128. https://doi.org/10.1093/nar/gks1243. PubMed PMID: 23197659; PMCID: PMC3531192.

7 McKee, A.E., Minet, E., Stern, C. et al. (2005). A genome-wide in situ hybridization map of RNA-binding proteins reveals anatomically restricted expression in the developing mouse brain. *BMC Dev Biol.* 5 (14) Epub 20050720. https://doi.org/10.1186/1471-213X-5-14: PubMed PMID: 16033648; PMCID: PMC1199591.

8 Galante, P.A., Sandhu, D., de Sousa, A.R. et al. (2009). A comprehensive in silico expression analysis of RNA binding proteins in normal and tumor tissue: Identification of potential players in tumor formation. *RNA Biol.* 6 (4): 426–433. Epub 20090924. https://doi.org/10.4161/rna.6.4.8841. PubMed PMID: 19458496; PMCID: PMC2935330.

9 Anantharaman, V., Koonin, E.V., and Aravind, L. (2002). Comparative genomics and evolution of proteins involved in RNA metabolism. *Nucleic Acids Res.* 30 (7): 1427–1464. https://doi.org/10.1093/nar/30.7.1427. PubMed PMID: 11917006; PMCID: PMC101826.

10 Corley, M., Burns, M.C., and Yeo, G.W. (2020). How RNA-binding proteins interact with RNA: molecules and mechanisms. *Mol Cell.* 78 (1): 9–29. https://

doi.org/10.1016/j.molcel.2020.03.011. PubMed PMID: 32243832; PMCID: PMC7202378.

11 McHugh, C.A., Russell, P., and Guttman, M. (2014). Methods for comprehensive experimental identification of RNA-protein interactions. *Genome Biol.* 15 (1): 203. Epub 20140127. https://doi.org/10.1186/gb4152. PubMed PMID: 24467948; PMCID: PMC4054858.

12 Van Nostrand, E.L., Freese, P., Pratt, G.A. et al. (2020). A large-scale binding and functional map of human RNA-binding proteins. *Nature.* 583 (7818): 711–719. https://doi.org/10.1038/s41586-020-2077-3.

13 Dreyfuss, G., Kim, V.N., and Kataoka, N. (2002). Messenger-RNA-binding proteins and the messages they carry. *Nat Rev Mol Cell Biol.* 3 (3): 195–205. https://doi.org/10.1038/nrm760. PubMed PMID: 11994740.

14 Clery, A., Blatter, M., and Allain, F.H. (2008). RNA recognition motifs: boring? Not quite. *Curr Opin Struct Biol.* 18 (3): 290–298. https://doi.org/10.1016/j.sbi.2008.04.002. PubMed PMID: 18515081.

15 Banerjee, S. and Barraud, P. (2014). Functions of double-stranded RNA-binding domains in nucleocytoplasmic transport. *RNA Biol.* 11 (10): 1226–1232. https://doi.org/10.4161/15476286.2014.972856. PubMed PMID: 25584639; PMCID: PMC4615638.

16 Hall, T.M. (2005). Multiple modes of RNA recognition by zinc finger proteins. *Curr Opin Struct Biol.* 15 (3): 367–373. https://doi.org/10.1016/j.sbi.2005.04.004. PubMed PMID: 15963892.

17 Valverde, R., Edwards, L., and Regan, L. (2008). Structure and function of KH domains. *FEBS J.* 275 (11): 2712–2726. Epub 20080415. https://doi.org/10.1111/j.1742-4658.2008.06411.x. PubMed PMID: 18422648.

18 Antoine Cléry FH-TA (2000-2013). *From Structure to Function of RNA Binding Domains.* Austin (TX): Landes Bioscience.

19 Jankowsky, E. and Harris, M.E. (2015). Specificity and nonspecificity in RNA–protein interactions. *Nature Reviews Molecular Cell Biology.* 16 (9): 533–544. https://doi.org/10.1038/nrm4032.

20 Jonas, S. and Izaurralde, E. (2013). The role of disordered protein regions in the assembly of decapping complexes and RNP granules. *Genes Dev.* 27 (24): 2628–2641. https://doi.org/10.1101/gad.227843.113. PubMed PMID: 24352420; PMCID: PMC3877753.

21 Teplova, M., Malinina, L., Darnell, J.C. et al. (2011). Protein-RNA and protein-protein recognition by dual KH1/2 domains of the neuronal splicing factor Nova-1. *Structure.* 19 (7): 930–944. https://doi.org/10.1016/j.str.2011.05.002. PubMed PMID: 21742260; PMCID: PMC3134789.

22 Cienikova, Z., Jayne, S., Damberger, F.F. et al. (2015). Evidence for cooperative tandem binding of hnRNP C RRMs in mRNA processing. *RNA* 21 (11): 1931–1942. Epub 20150914. https://doi.org/10.1261/rna.052373.115. PubMed PMID: 26370582; PMCID: PMC4604433.

23 MacNicol, A.M., Wilczynska, A., and MacNicol, M.C. (2008). Function and regulation of the mammalian Musashi mRNA translational regulator. *Biochem Soc*

Trans. 36 (Pt 3): 528–530. https://doi.org/10.1042/bst0360528. PubMed PMID: 18481998; PMCID: PMC2562719.

24 Geuens, T., Bouhy, D., and Timmerman, V. (2016). The hnRNP family: insights into their role in health and disease. *Hum Genet.* 135 (8): 851–867. Epub 20160523. https://doi.org/10.1007/s00439-016-1683-5. PubMed PMID: 27215579; PMCID: PMC4947485.

25 Bradley, T., Cook, M.E., and Blanchette, M. (2015). SR proteins control a complex network of RNA-processing events. *RNA* 21 (1): 75–92. Epub 20141120. https://doi.org/10.1261/rna.043893.113. PubMed PMID: 25414008; PMCID: PMC4274639.

26 Hinman, M.N. and Lou, H. (2008). Diverse molecular functions of Hu proteins. *Cell Mol Life Sci.* 65 (20): 3168–3181. https://doi.org/10.1007/s00018-008-8252-6. PubMed PMID: 18581050; PMCID: PMC2580827.

27 Heraud-Farlow, J.E. and Kiebler, M.A. (2014). The multifunctional Staufen proteins: conserved roles from neurogenesis to synaptic plasticity. *Trends Neurosci.* 37 (9): 470–479. Epub 20140707. https://doi.org/10.1016/j.tins.2014.05.009. PubMed PMID: 25012293; PMCID: PMC4156307.

28 Song, M.S. and Rossi, J.J. (2017). Molecular mechanisms of Dicer: endonuclease and enzymatic activity. *Biochem J.* 474 (10): 1603–1618. Epub 20170504. https://doi.org/10.1042/bcj20160759. PubMed PMID: 28473628; PMCID: PMC5415849.

29 Rybak-Wolf, A., Jens, M., Murakawa, Y. et al. (2014). A variety of dicer substrates in human and *C. elegans*. *Cell.* 159 (5): 1153–1167. https://doi.org/10.1016/j.cell.2014.10.040. PubMed PMID: 25416952.

30 Daniels, S.M. and Gatignol, A. (2012). The multiple functions of TRBP, at the hub of cell responses to viruses, stress, and cancer. *Microbiol Mol Biol Rev.* 76 (3): 652–666. https://doi.org/10.1128/mmbr.00012-12. PubMed PMID: 22933564; PMCID: PMC3429622.

31 Teplova, M. and Patel, D.J. (2008). Structural insights into RNA recognition by the alternative-splicing regulator muscleblind-like MBNL1. *Nat Struct Mol Biol.* 15 (12): 1343–1351. Epub 20081130. https://doi.org/10.1038/nsmb.1519. PubMed PMID: 19043415; PMCID: PMC4689322.

32 Tiedje, C., Diaz-Muñoz, M.D., Trulley, P. et al. (2016). The RNA-binding protein TTP is a global post-transcriptional regulator of feedback control in inflammation. *Nucleic Acids Res.* 44 (15): 7418–7440. Epub 20160524. https://doi.org/10.1093/nar/gkw474. PubMed PMID: 27220464; PMCID: PMC5009735.

33 Behrens, G. and Heissmeyer, V. (2022). Cooperation of RNA-binding proteins - a focus on roquin function in T cells. *Front Immunol.* 13: 839762. Epub 20220218. https://doi.org/10.3389/fimmu.2022.839762. PubMed PMID: 35251035; PMCID: PMC8894612.

34 Meyer, N.H., Tripsianes, K., Vincendeau, M. et al. (2010). Structural basis for homodimerization of the Src-associated during mitosis, 68-kDa protein (Sam68) Qua1 domain. *J Biol Chem.* 285 (37): 28893–28901. Epub 20100706. https://doi.org/10.1074/jbc.M110.126185. PubMed PMID: 20610388; PMCID: PMC2937916.

35 Quinn, L.M. (2017). FUBP/KH domain proteins in transcription: back to the future. *Transcription* 8 (3): 185–192. Epub 20170216. https://doi.org/10.1080/21541264.2017.1293595. PubMed PMID: 28301294; PMCID: PMC5501386.

36 Cheng, M.H. and Jansen, R.P. (2017). A jack of all trades: the RNA-binding protein vigilin. *Wiley Interdiscip Rev RNA* 8 (6) Epub 20171004. https://doi.org/10.1002/wrna.1448: PubMed PMID: 28975734.

37 Burmann, B.M. and Rösch, P. (2011). The role of E. coli Nus-factors in transcription regulation and transcription:translation coupling: from structure to mechanism. *Transcription.* 2 (3): 130–134. https://doi.org/10.4161/trns.2.3.15671. PubMed PMID: 21922055; PMCID: PMC3173649.

38 Budkina, K.S., Zlobin, N.E., Kononova, S.V. et al. (2020). Cold shock domain proteins: structure and interaction with nucleic acids. *Biochemistry (Mosc).* 85 (Suppl 1): S1–s19. https://doi.org/10.1134/s0006297920140011. PubMed PMID: 32087051.

39 Liao, J., Wei, Y., Liang, J. et al. (2022). Insight into the structure, physiological function, and role in cancer of m6A readers—YTH domain-containing proteins. *Cell Death Discovery.* 8 (1): 137. https://doi.org/10.1038/s41420-022-00947-0.

40 Wang, M., Ogé, L., Perez-Garcia, M.D. et al. (2018). The PUF protein family: overview on PUF RNA targets, biological functions, and post transcriptional regulation. *Int J Mol Sci.* 19 (2) Epub 20180130. https://doi.org/10.3390/ijms19020410: PubMed PMID: 29385744; PMCID: PMC5855632.

41 Maris, C., Dominguez, C., and Allain, F.H. (2005). The RNA recognition motif, a plastic RNA-binding platform to regulate post-transcriptional gene expression. *FEBS J.* 272 (9): 2118–2131. https://doi.org/10.1111/j.1742-4658.2005.04653.x. PubMed PMID: 15853797.

42 Venter, J.C., Adams, M.D., Myers, E.W. et al. (2001). The sequence of the human genome. *Science.* 291 (5507): 1304–1351. https://doi.org/10.1126/science.1058040. PubMed PMID: 11181995.

43 Dreyfuss, G., Swanson, M.S., and Pinol-Roma, S. (1988). Heterogeneous nuclear ribonucleoprotein particles and the pathway of mRNA formation. *Trends Biochem Sci.* 13 (3): 86–91. https://doi.org/10.1016/0968-0004(88)90046-1. PubMed PMID: 3072706.

44 Adam, S.A., Nakagawa, T., Swanson, M.S. et al. (1986). mRNA polyadenylate-binding protein: gene isolation and sequencing and identification of a ribonucleoprotein consensus sequence. *Mol Cell Biol.* 6 (8): 2932–2943. https://doi.org/10.1128/mcb.6.8.2932-2943.1986. PubMed PMID: 3537727; PMCID: PMC367862.

45 Swanson, M.S., Nakagawa, T.Y., LeVan, K., and Dreyfuss, G. (1987). Primary structure of human nuclear ribonucleoprotein particle C proteins: conservation of sequence and domain structures in heterogeneous nuclear RNA, mRNA, and pre-rRNA-binding proteins. *Mol Cell Biol.* 7 (5): 1731–1739. https://doi.org/10.1128/mcb.7.5.1731-1739.1987. PubMed PMID: 3110598; PMCID: PMC365274.

46 Kenan, D.J., Query, C.C., and Keene, J.D. (1991). RNA recognition: towards identifying determinants of specificity. *Trends Biochem Sci.* 16 (6): 214–220. https://doi.org/10.1016/0968-0004(91)90088-d. PubMed PMID: 1716386.

47 Birney, E., Kumar, S., and Krainer, A.R. (1993). Analysis of the RNA-recognition motif and RS and RGG domains: conservation in metazoan pre-mRNA splicing factors. *Nucleic Acids Res.* 21 (25): 5803–5816. https://doi.org/10.1093/nar/21.25.5803. PubMed PMID: 8290338; PMCID: PMC310458.

48 Skrisovska, L., Bourgeois, C.F., Stefl, R. et al. (2007). The testis-specific human protein RBMY recognizes RNA through a novel mode of interaction. *EMBO Rep.* 8 (4): 372–379. Epub 20070223. https://doi.org/10.1038/sj.embor.7400910. PubMed PMID: 17318228; PMCID: PMC1852761.

49 Volpon, L., D'Orso, I., Young, C.R. et al. (2005). NMR structural study of TcUBP1, a single RRM domain protein from *Trypanosoma cruzi*: contribution of a beta hairpin to RNA binding. *Biochemistry.* 44 (10): 3708–3717. https://doi.org/10.1021/bi047450e. PubMed PMID: 15751947.

50 Tintaru, A.M., Hautbergue, G.M., Hounslow, A.M. et al. (2007). Structural and functional analysis of RNA and TAP binding to SF2/ASF. *EMBO Rep.* 8 (8): 756–762. Epub 20070713. https://doi.org/10.1038/sj.embor.7401031. PubMed PMID: 17668007; PMCID: PMC1978082.

51 Dominguez, C. and Allain, F.H. (2006). NMR structure of the three quasi RNA recognition motifs (qRRMs) of human hnRNP F and interaction studies with Bcl-x G-tract RNA: a novel mode of RNA recognition. *Nucleic Acids Res.* 34 (13): 3634–3645. Epub 20060802. https://doi.org/10.1093/nar/gkl488. PubMed PMID: 16885237; PMCID: PMC1540728.

52 Stefl, R., Skrisovska, L., and Allain, F.H. (2005). RNA sequence- and shape-dependent recognition by proteins in the ribonucleoprotein particle. *EMBO Rep.* 6 (1): 33–38. https://doi.org/10.1038/sj.embor.7400325. PubMed PMID: 15643449; PMCID: PMC1299235.

53 Ryter, J.M. and Schultz, S.C. (1998). Molecular basis of double-stranded RNA-protein interactions: structure of a dsRNA-binding domain complexed with dsRNA. *EMBO J.* 17 (24): 7505–7513. https://doi.org/10.1093/emboj/17.24.7505. PubMed PMID: 9857205; PMCID: PMC1171094.

54 Stefl, R., Oberstrass, F.C., Hood, J.L. et al. (2010). The solution structure of the ADAR2 dsRBM-RNA complex reveals a sequence-specific readout of the minor groove. *Cell.* 143 (2): 225–237. https://doi.org/10.1016/j.cell.2010.09.026. PubMed PMID: 20946981; PMCID: PMC2956598.

55 Wang, Z., Hartman, E., Roy, K. et al. (2011). Structure of a yeast RNase III dsRBD complex with a noncanonical RNA substrate provides new insights into binding specificity of dsRBDs. *Structure.* 19 (7): 999–1010. https://doi.org/10.1016/j.str.2011.03.022. PubMed PMID: 21742266; PMCID: PMC3143303.

56 Barraud, P., Banerjee, S., Mohamed, W.I. et al. (2014). A bimodular nuclear localization signal assembled via an extended double-stranded RNA-binding domain acts as an RNA-sensing signal for transportin 1. *Proc Natl Acad Sci U S A.* 111 (18): E1852–E1861. Epub 20140421. https://doi.org/10.1073/pnas.1323698111. PubMed PMID: 24753571; PMCID: PMC4020056.

57 Chang, K.Y. and Ramos, A. (2005). The double-stranded RNA-binding motif, a versatile macromolecular docking platform. *FEBS J.* 272 (9): 2109–2117. https://doi.org/10.1111/j.1742-4658.2005.04652.x. PubMed PMID: 15853796.

58 Wolfe, S.A., Nekludova, L., and Pabo, C.O. (2000). DNA recognition by Cys2His2 zinc finger proteins. *Annu Rev Biophys Biomol Struct.* 29: 183–212. https://doi.org/10.1146/annurev.biophys.29.1.183. PubMed PMID: 10940247.

59 Pelham, H.R. and Brown, D.D. (1980). A specific transcription factor that can bind either the 5S RNA gene or 5S RNA. *Proc Natl Acad Sci U S A.* 77 (7): 4170–4174. https://doi.org/10.1073/pnas.77.7.4170. PubMed PMID: 7001457; PMCID: PMC349792.

60 Amarasinghe, G.K., De Guzman, R.N., Turner, R.B. et al. (2000). NMR structure of the HIV-1 nucleocapsid protein bound to stem-loop SL2 of the psi-RNA packaging signal. Implications for genome recognition. *J Mol Biol.* 301 (2): 491–511. https://doi.org/10.1006/jmbi.2000.3979. PubMed PMID: 10926523.

61 Hudson, B.P., Martinez-Yamout, M.A., Dyson, H.J., and Wright, P.E. (2004). Recognition of the mRNA AU-rich element by the zinc finger domain of TIS11d. *Nat Struct Mol Biol.* 11 (3): 257–264. Epub 20040208. https://doi.org/10.1038/nsmb738. PubMed PMID: 14981510.

62 Lu, D., Searles, M.A., and Klug, A. (2003). Crystal structure of a zinc-finger-RNA complex reveals two modes of molecular recognition. *Nature.* 426 (6962): 96–100. https://doi.org/10.1038/nature02088. PubMed PMID: 14603324.

63 Blackshear, P.J. (2002). Tristetraprolin and other CCCH tandem zinc-finger proteins in the regulation of mRNA turnover. *Biochem Soc Trans.* 30 (Pt 6): 945–952. https://doi.org/10.1042/bst0300945. PubMed PMID: 12440952.

64 Loughlin, F.E., Mansfield, R.E., Vaz, P.M. et al. (2009). The zinc fingers of the SR-like protein ZRANB2 are single-stranded RNA-binding domains that recognize 5' splice site-like sequences. *Proc Natl Acad Sci U S A.* 106 (14): 5581–5586. Epub 20090320. https://doi.org/10.1073/pnas.0802466106. PubMed PMID: 19304800; PMCID: PMC2667063.

65 Grishin, N.V. (2001). KH domain: one motif, two folds. *Nucleic Acids Res.* 29 (3): 638–643. https://doi.org/10.1093/nar/29.3.638. PubMed PMID: 11160884; PMCID: PMC30387.

66 Beuth, B., Pennell, S., Arnvig, K.B. et al. (2005). Structure of a *Mycobacterium tuberculosis* NusA-RNA complex. *EMBO J.* 24 (20): 3576–3587. Epub 20050929. https://doi.org/10.1038/sj.emboj.7600829. PubMed PMID: 16193062; PMCID: PMC1276712.

67 Amir, M., Kumar, V., Dohare, R. et al. (2018). Sequence, structure and evolutionary analysis of cold shock domain proteins, a member of OB fold family. *J Evol Biol.* 31 (12): 1903–1917. Epub 20181019. https://doi.org/10.1111/jeb.13382. PubMed PMID: 30267552.

68 Hazra, D., Chapat, C., and Graille, M. (2019). m(6)A mRNA destiny: chained to the rhYTHm by the YTH-containing proteins. *Genes (Basel).* 10 (1) Epub 20190115. https://doi.org/10.3390/genes10010049: PubMed PMID: 30650668; PMCID: PMC6356822.

69 Li, J., Xie, H., Ying, Y. et al. (2020). YTHDF2 mediates the mRNA degradation of the tumor suppressors to induce AKT phosphorylation in N6-methyladenosine-dependent way in prostate cancer. *Mol Cancer.* 19 (1):

152. Epub 20201029. https://doi.org/10.1186/s12943-020-01267-6. PubMed PMID: 33121495; PMCID: PMC7599101.

70 Chen, Z., Zhong, X., Xia, M., and Zhong, J. (2021). The roles and mechanisms of the m6A reader protein YTHDF1 in tumor biology and human diseases. *Mol Ther Nucleic Acids* 26: 1270–1279. Epub 20211104. https://doi.org/10.1016/j.omtn.2021.10.023. PubMed PMID: 34853726; PMCID: PMC8609105.

71 Thandapani, P., O'Connor, T.R., Bailey, T.L., and Richard, S. (2013). Defining the RGG/RG motif. *Mol Cell.* 50 (5): 613–623. https://doi.org/10.1016/j.molcel.2013.05.021. PubMed PMID: 23746349.

72 Dennis, G. Jr.,, Sherman, B.T., Hosack, D.A. et al. (2003). DAVID: database for annotation, visualization, and integrated discovery. *Genome Biol.* 4 (5): P3. Epub 20030403. PubMed PMID: 12734009.

73 Blackwell, E. and Ceman, S. (2011). A new regulatory function of the region proximal to the RGG box in the fragile X mental retardation protein. *J Cell Sci.* 124 (Pt 18): 3060–3065. Epub 20110824. https://doi.org/10.1242/jcs.086751. PubMed PMID: 21868366; PMCID: PMC3172185.

74 Ina, S., Tsunekawa, N., Nakamura, A., and Noce, T. (2003). Expression of the mouse Aven gene during spermatogenesis, analyzed by subtraction screening using Mvh-knockout mice. *Gene Expr Patterns.* 3 (5): 635–638. https://doi.org/10.1016/s1567-133x(03)00111-x. PubMed PMID: 12971998.

75 Matsuoka, S., Ballif, B.A., Smogorzewska, A. et al. (2007). ATM and ATR substrate analysis reveals extensive protein networks responsive to DNA damage. *Science.* 316 (5828): 1160–1166. https://doi.org/10.1126/science.1140321. PubMed PMID: 17525332.

76 Nissan, T., Rajyaguru, P., She, M. et al. (2010). Decapping activators in Saccharomyces cerevisiae act by multiple mechanisms. *Mol Cell.* 39 (5): 773–783. https://doi.org/10.1016/j.molcel.2010.08.025. PubMed PMID: 20832728; PMCID: PMC2946179.

77 Rajyaguru, P., She, M., and Parker, R. (2012). Scd6 targets eIF4G to repress translation: RGG motif proteins as a class of eIF4G-binding proteins. *Mol Cell.* 45 (2): 244–254. https://doi.org/10.1016/j.molcel.2011.11.026. PubMed PMID: 22284680; PMCID: PMC3277450.

78 Andrisani, O., Liu, Q., Kehn, P. et al. (2022). Biological functions of DEAD/DEAH-box RNA helicases in health and disease. *Nat Immunol.* 23 (3): 354–357. https://doi.org/10.1038/s41590-022-01149-7. PubMed PMID: 35194205.

79 Wickens, M., Bernstein, D.S., Kimble, J., and Parker, R. (2002). A PUF family portrait: 3'UTR regulation as a way of life. *Trends Genet.* 18 (3): 150–157. https://doi.org/10.1016/s0168-9525(01)02616-6. PubMed PMID: 11858839.

80 Chen, Y. and Varani, G. (2011). Finding the missing code of RNA recognition by PUF proteins. *Chem Biol.* 18 (7): 821–823. https://doi.org/10.1016/j.chembiol.2011.07.001. PubMed PMID: 21802002; PMCID: PMC3161827.

81 Tam, P.P., Barrette-Ng, I.H., Simon, D.M. et al. (2010). The Puf family of RNA-binding proteins in plants: phylogeny, structural modeling, activity and subcellular localization. *BMC Plant Biol.* 10: 44. Epub 20100309. https://doi.org/10.1186/1471-2229-10-44. PubMed PMID: 20214804; PMCID: PMC2848763.

82 Rissland, O.S. (2017). The organization and regulation of mRNA-protein complexes. *Wiley Interdiscip Rev RNA* 8 (1) Epub 20160621. https://doi.org/10.1002/wrna.1369: PubMed PMID: 27324829; PMCID: PMC5213448.
83 Ransohoff, J.D., Wei, Y., and Khavari, P.A. (2018). The functions and unique features of long intergenic non-coding RNA. *Nat Rev Mol Cell Biol.* 19 (3): 143–157. Epub 20171115. https://doi.org/10.1038/nrm.2017.104. PubMed PMID: 29138516; PMCID: PMC5889127.
84 Statello, L., Guo, C.J., Chen, L.L., and Huarte, M. (2021). Gene regulation by long non-coding RNAs and its biological functions. *Nat Rev Mol Cell Biol.* 22 (2): 96–118. Epub 20201222. https://doi.org/10.1038/s41580-020-00315-9. PubMed PMID: 33353982; PMCID: PMC7754182.
85 Treiber, T., Treiber, N., and Meister, G. (2019). Regulation of microRNA biogenesis and its crosstalk with other cellular pathways. *Nature Reviews Molecular Cell Biology.* 20 (1): 5–20. https://doi.org/10.1038/s41580-018-0059-1.
86 Wilkinson, E., Cui, Y.H., and He, Y.Y. (2022). Roles of RNA modifications in diverse cellular functions. *Front Cell Dev Biol.* 10: 828683. Epub 20220308. https://doi.org/10.3389/fcell.2022.828683. PubMed PMID: 35350378; PMCID: PMC8957929.
87 Shi, H., Chai, P., Jia, R., and Fan, X. (2020). Novel insight into the regulatory roles of diverse RNA modifications: Re-defining the bridge between transcription and translation. *Mol Cancer.* 19 (1): 78. Epub 20200417. https://doi.org/10.1186/s12943-020-01194-6. PubMed PMID: 32303268; PMCID: PMC7164178.
88 Katz, N., Cohen, R., Solomon, O. et al. (2018). RBP-RNA interactions in the 5' UTR lead to structural changes that alter translation. *bioRxiv.* 174888. https://doi.org/10.1101/174888.
89 Szostak, E. and Gebauer, F. (2013). Translational control by 3'-UTR-binding proteins. *Brief Funct Genomics* 12 (1): 58–65. Epub 20121128. https://doi.org/10.1093/bfgp/els056. PubMed PMID: 23196851; PMCID: PMC3548161.
90 Grzybowska, E.A. and Wakula, M. (2021). Protein binding to cis-motifs in mRNAs coding sequence is common and regulates transcript stability and the rate of translation. *Cells* 10 (11) Epub 20211027. https://doi.org/10.3390/cells10112910: PubMed PMID: 34831133; PMCID: PMC8616275.
91 Savisaar, R. and Hurst, L.D. (2017). Both maintenance and avoidance of RNA-binding protein interactions constrain coding sequence evolution. *Molecular Biology and Evolution.* 34 (5): 1110–1126. https://doi.org/10.1093/molbev/msx061.
92 Leppek, K., Das, R., and Barna, M. (2018). Functional 5' UTR mRNA structures in eukaryotic translation regulation and how to find them. *Nat Rev Mol Cell Biol.* 19 (3): 158–174. Epub 20171122. https://doi.org/10.1038/nrm.2017.103. PubMed PMID: 29165424; PMCID: PMC5820134.
93 Mignone, F., Gissi, C., Liuni, S., and Pesole, G. (2002). Untranslated regions of mRNAs. *Genome Biol.* 3 (3) Reviews0004. Epub 20020228. https://doi.org/10.1186/gb-2002-3-3-reviews0004: PubMed PMID: 11897027; PMCID: PMC139023.
94 Mayya, V.K. and Duchaine, T.F. (2019). Ciphers and executioners: how 3'-untranslated regions determine the fate of messenger RNAs. *Front Genet.*

10 (6) Epub 20190124. https://doi.org/10.3389/fgene.2019.00006: PubMed PMID: 30740123; PMCID: PMC6357968.

95 Kapeli, K., Martinez, F.J., and Yeo, G.W. (2017). Genetic mutations in RNA-binding proteins and their roles in ALS. *Hum Genet.* 136 (9): 1193–1214. Epub 20170731. https://doi.org/10.1007/s00439-017-1830-7. PubMed PMID: 28762175; PMCID: PMC5602095.

96 Khabar, K.S. (2017). Hallmarks of cancer and AU-rich elements. *Wiley Interdiscip Rev RNA* 8 (1) Epub 20160601. https://doi.org/10.1002/wrna.1368: PubMed PMID: 27251431; PMCID: PMC5215528.

97 Mir, C., Garcia-Mayea, Y., and ME LL (2022). Targeting the "undruggable": RNA-binding proteins in the spotlight in cancer therapy. *Semin Cancer Biol.* 86 (Pt 3): 69–83. Epub 20220627. https://doi.org/10.1016/j.semcancer.2022.06.008. PubMed PMID: 35772609.

98 Berson, A., Barbash, S., Shaltiel, G. et al. (2012). Cholinergic-associated loss of hnRNP-A/B in Alzheimer's disease impairs cortical splicing and cognitive function in mice. *EMBO Mol Med.* 4 (8): 730–742. Epub 20120525. https://doi.org/10.1002/emmm.201100995. PubMed PMID: 22628224; PMCID: PMC3494073.

99 Donev, R., Newall, A., Thome, J., and Sheer, D. (2007). A role for SC35 and hnRNPA1 in the determination of amyloid precursor protein isoforms. *Mol Psychiatry* 12 (7): 681–690. Epub 20070313. https://doi.org/10.1038/sj.mp.4001971. PubMed PMID: 17353911; PMCID: PMC2684093.

100 Kharas, M.G. and Lengner, C.J. (2017). Stem cells, cancer, and MUSASHI in blood and guts. *Trends in Cancer.* 3 (5): 347–356. https://doi.org/10.1016/j.trecan.2017.03.007.

101 Sakakibara, S. and Okano, H. (1997). Expression of neural RNA-binding proteins in the postnatal CNS: implications of their roles in neuronal and glial cell development. *J Neurosci.* 17 (21): 8300–8312. https://doi.org/10.1523/jneurosci.17-21-08300.1997. PubMed PMID: 9334405; PMCID: PMC6573750.

102 Imai, T., Tokunaga, A., Yoshida, T. et al. (2001). The neural RNA-binding protein Musashi1 translationally regulates mammalian numb gene expression by interacting with its mRNA. *Mol Cell Biol.* 21 (12): 3888–3900. https://doi.org/10.1128/mcb.21.12.3888-3900.2001. PubMed PMID: 11359897; PMCID: PMC87052.

103 Gulino, A., Di Marcotullio, L., and Screpanti, I. (2010). The multiple functions of Numb. *Experimental Cell Research.* 316 (6): 900–906. https://doi.org/10.1016/j.yexcr.2009.11.017.

104 Bentley, D.L. (2014). Coupling mRNA processing with transcription in time and space. *Nature Reviews Genetics.* 15 (3): 163–175. https://doi.org/10.1038/nrg3662.

105 Fredericks, A.M., Cygan, K.J., Brown, B.A., and Fairbrother, W.G. (2015). RNA-binding proteins: splicing factors and disease. *Biomolecules* 5 (2): 893–909. Epub 20150513. https://doi.org/10.3390/biom5020893. PubMed PMID: 25985083; PMCID: PMC4496701.

106 Jeong, S. (2017). SR proteins: binders, regulators, and connectors of RNA. *Mol Cells.* 40 (1): 1–9. Epub 20170126. https://doi.org/10.14348/molcells.2017.2319. PubMed PMID: 28152302; PMCID: PMC5303883.

107 Chou, M.Y., Rooke, N., Turck, C.W., and Black, D.L. (1999). hnRNP H is a component of a splicing enhancer complex that activates a c-src alternative exon in neuronal cells. *Mol Cell Biol.* 19 (1): 69–77. https://doi.org/10.1128/mcb.19.1.69. PubMed PMID: 9858532; PMCID: PMC83866.

108 Zhang, J. and Manley, J.L. (2013). Misregulation of pre-mRNA alternative splicing in cancer. *Cancer Discov.* 3 (11): 1228–1237. Epub 20131021. https://doi.org/10.1158/2159-8290.Cd-13-0253. PubMed PMID: 24145039; PMCID: PMC3823817.

109 Anczuków, O., Rosenberg, A.Z., Akerman, M. et al. (2012). The splicing factor SRSF1 regulates apoptosis and proliferation to promote mammary epithelial cell transformation. *Nat Struct Mol Biol.* 19 (2): 220–228. Epub 20120115. https://doi.org/10.1038/nsmb.2207. PubMed PMID: 22245967; PMCID: PMC3272117.

110 Arnold, E.S., Ling, S.C., Huelga, S.C. et al. (2013). ALS-linked TDP-43 mutations produce aberrant RNA splicing and adult-onset motor neuron disease without aggregation or loss of nuclear TDP-43. *Proc Natl Acad Sci U S A* 110 (8): E736–E745. Epub 20130204. https://doi.org/10.1073/pnas.1222809110. PubMed PMID: 23382207; PMCID: PMC3581922.

111 Fogel, B.L., Wexler, E., Wahnich, A. et al. (2012). RBFOX1 regulates both splicing and transcriptional networks in human neuronal development. *Hum Mol Genet.* 21 (19): 4171–4186. Epub 20120623. https://doi.org/10.1093/hmg/dds240. PubMed PMID: 22730494; PMCID: PMC3441119.

112 Wang, E.T., Cody, N.A., Jog, S. et al. (2012). Transcriptome-wide regulation of pre-mRNA splicing and mRNA localization by muscleblind proteins. *Cell.* 150 (4): 710–724. https://doi.org/10.1016/j.cell.2012.06.041. PubMed PMID: 22901804; PMCID: PMC3428802.

113 Bradley, R.K. and Anczuków, O. (2023). RNA splicing dysregulation and the hallmarks of cancer. *Nature Reviews Cancer.* 23 (3): 135–155. https://doi.org/10.1038/s41568-022-00541-7.

114 Borden, K.L.B. (2020). The Nuclear Pore Complex and mRNA Export in Cancer. *Cancers (Basel).* 13 (1) Epub 20201225. https://doi.org/10.3390/cancers13010042: PubMed PMID: 33375634; PMCID: PMC7796397.

115 Hurt, J.A. and Silver, P.A. (2008). mRNA nuclear export and human disease. *Dis Model Mech.* 1 (2-3): 103–108. https://doi.org/10.1242/dmm.000745. PubMed PMID: 19048072; PMCID: PMC2562179.

116 Chau, A. and Kalsotra, A. (2015). Developmental insights into the pathology of and therapeutic strategies for DM1: Back to the basics. *Dev Dyn.* 244 (3): 377–390. Epub 20150113. https://doi.org/10.1002/dvdy.24240. PubMed PMID: 25504326.

117 Pettersson, O.J., Aagaard, L., Jensen, T.G., and Damgaard, C.K. (2015). Molecular mechanisms in DM1 - a focus on foci. *Nucleic Acids Res.* 43 (4): 2433–2441. Epub 20150120. https://doi.org/10.1093/nar/gkv029. PubMed PMID: 25605794; PMCID: PMC4344492.

118 Brook, J.D., McCurrach, M.E., Harley, H.G. et al. (1992). Molecular basis of myotonic dystrophy: expansion of a trinucleotide (CTG) repeat at the 3' end of a transcript encoding a protein kinase family member. *Cell.* 68 (4): 799–808. https://doi.org/10.1016/0092-8674(92)90154-5. PubMed PMID: 1310900.

119 Buxton, J., Shelbourne, P., Davies, J. et al. (1992). Detection of an unstable fragment of DNA specific to individuals with myotonic dystrophy. *Nature.* 355 (6360): 547–548. https://doi.org/10.1038/355547a0. PubMed PMID: 1346924.

120 Fu, Y.H., Pizzuti, A., Fenwick, R.G. Jr., et al. (1992). An unstable triplet repeat in a gene related to myotonic muscular dystrophy. *Science.* 255 (5049): 1256–1258. https://doi.org/10.1126/science.1546326. PubMed PMID: 1546326.

121 Harley, H.G., Brook, J.D., Rundle, S.A. et al. (1992). Expansion of an unstable DNA region and phenotypic variation in myotonic dystrophy. *Nature.* 355 (6360): 545–546. https://doi.org/10.1038/355545a0. PubMed PMID: 1346923.

122 Mahadevan, M., Tsilfidis, C., Sabourin, L. et al. (1992). Myotonic dystrophy mutation: an unstable CTG repeat in the 3' untranslated region of the gene. *Science.* 255 (5049): 1253–1255. https://doi.org/10.1126/science.1546325. PubMed PMID: 1546325.

123 Paulson, H. (2018). Repeat expansion diseases. *Handb Clin Neurol.* 147: 105–123. https://doi.org/10.1016/b978-0-444-63233-3.00009-9. PubMed PMID: 29325606; PMCID: PMC6485936.

124 Johnson, B.S., Snead, D., Lee, J.J. et al. (2009). TDP-43 is intrinsically aggregation-prone, and amyotrophic lateral sclerosis-linked mutations accelerate aggregation and increase toxicity. *J Biol Chem.* 284 (30): 20329–20339. Epub 20090522. https://doi.org/10.1074/jbc.M109.010264. PubMed PMID: 19465477; PMCID: PMC2740458.

125 Barmada, S.J., Skibinski, G., Korb, E. et al. (2010). Cytoplasmic mislocalization of TDP-43 is toxic to neurons and enhanced by a mutation associated with familial amyotrophic lateral sclerosis. *J Neurosci.* 30 (2): 639–649. https://doi.org/10.1523/jneurosci.4988-09.2010. PubMed PMID: 20071528; PMCID: PMC2821110.

126 Wang, W., Wang, L., Lu, J. et al. (2016). The inhibition of TDP-43 mitochondrial localization blocks its neuronal toxicity. *Nat Med.* 22 (8): 869–878. Epub 20160627. https://doi.org/10.1038/nm.4130. PubMed PMID: 27348499; PMCID: PMC4974139.

127 Paronetto, M.P., Messina, V., Bianchi, E. et al. (2009). Sam68 regulates translation of target mRNAs in male germ cells, necessary for mouse spermatogenesis. *Journal of Cell Biology.* 185 (2): 235–249. https://doi.org/10.1083/jcb.200811138.

128 Paronetto, M.P., Zalfa, F., Botti, F. et al. (2006). The nuclear RNA-binding protein Sam68 translocates to the cytoplasm and associates with the polysomes in mouse spermatocytes. *Mol Biol Cell.* 17 (1): 14–24. Epub 20051012. https://doi.org/10.1091/mbc.e05-06-0548. PubMed PMID: 16221888; PMCID: PMC1345642.

129 Frisone, P., Pradella, D., Di Matteo, A. et al. (2015). SAM68: Signal Transduction and RNA Metabolism in Human Cancer. *Biomed Res Int.* 2015: 528954. Epub 20150726. https://doi.org/10.1155/2015/528954. PubMed PMID: 26273626; PMCID: PMC4529925.

130 Zhang, Z., Li, J., Zheng, H. et al. (2009). Expression and cytoplasmic localization of SAM68 is a significant and independent prognostic marker for renal cell carcinoma. *Cancer Epidemiol Biomarkers Prev.* 18 (10): 2685–2693. Epub 20090915. https://doi.org/10.1158/1055-9965.Epi-09-0097. PubMed PMID: 19755649.

131 Song, L., Wang, L., Li, Y. et al. (2010). Sam68 up-regulation correlates with, and its down-regulation inhibits, proliferation and tumourigenicity of breast cancer cells. *J Pathol.* 222 (3): 227–237. https://doi.org/10.1002/path.2751. PubMed PMID: 20662004.

132 Almasi, S. and Jasmin, B.J. (2021). The multifunctional RNA-binding protein Staufen1: an emerging regulator of oncogenesis through its various roles in key cellular events. *Cellular and Molecular Life Sciences.* 78 (23): 7145–7160. https://doi.org/10.1007/s00018-021-03965-w.

133 Wickham, L., Duchaîne, T., Luo, M. et al. (1999). Mammalian staufen is a double-stranded-RNA- and tubulin-binding protein which localizes to the rough endoplasmic reticulum. *Mol Cell Biol.* 19 (3): 2220–2230. https://doi.org/10.1128/mcb.19.3.2220. PubMed PMID: 10022909; PMCID: PMC84015.

134 Liu, H., Luo, M., and Wen, J.K. (2014). mRNA stability in the nucleus. *J Zhejiang Univ Sci B.* 15 (5): 444–454. https://doi.org/10.1631/jzus.B1400088. PubMed PMID: 24793762; PMCID: PMC4076601.

135 Yamaguchi, Y., Naiki, T., and Irie, K. (2012). Stau1 regulates Dvl2 expression during myoblast differentiation. *Biochem Biophys Res Commun.* 417 (1): 427–432. Epub 20111207. https://doi.org/10.1016/j.bbrc.2011.11.133. PubMed PMID: 22166206.

136 Kim, Y.K., Furic, L., Desgroseillers, L., and Maquat, L.E. (2005). Mammalian Staufen1 recruits Upf1 to specific mRNA 3'UTRs so as to elicit mRNA decay. *Cell.* 120 (2): 195–208. https://doi.org/10.1016/j.cell.2004.11.050. PubMed PMID: 15680326.

137 Yu, Z., Fan, D., Gui, B. et al. (2012). Neurodegeneration-associated TDP-43 interacts with fragile X mental retardation protein (FMRP)/Staufen (STAU1) and regulates SIRT1 expression in neuronal cells. *J Biol Chem.* 287 (27): 22560–22572. Epub 20120514. https://doi.org/10.1074/jbc.M112.357582. PubMed PMID: 22584570; PMCID: PMC3391095.

138 Jing, F., Ruan, X., Liu, X. et al. (2020). The PABPC5/HCG15/ZNF331 feedback loop regulates vasculogenic mimicry of glioma via STAU1-mediated mRNA decay. *Mol Ther Oncolytics.* 17: 216–231. Epub 20200330. https://doi.org/10.1016/j.omto.2020.03.017. PubMed PMID: 32346611; PMCID: PMC7183103.

139 Su, R., Ma, J., Zheng, J. et al. (2020). PABPC1-induced stabilization of BDNF-AS inhibits malignant progression of glioblastoma cells through STAU1-mediated decay. *Cell Death Dis.* 11 (2): 81. Epub 20200203. https://doi.org/10.1038/s41419-020-2267-9. PubMed PMID: 32015336; PMCID: PMC6997171.

140 Cushman, M., Johnson, B.S., King, O.D. et al. (2010). Prion-like disorders: blurring the divide between transmissibility and infectivity. *J Cell Sci.* 123 (Pt 8): 1191–1201. https://doi.org/10.1242/jcs.051672. PubMed PMID: 20356930; PMCID: PMC2848109.

141 Vance, C., Scotter, E.L., Nishimura, A.L. et al. (2013). ALS mutant FUS disrupts nuclear localization and sequesters wild-type FUS within cytoplasmic stress granules. *Hum Mol Genet.* 22 (13): 2676–2688. Epub 20130307. https://doi.org/10.1093/hmg/ddt117. PubMed PMID: 23474818; PMCID: PMC3674807.

142 Gebauer, F., Schwarzl, T., Valcarcel, J., and Hentze, M.W. (2021). RNA-binding proteins in human genetic disease. *Nat Rev Genet.* 22 (3): 185–198. Epub 20201124. https://doi.org/10.1038/s41576-020-00302-y. PubMed PMID: 33235359.

143 Aguzzi, A. and Altmeyer, M. (2016). Phase separation: linking cellular compartmentalization to disease. *Trends Cell Biol.* 26 (7): 547–558. Epub 20160401. https://doi.org/10.1016/j.tcb.2016.03.004. PubMed PMID: 27051975.

144 Kato, M., Han, T.W., Xie, S. et al. (2012). Cell-free formation of RNA granules: low complexity sequence domains form dynamic fibers within hydrogels. *Cell.* 149 (4): 753–767. https://doi.org/10.1016/j.cell.2012.04.017. PubMed PMID: 22579281; PMCID: PMC6347373.

145 Lin, Y., Protter, D.S., Rosen, M.K., and Parker, R. (2015). Formation and maturation of phase-separated liquid droplets by RNA-binding proteins. *Mol Cell.* 60 (2): 208–219. Epub 20150924. https://doi.org/10.1016/j.molcel.2015.08.018. PubMed PMID: 26412307; PMCID: PMC4609299.

146 Guillén-Boixet, J., Kopach, A., Holehouse, A.S. et al. (2020). RNA-induced conformational switching and clustering of G3BP drive stress granule assembly by condensation. *Cell.* 181 (2): 346–61.e17. https://doi.org/10.1016/j.cell.2020.03.049. PubMed PMID: 32302572; PMCID: PMC7181197.

147 Yang, P., Mathieu, C., Kolaitis, R.M. et al. (2020). G3BP1 is a tunable switch that triggers phase separation to assemble stress granules. *Cell.* 181 (2): 325–45.e28. https://doi.org/10.1016/j.cell.2020.03.046. PubMed PMID: 32302571; PMCID: PMC7448383.

148 Sanders, D.W., Kedersha, N., Lee, D.S.W. et al. (2020). Competing protein-RNA interaction networks control multiphase intracellular organization. *Cell.* 181 (2): 306–24.e28. https://doi.org/10.1016/j.cell.2020.03.050. PubMed PMID: 32302570; PMCID: PMC7816278.

149 Mittag, T. and Parker, R. (2018). Multiple modes of protein-protein interactions promote RNP granule assembly. *J Mol Biol.* 430 (23): 4636–4649. Epub 20180809. https://doi.org/10.1016/j.jmb.2018.08.005. PubMed PMID: 30099026; PMCID: PMC6204294.

150 Patel, A., Lee, H.O., Jawerth, L. et al. (2015). A liquid-to-solid phase transition of the ALS protein FUS accelerated by disease mutation. *Cell.* 162 (5): 1066–1077. https://doi.org/10.1016/j.cell.2015.07.047. PubMed PMID: 26317470.

151 Bogaert, E., Boeynaems, S., Kato, M. et al. (2018). Molecular dissection of FUS points at synergistic effect of low-complexity domains in toxicity. *Cell Rep.* 24 (3): 529–37.e4. https://doi.org/10.1016/j.celrep.2018.06.070. PubMed PMID: 30021151; PMCID: PMC6077250.

152 Yu, A.M., Choi, Y.H., and Tu, M.J. (2020). RNA drugs and RNA targets for small molecules: principles, progress, and challenges. *Pharmacol Rev.* 72 (4): 862–898. https://doi.org/10.1124/pr.120.019554. PubMed PMID: 32929000; PMCID: PMC7495341.

153 Yang, Y., Wang, Q., and Guo, D. (2008). A novel strategy for analyzing RNA-protein interactions by surface plasmon resonance biosensor. *Mol Biotechnol.* 40 (1): 87–93. Epub 20080509. https://doi.org/10.1007/s12033-008-9066-3. PubMed PMID: 18465270; PMCID: PMC7090661.

154 Feig, A.L. (2009). Studying RNA-RNA and RNA-protein interactions by isothermal titration calorimetry. *Methods Enzymol.* 468: 409–422. https://doi.org/10.1016/S0076-6879(09)68019-8. PubMed PMID: 20946780; PMCID: PMC3035487.

155 Katsamba, P.S., Park, S., and Laird-Offringa, I.A. (2002). Kinetic studies of RNA-protein interactions using surface plasmon resonance. *Methods.* 26 (2): 95–104. https://doi.org/10.1016/S1046-2023(02)00012-9. PubMed PMID: 12054886.

156 von Hacht, A., Seifert, O., Menger, M. et al. (2014). Identification and characterization of RNA guanine-quadruplex binding proteins. *Nucleic Acids Res.* 42 (10): 6630–6644. Epub 20140425. https://doi.org/10.1093/nar/gku290. PubMed PMID: 24771345; PMCID: PMC4041461.

157 Baker, J.D., Uhrich, R.L., Strovas, T.J. et al. (2020). Targeting pathological tau by small molecule inhibition of the poly(A):MSUT2 RNA-protein interaction. *ACS Chem Neurosci.* 11 (15): 2277–2285. Epub 20200709. https://doi.org/10.1021/acschemneuro.0c00214. PubMed PMID: 32589834; PMCID: PMC8629322.

158 Lightfoot, H.L., Miska, E.A., and Balasubramanian, S. (2016). Identification of small molecule inhibitors of the Lin28-mediated blockage of pre-let-7g processing. *Org Biomol Chem.* 14 (43): 10208–10216. https://doi.org/10.1039/c6ob01945e. PubMed PMID: 27731469; PMCID: PMC5433426.

159 Wang, L., Rowe, R.G., Jaimes, A. et al. (2018). Small-molecule inhibitors disrupt let-7 oligouridylation and release the selective blockade of let-7 processing by LIN28. *Cell Rep.* 23 (10): 3091–3101. https://doi.org/10.1016/j.celrep.2018.04.116. PubMed PMID: 29874593; PMCID: PMC6511231.

160 Moerke, N.J., Aktas, H., Chen, H. et al. (2007). Small-molecule inhibition of the interaction between the translation initiation factors eIF4E and eIF4G. *Cell.* 128 (2): 257–267. https://doi.org/10.1016/j.cell.2006.11.046. PubMed PMID: 17254965.

161 Minuesa, G., Antczak, C., Shum, D. et al. (2014). A 1536-well fluorescence polarization assay to screen for modulators of the MUSASHI family of RNA-binding proteins. *Comb Chem High Throughput Screen.* 17 (7): 596–609. https://doi.org/10.2174/1386207317666140609122714. PubMed PMID: 24912481; PMCID: PMC4135234.

162 Wu, X., Gardashova, G., Lan, L. et al. (2020). Targeting the interaction between RNA-binding protein HuR and FOXQ1 suppresses breast cancer invasion and metastasis. *Commun Biol.* 3 (1): 193. Epub 20200424. https://doi.org/10.1038/s42003-020-0933-1. PubMed PMID: 32332873; PMCID: PMC7181695.

163 Roos, M., Pradere, U., Ngondo, R.P. et al. (2016). A small-molecule inhibitor of Lin28. *ACS Chem Biol.* 11 (10): 2773–2781. Epub 20160822. https://doi.org/10.1021/acschembio.6b00232. PubMed PMID: 27548809.

164 Lim, D., Byun, W.G., Koo, J.Y. et al. (2016). Discovery of a small-molecule inhibitor of protein-MicroRNA interaction using binding assay with a site-specifically labeled Lin28. *J Am Chem Soc.* 138 (41): 13630–13638. Epub 20161007. https://doi.org/10.1021/jacs.6b06965. PubMed PMID: 27668966.

165 Diouf, B., Lin, W., Goktug, A. et al. (2018). Alteration of RNA splicing by small-molecule inhibitors of the interaction between NHP2L1 and U4. *SLAS Discov.* 23 (2): 164–173. Epub 20171006. https://doi.org/10.1177/2472555217735035. PubMed PMID: 28985478; PMCID: PMC5783296.

166 Borgelt, L., Li, F., Hommen, P. et al. (2021). Trisubstituted pyrrolinones as small-molecule inhibitors disrupting the protein–RNA interaction of LIN28 and Let-7. *ACS Medicinal Chemistry Letters.* 12 (6): 893–898. https://doi.org/10.1021/acsmedchemlett.0c00546.

167 Minuesa, G., Albanese, S.K., Xie, W. et al. (2019). Small-molecule targeting of MUSASHI RNA-binding activity in acute myeloid leukemia. *Nature Communications.* 10 (1): 2691. https://doi.org/10.1038/s41467-019-10523-3.

168 Sperry, S., Xiang, A., Ernst, J., et al., inventors; eFFECTOR Therapeutics, Inc., assignee. (2021) EIF4E-inhibiting 4-oxo-3,4-dihydropyrido[3,4-d]pyrimidine compounds.

169 Wade, M., Mendez, J., Coussens, N.P. et al. (2004). Inhibition of protein-protein interactions: cell-based assays. In: *Assay Guidance Manual* (ed. S. Markossian, A. Grossman, K. Brimacombe, et al.). Bethesda (MD).

170 Garner, A.L. (2018). cat-ELCCA: catalyzing drug discovery through click chemistry. *Chem Commun (Camb).* 54 (50): 6531–6539. https://doi.org/10.1039/c8cc02332h. PubMed PMID: 29781014; PMCID: PMC6008226.

171 Sherman, E.J., Lorenz, D.A., and Garner, A.L. (2019). Click chemistry-mediated complementation assay for RNA-protein interactions. *ACS Comb Sci.* 21 (7): 522–527. Epub 20190607. https://doi.org/10.1021/acscombsci.9b00071. PubMed PMID: 31181888.

172 Garner, A.L. and Janda, K.D. (2010). cat-ELCCA: a robust method to monitor the fatty acid acyltransferase activity of ghrelin O-acyltransferase (GOAT). *Angew Chem, Int Ed.* 49: 9630–9634.

173 Lorenz, D.A., Song, J.M., and Garner, A.L. (2015). High-throughput platform assay technology for the discovery of pre-microRNA-selective small molecule probes. *Bioconj Chem.* 26: 19–23.

174 Lorenz, D.A. and Garner, A.L. (2016). A click chemistry-based microRNA maturation assay optimized for high-throughput screening. *Chem Commun.* 52: 8267–8270.

175 Lorenz, D.A., Vander Roest, S., Larsen, M.J., and Garner, A.L. (2018). Development and implementation of an HTS-compatible assay for the discovery of selective small-molecule ligands for pre-microRNAs. *SLAS Disc.* 23: 47–54.

176 Lorenz, D.A., Kaur, T., Kerk, S.A. et al. (2018). Expansion of cat-ELCCA for the discovery of small molecule inhibitors of the Pre-let-7–Lin28 RNA–protein interaction. *ACS Medicinal Chemistry Letters.* 9 (6): 517–521. https://doi.org/10.1021/acsmedchemlett.8b00126.

177 Song, J.M., Menon, A., Mitchell, D.C. et al. (2017). High-throughput chemical probing of full-length protein-protein interactions. *ACS Comb Sci.* 19: 763–769.

178 Dixon, A.S., Schwinn, M.K., Hall, M.P. et al. (2016). NanoLuc complementation reporter optimized for accurate measurement of protein interactions in cells. *ACS Chem Biol.* 11 (2): 400–408. Epub 20151210. https://doi.org/10.1021/acschembio.5b00753. PubMed PMID: 26569370.

179 Los, G.V., Encell, L.P., McDougall, M.G. et al. (2008). HaloTag: a novel protein labeling technology for cell imaging and protein analysis. *ACS Chem Biol.* 3 (6): 373–382. https://doi.org/10.1021/cb800025k. PubMed PMID: 18533659.

180 Brannan, K.W., Jin, W., Huelga, S.C. et al. (2016). SONAR discovers RNA-binding proteins from analysis of large-scale protein-protein interactomes. *Mol Cell.* 64 (2): 282–293. Epub 20161006. https://doi.org/10.1016/j.molcel.2016.09.003. PubMed PMID: 27720645; PMCID: PMC5074894.

181 Castello, A., Fischer, B., Frese, C.K. et al. (2016). Comprehensive identification of RNA-binding domains in human cells. *Mol Cell.* 63 (4): 696–710. Epub 20160721. https://doi.org/10.1016/j.molcel.2016.06.029. PubMed PMID: 27453046; PMCID: PMC5003815.

182 Urbanek, M.O., Galka-Marciniak, P., Olejniczak, M., and Krzyzosiak, W.J. (2014). RNA imaging in living cells - methods and applications. *RNA Biol.* 11 (8): 1083–1095. https://doi.org/10.4161/rna.35506. PubMed PMID: 25483044; PMCID: PMC4615301.

183 Lorenz, M. (2009). Visualizing protein-RNA interactions inside cells by fluorescence resonance energy transfer. *RNA* 15 (1): 97–103. Epub 20081125. https://doi.org/10.1261/rna.1307809. PubMed PMID: 19033374; PMCID: PMC2612761.

184 Huranova, M., Jablonski, J.A., Benda, A. et al. (2009). In vivo detection of RNA-binding protein interactions with cognate RNA sequences by fluorescence resonance energy transfer. *RNA* 15 (11): 2063–2071. Epub 20090918. https://doi.org/10.1261/rna.1678209. PubMed PMID: 19767419; PMCID: PMC2764471.

185 Jazurek, M., Ciesiolka, A., Starega-Roslan, J. et al. (2016). Identifying proteins that bind to specific RNAs - focus on simple repeat expansion diseases. *Nucleic Acids Res.* 44 (19): 9050–9070. Epub 20160912. https://doi.org/10.1093/nar/gkw803. PubMed PMID: 27625393; PMCID: PMC5100574.

186 ENCODE: Encyclopedia of DNA Elements.

187 Yin, J., Zhu, D., Zhang, Z. et al. (2013). Imaging of mRNA-protein interactions in live cells using novel mCherry trimolecular fluorescence complementation systems. *PLoS One.* 8 (11): e80851. Epub 20131115. https://doi.org/10.1371/journal.pone.0080851. PubMed PMID: 24260494; PMCID: PMC3829953.

188 Han, Y., Wang, S., Zhang, Z. et al. (2014). In vivo imaging of protein-protein and RNA-protein interactions using novel far-red fluorescence complementation systems. *Nucleic Acids Res.* 42 (13): e103. Epub 20140509. https://doi.org/10.1093/nar/gku408. PubMed PMID: 24813442; PMCID: PMC4117741.

189 Gelderman, G., Sivakumar, A., Lipp, S., and Contreras, L. (2015). Adaptation of Tri-molecular fluorescence complementation allows assaying of regulatory Csr RNA-protein interactions in bacteria. *Biotechnol Bioeng.* 112 (2): 365–375. Epub 20140926. https://doi.org/10.1002/bit.25351. PubMed PMID: 25080893.

190 Porter, J.R., Stains, C.I., Jester, B.W., and Ghosh, I. (2008). A general and rapid cell-free approach for the interrogation of protein-protein, protein-DNA, and protein-RNA interactions and their antagonists utilizing split-protein reporters. *J Am Chem Soc* 130 (20): 6488–6497. Epub 20080429. https://doi.org/10.1021/ja7114579. PubMed PMID: 18444624.

191 Peabody, D.S. (1993). The RNA binding site of bacteriophage MS2 coat protein. *EMBO J.* 12 (2): 595–600. https://doi.org/10.1002/j.1460-2075.1993.tb05691.x. PubMed PMID: 8440248; PMCID: PMC413242.

192 D'Agostino, V.G., Sighel, D., Zucal, C. et al. (2019). Screening approaches for targeting ribonucleoprotein complexes: a new dimension for drug discovery. *SLAS Discov.* 24 (3): 314–331. Epub 20190107. https://doi.org/10.1177/2472555218818065. PubMed PMID: 30616427.

193 Duan, N., Arroyo, M., Deng, W. et al. (2021). Visualization and characterization of RNA-protein interactions in living cells. *Nucleic Acids Res.* 49 (18): e107. https://doi.org/10.1093/nar/gkab614. PubMed PMID: 34313753; PMCID: PMC8501972.

194 Rosenblum, S.L., Lorenz, D.A., and Garner, A.L. (2021). A live-cell assay for the detection of pre-microRNA-protein interactions. *RSC Chem Biol.* 2 (1): 241–247. Epub 20201208. https://doi.org/10.1039/d0cb00055h. PubMed PMID: 33817642; PMCID: PMC8006716.

195 Rosenblum, S.L. and Garner, A.L. (2022). RiPCA: an assay for the detection of RNA-protein interactions in live cells. *Curr Protoc.* 2 (2): e358. https://doi.org/10.1002/cpz1.358. PubMed PMID: 35113480; PMCID: PMC8852372.

196 Rosenblum, S. and Garner, A.L. (2022. Epub 20221102. https://doi.org/10.1002/cbic.202200508). Optimization of RiPCA for the live-cell detection of pre-microRNA-protein interactions. *Chembiochem* PubMed PMID: 36322053.

12

Drugging the Epitranscriptome

Tanner W. Eggert and Ralph E. Kleiner

Frick Chemistry Laboratory, Department of Chemistry, Princeton University, Washington Road, Princeton, NJ 08544, USA

12.1 Introduction

The properties of cellular RNA are modulated by a diverse array of post-transcriptional modifications. The study of these modifications, collectively known as the RNA epitranscriptome, dates back to the discovery of pseudouridine in 1951 [1], and work in subsequent decades has led to the characterization of the chemical structure of numerous abundant RNA modifications on tRNAs from model organisms (e.g. *E. coli* and yeast) [2, 3]. However, studies of the biological role of modified nucleotides *en masse* awaited the genomic era and the discovery of genes for associated RNA-modifying enzymes or "writers." The biology of some RNA modifications is also regulated by proteins known as "readers" and "erasers," which bind and remove modifications, respectively. In recent years, the investigation of RNA modification chemistry and biology has enjoyed a renaissance – in large part driven by technological advances in liquid chromatography-mass spectrometry (LC-MS) and high-throughput RNA sequencing that have alleviated some of the analytical challenges in characterizing modification sites across the transcriptome – but also propelled by the demonstration that RNA modifications can be dynamic [4–6] and serve to regulate biological processes in response to endogenous and external cues [7–10]. Further, while significant gaps exist in our fundamental understanding of RNA modification biology, numerous studies have identified connections between RNA modifications, RNA-modifying enzymes, and human disease [11–20], spurring interest from the pharmaceutical and biotechnology industries.

Over 170 structurally distinct RNA modifications have been identified in nature [21] and occur in all classes of RNA and all kingdoms of life [22]. Modifications range from simple changes such as methylation on the nucleobases or the ribose 2′-OH, isomerization, deamination, or hydrogenation, to more complex modifications involving the addition of amino acids or other small-molecule metabolites, which can require multiple biosynthetic enzymes. The function of RNA modifications is determined by their specific chemical structure and molecular context, but generally, they can impact RNA structure through modulation of

RNA as a Drug Target: The Next Frontier for Medicinal Chemistry, First Edition.
Edited by John Schneekloth and Martin Pettersson.

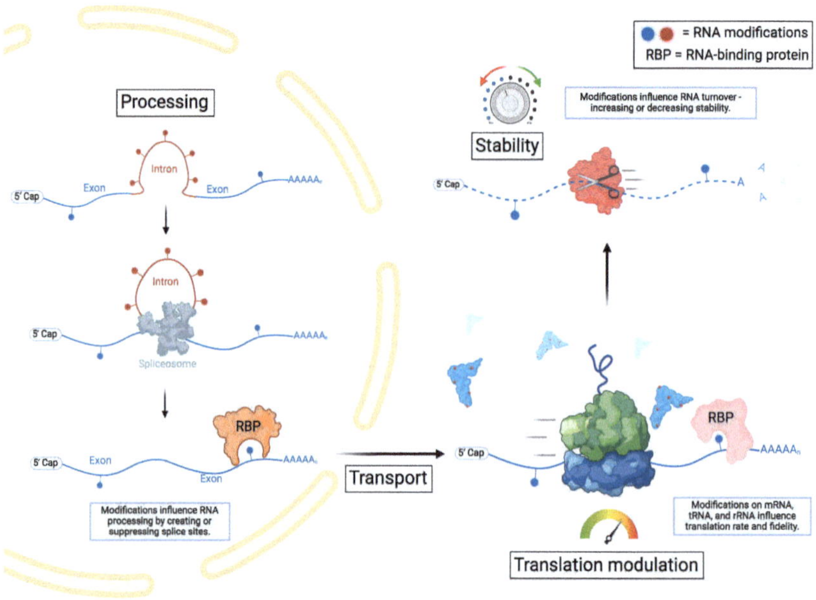

Figure 12.1 Roles of mRNA modifications.

hydrogen bonding (i.e. base pairing), base stacking, and nucleotide conformation. In addition, modifications can directly or indirectly impact functionally significant RNA–protein interactions [23–25]. These molecular mechanisms underlie the effects of RNA modifications on coding and non-coding RNA transcripts, which in turn can affect RNA metabolism [26, 27], splicing [28], and trafficking [24, 25, 29], as well as protein translation [30–33] (Figure 12.1). RNA modification-dependent perturbations in gene expression programs have been shown to impact embryonic development [34–36], learning and memory [37], and immune system function [16, 38]. The absence of specific RNA modifications has been associated with mitochondrial [39–42] and neurological disorders [43–47], while dysregulated RNA modification pathways (often resulting from perturbations in RNA modification-associated proteins) can contribute to cancer pathogenesis.

In this chapter, we highlight some of the most well-studied RNA modifications on mRNA, tRNA, and rRNA (Figure 12.2), discuss their roles in disease, and touch upon the therapeutic approaches in motion to target and exploit RNA modification pathways. Our goal is not to provide a comprehensive treatment of RNA modifications – many excellent reviews have emerged on this topic in recent years [11–18, 20, 43, 48–59]. We seek to provide a brief account of the state of inhibitor development and therapeutic use cases for modifying enzymes, identify areas for further study, and speculate on the future of pharmaceutical development in the field of epitranscriptomics. Several biotechnology companies have been established in the last 5+ years to develop drugs to target RNA modification writers. Others are developing strategies to repurpose endogenous RNA-modifying enzymes or tRNAs to facilitate transcript recoding (Table 12.1). If successful, these approaches will represent new modalities for disease treatment.

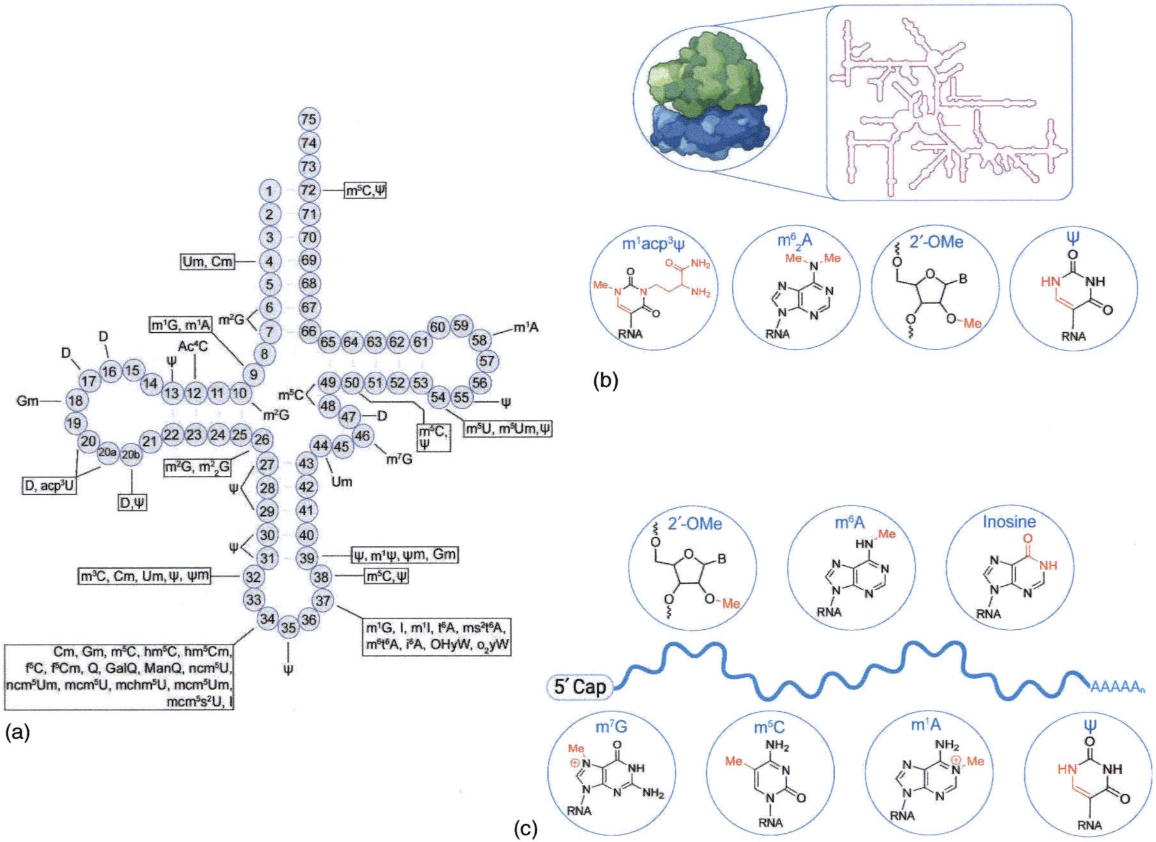

Figure 12.2 Human RNA modifications on tRNA, rRNA, and mRNA. (a) Human tRNA modifications and the positions where they occur. (b) Select rRNA modification structures. (c) Select mRNA modification structures.

Table 12.1 Companies targeting or exploiting RNA modifications.

Company	Est.	Disease Area(s)	Target(s)	Approach	Status
Accent Tx	2017	Oncology (CRC, endometrial, gastric)	DHX9	Small molecule	Pre-clinical
		Oncology (AML)	METTL3	Small molecule	Pre-clinical
		Oncology (HNSCC, NSCLC, PD-(L)1)	ADAR1	Small molecule	Pre-clinical
ADARx Pharmaceuticals	2019	alpha-1 antitrypsin deficiency	ADAR1	Oligo-based ADAR recruitment	N/A
A2I Tx/AtomWise	2020	Immuno-oncology (NSCLC, TNBC)	ADAR1	Small molecule	N/A
Covant Tx/Boehringer Ingelheim	2017	Immuno-oncology	ADAR1	Small molecule	N/A
Edigene	2015	Usher syndrome type 2, Hurler syndrome	ADAR1	Oligo-based ADAR recruitment	Discovery
EPICS Tx	2018	Oncology (AML, solid tumors)	METTL3	Small molecule	Pre-clinical
Gotham Tx (858 Tx)	2017	Oncology	METTL3	Small molecule	N/A
Gossamer Bio	2015	Immuno-oncology	ADAR1	Small molecule	Discovery
Korro Bio/Genevant	2018	alpha-1 antitrypsin deficiency	ADAR1	Oligo-based ADAR recruitment	Discovery
ProQR/Eli lilly	2012	Cholestatic disorders, cardiovascular, metabolic, neurodegenerative	ADAR1	Oligo-based ADAR recruitment	Pre-clinical
Shape Tx	2018	Parkinson's, Alzheimer's, alpha-1 antitrypsin deficiency, Rett syndrome	ADAR1 mRNA	Oligo-based ADAR recruitment	N/A
			Premature stop codons	Engineered suppressor tRNAs	N/A
			Gene replacement	Tailored gene expression	N/A
STORM Tx/Exelixis	2015	Oncology (solid tumors)	METTL3	Small molecule	Phase 1
		Oncology (solid tumors)	ADAR1	Small molecule	N/A
Wave Life Sciences	2012	alpha-1 antitrypsin deficiency	ADAR1	Oligo-based ADAR recruitment	Pre-clinical
858 Tx	2019	Oncology (solid tumors)	ADAR1	Small molecule	Pre-clinical

12.2 Modifications on mRNA: N^6-Methyladenosine, Pseudouridine, and Inosine

Modifications on mRNA (Figure 12.2) are less abundant and diverse than those on non-coding RNAs but have attracted significant attention in the last 10+ years as advances in sequencing strategies have enabled the characterization of modification sites across the transcriptome [60–63]. It is now well appreciated that several modified nucleotides are commonly found in coding transcripts [7, 60, 62–65]. In this section, we will avoid discussing post-transcriptional mRNA modifications involved in transcript processing such as polyadenylation, 5′-cap, and splicing, which have been reviewed extensively elsewhere [66–70], and will focus instead on the most abundant internal mRNA modifications – N^6-methyladenosine (m^6A), pseudouridine (Ψ), and inosine (I).

12.2.1 N^6-Methyladenosine (m^6A)

The most abundant internal mRNA modification in eukaryotes is N^6-methyladenosine (m^6A), which occurs at a frequency of 1 in 200 adenosines or about 0.5% in mammals [71]. Despite its discovery in 1974 [71, 72], there were few studies of m^6A until the development of m^6A-specific sequencing technologies in 2012 (MeRIP-seq and m^6A-seq) [60, 73], which enabled the mapping of individual m^6A-modified transcripts and modification sites across the transcriptome, revealing its enrichment in the 3′-UTR and at characteristic GG(m^6A)CU sequence motifs. These early approaches have since been superseded by methods that can more efficiently map m^6A sites at single-nucleotide resolution and measure modification stoichiometry [74–78], and analogous approaches have been developed or are in development for other epitranscriptomic mRNA modifications [62, 63, 79–82].

Installation of m^6A on mRNA is catalyzed by the METTL3/METTL14 core methyltransferase complex together with a host of adaptor proteins (i.e. WTAP and RBM15) [83–85]. Oxidative demethylase eraser enzymes fat mass and obesity-associated (FTO) and AlkB homolog 5 (ALKBH5) can convert m^6A back to A [4, 5]. Knockdown of METTL3 is embryonic lethal in mice and significantly impacts the viability of cultured cells [86]. Levels of m^6A are dynamic and fluctuate in response to cellular state [60, 87], but the mechanisms underlying this regulation are still poorly understood. Notably, recent studies have suggested that deposition of m^6A on mRNA is primarily controlled by the exon–junction complex (EJC) through a steric occlusion model [88–90], explaining its enrichment in long exons and near stop codons (terminal exons tend to be longer).

The function of m^6A on mRNA has been studied extensively by multiple groups, and consensus has emerged on a role for m^6A in accelerating the turnover of modified transcripts [26, 27, 91], which is important in multiple biological processes [34, 35]. In addition, roles in splicing [28], nuclear export [25], translation [27, 31, 32, 92], and cytosolic trafficking [29] have been reported. A further role for m^6A involves m^6A-modified chromatin-associated regulatory RNAs (carRNAs), which can modulate chromatin accessibility and transcription [93]. The mechanism for m^{6}A function is thought to primarily involve recognition of this mark by reader proteins, predominantly YTH-domain proteins YTHDF1-3 [27, 29, 32, 37, 91, 94] and YTHDC1-2 [28, 31], but also other reported readers such as IGF2BP1-3 [92] and FMR1 [95, 96]. Canonical RNA structure is also perturbed by m^{6}A, although W-C pairing is still possible [97].

Given the abundance of m^{6}A and its effects on mRNA transcript behavior, it is perhaps unsurprising that aberrant levels of this modification have been associated with disease pathogenesis and progression. These include over a dozen types of cancer, such as glioblastoma [56, 98, 99], breast [100–104], lung [105–107], blood [108, 109], and pancreatic cancers [110–114]; neurological disorders like depression [115, 116], Attention Deficit Hyperactivity Disorder (ADHD) [117], and Alzheimer's [118]; osteoporosis [119], viral infections [120, 121], metabolic disorders [12, 122–124], and cardiovascular diseases [12, 51]. Considerable research efforts have been devoted to exploring m^{6}A in cancer, and this work has been reviewed elsewhere [14, 54, 56, 103–105, 124–128]. Here, we will discuss some of the approaches taken to drug the m^{6}A machinery to treat cancer.

Overexpression of m^{6}A methyltransferase METTL3 is implicated in at least eight types of cancer where it behaves as an oncogene [107, 109, 114], but this is not strictly the case as METTL3 can also act as a tumor suppressor [129–131]. Mechanisms of METTL3-mediated oncogenesis vary across different cancers. For example, in acute myeloid leukemia (AML), METTL3 promotes the translation of MYC, BCL2, and PTEN mRNAs [109]. In glioblastoma, METTL3 promotes the stability of SOX2 mRNA [132]. Numerous small-molecule inhibitors of METTL3 have been reported in the literature [133–136], and at least three private companies are working to develop METTL3 inhibitor drugs (Table 12.1). STORM Therapeutics (Cambridge, UK) has announced a clinical trial for its compound, STC-15, an orally available small-molecule inhibitor of METTL3. STC-15 has shown efficacy in AML models [137]; however, the phase 1 study, which began in late 2022, will evaluate activity in solid tumors, rather than AML [138]. The precursor to STC-15, STM-2457, was developed by STORM Therapeutics together with the Kouzarides and Tzelepis groups [133]. STM-2457 was identified in a high-throughput screen and inhibits METTL3 catalytic activity (IC_{50} = 16.9 nM) by competing with the *S*-adenosyl-methionine (SAM) co-factor. Despite engaging the SAM-binding site, STM-2457 is highly specific for METTL3, demonstrating 1000-fold selectivity over 45 other DNA, RNA, and protein methyltransferases. The molecular selectivity likely arises from divergence in SAM-binding sites among methyltransferase enzymes, the dissimilarity of STM-2457 to SAM and other known methyltransferase inhibitors, and structural reorganization in the enzyme active site upon compound binding. STM-2457 potently inhibits METTL3 in cells and mice and reduces m^{6}A levels in a dose-dependent fashion. It selectively inhibits the growth of AML cell lines over non-leukemic cells, consistent with the importance of METTL3 catalytic function for leukemia growth. Mechanistically, STM-2457 reduces the m^{6}A level and translational efficiency of METTL3-dependent leukemogenic mRNAs, impairing AML stem cell self-renewal. Studies with STM-2457 in human AML-derived xenografts prolonged mouse lifespan by 75% or more, with mechanistic effects mirroring *in vitro* observations and showing minimal off-target toxicity. In addition to STORM Therapeutics, other companies developing METTL3 inhibitors include Gotham Therapeutics, Accent Therapeutics, and EPICS Therapeutics (Table 12.1). Gotham Therapeutics, acquired by 858 Therapeutics in 2021, is evaluating undisclosed solid tumor targets. Accent Therapeutics is also targeting METTL3 in AML in partnership with Ipsen [139], and has partnered with AstraZeneca to develop inhibitors for undisclosed RNA-modifying enzymes [140]. The outcome of STORM's STC-15 trial and whether other METTL3 inhibitors make it to clinical trials soon will be significant milestones for the epitranscriptomics field.

Perturbation of m^6A levels for therapeutic benefit can also be accomplished by targeting m^6A eraser enzymes. FTO and ALKBH5 are the major m^6A demethylases [4, 5] and belong to the Fe^{2+}, O_2, alpha-ketoglutarate-dependent dioxygenase family. FTO can also demethylate N^6, 2′-*O*-dimethyladenosine (m^6A_m) and m^1A on tRNA [141]. Like METTL3, FTO and ALKBH5 dysregulation is associated with various diseases such as obesity [142–146], multiple malignancies [98, 102, 106, 108, 111, 113, 147–152], neurological disease [43, 153–155], metabolic disease [156], and developmental disorders [157, 158]. Much of the early research around FTO focused on the enzyme's role in obesity-related phenotypes [145, 146]. Studies have also shown that FTO plays an important role in tumorigenesis, serving both oncogenic and tumor suppressor functions. For example, in AML, FTO overexpression leads to m^6A-dependent destabilization of ASB2 and RARA mRNAs and stabilization of MYC and CEBPA mRNAs which promotes leukemogenesis [108]. Similar mechanisms of oncogenesis occur in other cancers, affecting a variety of target transcripts and associated biological processes [144, 145, 159]. In contrast, in ovarian cancer stem cells, FTO acts as a tumor suppressor by regulating m^6A levels on two phosphodiesterase transcripts [148]. Similar to FTO, ALKBH5 has also been implicated as an oncogene in a wide variety of cancers and as a tumor suppressor in a few others [151, 152]. Thus far, reported FTO inhibitors have been shown to exhibit anti-cancer activities in AML [160–162], glioblastoma [99], esophageal cancer [163], and breast cancer [101, 164]. ALKBH5 inhibitors have also been developed and show some anti-cancer activity in glioblastoma cells [149, 165] and leukemia cells [166]. Many reported compounds for both enzymes suffer from poor potency, selectivity, or both. Due to the similarity among Fe^{2+}, α-KG-dependent enzymes, a major challenge in the development of effective compounds is achieving selectivity. To our knowledge, as of July 2023, no small-molecule drug for FTO or ALKBH5 is currently in clinical development.

12.2.2 Pseudouridine (Ψ)

The abundance of pseudouridine (Ψ) on mRNA is similar to m^6A, accounting for ~0.3% of all uridine (U) residues [167]. Ψ is an isomer of U (Figure 12.2) containing a C5-glycosyl linkage and an extra N^1-hydrogen bond. Ψ possesses enhanced base-stacking and base-pairing ability over U [168, 169]. It was the first RNA modification discovered and was initially shown to exist at specific sites in tRNA [1, 170, 171] and rRNA [172, 173]. Its presence in mRNA was not known until 2014

[62, 63]. Since Ψ base pairs similarly to U, mapping is performed through chemical derivatization of RNA to generate Ψ-based adducts that induce reverse transcription termination or misincorporation [62, 63]. Early approaches used the enhanced reactivity of Ψ toward the carbodiimide compound CMC [173], but more recently, methods based upon bisulfite reactivity have been used successfully [167, 174]. The biological role of Ψ in mRNA is still poorly understood, but sites primarily occur in coding regions and the 3′-UTR [62, 63] and show dynamic regulation [175]. Multiple studies have implicated Ψ in translational control [176]. Some Ψ sites can promote stop-codon readthrough [177, 178], and *in vitro* translation assays have indicated that Ψ slows ribosomal elongation and promotes misincorporation at certain codons [179]. Roles of Ψ in transcript stability [180] and pre-mRNA splicing [181] have also been reported, although the mechanisms are unknown.

Ψ is installed by pseudouridine synthase (PUS) enzymes, of which there are 13 in humans. These fall into two categories: RNA-dependent (those that utilize an RNA guide strand) and RNA-independent stand-alone enzymes [182]. Ψ is widespread on all types of RNA, and therefore it is no surprise that Ψ and PUS enzymes have broad disease relevance and have been shown to be dysregulated in cancer [183, 184], mitochondrial and metabolic disorders [185, 186], and neurodevelopmental disorders [187–189], and even influence HIV pathology [190]. These diseases often harbor mutated PUS genes, such as in mitochondrial myopathy, which results from mutations in PUS1 [185] and dyskeratosis congenita and Hoyeraal–Hreidarsson syndrome, which results from mutations in DKC1 [191], an RNA-dependent PUS. Recently, PUS7 was implicated in glioblastoma through a tRNA-pseudouridylation mechanism, and small-molecule inhibitors of the enzyme were shown to impede tumorigenesis [192]. While there is still much to learn about the role of Ψ in normal and disease biology, therapeutic targeting of specific Ψ sites will likely prove challenging due to the large number of related PUS enzymes and their promiscuous activity on coding and non-coding RNA transcripts (in some cases, individual PUS enzymes appear to modify different classes of RNA substrates [193]); therefore, even targeted efforts will likely have collateral effects. Further, PUS enzymes do not possess a co-factor binding site that can be readily exploited for small-molecule targeting. While we are not aware of therapeutic programs to develop PUS-inhibiting compounds, Ψ and its derivatives are exploited therapeutically. The ability of artificial Ψ modifications to suppress innate immune activation via Toll-like receptors (TLRs) [38, 180] and other pattern recognition receptors is used widely in mRNA therapeutic development including the recent SARS-CoV-2 mRNA vaccines, which employ a Ψ derivative, N^1-Me-Ψ, at all U positions to achieve two functions: (i) suppress TLR immune stimulation and protein kinase R (PKR) activation [194–196], and (ii) enhance protein production by boosting ribosome loading [197–199].

12.2.3 Inosine (I)

Inosine (I) is an abundant RNA modification first discovered at the wobble position of yeast $tRNA^{Ala}$ in 1965 [171]. Its discovery in mRNA came several decades later

[64, 200]. Inosine is installed by ADARs (adenosine deaminase acting on RNA) and the tRNA-specific ADATs. Three ADARs exist in humans, ADAR1-3, and ADAR3 is catalytically inactive. These enzymes hydrolytically deaminate the N^6-position of adenosine (A) to yield inosine in a process referred to as A-to-I editing or simply RNA editing. Inosine exhibits base-pairing properties distinct from A. Inosine on tRNA facilitates wobble decoding, while inosine on mRNA is read as G during translation and reverse transcription, effectively recoding the sequence information in an mRNA transcript.

As with any modification, understanding its prevalence and distribution is critical to understanding its function. Sequencing technologies for inosine capitalize on its interpretation as G by biological machinery, and putative sites can be identified as A-to-G mutations when comparing whole transcriptome RNA-seq data to a reference genome [201, 202]. Stringent bioinformatic pipelines have been developed to reliably identify high-confidence inosine sites [203], and chemoenzymatic methods for inosine detection have also been utilized [80, 200, 204]. Inosine on mRNA serves two primary roles in mammals: (i) mRNA recoding, and (ii) regulation of innate immune activation. Estimates for inosine sites in human mRNA range from 15,000 to 36,000 [201, 205], with the vast majority occurring in repetitive Alu repeats, and roughly 50–200 recoding sites occurring in non-repetitive sequences [202, 206–208]. RNA editing is critical in the nervous system, where several inosine-mediated recoding events are important for protein function, including editing sites in GluR-B receptor [209–215] and serotonin 2C receptor [216]. Defective editing on these and other substrates can lead to neurodegenerative [217, 218] and neuropsychiatric disorders [219]. Recoding events are less common outside of the nervous system, but have been characterized in NEIL1 [220, 221], a DNA repair protein, and Filamin A, an actin crosslinking protein [222, 223]. Emerging evidence suggests that recoding sites may number over 1,000 and contribute to diversity across cellular subpopulations [203, 224], although most sites are weakly edited, and their functional relevance needs to be further interrogated. Protein recoding through programmable RNA editing has become an active area in pharmaceutical drug development, and several companies aim to harness endogenous ADAR activity for this purpose (Table 12.1), but an extensive commentary on this approach is outside the scope of this chapter [225].

Many inosine sites occur in double-stranded RNA (dsRNA), which plays an important role in regulating the innate immune response. DsRNAs are characteristic of viral infection and are recognized by the cytosolic nucleic acid sensor MDA5 to induce a type I interferon response [226]. Editing of endogenous dsRNAs by ADAR1 prevents their recognition by MDA5 and induction of an auto-immune response [227, 228]. Consistent with this function, ADAR1-deficient mice do not survive embryonic development and display activated interferon and nucleic acid sensing pathways [229] – embryonic lethality is rescued by concurrent knockout of MDA5 [230]. In humans, loss-of-function mutations in ADAR1 lead to autoimmune diseases [231]. On the other hand, some cancers appear to be "addicted" to ADAR1 activity to suppress immune surveillance, and these cancers are susceptible to ADAR1 inhibition [232, 233]. Therefore, ADAR1 inhibition has emerged as a promising strategy for treating cancers directly or sensitizing them to immunotherapy [232, 234–238].

Efforts to develop small-molecule ADAR1 inhibitors are still in the early stages. The earliest reported inhibitors of ADAR1 were the adenosine analogs 8-chloroadenosine and 8-azadenosine, although recent data has indicated that these compounds are broadly cytotoxic rather than specific ADAR1 inhibitors [239]. In 2021, a pre-print article reported that the compound ZYS-1 (2-fluoro, 5′-chloro-adenosine) inhibited ADAR1 with an IC_{50} of 866 nM and suppressed the growth of prostate cancer cells [240], demonstrating that nucleoside-based scaffolds may provide fruitful starting points for ADAR1 inhibitors. Nucleoside analogs can be incorporated into synthetic dsRNA duplexes to inhibit ADAR1, relying upon its preference for binding to dsRNA [241]. These modified oligos are useful for biochemical and structural studies of the enzyme but are likely of limited utility as therapeutic agents due to delivery/bioavailability challenges. Interestingly, a recent report [242] identified a macrolide ADAR1 inhibitor, Rebecsinib, which functions by altering splicing and expression of the malignant ADAR1 p150 isoform, rather than direct protein engagement. Rebecsinib inhibits leukemic stem cell (LSC) self-renewal and prolongs survival in a humanized LSC mouse model. In addition to reports from academic groups, multiple industrial efforts to develop ADAR1-inhibiting compounds are underway. STORM Therapeutics (in partnership with Exelixis), Accent Therapeutics, Covant Therapeutics (in partnership with Boehringer Ingelheim), A2I Therapeutics (in partnership with Atomwise), and 858 Therapeutics all have ongoing ADAR1 programs (Table 12.1), although few details regarding these efforts are publicly available. Gossamer Bio has developed an ADAR1 inhibitor, GB-10037 (IC_{50} of 259 nM), and is pursuing this compound for immuno-oncology [243]. Given the amount of interest in the pharmaceutical and biotechnology industries, it is likely that promising ADAR1 inhibitors will begin to undergo pre-clinical/clinical evaluation in the near future.

12.3 Modifications on tRNA and rRNA

While much of the recent effort in studying and targeting epitranscriptomic pathways has focused on mRNA modifications (particularly m^6A and inosine), RNA modifications are considerably more diverse and abundant on non-coding RNAs. In particular, tRNAs are the most heavily modified RNA species with an average of 13 modifications per tRNA molecule [244], and tRNA modifications were the first to be identified and characterized [170, 171] (Figure 12.2). Modifications play important roles in tRNA and rRNA biology, and dysregulation of non-coding RNA modifications has been implicated in a wide variety of human diseases, as discussed below.

12.3.1 tRNA Modifications

Modifications on tRNA were first identified in yeast with Holley's elucidation of the chemical structure of yeast $tRNA^{Ala}$, which revealed multiple modified nucleotides distributed throughout the sequence including inosine, dihydrouridine, pseudouridine, 5-methyluridine (ribothymidine), and methylated guanosine [171]. Notably, Holley's identification of inosine in the anticodon motivated Crick's formulation of the "wobble hypothesis" [245]. Indeed, modifications in the anticodon stem-loop (ASL) are among the most prevalent and serve to facilitate proper codon-anticodon pairing, recognition by the ribosome and aminoacyl-tRNA synthetases, and maintenance of reading frame [246–248]. Studies of individual tRNAs from different organisms revealed that a subset of modifications were broadly conserved across many different tRNA species and throughout evolution, whereas others were tRNA and/or species-specific. For example, modifications in the D arm and T arm – dihydrouridine, ribothymidine, and pseudouridine – are found broadly across different tRNAs and different kingdoms of life [22, 249], whereas lysidine is a modification only present in bacteria [250]. While the full complement of tRNA modifications has been largely known for multiple decades, particularly in model organisms such as *E. coli* and yeast [2], the function of many tRNA modifications is still mysterious since the corresponding tRNA-modifying enzymes have been characterized much more recently, or are largely uncharacterized, as is the case with many mammalian tRNA-modifying enzymes. Further, characterizing the global distribution, stoichiometry, and dynamics of modifications across all cellular tRNA species is still a major challenge but has benefited from advances in high-throughput [251, 252] and single-molecule [253–258] RNA sequencing technologies and advanced mass spectrometry methods [251, 259].

RNA modifications play a vital role in tRNA function and can regulate tRNA folding, stability, aminoacylation ("charging"), and decoding ability [11, 13, 244, 246, 248] (Figure 12.3). These properties affect the translation of corresponding gene products in a codon-specific manner. Historically, tRNAs and their modifications were viewed as static entities relegated to a fundamental housekeeping role; however, it is now appreciated that the tRNA pool is dynamic and can regulate translational programs in response to cellular state or environmental cues [260–262]. In addition, tRNAs can be cleaved to generate tRNA-derived fragments (tRFs) that can play a gene regulatory role [263–265].

Deficiencies in tRNA modifications impair tRNA function and are associated with many human diseases, termed "tRNA modopathies." Comprehensive reviews of tRNA modifications [11, 246, 248] and tRNA modopathies [11, 13, 17–20, 41, 47, 266] have been published elsewhere, and we refer the reader to these resources. Here, we provide a summary of major findings.

Dysregulation of tRNA modifications most commonly manifests as diseases of the brain (e.g. microcephaly and intellectual disabilities), but also is associated with disorders of the mitochondria, kidneys, and cancer [11, 13, 17–20, 41, 47, 266]. Mutation or altered expression of 54 tRNA-modifying enzymes is associated with tRNA modopathies [13]; however, the precise biochemical mechanisms of pathogenesis have only been worked out for a few of these diseases. Generally, tRNA modopathies result from alterations in codon-specific translation corresponding to the aberrantly modified tRNA species, although other mechanisms are possible, such as alterations in the production of tRNA-derived fragments. In neurological

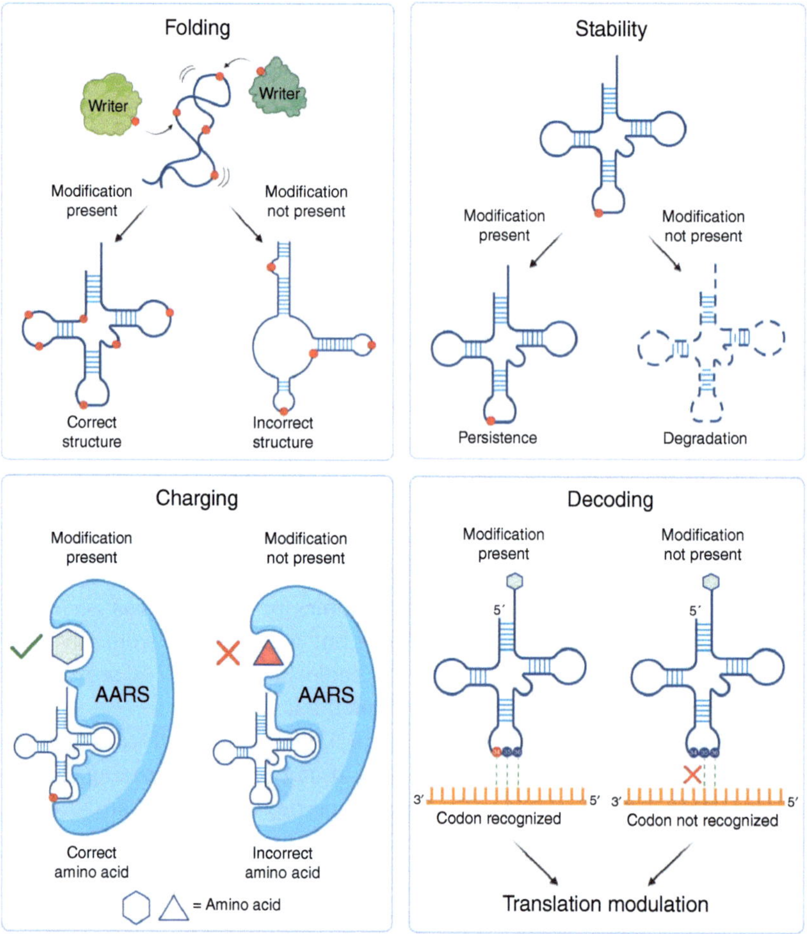

Figure 12.3 Roles of tRNA modifications.

and mitochondrial disorders, modification levels are often reduced through mutation or reduced expression of the modification writer, whereas in cancer, writers are often overexpressed or hyperactive, leading to increased modification levels [11, 13, 17–20, 41, 47, 266].

tRNA modifications such as m^1A, m^5C, m^3C, m^7G, Ψ, and mcm^5s^2U have been implicated in over a dozen cancers. Among the best characterized cancer-associated modifications are the wobble uridine modifications (e.g. mcm^5s^2U) installed by an enzyme cascade involving the Elongator complex, the CTU1/2 complex, and ALKBH8 [267]. Wobble uridine modifications are present on 11 tRNAs and play important roles in maintaining efficient translation and preventing protein misfolding [267–269]. In cancers, these modifications drive specific translational programs that induce malignant transformation. For example, mcm^5s^2U maintains translation of HIF1α protein to promote glycolysis in melanoma [268]. In breast cancer, translation of the oncoprotein DEK relies upon wobble uridine modification [270]. METTL1-WDR4, which installs m^7G46 on certain tRNAs, can also contribute to tumorigenesis through translational reprogramming [271–273]. Overexpression of many other tRNA-modifying enzymes [13] has been associated with cancer, although mechanistic links are often lacking.

Aberrant tRNA modification has been shown to play a role in many neurological disorders including microcephaly, autism, cerebellar ataxia, amyotrophic lateral sclerosis (ALS), and general intellectual disability [11, 13, 45, 47]. Mutations in the methyltransferase TRMT1, which installs $m^2{}_2G26$ on multiple tRNAs, have been linked to microcephaly and intellectual disability [274]. TRMT1-deficient cells exhibit increased reactive oxygen species (ROS) levels, decreased growth rates, and altered protein synthesis [275]. Proposed roles for $m^2{}_2G$ include facilitating proper tRNA folding and recognition by the ribosome [275]. Mutations in NSUN2, which installs m^5C at positions 48–50 in tRNAs, result in hypomodification and the accumulation of angiogenin-produced tRNA fragments, reducing protein translation rates and activating stress responses [45]. This leads to the apoptotic death of striatal, cortical, and hippocampal neurons and leads to Dubowitz syndrome [46], characterized by microcephaly, short stature, and growth and mental retardation. Mutations in WDR4/METTL1, described above in relation to cancer, also have neuronal phenotypes and have been linked to primordial dwarfism and brain malformation [276].

Mitochondria encode their own set of tRNAs, which possess both common and unique modifications compared to nuclear-encoded tRNAs [277]. Two of the most well-studied mitochondrial disorders connected to tRNA modification levels include MELAS (mitochondrial encephalomyopathy, lactate acidosis, and stroke-like episodes) and MERRF (myoclonus epilepsy associated with ragged-red fibers), which result from 5-taurinomethyl (MELAS) and 5-taurinomethyl-2-thio (MERRF) hypomodification at U34 in the ASL of mt-$tRNA^{Leu(UUR)}$ and mt-$tRNA^{Lys}$ [41]. This modification is installed by the MTO1-GTPBP3 complex [278, 279], and MTO1 knockout is embryonic lethal in mice [39]. Taurine modification deficiency results in mitochondrial structure abnormalities, decreased mitochondrial protein synthesis, and reduced oxidative phosphorylation activity. Patients with these diseases typically possess mutations in the mt-tRNA genes, which reduce modification levels at U34 [42], or mutations in MTO1 and GTPBP3 [40].

There are treatment options for MELAS patients. The first is simply high-dose oral administration of taurine [280, 281], which was shown to marginally increase the level of taurinomethyl modification at U34 in mt-$tRNA^{Leu(UUR)}$ [282]. The second treatment, not yet shown to be efficacious in treating mitochondrial disease but being tested in humans for other diseases, is tauroursodeoxycholic acid. This compound acts as a chemical chaperone to improve protein folding and prevent aggregation, compensating for translational defects observed in MELAS patients [39]. A genetic editing approach using TALEN was demonstrated to have some restorative function in cells [283], but applying this technique in humans would require editing of mitochondrial DNA in oocytes. Gene- and peptide-mediated therapies have been explored in both MELAS and MERRF *in cellulo* with some success [284]. For both MELAS and MERRF, treatments largely focus on symptom management such as prescribing anticonvulsants for seizures and physical therapy for impaired motor function. However, some patients have responded modestly to vitamins and supplements which improve mitochondrial function [285].

At the time of writing, there are limited approved therapies for treating tRNA modopathies. In diseases caused by hypomodification of tRNA, enzyme reactivation or replacement would be required to address the molecular basis of the disorder. Notably, several companies are attempting to use tRNA as a therapeutic (Table 12.1). For example, Tevard Biosciences is developing suppressor tRNAs to treat diseases caused by premature stop codons, including Dravet syndrome and Duchenne muscular dystrophy (in partnership with Vertex). Additionally, they are working to deliver specific tRNAs to diseased cells caused by haploinsufficiency to compensate for the reduced levels of those specific tRNAs. Other companies like hC Bioscience, Alltrna, and Shape Therapeutics are developing similar tRNA therapies. These approaches are not designed to correct aberrant tRNA modification levels, per se, but may be able to compensate for defects in tRNA function caused by hypomodification. Further, given that these tRNAs will be expressed in human cells, they are likely to accumulate native modifications which will affect their function.

12.3.2 rRNA Modifications

Ribosomal RNA (rRNA) is the most abundant RNA species. The scope of rRNA modifications is narrower than those that occur on tRNAs and includes Ψ and ribose 2′-*O*-methylation [286]. There are some unique modifications to rRNA, such as $m^1acp^3\Psi$ [287] and $m^6{}_2A$ [286] (Figure 12.2). Collectively, these affect ribosome structure, translational rate, and fidelity [286]. Several modifications have important roles in rRNA processing [286]. Ribosomal RNA modifications are installed by standalone enzymes and by small nucleolar ribonucleoproteins (snoRNPs). These complexes consist of a short RNA molecule that hybridizes with the rRNA to site-specifically direct the catalytic machinery. Modifications on rRNA are clustered around important functional sites in the ribosome i.e. the tRNA-binding sites, peptidyltransferase center, and the 40S/60S subunit interface. Interestingly, the loss of some modifications is not critical to ribosome function, and deleterious phenotypic effects are sometimes only observed when multiple modifications are lost simultaneously, but this is not universal [286].

Diseases can result from the dysregulation of rRNA modifications. For example, a single-point mutation in the EMG1 gene, an 18S rRNA Ψ methyltransferase that generates $m^1\Psi$, results in Bowen–Conradi syndrome [288], a very rare disease characterized by moderate-to-severe pre- and post-natal growth retardation, microcephaly, developmental malformations, and is typically lethal during infancy. Other examples include Williams–Beuren syndrome resulting from deletions of WBSCR22 and NSUN5, both of which are methyltransferases [289]. Mutations or changes in the expression of snoRNP components have been implicated in cancers such as Burkitt's lymphoma [290] and metastatic melanoma [291–293]. X-linked dyskeratosis congenita is connected to aberrant Ψ modification levels on rRNA [184, 191, 294]. 2′-*O*-methylation levels have also been linked to multiple cancers.

Overexpression of the methyltransferase fibrillarin results in increased levels of 2′-*O*-Me modifications, decreased translational quality control, and increased internal ribosome entry site (IRES)-mediated translation of cancer-related genes [295]. Ribosome biogenesis has become an attractive anti-cancer target, and multiple compounds exist that inhibit rRNA transcription, processing, or ribosome assembly [296]. These drugs include platinum-based compounds, the RNA polymerase I inhibitor actinomycin D, 5-fluorouridine, and poly-ADP ribose polymerase (PARP) inhibitors. A newer promising drug, CX-5461 [297], has been shown to inhibit Pol I transcription and has already completed a phase 1 clinical trial. To the best of our knowledge, no treatments are yet in development that target specific rRNA-modifying enzymes or snoRNP levels; however, such compounds could conceivably be added to the arsenal of ribosome biogenesis inhibitors.

12.4 Concluding Remarks

The study of RNA modifications has emerged as a major area in biomedical research. As highlighted in this chapter, there is a large diversity of post-transcriptional modifications occurring on all types of RNA. These modifications regulate gene expression through different mechanisms and play an important role in biology. Clear links to human disease resulting from absence or dysregulation of modifications have been established, and therapeutics targeting RNA modification-associated proteins, or exploiting modification pathways, are in active development. Arguably, we have only scratched the surface of the ~170 different modified nucleotides that are known in biological systems.

With expanding studies of RNA modification biology and disease-associated phenotypes, we urge caution in interpreting the effects of modification pathways given the significant gaps in the characterization of RNA modification sites and associated molecular mechanisms. RNA modification mapping is still largely a cottage industry [252], and we lack unified approaches for characterizing the distribution and stoichiometry of multiple RNA modifications transcriptome-wide in a single biological sample. Recently, direct RNA sequencing technologies such as nanopore sequencing (commercialized by Oxford Nanopore Technologies) offer the promise of quantitative modification sequencing across multiple modification types [253]; however, it is becoming apparent that only a subset of epitranscriptomic modifications can be readily detected using this technology in its current implementation [298]. In addition to modification mapping, identification and characterization of relevant RNA-modifying enzymes is still incomplete in many organisms. Continued innovation in technologies for mapping RNA modifications [167, 299] and identifying and characterizing RNA-modifying enzymes [65, 300] are likely to have a considerable impact on the future of the epitranscriptomics field. Once these methods are in place and widely accessible, functional studies of individual modification sites, connecting observations in defined *in vitro* systems with cell biological and organismal phenotypes, should enable the development of rigorous molecular frameworks for understanding RNA modification biology.

Finally, despite the rapid development of METTL3 inhibitors, there are currently few available small-molecule modulators of RNA-modifying enzymes. While nucleic-acid-modifying enzymes do present some unique molecular challenges compared to more traditional protein targets, the success with METTL3 and the recent emergence of ADAR1 inhibitors suggest that the standard tools of small-molecule discovery and medicinal chemistry can be readily applied to this class of proteins. Therefore, leveraging advances in chemical biology, structural biology, medicinal chemistry, and *in silico* screening, among other approaches, will likely yield promising starting points for small-molecule probes. Such compounds will not only accelerate therapeutic development but can also serve as tool compounds to facilitate the chemical genetic exploration of the diverse biological role(s) of RNA modification-associated proteins.

References

1 Cohn, W.E. and Volkin, E. (1951). Nucleoside-5′-phosphates from ribonucleic acid. *Nature* 167: 483–484.

2 de Crécy-Lagard, V. and Jaroch, M. (2021). Functions of bacterial tRNA modifications: from ubiquity to diversity. *Trends Microbiol.* 29: 41–53.

3 de Crecy-Lagard, V., Boccaletto, P., Mangleburg, C.G. et al. (2019). Matching tRNA modifications in humans to their known and predicted enzymes. *Nucleic Acids Res.* 47: 2143–2159.

4 Jia, G., Fu, Y.E., Zhao, X.U. et al. (2011). N^6-Methyladenosine in nuclear RNA is a major substrate of the obesity-associated FTO. *Nat. Chem. Biol.* 7: 885–887.

5 Zheng, G., Dahl, J.A., Niu, Y. et al. (2013). ALKBH5 is a mammalian RNA demethylase that impacts RNA metabolism and mouse fertility. *Mol. Cell* 49: 18–29.

6 Jia, G., Yang, C.G., Yang, S. et al. (2008). Oxidative demethylation of 3-methylthymine and 3-methyluracil in single-stranded DNA and RNA by mouse and human FTO. *FEBS Lett.* 582: 3313–3319.

7 Dominissini, D. et al. (2016). The dynamic N(1)-methyladenosine methylome in eukaryotic messenger RNA. *Nature* 530: 441–446.

8 Li, X., Xiong, X., Wang, K. et al. (2016). Transcriptome-wide mapping reveals reversible and dynamic N(1)-methyladenosine methylome. *Nat. Chem. Biol.* 12: 311–316.

9 Roundtree, I.A., Evans, M.E., Pan, T., and He, C. (2017). Dynamic RNA modifications in gene expression regulation. *Cell* 169: 1187–1200.

10 Liu, F., Clark, W., Luo, G. et al. (2016). ALKBH1-mediated tRNA demethylation regulates translation. *Cell* 167: 816–828.e816.

11 Suzuki, T. (2021). The expanding world of tRNA modifications and their disease relevance. *Nat. Rev. Mol. Cell Biol.* 22: 375–392.

12 Yang, C., Hu, Y., Zhou, B. et al. (2020). The role of m^6A modification in physiology and disease. *Cell Death Dis.* 11: 960.

13 Chujo, T. and Tomizawa, K. (2021). Human transfer RNA modopathies: diseases caused by aberrations in transfer RNA modifications. *FEBS J.* 288: 7096–7122.

14 Nombela, P., Miguel-López, B., and Blanco, S. (2021). The role of m^6A, m^5C and Ψ RNA modifications in cancer: novel therapeutic opportunities. *Mol. Cancer* 20: 18.

15 Konno, M. and Ishii, H. (2021). *Epitranscriptomics* (ed. S. Jurga and J. Barciszewski), 121–140. Cham: Springer International Publishing.

16 Cui, L., Ma, R., Cai, J. et al. (2022). RNA modifications: importance in immune cell biology and related diseases. *Signal Transduction Targeted Ther.* 7: 334.

17 Pereira, M., Francisco, S., Varanda, A.S. et al. (2018). Impact of tRNA modifications and tRNA-modifying enzymes on proteostasis and human disease. *Int. J. Mol. Sci.* 19: 3738.

18 Torres, A.G., Batlle, E., and Ribas de Pouplana, L. (2014). Role of tRNA modifications in human diseases. *Trends Mol. Med.* 20: 306–314.

19 Sarin, L.P. and Leidel, S.A. (2014). Modify or die? – RNA modification defects in metazoans. *RNA Biol.* 11: 1555–1567.

20 Jonkhout, N., Tran, J., Smith, M.A. et al. (2017). The RNA modification landscape in human disease. *RNA* 23: 1754–1769.

21 Boccaletto, P., Stefaniak, F., Ray, A. et al. (2021). MODOMICS: a database of RNA modification pathways. 2021 update. *Nucleic Acids Res.* 50: D231–D235.

22 Höfer, K. and Jäschke, A. (2018). Epitranscriptomics: RNA modifications in bacteria and archaea. *Microbiol. Spectrum* 6, https://doi.org/10.1128/microbiolspec.rwr-0015-2017.

23 Arguello, A.E., DeLiberto, A.N., and Kleiner, R.E. (2017). RNA chemical proteomics reveals the N^6-methyladenosine (m^6A)-regulated protein–RNA interactome. *JACS* 139: 17249–17252.

24 Yang, X., Yang, Y., Sun, B.F. et al. (2017). 5-methylcytosine promotes mRNA export — NSUN2 as the methyltransferase and ALYREF as an m5C reader. *Cell Res.* 27: 606–625.

25 Roundtree, I.A., Luo, G.Z., Zhang, Z. et al. (2017). YTHDC1 mediates nuclear export of N^6-methyladenosine methylated mRNAs. *eLife* 6: e31311.

26 Wang, X., Lu, Z., Gomez, A. et al. (2014). N^6-methyladenosine-dependent regulation of messenger RNA stability. *Nature* 505: 117–120.

27 Shi, H., Wang, X., Lu, Z. et al. (2017). YTHDF3 facilitates translation and decay of N^6-methyladenosine-modified RNA. *Cell Res.* 27: 315–328.

28 Xiao, W., Adhikari, S., Dahal, U. et al. (2016). Nuclear m^6A reader YTHDC1 regulates mRNA splicing. *Mol. Cell* 61: 507–519.

29 Fu, Y. and Zhuang, X. (2020). m(6)A-binding YTHDF proteins promote stress granule formation. *Nat. Chem. Biol.* 16: 955–963.

30 Meyer, K.D., Patil, D.P., Zhou, J. et al. (2015). 5′ UTR m^6A promotes cap-independent translation. *Cell* 163: 999–1010.

31 Mao, Y., Dong, L., Liu, X.M. et al. (2019). m^6A in mRNA coding regions promotes translation via the RNA helicase-containing YTHDC2. *Nat. Commun.* 10: 5332.

32 Li, A., Chen, Y.S., Ping, X.L. et al. (2017). Cytoplasmic m^6A reader YTHDF3 promotes mRNA translation. *Cell Res.* 27: 444–447.

33 Wang, X., Zhao, B.S., Roundtree, I.A. et al. (2015). N^6-methyladenosine modulates messenger RNA translation efficiency. *Cell* 161: 1388–1399.

34 Frye, M., Harada, B.T., Behm, M., and He, C. (2018). RNA modifications modulate gene expression during development. *Science* 361: 1346–1349.

35 Wang, Y., Li, Y., Toth, J.I. et al. (2014). N 6-methyladenosine modification destabilizes developmental regulators in embryonic stem cells. *Nat. Cell Biol.* 16: 191–198.

36 Liu, J., Huang, T., Chen, W. et al. (2022). Developmental mRNA m5C landscape and regulatory innovations of massive m5C modification of maternal mRNAs in animals. *Nat. Commun.* 13: 2484.

37 Shi, H., Zhang, X., Weng, Y.L. et al. (2018). m^6A facilitates hippocampus-dependent learning and memory through YTHDF1. *Nature* 563: 249–253.

38 Karikó, K., Buckstein, M., Ni, H., and Weissman, D. (2005). Suppression of RNA recognition by toll-like receptors: the impact of nucleoside modification and the evolutionary origin of RNA. *Immunity* 23: 165–175.

39 Fakruddin, M., Wei, F.Y., Suzuki, T. et al. (2018). Defective mitochondrial tRNA taurine modification activates global proteostress and leads to mitochondrial disease. *Cell Rep.* 22: 482–496.

40 Ghezzi, D. et al. (2012). Mutations of the mitochondrial-tRNA modifier MTO1 cause hypertrophic cardiomyopathy and lactic acidosis. *Am. J. Hum. Genet.* 90: 1079–1087.

41 Kazuhito, T. and Wei, F.-Y. (2020). Posttranscriptional modifications in mitochondrial tRNA and its implication in mitochondrial translation and disease. *J. Biochem.* 168: 435–444.

42 Kirino, Y., Yasukawa, T., Ohta, S. et al. (2004). Codon-specific translational defect caused by a wobble modification deficiency in mutant tRNA from a human mitochondrial disease. *PNAS* 101: 15070–15075.

43 Annapoorna, P.K., Iyer, H., Parnaik, T. et al. (2019). FTO: an emerging molecular player in neuropsychiatric diseases. *Neuroscience* 418: 15–24.

44 Bento-Abreu, A., Jager, G., Swinnen, B. et al. (2018). Elongator subunit 3 (ELP3) modifies ALS through tRNA modification. *Hum. Mol. Genet.* 27: 1276–1289.

45 Blanco, S., Dietmann, S., Flores, J.V. et al. (2014). Aberrant methylation of tRNAs links cellular stress to neuro-developmental disorders. *Embo J.* 33: 2020–2039.

46 Martinez, F.J., Lee, J.H., Lee, J.E. et al. (2012). Whole exome sequencing identifies a splicing mutation in NSUN2 as a cause of a Dubowitz-like syndrome. *J. Med. Genet.* 49: 380–385.

47 Ramos, J. and Fu, D. (2019). The emerging impact of tRNA modifications in the brain and nervous system. *Biochim. Biophys. Acta, Gene Regul.* 1862: 412–428.

48 Barbieri, I. and Kouzarides, T. (2020). Role of RNA modifications in cancer. *Nat. Rev. Cancer* 20: 303–322.

49 Christofi, T. and Zaravinos, A. (2019). RNA editing in the forefront of epitranscriptomics and human health. *J. Transl. Med.* 17: 319.

50 Leptidis, S., Papakonstantinou, E., Diakou, K.I. et al. (2022). Epitranscriptomics of cardiovascular diseases (review). *Int. J. Mol. Med.* 49: 9.

51 Qin, Y., Li, L., Luo, E. et al. (2020). Role of m^6A RNA methylation in cardiovascular disease (review). *Int. J. Mol. Med.* 46: 1958–1972.

52 Shafik, A.M., Allen, E.G., and Jin, P. (2020). Dynamic N^6-methyladenosine RNA methylation in brain and diseases. *Epigenomics* 12: 371–380.

53 Song, H., Zhang, J., Liu, B. et al. (2022). Biological roles of RNA m(5)C modification and its implications in cancer immunotherapy. *Biomarker Res.* 10: 15.

54 Wang, T., Kong, S., Tao, M., and Ju, S. (2020). The potential role of RNA N^6-methyladenosine in Cancer progression. *Mol. Cancer* 19: 88.

55 Yen, Y.P. and Chen, J.A. (2021). The m(6)A epitranscriptome on neural development and degeneration. *J. Biomed. Sci.* 28: 40.

56 Zhang, Y., Geng, X., Li, Q. et al. (2020). m^6A modification in RNA: biogenesis, functions and roles in gliomas. *J. Exp. Clin. Cancer Res.* 39: 192.

57 Trixl, L. and Lusser, A. (2019). The dynamic RNA modification 5-methylcytosine and its emerging role as an epitranscriptomic mark. *Wiley Interdiscip. Rev.: RNA* 10: e1510.

58 Kumar, S. and Mohapatra, T. (2021). Deciphering epitranscriptome: modification of mRNA bases provides a new perspective for post-transcriptional regulation of gene expression. *Front. Cell Dev. Biol.* 9.

59 Boo, S.H. and Kim, Y.K. (2020). The emerging role of RNA modifications in the regulation of mRNA stability. *Exp. Mol. Med.* 52: 400–408.

60 Dominissini, D., Moshitch-Moshkovitz, S., Schwartz, S. et al. (2012). Topology of the human and mouse m^6A RNA methylomes revealed by m^6A-seq. *Nature* 485: 201–206.

61 Dominissini, D., Moshitch-Moshkovitz, S., Salmon-Divon, M. et al. (2013). Transcriptome-wide mapping of N^6-methyladenosine by m^6A-seq based on immunocapturing and massively parallel sequencing. *Nat. Protoc.* 8: 176–189.

62 Schwartz, S., Bernstein, D.A., Mumbach, M.R. et al. (2014). Transcriptome-wide mapping reveals widespread dynamic-regulated pseudouridylation of ncRNA and mRNA. *Cell* 159: 148–162.

63 Carlile, T.M., Rojas-Duran, M.F., Zinshteyn, B. et al. (2014). Pseudouridine profiling reveals regulated mRNA pseudouridylation in yeast and human cells. *Nature* 515: 143–146.

64 Paul, M.S. and Bass, B.L. (1998). Inosine exists in mRNA at tissue-specific levels and is most abundant in brain mRNA. *Embo J.* 17: 1120–1127.

65 Arguello, A.E., Li, A., Sun, X. et al. (2022). Reactivity-dependent profiling of RNA 5-methylcytidine dioxygenases. *Nat. Commun.* 13: 4176.

66 Colgan, D.F. and Manley, J.L. (1997). Mechanism and regulation of mRNA polyadenylation. *Genes Dev.* 11: 2755–2766.

67 Di Giammartino, D.C., Nishida, K., and Manley, J.L. (2011). Mechanisms and consequences of alternative polyadenylation. *Mol. Cell* 43: 853–866.

68 Galloway, A. and Cowling, V.H. (2019). mRNA cap regulation in mammalian cell function and fate. *Biochim. Biophys. Acta, Gene Regul. Mech.* 1862: 270–279.

69 Ramanathan, A., Robb, G.B., and Chan, S.H. (2016). mRNA capping: biological functions and applications. *Nucleic Acids Res.* 44: 7511–7526.

70 Rogalska, M.E., Vivori, C., and Valcárcel, J. (2023). Regulation of pre-mRNA splicing: roles in physiology and disease, and therapeutic prospects. *Nat. Rev. Genet.* 24: 251–269.

71 Perry, R.P. and Kelley, D.E. (1974). Existence of methylated messenger RNA in mouse L cells. *Cell* 1: 37–42.

72 Desrosiers, R., Friderici, K., and Rottman, F. (1974). Identification of methylated nucleosides in messenger RNA from Novikoff hepatoma cells. *Proc. Natl. Acad. Sci.* 71: 3971–3975.

73 Meyer, K.D., Saletore, Y., Zumbo, P. et al. (2012). Comprehensive analysis of mRNA methylation reveals enrichment in 3' UTRs and near stop codons. *Cell* 149: 1635–1646.

74 Meyer, K.D. (2019). DART-seq: an antibody-free method for global m(6)A detection. *Nat. Methods* 16: 1275–1280.

75 Zhang, Z., Chen, L.Q., Zhao, Y.L. et al. (2019). Single-base mapping of m^6A by an antibody-independent method. *Sci. Adv.* 5: eaax0250.

76 Garcia-Campos, M.A., Edelheit, S., Toth, U. et al. (2019). Deciphering the "m^6A code" via antibody-independent quantitative profiling. *Cell* 178: 731–747. e716.

77 Chen, K., Lu, Z., Wang, X. et al. (2015). High-resolution N(6) -methyladenosine (m(6)A) map using photo-crosslinking-assisted m(6)A sequencing. *Angew. Chem. Int. Ed.* 54: 1587–1590.

78 Hu, L., Liu, S., Peng, Y. et al. (2022). m^6A RNA modifications are measured at single-base resolution across the mammalian transcriptome. *Nat. Biotechnol.* 40: 1210–1219.

79 Schaefer, M., Pollex, T., Hanna, K., and Lyko, F. (2009). RNA cytosine methylation analysis by bisulfite sequencing. *Nucleic Acids Res.* 37: e12.

80 Suzuki, T., Ueda, H., Okada, S., and Sakurai, M. (2015). Transcriptome-wide identification of adenosine-to-inosine editing using the ICE-seq method. *Nat. Protoc.* 10: 715–732.

81 Li, A., Sun, X., Arguello, A.E., and Kleiner, R.E. (2022). Chemical method to sequence 5-formylcytosine on RNA. *ACS Chem. Biol.* 17: 503–508.

82 Li, X., Xiong, X., Zhang, M. et al. (2017). Base-resolution mapping reveals distinct m(1)A methylome in nuclear- and mitochondrial-encoded transcripts. *Mol. Cell* 68: 993–1005.e1009.

83 Liu, J., Yue, Y., Han, D. et al. (2014). A METTL3–METTL14 complex mediates mammalian nuclear RNA N^6-adenosine methylation. *Nat. Chem. Biol.* 10: 93–95.

84 Wang, X., Feng, J., Xue, Y. et al. (2016). Structural basis of N 6-adenosine methylation by the METTL3–METTL14 complex. *Nature* 534: 575–578.

85 Ping, X.-L., Sun, B.F., Wang, L.U. et al. (2014). Mammalian WTAP is a regulatory subunit of the RNA N^6-methyladenosine methyltransferase. *Cell Res.* 24: 177–189.

86 Geula, S., Moshitch-Moshkovitz, S., Dominissini, D. et al. (2015). m^6A mRNA methylation facilitates resolution of naïve pluripotency toward differentiation. *Science* 347: 1002–1006.

87 Zhou, J., Wan, J., Gao, X. et al. (2015). Dynamic m(6)A mRNA methylation directs translational control of heat shock response. *Nature* 526: 591–594.

88 Yang, X., Triboulet, R., Liu, Q. et al. (2022). Exon junction complex shapes the m^6A epitranscriptome. *Nat. Commun.* 13: 7904.

89 Uzonyi, A., Dierks, D., Nir, R. et al. (2023). Exclusion of m^6A from splice-site proximal regions by the exon junction complex dictates m^6A topologies and mRNA stability. *Mol. Cell* 83: 237–251.e237.

90 He, P.C., Wei, J., Dou, X. et al. (2023). Exon architecture controls mRNA m(6)a suppression and gene expression. *Science* 379: 677–682.

91 Du, H., Zhao, Y., He, J. et al. (2016). YTHDF2 destabilizes m^6A-containing RNA through direct recruitment of the CCR4–NOT deadenylase complex. *Nat. Commun.* 7: 12626.

92 Huang, H., Weng, H., Sun, W. et al. (2018). Recognition of RNA N(6)-methyladenosine by IGF2BP proteins enhances mRNA stability and translation. *Nat. Cell Biol.* 20: 285–295.

93 Liu, J., Dou, X., Chen, C. et al. (2020). N(6)-methyladenosine of chromosome-associated regulatory RNA regulates chromatin state and transcription. *Science* 367: 580–586.

94 Zaccara, S. and Jaffrey, S.R. (2020). A unified model for the function of YTHDF proteins in regulating m^6A-modified mRNA. *Cell* 181: 1582–1595.e1518.

95 Zhang, F., Kang, Y., Wang, M. et al. (2018). Fragile X mental retardation protein modulates the stability of its m^6A-marked messenger RNA targets. *Hum. Mol. Genet.* 27: 3936–3950.

96 Zhang, G., Xu, Y., Wang, X. et al. (2022). Dynamic FMR1 granule phase switch instructed by m^6A modification contributes to maternal RNA decay. *Nat. Commun.* 13: 859.

97 Roost, C., Lynch, S.R., Batista, P.J. et al. (2015). Structure and thermodynamics of N^6-methyladenosine in RNA: a spring-Loaded Base modification. *JACS* 137: 2107–2115.

98 Dixit, D., Xie, Q., Rich, J.N., and Zhao, J.C. (2017). Messenger RNA methylation regulates glioblastoma tumorigenesis. *Cancer Cell* 31: 474–475.

99 Huff, S., Tiwari, S.K., Gonzalez, G.M. et al. (2021). m^6A-RNA demethylase FTO inhibitors impair self-renewal in glioblastoma stem cells. *ACS Chem. Biol.* 16: 324–333.

100 He, X., Tan, L., Ni, J., and Shen, G. (2021). Expression pattern of m^6A regulators is significantly correlated with malignancy and antitumor immune response of breast cancer. *Cancer Gene Ther.* 28: 188–196.

101 Singh, B., Kinne, H.E., Milligan, R.D. et al. (2016). Important role of FTO in the survival of rare panresistant triple-negative inflammatory breast cancer cells facing a severe metabolic challenge. *PLoS One* 11: e0159072.

102 Xu, Y., Kinne, H.E., Milligan, R.D. et al. (2020). The FTO/miR-181b-3p/ARL5B signaling pathway regulates cell migration and invasion in breast cancer. *Cancer Commun. (Lond)* 40: 484–500.

103 Zheng, F., Du, F., Zhao, J. et al. (2021). The emerging role of RNA N^6-methyladenosine methylation in breast cancer. *Biomarker Res.* 9: 39.

104 Zhou, M., Dong, M., Yang, X. et al. (2022). The emerging roles and mechanism of m^6A in breast cancer progression. *Front. Genet.* 13.

105 Diao, M.-N., Zhang, X.-J., and Zhang, Y.-F. (2023). The critical roles of m^6A RNA methylation in lung cancer: from mechanism to prognosis and therapy. *Br. J. Cancer* 129: 8–23.

106 Li, J., Han, Y., Zhang, H. et al. (2019). The m^6A demethylase FTO promotes the growth of lung cancer cells by regulating the m^6A level of USP7 mRNA. *Biochem. Biophys. Res. Commun.* 512: 479–485.

107 Wanna-Udom, S., Terashima, M., Lyu, H. et al. (2020). The m^6A methyltransferase METTL3 contributes to transforming growth factor-beta-induced epithelial-mesenchymal transition of lung cancer cells through the regulation of JUNB. *Biochem. Biophys. Res. Commun.* 524: 150–155.

108 Li, Z., Weng, H., Su, R. et al. (2017). FTO plays an oncogenic role in acute myeloid Leukemia as a N(6)-methyladenosine RNA demethylase. *Cancer Cell* 31: 127–141.

109 Vu, L.P., Pickering, B.F., Cheng, Y. et al. (2017). The N^6-methyladenosine (m^6A)-forming enzyme METTL3 controls myeloid differentiation of normal hematopoietic and leukemia cells. *Nat. Med.* 23: 1369–1376.

110 Geng, Y., Guan, R., Hong, W. et al. (2020). Identification of m^6A-related genes and m^6A RNA methylation regulators in pancreatic cancer and their association with survival. *Ann. Transl. Med.* 8.

111 Guo, X., Li, K., Jiang, W. et al. (2020). RNA demethylase ALKBH5 prevents pancreatic cancer progression by posttranscriptional activation of PER1 in an m^6A-YTHDF2-dependent manner. *Mol. Cancer* 19: 1–19.

112 Taketo, K., Konno, M., Asai, A. et al. (2018). The epitranscriptome m^6A writer METTL3 promotes chemo-and radioresistance in pancreatic cancer cells. *Int. J. Oncol.* 52: 621–629.

113 Tang, B., Yang, Y., Kang, M. et al. (2020). m^6A demethylase ALKBH5 inhibits pancreatic cancer tumorigenesis by decreasing WIF-1 RNA methylation and mediating Wnt signaling. *Mol. Cancer* 19: 1–15.

114 Xia, T., Wu, X., Cao, M. et al. (2019). The RNA m^6A methyltransferase METTL3 promotes pancreatic cancer cell proliferation and invasion. *Pathol. Res. Pract.* 215: 152666.

115 Niu, J., Wang, B., Wang, T., and Zhou, T. (2022). Mechanism of METTL3-mediated m^6A modification in depression-induced cognitive deficits. *Am. J. Med. Genet. Part B: Neuropsychiatr. Genet.* 189: 86–99.

116 Chokkalla, A.K., Mehta, S.L., and Vemuganti, R. (2020). Epitranscriptomic regulation by m^6A RNA methylation in brain development and diseases. *J. Cereb. Blood Flow Metab.* 40: 2331–2349.

117 Choudhry, Z., Sengupta, S.M., Grizenko, N. et al. (2013). Association between obesity-related gene FTO and ADHD. *Obesity* 21: E738–E744.

118 Han, M., Liu, Z., Xu, Y. et al. (2020). Abnormality of m^6A mRNA methylation is involved in Alzheimer's disease. *Front. Neurosci.* 14: 98.

119 Wu, Y., Xie, L., Wang, M. et al. (2018). Mettl3-mediated m^6A RNA methylation regulates the fate of bone marrow mesenchymal stem cells and osteoporosis. *Nat. Commun.* 9: 4772.

120 Winkler, R., Gillis, E., Lasman, L. et al. (2019). m^6A modification controls the innate immune response to infection by targeting type I interferons. *Nat. Immunol.* 20: 173–182.

121 Tan, B. and Gao, S.J. (2018). RNA epitranscriptomics: regulation of infection of RNA and DNA viruses by N^6-methyladenosine (m^6A). *Rev. Med. Virol.* 28: e1983.

122 Wang, Y., Wang, Y., Gu, J. et al. (2022). The role of RNA m^6A methylation in lipid metabolism. *Front. Endocrinol.* 13: 866116.

123 Zhang, Y., Chen, W., Zheng, X. et al. (2021). Regulatory role and mechanism of m(6)A RNA modification in human metabolic diseases. *Mol. Ther. Oncolytics* 22: 52–63.

124 An, Y. and Duan, H. (2022). The role of m^6A RNA methylation in cancer metabolism. *Mol. Cancer* 21: 14.

125 Zeng, C., Huang, W., Li, Y., and Weng, H. (2020). Roles of METTL3 in cancer: mechanisms and therapeutic targeting. *J. Hematol. Oncol.* 13: 117.

126 Deng, L.J., Deng, W.Q., Fan, S.R. et al. (2022). m^6A modification: recent advances, anticancer targeted drug discovery and beyond. *Mol. Cancer* 21: 52.

127 Huang, W., Chen, T.Q., Fang, K. et al. (2021). N^6-methyladenosine methyltransferases: functions, regulation, and clinical potential. *J. Hematol. Oncol.* 14: 117.

128 Lan, Q., Liu, P.Y., Haase, J. et al. (2019). The critical role of RNA m^6A methylation in cancer. *Cancer Res.* 79: 1285–1292.

129 Li, X., Tang, J., Huang, W. et al. (2017). The M6A methyltransferase METTL3: acting as a tumor suppressor in renal cell carcinoma. *Oncotarget* 8: 96103–96116.

130 Liu, J., Eckert, M.A., Harada, B.T. et al. (2018). m^6A mRNA methylation regulates AKT activity to promote the proliferation and tumorigenicity of endometrial cancer. *Nat. Cell Biol.* 20: 1074–1083.

131 Deng, R., Cheng, Y., Ye, S. et al. (2019). m^6A methyltransferase METTL3 suppresses colorectal cancer proliferation and migration through p38/ERK pathways. *OncoTargets Ther.* 12: 4391.

132 Visvanathan, A., Patil, V., Arora, A. et al. (2018). Essential role of METTL3-mediated m(6)A modification in glioma stem-like cells maintenance and radioresistance. *Oncogene* 37: 522–533.

133 Yankova, E., Blackaby, W., Albertella, M. et al. (2021). Small-molecule inhibition of METTL3 as a strategy against myeloid leukaemia. *Nature* 593: 597–601.

134 Dolbois, A., Bedi, R.K., Bochenkova, E. et al. (2021). 1,4,9-Triazaspiro[5.5]undecan-2-one derivatives as potent and selective METTL3 inhibitors. *J. Med. Chem.* 64: 12738–12760.

135 Moroz-Omori, E.V., Huang, D., Bedi, R.K. et al. (2021). METTL3 inhibitors for epitranscriptomic modulation of cellular processes. *ChemMedChem* 16: 3035–3043.

136 Bedi, R.K., Huang, D., Eberle, S.A. et al. (2020). Small-molecule inhibitors of METTL3, the major human epitranscriptomic writer. *ChemMedChem* 15: 744–748.

137 STORM Therapeutics (2023). STORM Therapeutics Presents STC-15 Preclinical Data Supporting Treatment of Patients with AML at the AACR Acute Myeloid Leukemia and Myelodysplastic Syndrome Conference. Retrieved September 7, 2023, from https://www.stormtherapeutics.com/media/news/storm-therapeutics-presents-stc-15-preclinical-data-supporting-treatment-of-patients-with-aml-at-the-aacr-acute-myeloid.

138 STORM Therapeutics (2022). STORM Therapeutics doses first patient with oral METTL3 targeting drug candidate in a solid tumor Phase 1 study. Retrieved September 7, 2023, from https://www.stormtherapeutics.com/media/news/storm-therapeutics-doses-first-patient-with-oral-mettl3-targeting-drug-candidate-in-a-solid-tumor-phase-1-study.

139 Ipsen. (2021) Ipsen adds another program into its pre-clinical R&D Oncology pipeline through an exclusive worldwide collaboration with Accent Therapeutics, targeting the RNA modifying protein, METTL3. Retrieved September 7, 2023, from https://www.ipsen.com/websites/Ipsen_Online/wp-content/uploads/2021/10/17165818/Ipsen-Accent-collaboration-18-October-2021.pdf.

140 Idrus, A.A. (2020). Fierce Biotech.

141 Wei, J., Liu, F., Lu, Z. et al. (2018). Differential m^6A, m^6Am, and m^1A demethylation mediated by FTO in the cell nucleus and cytoplasm. *Mol. Cell* 71: 973–985.e975.

142 Dina, C., Meyre, D., Gallina, S. et al. (2007). Variation in FTO contributes to childhood obesity and severe adult obesity. *Nat. Genet.* 39: 724–726.

143 Fischer, J., Koch, L., Emmerling, C. et al. (2009). Inactivation of the FTO gene protects from obesity. *Nature* 458: 894–898.

144 Deng, X., Su, R., Stanford, S., and Chen, J. (2018). Critical enzymatic functions of FTO in obesity and cancer. *Front. Endocrinol.* 9.

145 Lan, N., Lu, Y., Zhang, Y. et al. (2020). FTO – a common genetic basis for obesity and cancer. *Front. Genet.* 11.

146 Fawcett, K.A. and Barroso, I. (2010). The genetics of obesity: FTO leads the way. *Trends Genet.* 26: 266–274.

147 Zhou, S., Bai, Z.L., Xia, D. et al. (2018). FTO regulates the chemo-radiotherapy resistance of cervical squamous cell carcinoma (CSCC) by targeting β-catenin through mRNA demethylation. *Mol. Carcinog.* 57: 590–597.

148 Huang, H., Wang, Y., Kandpal, M. et al. (2020). FTO-dependent N (6)-methyladenosine modifications inhibit ovarian cancer stem cell self-renewal by blocking cAMP signaling. *Cancer Res.* 80: 3200–3214.

149 Malacrida, A. et al. (2020). 3D proteome-wide scale screening and activity evaluation of a new ALKBH5 inhibitor in U87 glioblastoma cell line. *Bioorg. Med. Chem.* 28: 115300.

150 Yuan, Y., Rivara, M., Di Domizio, A. et al. (2021). ALKBH5 suppresses tumor progression via an m^{6}A-dependent epigenetic silencing of pre-miR-181b-1/YAP signaling axis in osteosarcoma. *Cell Death Dis.* 12: 60.

151 Wei, C. et al. (2022). Pan-Cancer analysis shows that ALKBH5 is a potential prognostic and immunotherapeutic biomarker for multiple cancer types including gliomas. *Front. Immunol.* 13.

152 Qu, J., Yan, H., Hou, Y. et al. (2022). RNA demethylase ALKBH5 in cancer: from mechanisms to therapeutic potential. *J. Hematol. Oncol.* 15: 8.

153 Hess, M.E., Hess, S., Meyer, K.D. et al. (2013). The fat mass and obesity associated gene (FTO) regulates activity of the dopaminergic midbrain circuitry. *Nat. Neurosci.* 16: 1042–1048.

154 Chang, R., Huang, Z., Zhao, S. et al. (2022). Emerging roles of FTO in neuropsychiatric disorders. *Biomed Res. Int.* 2022: 2677312.

155 Wang, B., Fang, X., Sun, X. et al. (2021). m(6)A demethylase ALKBH5 suppresses proliferation and migration of enteric neural crest cells by regulating TAGLN in Hirschsprung's disease. *Life Sci.* 278: 119577.

156 Bego, T., Čaušević, A., Dujić, T. et al. (2019). Association of FTO gene variant (rs8050136) with type 2 diabetes and markers of obesity, glycaemic control and inflammation. *J. Med. Biochem.* 38: 153–163.

157 Daoud, H., Zhang, F.M.M. et al. (2016). Identification of a pathogenic FTO mutation by next-generation sequencing in a newborn with growth retardation and developmental delay. *J. Med. Genet.* 53: 200–207.

158 Kim, H., Lee, Y., Kim, S.M. et al. (2021). RNA demethylation by FTO stabilizes the FOXJ1 mRNA for proper motile ciliogenesis. *Dev. Cell* 56: 1118–1130. e1116.

159 Azzam, S.K., Alsafar, H., and Sajini, A.A. (2022). FTO m^{6}A demethylase in obesity and cancer: implications and underlying molecular mechanisms. *Int. J. Mol. Sci.* 23.

160 Su, R., Dong, L., Li, Y. et al. (2020). Targeting FTO suppresses cancer stem cell maintenance and immune evasion. *Cancer Cell* 38: 79–96.e11.

161 Huang, Y., Su, R., Sheng, Y. et al. (2019). Small-molecule targeting of oncogenic FTO demethylase in acute myeloid leukemia. *Cancer Cell* 35: 677–691.e610.

162 Sun, K., Du, Y., Hou, Y. et al. (2021). Saikosaponin D exhibits anti-leukemic activity by targeting FTO/m(6)A signaling. *Theranostics* 11: 5831–5846.

163 Qin, B., Bai, Q., Yan, D. et al. (2022). Discovery of novel mRNA demethylase FTO inhibitors against esophageal cancer. *J. Enzyme Inhib. Med. Chem.* 37: 1995–2003.

164 Xie, G., Wu, X.N., Ling, Y. et al. (2022). A novel inhibitor of N^6-methyladenosine demethylase FTO induces mRNA methylation and shows anti-cancer activities. *Acta Pharm. Sin. B* 12: 853–866.

165 Takahashi, H., Hase, H., Yoshida, T. et al. (2022). Discovery of two novel ALKBH5 selective inhibitors that exhibit uncompetitive or competitive type and suppress the growth activity of glioblastoma multiforme. *Chem. Biol. Drug Design* 100: 1–12.

166 Selberg, S., Seli, N., Kankuri, E., and Karelson, M. (2021). Rational design of novel anticancer small-molecule RNA m^6A demethylase ALKBH5 inhibitors. *ACS Omega* 6: 13310–13320.

167 Dai, Q., Zhang, L.S., Sun, H.L. et al. (2023). Quantitative sequencing using BID-seq uncovers abundant pseudouridines in mammalian mRNA at base resolution. *Nat. Biotechnol.* 41: 344–354.

168 Davis, D.R. (1995). Stabilization of RNA stacking by pseudouridine. *Nucleic Acids Res.* 23: 5020–5026.

169 Kierzek, E., Malgowska, M., Lisowiec, J. et al. (2014). The contribution of pseudouridine to stabilities and structure of RNAs. *Nucleic Acids Res.* 42: 3492–3501.

170 Davis, F.F. and Allen, F.W. (1957). Ribonucleic acids from yeast which contain a fifth nucleotide. *J. Biol. Chem.* 227: 907–915.

171 Holley, R.W., Apgar, J., Everett, G.A. et al. (1965). Structure of a ribonucleic acid. *Science* 147: 1462–1465.

172 Lane, B.G., Ofengand, J., and Gray, M.W. (1992). Pseudouridine in the large-subunit (23 S-like) ribosomal RNA. The site of peptidyl transfer in the ribosome? *FEBS Lett.* 302: 1–4.

173 Bakin, A. and Ofengand, J. (1993). Four newly located pseudouridylate residues in *Escherichia coli* 23S ribosomal RNA are all at the peptidyltransferase center: analysis by the application of a new sequencing technique. *Biochemistry* 32: 9754–9762.

174 Khoddami, V., Yerra, A., Mosbruger, T.L. et al. (2019). Transcriptome-wide profiling of multiple RNA modifications simultaneously at single-base resolution. *Proc. Natl. Acad. Sci.* 116: 6784–6789.

175 Li, X., Zhu, P., Ma, S. et al. (2015). Chemical pulldown reveals dynamic pseudouridylation of the mammalian transcriptome. *Nat. Chem. Biol.* 11: 592–597.

176 Eyler, D.E., Franco, M.K., Batool, Z. et al. (2019). Pseudouridinylation of mRNA coding sequences alters translation. *PNAS* 116: 23068–23074.

177 Adachi, H. and Yu, Y.T. (2020). Pseudouridine-mediated stop codon readthrough in *S. cerevisiae* is sequence context-independent. *RNA* 26: 1247–1256.

178 Karijolich, J. and Yu, Y.-T. (2011). Converting nonsense codons into sense codons by targeted pseudouridylation. *Nature* 474: 395–398.

179 Levi, O. and Arava, Y.S. (2021). Pseudouridine-mediated translation control of mRNA by methionine aminoacyl tRNA synthetase. *Nucleic Acids Res.* 49: 432–443.

180 Karikó, K., Muramatsu, H., Welsh, F.A. et al. (2008). Incorporation of pseudouridine into mRNA yields superior nonimmunogenic vector with increased translational capacity and biological stability. *Mol. Ther.* 16: 1833–1840.

181 Martinez, N.M., Su, A., Burns, M.C. et al. (2022). Pseudouridine synthases modify human pre-mRNA co-transcriptionally and affect pre-mRNA processing. *Mol. Cell* 82: 645–659.e649.

182 Hamma, T. and Ferré-D'Amaré, A.R. (2006). Pseudouridine synthases. *Chem. Biol.* 13: 1125–1135.

183 Liu, B., Zhang, J., Huang, C., and Liu, H. (2012). Dyskerin overexpression in human hepatocellular carcinoma is associated with advanced clinical stage and poor patient prognosis. *PLoS One* 7: e43147.

184 Montanaro, L., Brigotti, M., Clohessy, J. et al. (2006). Dyskerin expression influences the level of ribosomal RNA pseudo-uridylation and telomerase RNA component in human breast cancer. *J. Pathol.* 210: 10–18.

185 Bykhovskaya, Y., Casas, K., Mengesha, E. et al. (2004). Missense mutation in pseudouridine synthase 1 (PUS1) causes mitochondrial myopathy and sideroblastic anemia (MLASA). *Am. J. Human Genet.* 74: 1303–1308.

186 Patton, J.R., Bykhovskaya, Y., Mengesha, E. et al. (2005). Mitochondrial myopathy and sideroblastic anemia (MLASA): missense mutation in the pseudouridine synthase 1 (PUS1) gene is associated with the loss of tRNA pseudouridylation. *J. Biol. Chem.* 280: 19823–19828.

187 Han, S.T., Kim, A.C., Garcia, K. et al. (2022). PUS7 deficiency in human patients causes profound neurodevelopmental phenotype by dysregulating protein translation. *Mol. Genet. Metab.* 135: 221–229.

188 Shaheen, R., Tasak, M., Maddirevula, S. et al. (2019). PUS7 mutations impair pseudouridylation in humans and cause intellectual disability and microcephaly. *Hum. Genet.* 138: 231–239.

189 Shaheen, R., Han, L., Faqeih, E. et al. (2016). A homozygous truncating mutation in PUS3 expands the role of tRNA modification in normal cognition. *Hum. Genet.* 135: 707–713.

190 Zhao, Y., Karijolich, J., Glaunsinger, B., and Zhou, Q. (2016). Pseudouridylation of 7SK snRNA promotes 7SK snRNP formation to suppress HIV-1 transcription and escape from latency. *EMBO Rep.* 17: 1441–1451.

191 Heiss, N.S., Knight, S.W., Vulliamy, T.J. et al. (1998). X-linked dyskeratosis congenita is caused by mutations in a highly conserved gene with putative nucleolar functions. *Nat. Genet.* 19: 32–38.

192 Cui, Q., Yin, K., Zhang, X. et al. (2021). Targeting PUS7 suppresses tRNA pseudouridylation and glioblastoma tumorigenesis. *Nat. Cancer* 2: 932–949.

193 Purchal, M.K., Eyler, D.E., Tardu, M. et al. (2022). Pseudouridine synthase 7 is an opportunistic enzyme that binds and modifies substrates with diverse sequences and structures. *Proc. Natl. Acad. Sci.* 119: e2109708119.

194 Andries, O., Cafferty, S.M., De Smedt, S.C. et al. (2015). N(1)-methylpseudouridine-incorporated mRNA outperforms pseudouridine-incorporated mRNA by providing enhanced protein expression and reduced immunogenicity in mammalian cell lines and mice. *J. Controlled Release* 217: 337–344.

195 Mauger, D.M., Cabral, B.J., Presnyak, V. et al. (2019). mRNA structure regulates protein expression through changes in functional half-life. *PNAS* 116: 24075–24083.

196 Anderson, B.R., Muramatsu, H., Nallagatla, S.R. et al. (2010). Incorporation of pseudouridine into mRNA enhances translation by diminishing PKR activation. *Nucleic Acids Res.* 38: 5884–5892.

197 Svitkin, Y.V., Cheng, Y.M., Chakraborty, T. et al. (2017). N^1-methyl-pseudouridine in mRNA enhances translation through eIF2α-dependent and independent mechanisms by increasing ribosome density. *Nucleic Acids Res.* 45: 6023–6036.

198 Nance, K.D. and Meier, J.L. (2021). Modifications in an emergency: the role of N^1-Methylpseudouridine in COVID-19 vaccines. *ACS Cent. Sci.* 7: 748–756.

199 Morais, P., Adachi, H., and Yu, Y.-T. (2021). The critical contribution of pseudouridine to mRNA COVID-19 vaccines. *Front. Cell Dev. Biol.* 9.

200 Morse, D.P. and Bass, B.L. (1997). Detection of inosine in messenger RNA by inosine-specific cleavage. *Biochemistry* 36: 8429–8434.

201 Li, J.B., Levanon, E.Y., Yoon, J.K. et al. (2009). Genome-wide identification of human RNA editing sites by parallel DNA capturing and sequencing. *Science* 324: 1210–1213.

202 Levanon, E.Y., Eisenberg, E., Yelin, R. et al. (2004). Systematic identification of abundant A-to-I editing sites in the human transcriptome. *Nat. Biotechnol.* 22: 1001–1005.

203 Gabay, O., Shoshan, Y., Kopel, E. et al. (2022). Landscape of adenosine-to-inosine RNA recoding across human tissues. *Nat. Commun.* 13: 1184.

204 Morita, Y., Shibutani, T., Nakanishi, N. et al. (2013). Human endonuclease V is a ribonuclease specific for inosine-containing RNA. *Nat. Commun.* 4: 2273.

205 Sakurai, M., Ueda, H., Yano, T. et al. (2014). A biochemical landscape of A-to-I RNA editing in the human brain transcriptome. *Genome Res.* 24: 522–534.

206 Bahn, J.H., Lee, J.H., Li, G. et al. (2012). Accurate identification of A-to-I RNA editing in human by transcriptome sequencing. *Genome Res.* 22: 142–150.

207 Peng, Z., Cheng, Y., Tan, B.C.M. et al. (2012). Comprehensive analysis of RNA-Seq data reveals extensive RNA editing in a human transcriptome. *Nat. Biotechnol.* 30: 253–260.

208 Bazak, L., Haviv, A., Barak, M. et al. (2014). A-to-I RNA editing occurs at over a hundred million genomic sites, located in a majority of human genes. *Genome Res.* 24: 365–376.

209 Maas, S., Patt, S., Schrey, M., and Rich, A. (2001). Underediting of glutamate receptor GluR-B mRNA in malignant gliomas. *PNAS* 98: 14687–14692.

210 Higuchi, M., Single, F.N., Köhler, M. et al. (1993). RNA editing of AMPA receptor subunit GluR-B: a base-paired intron-exon structure determines position and efficiency. *Cell* 75: 1361–1370.

211 Rueter, S.M., Burns, C.M., Coode, S.A. et al. (1995). Glutamate receptor RNA editing in vitro by enzymatic conversion of adenosine to inosine. *Science* 267: 1491–1494.

212 Yang, J.H., Sklar, P., Axel, R., and Maniatis, T. (1995). Editing of glutamate receptor subunit B pre-mRNA in vitro by site-specific deamination of adenosine. *Nature* 374: 77–81.

213 Sommer, B., Köhler, M., Sprengel, R., and Seeburg, P.H. (1991). RNA editing in brain controls a determinant of ion flow in glutamate-gated channels. *Cell* 67: 11–19.

214 Brusa, R., Zimmermann, F., Koh, D.S. et al. (1995). Early-onset epilepsy and postnatal lethality associated with an editing-deficient GluR-B allele in mice. *Science* 270: 1677–1680.

215 Feldmeyer, D., Kask, K., Brusa, R. et al. (1999). Neurological dysfunctions in mice expressing different levels of the Q/R site-unedited AMPAR subunit GluR-B. *Nat. Neurosci.* 2: 57–64.

216 Burns, C.M., Chu, H., Rueter, S.M. et al. (1997). Regulation of serotonin-2C receptor G-protein coupling by RNA editing. *Nature* 387: 303–308.

217 Alonso-Andrés, P., Albasanz, J.L., Ferrer, I., and Martín, M. (2018). Purine-related metabolites and their converting enzymes are altered in frontal, parietal and temporal cortex at early stages of Alzheimer's disease pathology. *Brain Pathol.* 28: 933–946.

218 Basile, M.S., Bramanti, P., and Mazzon, E. (2022). Inosine in neurodegenerative diseases: from the bench to the bedside. *Molecules* 27.

219 Gurevich, I., Tamir, H., Arango, V. et al. (2002). Altered editing of serotonin 2C receptor pre-mRNA in the prefrontal cortex of depressed suicide victims. *Neuron* 34: 349–356.

220 Lotsof, E.R., Krajewski, A.E., Anderson-Steele, B. et al. (2022). NEIL1 recoding due to RNA editing impacts lesion-specific recognition and excision. *JACS* 144: 14578–14589.

221 Yeo, J., Goodman, R.A., Schirle, N.T. et al. (2010). RNA editing changes the lesion specificity for the DNA repair enzyme NEIL1. *Proc. Natl. Acad. Sci.* 107: 20715–20719.

222 Jain, M., Manjaly, G., Maly, K. et al. (2022). Filamin a pre-mRNA editing modulates vascularization and tumor growth. *Mol. Ther. Nucleic Acids* 30: 522–534.

223 Jain, M., Mann, T.D., Stulić, M. et al. (2018). RNA editing of filamin a pre-mRNA regulates vascular contraction and diastolic blood pressure. *Embo J.* 37.

224 Rafels-Ybern, À., Torres, A.G., Camacho, N. et al. (2018). The expansion of inosine at the wobble position of tRNAs, and its role in the evolution of proteomes. *Mol. Biol. Evol.* 36: 650–662.

225 Diaz Quiroz, J.F., Siskel, L.D., and Rosenthal, J.J.C. (2023). Site-directed A → I RNA editing as a therapeutic tool: moving beyond genetic mutations. *RNA* 29: 498–505.

226 Kato, H., Takeuchi, O., Sato, S. et al. (2006). Differential roles of MDA5 and RIG-I helicases in the recognition of RNA viruses. *Nature* 441: 101–105.

227 Chung, H., Calis, J.J.A., Wu, X. et al. (2018). Human ADAR1 prevents endogenous RNA from triggering translational shutdown. *Cell* 172: 811–824.e814.

228 Liddicoat, B.J., Piskol, R., Chalk, A.M. et al. (2015). RNA editing by ADAR1 prevents MDA5 sensing of endogenous dsRNA as nonself. *Science* 349: 1115–1120.

229 Hartner, J.C., Schmittwolf, C., Kispert, A. et al. (2004). Liver disintegration in the mouse embryo caused by deficiency in the RNA-editing enzyme ADAR1. *J. Biol. Chem.* 279: 4894–4902.

230 Pestal, K., Funk, C.C., Snyder, J.M. et al. (2015). Isoforms of RNA-editing enzyme ADAR1 independently control nucleic acid sensor MDA5-driven autoimmunity and multi-organ development. *Immunity* 43: 933–944.

231 Rice, G.I., Kasher, P.R., Forte, G.M.A. et al. (2012). Mutations in ADAR1 cause Aicardi-Goutières syndrome associated with a type I interferon signature. *Nat. Genet.* 44: 1243–1248.

232 Kung, C.-P., Cottrell, K.A., Ryu, S. et al. (2021). Evaluating the therapeutic potential of ADAR1 inhibition for triple-negative breast cancer. *Oncogene* 40: 189–202.

233 Galore-Haskel, G., Nemlich, Y., Greenberg, E. et al. (2015). A novel immune resistance mechanism of melanoma cells controlled by the ADAR1 enzyme. *Oncotarget* 6: 28999–29015.

234 Fritzell, K., Xu, L.D., Lagergren, J., and Öhman, M. (2018). ADARs and editing: the role of A-to-I RNA modification in cancer progression. *Semin. Cell Dev. Biol.* 79: 123–130.

235 Gannon, H.S., Zou, T., Kiessling, M.K. et al. (2018). Identification of ADAR1 adenosine deaminase dependency in a subset of cancer cells. *Nat. Commun.* 9: 5450.

236 Liu, H., Golji, J., Brodeur, L.K. et al. (2019). Tumor-derived IFN triggers chronic pathway agonism and sensitivity to ADAR loss. *Nat. Med.* 25: 95–102.

237 Ishizuka, J.J., Manguso, R.T., Cheruiyot, C.K. et al. (2019). Loss of ADAR1 in tumours overcomes resistance to immune checkpoint blockade. *Nature* 565: 43–48.

238 Bhate, A., Sun, T., and Li, J.B. (2019). ADAR1: a new target for immuno-oncology therapy. *Mol. Cell* 73: 866–868.

239 Cottrell, K.A., Torres, L.S., Dizon, M.G., and Weber, J.D. (2021). 8-Azaadenosine and 8-chloroadenosine are not selective inhibitors of ADAR. *Cancer Res. Commun.* 1: 56–64.

240 Wang, X., Li, J., Zhu, Y. et al. (2021). Targeting ADAR1 with a novel small-molecule for the treatment of prostate cancer. *Res. Square* https://doi.org/10.21203/rs.3.rs-879741/v1.

241 Mendoza, H.G., Matos, V.J., Park, S. et al. (2023). Selective inhibition of ADAR1 using 8-azanebularine-modified RNA duplexes. *Biochemistry* 62: 1376–1387.

242 Crews, L.A., Ma, W., Ladel, L. et al. (2023). Reversal of malignant ADAR1 splice isoform switching with rebecsinib. *Cell Stem Cell* 30: 250–263.e256.

243 Guimond, D.S., Theodore, Joseph, G. et al. (2022). Gossamer Bio, 27th Annual Meeting of the RNA Society.

244 Pan, T. (2018). Modifications and functional genomics of human transfer RNA. *Cell Res.* 28: 395–404.

245 Crick, F.H.C. (1966). Codon—anticodon pairing: the wobble hypothesis. *J. Mol. Biol.* 19: 548–555.

246 Lorenz, C., Lünse, C.E., and Mörl, M. (2017). tRNA modifications: impact on structure and thermal adaptation. *Biomolecules* 7: 35.

247 Han, L. and Phizicky, E.M. (2018). A rationale for tRNA modification circuits in the anticodon loop. *RNA* 24: 1277–1284.

248 Motorin, Y. and Helm, M. (2010). tRNA stabilization by modified nucleotides. *Biochemistry* 49: 4934–4944.

249 Brégeon, D., Pecqueur, L., Toubdji, S. et al. (2022). Dihydrouridine in the transcriptome: new life for this ancient RNA chemical modification. *ACS Chem. Biol.* 17: 1638–1657.

250 Muramatsu, T., Yokoyama, S., Horie, N. et al. (1988). A novel lysine-substituted nucleoside in the first position of the anticodon of minor isoleucine tRNA from *Escherichia coli*. *J. Biol. Chem.* 263: 9261–9267.

251 Moshitch-Moshkovitz, S., Dominissini, D., and Rechavi, G. (2022). The epitranscriptome toolbox. *Cell* 185: 764–776.

252 Li, X., Xiong, X., and Yi, C. (2017). Epitranscriptome sequencing technologies: decoding RNA modifications. *Nat. Methods* 14: 23–31.

253 Jain, M., Abu-Shumays, R., Olsen, H.E., and Akeson, M. (2022). Advances in nanopore direct RNA sequencing. *Nat. Methods* 19: 1160–1164.

254 Pratanwanich, P.N., Yao, F., Chen, Y. et al. (2021). Identification of differential RNA modifications from nanopore direct RNA sequencing with xPore. *Nat. Biotechnol.* 39: 1394–1402.

255 Workman, R.E., Tang, A.D., Tang, P.S. et al. (2019). Nanopore native RNA sequencing of a human poly(A) transcriptome. *Nat. Methods* 16: 1297–1305.

256 Begik, O., Lucas, M.C., Pryszcz, L.P. et al. (2021). Quantitative profiling of pseudouridylation dynamics in native RNAs with nanopore sequencing. *Nat. Biotechnol.* 39: 1278–1291.

257 Liu, H., Begik, O., Lucas, M.C. et al. (2019). Accurate detection of m^6A RNA modifications in native RNA sequences. *Nat. Commun.* 10: 4079.

258 Leger, A., Amaral, P.P., Pandolfini, L. et al. (2021). RNA modifications detection by comparative nanopore direct RNA sequencing. *Nat. Commun.* 12: 7198.

259 Su, D., Chan, C.T.Y., Gu, C. et al. (2014). Quantitative analysis of ribonucleoside modifications in tRNA by HPLC-coupled mass spectrometry. *Nat. Protoc.* 9: 828–841.

260 Gu, C., Begley, T.J., and Dedon, P.C. (2014). tRNA modifications regulate translation during cellular stress. *FEBS Lett.* 588: 4287–4296.

261 Chan, C.T., Pang, Y.L.J., Deng, W. et al. (2012). Reprogramming of tRNA modifications controls the oxidative stress response by codon-biased translation of proteins. *Nat. Commun.* 3: 937.

262 Candiracci, J., Migeot, V., Chionh, Y.H. et al. (2019). Reciprocal regulation of TORC signaling and tRNA modifications by elongator enforces nutrient-dependent cell fate. *Sci. Adv.* 5: eaav0184.

263 Keam, S.P. and Hutvagner, G. (2015). tRNA-derived fragments (tRFs): emerging new roles for an ancient RNA in the regulation of gene expression. *Life* 5: 1638–1651.

264 Krishna, S., Raghavan, S., DasGupta, R., and Palakodeti, D. (2021). tRNA-derived fragments (tRFs): establishing their turf in post-transcriptional gene regulation. *Cell. Mol. Life Sci.* 78: 2607–2619.

265 Zhu, L., Ge, J., Li, T. et al. (2019). tRNA-derived fragments and tRNA halves: the new players in cancers. *Cancer Lett.* 452: 31–37.

266 Wang, Y., Tao, E.W., Tan, J. et al. tRNA modifications: insights into their role in human cancers. *Trends Cell Biol.*

267 Schaffrath, R. and Leidel, S.A. (2017). Wobble uridine modifications-a reason to live, a reason to die?! *RNA Biol.* 14: 1209–1222.

268 Rapino, F., Delaunay, S., Rambow, F. et al. (2018). Codon-specific translation reprogramming promotes resistance to targeted therapy. *Nature* 558: 605–609.

269 Nedialkova, D.D. and Leidel, S.A. (2015). Optimization of codon translation rates via tRNA modifications maintains proteome integrity. *Cell* 161: 1606–1618.

270 Delaunay, S., Rapino, F., Tharun, L. et al. (2016). Elp3 links tRNA modification to IRES-dependent translation of LEF1 to sustain metastasis in breast cancer. *J. Exp. Med.* 213: 2503–2523.

271 Katsara, O. and Schneider, R.J. (2021). m7G tRNA modification reveals new secrets in the translational regulation of cancer development. *Mol. Cell* 81: 3243–3245.

272 Orellana, E.A., Liu, Q., Yankova, E. et al. (2021). METTL1-mediated m7G modification of Arg-TCT tRNA drives oncogenic transformation. *Mol. Cell* 81: 3323–3338.e3314.

273 Dai, Z., Liu, H., Liao, J. et al. (2021). N^7-Methylguanosine tRNA modification enhances oncogenic mRNA translation and promotes intrahepatic cholangiocarcinoma progression. *Mol. Cell* 81: 3339–3355.e3338.

274 Blaesius, K., Abbasi, A.A., Tahir, T.H. et al. (2018). Mutations in the tRNA methyltransferase 1 gene TRMT1 cause congenital microcephaly, isolated inferior vermian hypoplasia and cystic leukomalacia in addition to intellectual disability. *Am. J. Med. Genet. A* 176: 2517–2521.

275 Dewe, J.M., Fuller, B.L., Lentini, J.M. et al. (2017). TRMT1-catalyzed tRNA modifications are required for redox homeostasis to ensure proper cellular proliferation and oxidative stress survival. *Mol. Cell. Biol.* 37.

276 Lin, S., Liu, Q., Lelyveld, V.S. et al. (2018). Mettl1/Wdr4-mediated m(7)G tRNA methylome is required for normal mRNA translation and embryonic stem cell self-renewal and differentiation. *Mol. Cell* 71: 244–255.e245.

277 Suzuki, T., Yashiro, Y., Kikuchi, I. et al. (2020). Complete chemical structures of human mitochondrial tRNAs. *Nat. Commun.* 11: 4269.

278 Asano, K., Suzuki, T., Saito, A. et al. (2018). Metabolic and chemical regulation of tRNA modification associated with taurine deficiency and human disease. *Nucleic Acids Res.* 46: 1565–1583.

279 Morscher, R.J., Ducker, G.S., Li, S.H.J. et al. (2018). Mitochondrial translation requires folate-dependent tRNA methylation. *Nature* 554: 128–132.

280 Becker, L., Kling, E., Schiller, E. et al. (2014). MTO1-deficient mouse model mirrors the human phenotype showing complex I defect and cardiomyopathy. *PLoS One* 9: e114918.

281 Rikimaru, M., Ohsawa, Y., Wolf, A.M. et al. (2012). Taurine ameliorates impaired the mitochondrial function and prevents stroke-like episodes in patients with MELAS. *Intern. Med.* 51: 3351–3357.

282 Ohsawa, Y., Hagiwara, H., Nishimatsu, S. et al. (2019). Taurine supplementation for prevention of stroke-like episodes in MELAS: a multicentre, open-label, 52-week phase III trial. *J. Neurol. Neurosurg. Psychiatry* 90: 529–536.

283 Bacman, S.R., Williams, S.L., Pinto, M. et al. (2013). Specific elimination of mutant mitochondrial genomes in patient-derived cells by mitoTALENs. *Nat. Med.* 19: 1111–1113.

284 Ciara Ann, A., Penelope Nicole, H., and Peter, T. (2018). MERRF and MELAS: current gene therapy trends and approaches. 2: 9.

285 Velez-Bartolomei, F., Lee, C., and Enns, G. MERRF. *GeneReviews*.

286 Sloan, K.E., Warda, A.S., Sharma, S. et al. (2017). Tuning the ribosome: the influence of rRNA modification on eukaryotic ribosome biogenesis and function. *RNA Biol.* 14: 1138–1152.

287 Babaian, A., Rothe, K., Girodat, D. et al. (2020). Loss of m1acp3Ψ ribosomal RNA modification is a major feature of cancer. *Cell Rep.* 31: 107611.

288 Armistead, J., Khatkar, S., Meyer, B. et al. (2009). Mutation of a gene essential for ribosome biogenesis, EMG1, causes Bowen-Conradi syndrome. *Am. J. Human Genet.* 84: 728–739.

289 Doll, A. and Grzeschik, K.-H. (2001). Characterization of two novel genes, WBSCR20 and WBSCR22, deleted in Williams-Beuren syndrome. *Cytogenet. Cell Genet.* 95: 20–27.

290 Cowling, V.H., Turner, S.A., and Cole, M.D. (2014). Burkitt's lymphoma-associated c-Myc mutations converge on a dramatically altered target gene response and implicate Nol5a/Nop56 in oncogenesis. *Oncogene* 33: 3519–3527.

291 Ito, A., Watabe, K., Koma, Y. et al. (2001). Increased expression of a nucleolar Nop5/Sik family member in metastatic melanoma cells: evidence for its role in nucleolar sizing and function. *Am. J. Pathol.* 159: 1363–1374.

292 Williams, G.T. and Farzaneh, F. (2012). Are snoRNAs and snoRNA host genes new players in cancer? *Nat. Rev. Cancer* 12: 84–88.

293 Mannoor, K., Liao, J., and Jiang, F. (2012). Small nucleolar RNAs in cancer. *Biochim. Biophys. Acta* 1826: 121–128.

294 Ruggero, D., Grisendi, S., Piazza, F. et al. (2003). Dyskeratosis congenita and cancer in mice deficient in ribosomal RNA modification. *Science* 299: 259–262.

295 Marcel, V., Ghayad, S.E., Belin, S. et al. (2013). p53 acts as a safeguard of translational control by regulating fibrillarin and rRNA methylation in cancer. *Cancer Cell* 24: 318–330.

296 Catez, F., Venezia, N.D., Marcel, V. et al. (2019). Ribosome biogenesis: an emerging druggable pathway for cancer therapeutics. *Biochem. Pharmacol.* 159: 74–81.

297 Drygin, D., Lin, A., Bliesath, J. et al. (2011). Targeting RNA polymerase I with an oral small molecule CX-5461 inhibits ribosomal RNA synthesis and solid tumor growth. *Cancer Res.* 71: 1418–1430.

298 Lucas, M.C., Pryszcz, L.P., Medina, R. et al. (2023). Quantitative analysis of tRNA abundance and modifications by nanopore RNA sequencing. *Nat. Biotechnol.* 1–15.

299 Liu, C., Sun, H., Yi, Y. et al. (2023). Absolute quantification of single-base m(6)A methylation in the mammalian transcriptome using GLORI. *Nat. Biotechnol.* 41: 355–366.

300 Dai, W., Li, A., Yu, N.J. et al. (2021). Activity-based RNA-modifying enzyme probing reveals DUS3L-mediated dihydrouridylation. *Nat. Chem. Biol.*

13

Outlook

A Perspective on RNA: The Next Frontier for Small Molecule Therapeutics

Christopher R. Fullenkamp[1], *Xiao Liang*[1], *Martin Pettersson*[2], *and John Schneekloth Jr.*[1]

[1] *National Cancer Institute, Chemical Biology Laboratory, Frederick, MD 21702 USA*
[2] *Promedigen, Daejeon, 34050 Republic of Korea*

13.1 Introduction

RNA has historically been regarded as the central medium to translate genetic information encoded in DNA into protein sequences [1]. However, it has become clear that many RNAs have essential regulatory roles in diverse biological processes independent of translating genetic material into polypeptide sequences [2], establishing a central role for RNA in many areas of biology. Mutations in RNA can be disease-causing even when not resulting in altered protein sequence [3], and diverse non-coding RNAs (ncRNAs) are reported to modulate cellular homeostasis and disease phenotypes [4]. For example, non-coding mutations in mRNAs can drive splicing defects, resulting in tissue-specific pathogenesis [3]. Development of small molecule–RNA therapeutics has seen an increase in interest from academia and industry in recent years due partly to the revelation that >85% of the human genome is transcribed into RNA, whereas only ~2% encodes proteins. In addition, the growing evidence that supports RNA as a driver of multiple diseases, coupled with the recent approval of the mRNA splice modulator risdiplam, has further invigorated the investment in novel technologies to probe and identify small molecule modulators of RNA structure and function. Thus, a central promise of this approach is that targeting RNA could open up new target space to provide novel therapeutic intervention points and lead to the development of medicines for diseases with no cure.

The discovery process for identifying protein-interacting small molecules has been extensively optimized and standardized across academia and industry, and new and innovative techniques and modalities continue to emerge. In contrast, the target-based discovery of small molecules modulating RNA is still in its infancy, and standardized methods for the prediction and identification of structured regions in RNA, high-throughput screening assays, biophysical characterization methods, RNA–small molecule target engagement, functional effects, and lead optimization

RNA as a Drug Target: The Next Frontier for Medicinal Chemistry, First Edition.
Edited by John Schneekloth and Martin Pettersson.

are needed to accelerate the field. To date, numerous methods have been developed for screening small molecules against RNA targets. These include small molecule microarrays [5, 6], two-dimensional combinatorial screening (2DCS) [7], affinity selection mass spectrometry (AS-MS, automated ligand identification system [ALIS]) [8, 9], DNA-encoded libraries [10–12], catalytic enzyme-linked click chemistry assay (cat-ELCCA) [13–15], nuclear magnetic resonance (NMR) [16–19], and phenotypic screens [20–23], among others [24] (Figure 13.1). For a comprehensive overview of different screening methods, the reader is directed to the following reviews [1, 25–27] and Chapter 4 in this book. In contrast to numerous screening methods, techniques for biophysical interrogation of small molecule–RNA binding events, direct target engagement, and mapping of RNA–small molecule binding sites are in their infancy. Additionally, methods to overcome the unique

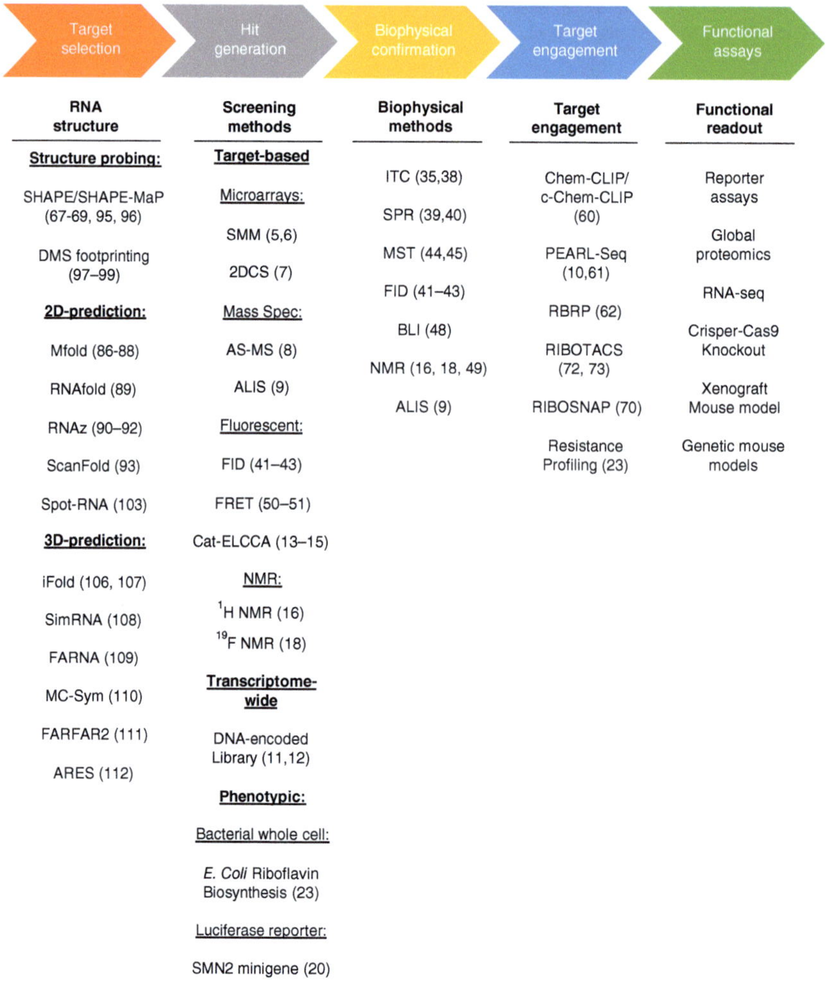

Figure 13.1 Overview of the current techniques and methods used for lead generation of RNA-targeting small molecules.

challenges of developing relevant and accurate functional assays and computational tools for RNA-targeting small molecules are underdeveloped compared to those used for protein-targeted drug discovery.

This chapter will discuss the current challenges in the field and highlight development opportunities with the potential to improve the discovery process of novel small molecule-based RNA therapeutics. Target selection, biophysical characterization, and target engagement studies will be emphasized, and the unique challenges of developing relevant and accurate functional assays for RNA targets will be addressed. In addition, an analysis of current computational tools used for structure prediction, docking, and molecular dynamics will be discussed in the context of how the limited number of available high-quality atomic resolution RNA structures is hindering the development and implementation of these tools. Furthermore, a discussion on the benefits of depositing RNA–small molecule screening, functional assay, and sequencing data in publicly accessible datasets can have on developing novel technologies to study RNA as a target for small molecules is included. For further insights into the challenges and opportunities of developing small molecules that target RNA, we direct the readers to this recent perspective [28].

13.2 Target Selection: Identification of the Most Promising RNA Intervention Points

From the perspective of medicinal chemists and drug hunters focused on designing and developing molecules against protein targets, it is well understood that different target classes involve various degrees of difficulty and often require diverging strategies. For example, the challenges and drug discovery strategies associated with targeting transporters, ion channels, G protein-coupled receptors (GPCRs) (agonist vs. antagonist), enzymes, protein–protein interactions, and transcription factors can vary significantly. Not only are different technologies often employed for hit generation and lead optimization, but the profile of the final drug candidate can also vary substantially, including physicochemical property space, potency, pharmacokinetic profile, and the exposure multiples (the ratio of unbound plasma drug concentration compared to *in vitro* IC_{50} value) required for *in vivo* efficacy. For example, while low exposure multiples may be sufficient for some nuclear hormone receptor agonists, higher exposure multiples are often required for enzymes such as kinases [29], and this has contributed to the emergence of covalent inhibitors as a useful strategy for this target class [30]. Similarly, targeting viral enzymes such as the severe acute respiratory syndrome coronavirus 2 (SARS CoV-2) protease C3Lpro typically requires targeting an IC_{90} at the minimum plasma concentration (C_{min}), directly impacting the requirements for oral bioavailability, half-life, and therapeutic dose [31]. It is conceivable that different "RNA target classes" will emerge that not only require different medicinal chemistry strategies but also are associated with various degrees of difficulty, where some RNA intervention points are more readily amenable to pharmacological intervention than others.

For example, different RNA target classes may include targeting maturation micro-RNA (blocking Drosha/Dicer processing of pri- and pre-mRNA) [15, 32, 33], binding and stabilizing the 3′ or 5′ untranslated region (UTR) of mRNA to reduce/inhibit translation and/or stability [34], targeting riboswitches [35, 36], tRNA, repeat expansions for particular genetic diseases [37], inhibiting cap-independent translation through targeting internal ribosome entry sites (IRES), and binding at the interface of pre-mRNA and the spliceosome to affect splice modulation (some of which have been discussed in detail in previous chapters of this book). Clearly, these therapeutic intervention points are not created equal, and similar to how knowledge for drugging different protein target classes has emerged over multiple decades, expansion of the toolbox for various RNA target classes will be needed to accelerate the field. This will also enable drug discovery teams to make high-quality decisions around target selection and appropriate lead-generation strategies.

13.3 Development of Robust Biophysical Methods, Alternative Strategies for Target Engagement, and Accurate and Reliable Functional Models

An early bottleneck when developing new RNA-targeting small molecules is the limitations of the available biophysical methods, which were initially developed for targeting proteins. These limitations contribute to challenges in hit validation and demonstration of target engagement. After identifying small molecules from hit-generation screens, direct binding to the target needs to be confirmed through orthogonal biophysical measurements. Each available method's strengths, weaknesses, and feasibility should be considered before choosing a technique. Following confirmation of direct target binding, confirmation of cellular target engagement and linking the small molecule–RNA interaction to functional activity is required. Traditionally, *in vitro* assays, such as reporter assays, analysis of mRNA and protein levels, phenotypic changes, and cytotoxicity, are commonly used to demonstrate functional activity for small molecules. Once compound binding has been linked to a relevant functional outcome in cells, attention is directed toward establishing appropriate preclinical and animal models to assess the impact of the small molecule *in vivo*. The development of widely applicable and accessible biophysical assays, alternative target engagement methods, and accurate functional assays that address the unique challenges of RNA targets is needed to streamline the discovery process for novel small molecule RNA-targeting therapeutics.

13.3.1 Biophysical Methods for Interrogating Small Molecule–RNA Interactions

Biophysical analysis of small molecule–RNA binding interactions can be challenging due to the dynamic structure of RNA. Therefore, several methods have been developed, including isothermal calorimetry (ITC) [35, 38], surface plasmon resonance (SPR) [39, 40], fluorescent indicator displacement (FID) [41–43], and microscale thermophoresis (MST) [44, 45] (Figure 13.1). However, typically, no individual biophysical assay is compatible with all RNA–small molecule systems, and it is common to evaluate several assays before a suitable technique is identified.

Currently, ITC and surface plasmon resonance (SPR) are the gold-standard biophysical methods to interrogate RNA–ligand interactions. ITC is a label-free method that allows for direct determination of stoichiometry (N), binding affinity (K_D), and change in enthalpy (ΔH) of the binding interaction. However, ITC requires a large amount of RNA and high aqueous solubility of the small molecules being investigated. Whereas SPR does not require a large quantity of RNA, the RNA must be labeled with biotin and immobilized on the surface of a sensor chip, which can result in altered folding and dynamics [39]. SPR experiments are highly amenable to automation and allow simultaneous analysis of multiple RNA targets with small molecules in the same experiment, greatly improving the throughput compared to ITC. In addition, kinetic parameters K_{on} and K_{off} can be acquired in conjunction with a binding affinity (K_D). However, the presence of avidin proteins and the negative charges on the surface of the chip can introduce non-specific interactions of the small molecule, resulting in non-saturable binding curves. A recent study by Arney and Weeks demonstrated a potential solution for subtracting non-specific interactions using a mutated non-binding RNA aptamer as the reference channel [40]. In addition, since SPR relies on a difference in molecular weight, it is challenging (if not prohibitive) to measure the binding of low-molecular-weight compounds to larger RNAs unless a significant conformational change is induced upon binding. For proteins, high immobilization on the chip has been used to overcome this limitation; however, for RNA, high immobilization can affect RNA structure and increase the non-specific binding of ligands, thus limiting the utility of SPR for large RNAs.

In addition to the techniques mentioned above, fluorescence-based methods such as FID assays [41] and MST [44] have also been successfully applied to measuring small molecule–RNA interactions. FID and MST are solution-based methods, unlike SPR, and differ from ITC by not requiring a large quantity of RNA. FID is a high-throughput solution-based assay that monitors the displacement of a fluorescent indicator from the RNA with increasing ligand concentration. It can be run on widely available plate readers, increasing its accessibility compared to SPR. However, for novel RNA aptamers, highly validated and characterized fluorescent indicators still need to be developed, which requires initial optimization and characterization of a new fluorescent indicator before FID can be used. Another emerging fluorescent technique is MST [44, 45], which works by utilizing the movement of fluorescent molecules along a temperature gradient or the thermophoretic effect [46, 47]. MST has become a valuable tool for affinity measurements when immobilization of the target RNA or obtaining large enough quantities of RNA is not feasible. However, not all RNA–ligand interactions result in a significant change in thermophoresis. Therefore, the method has been limited to systems with significant conformational changes, such as riboswitches or RNA–protein interactions [44]. As with other techniques, the success of fluorescence-based methods is highly system dependent and can require considerable assay development to implement successfully. In addition to the biophysical techniques highlighted above, other methods such as biolayer interferometry (BLI) [48], NMR [49], Förster Resonance Energy Transfer (FRET) [50, 51], electrospray ionization mass spectrometry (ESI-MS) [52], and AS-MS (ALIS) [8, 53, 54] have also been used to interrogate RNA–small molecule interactions. For a comprehensive review of the different biophysical methods (Figure 13.1) used to probe RNA–small molecules, the reader is directed to the numerous reviews published on targeting RNA with small molecules [1, 25–27, 55] and Chapter 4 in this book.

Notably, despite the extensive work that has gone into developing biophysical methods to study RNA–ligand interactions, there are remarkably few techniques capable of quantitatively measuring the binding of small ligands to larger RNAs. There is a considerable need for reliable assays that can be used to rank order hits from screens and for the optimization of a series of ligands through medicinal chemistry efforts. As the field advances, we must think deeply about developing next-generation biophysical methods to interrogate small molecule–RNA interactions. Ideally, new techniques would be robust and widely applicable to diverse RNA–ligand systems, emphasizing the need to preserve the RNA's physiologically or functionally relevant structure and dynamics.

13.3.2 Cellular Target Engagement Methods

Because many factors can influence phenotypic responses to drug treatment, target engagement assays are critical to demonstrating the on-target activity of any RNA-binding small molecule. Following confirmation of RNA–ligand binding and ligand optimization, direct target engagement in cells is needed to validate the RNA–small molecule interaction. Currently, methods to identify small molecule–protein engagement are more developed than those used for RNA–small molecule engagement. Some widely used techniques for protein target engagement include activity-based profiling [56] and chemoproteomic analysis using chemical crosslinking of small molecules to proteins via either electrophilic [57] or photoactivatable [58, 59] reactive groups and identification by mass spectrometry. In addition, cellular thermal shift assays (CETSA) provide a label-free approach to identifying direct interactions between small molecules and target proteins. In practice, a cellular thermal shift assay (CESTA)-type assay for RNA has yet to be developed, though such an assay could prove highly valuable if successfully realized. The unique challenges associated with target engagement studies with RNA include highly context-dependent expression and folding of RNA structures (i.e. co-transcriptional folding, protein-based conformation switching, etc.), high turnover of RNA, and the highly dynamic ensembles of RNA structures.

To date, several related methodologies have been described for the direct detection of small molecule–RNA engagement: chemical cross-linking and isolation by pull-down (Chem-CLIP, C-Chem-CLIP) [60], photoaffinity evaluation of RNA ligation-sequencing (PEARL-seq) [10, 61], and reactivity-based RNA profiling (RBRP) [62]. Direct target engagement through chemical crosslinking and enrichment allows for probing of small molecule–RNA interactions in cells and in a transcriptome-wide manner to identify and characterize all small molecule–RNA interactions and probe ligand selectivity. Approaches that use enrichment of the target RNA are powerful in that they enable the detection of targets with low levels of expression. However, other strategies might avoid artifactual error propagation or introduction of systematic biases. Current crosslinking and enrichment methods all follow a similar protocol and were developed in parallel by multiple academic and industry labs. The general outline of these methods is highlighted in (Figure 13.2b). Briefly, the first step is the synthesis of the ligand of interest with a reactive handle, either electrophilic or photoactivatable, and an affinity purification handle (Figure 13.2a). The second step involves incubation of the modified probe molecule *in vitro* or *in cellulo* to allow binding and proximity-based crosslinking of the probe molecule to the RNA. The third step is the enrichment of crosslinked RNA by magnetic avidin bead pulldown. If the target RNA is known, gene-specific reverse transcription-quantitative polymerase chain reaction (RT-qPCR) is completed after enrichment of the crosslinked RNA. If the RNA target is unknown, next-generation sequencing is conducted to identify the putative RNA targets (Figure 13.2b). In addition, ligand-target selectivity can be accessed by parallel incubation with a negative control nonspecific crosslinking ligand and competition experiments with the unmodified parent ligand [10, 60–62].

The first reported chemical crosslinking target engagement method was termed chemical crosslinking and isolation by pull-down (Chem-CLIP) by Guan and Disney in 2013 [60]. In 2015, Yang et al. elaborated upon the Chem-CLIP protocol to enable the mapping of small molecule binding sites with the development of Chem-CLIP-Map [63]. However, a significant drawback of the original Chem-CLIP protocols was the high reactivity of the chlorambucil electrophilic warhead. This led to a high background of nonspecific crosslinking events, making transcriptome-wide or *in cellulo* target engagement determination challenging. In addition, the identity of the RNA target had to be known before the crosslinking experiments for gene-specific RT-qPCR identification, which limits the applicability of this method. In 2018, two independent studies by Mortison et al. and Wang et al. developed similar approaches to Chem-CLIP for the RNA-target identification of tetracyclines, Col-3 and doxycycline, and SMN2 splicing modulator SMN-C2 [64, 65]. These improved methods replaced the previously used chlorambucil group with photoactivatable diazirine. The diazirine moiety has been used extensively in small molecule–protein target engagement studies [58, 59] and later with RNA. The replacement of chlorambucil with a diazirine enabled light-dependent crosslinking, reducing background crosslinking events and facilitating target identification by next-generation sequencing. Next-generation sequencing facilitates detecting RNA–probe interactions and determining the identified interactions' selectivity in a transcriptome-wide manner. However, these methods were not generalizable to all RNA–small molecule targets, and each study required unique analysis pipelines to identify the target RNAs.

In 2020, scientists at Arrakis Therapeutics described a generalized protocol and analysis pipeline called Photoaffinity Evaluation of the RNA Ligation-Sequencing or PEARL-seq [10, 61], which is a combination of the above-mentioned techniques.

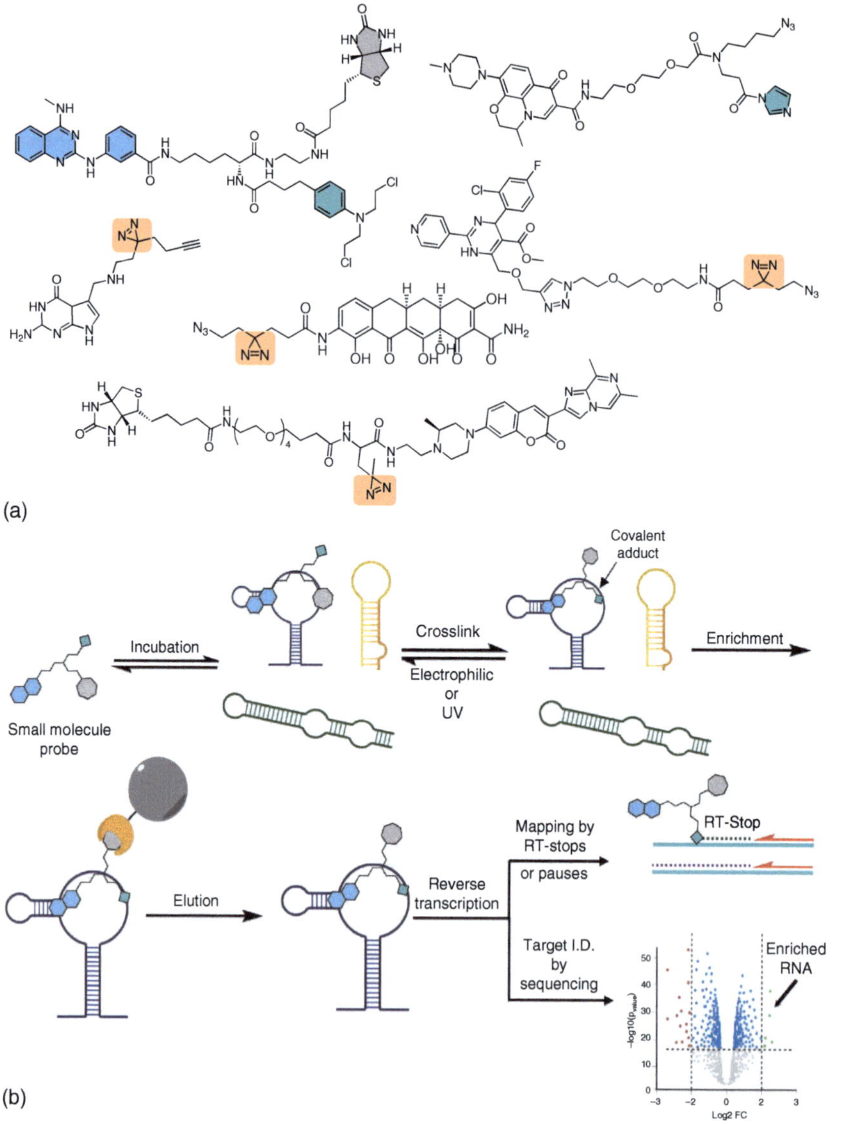

Figure 13.2 Selected examples of Chem-CLIP and RBRP probes and a general workflow. (a) Selected examples of electrophilic (teal color ring-fill) and photoactivatable (highlighted in an orange box) small molecule crosslinking probes. The structure at the top left has the cognate ligand (blue), the affinity purification handle, biotin (gray), and crosslinking moiety (teal) identified by the indicated ring-fill colors. (b) General workflow for Chem-CLIP methodology: First, the crosslinking probe is introduced to total RNA or cell lysates and allowed to bind. Second, proximity-based electrophilic crosslinking or photoactivation with ultraviolent light affords a covalent adduct of the ligand and RNA. Click reaction with biotin-azide and isolation with streptavidin-coated magnetic beads affords enriched crosslinked RNAs. If the RNA target is known, gene-specific RT-qPCR and RT-stop mapping is performed to confirm the RNA target and map the binding site. If the RNA target is unknown, ssDNA or cDNA libraries are prepared, followed by next-generation sequencing to identify RNA targets transcriptome-wide.

PEARL-seq combines photoactivable diazirine- and phenyl azide-based crosslinking probes with deep sequencing for target identification and RT-pausing analysis for mapping the ligand-binding site. Also, in 2020, work from our group demonstrated the power of next-generation sequencing-based Chem-CLIP methods for determining small molecule–RNA selectivity transcriptome-wide with a diazirine-appended PreQ1 ligand and enabled the identification of putative $PreQ_1$ RNA aptamers in human transcripts [66].

In 2021, work from Fang et al. developed a RBRP methodology to identify potential off-target RNA interactions of the United States Food and Drug Administration (FDA)-approved drugs hydroxychloroquine, dasatinib, and levofloxacin [62]. The RBRP methodology took inspiration from selective 2′-hydroxyl acylation analyzed by primer extension and mutational profiling (SHAPE-MaP) methods that have been used extensively for RNA structure probing experiments [67–69] and adopted an acyl imidazole reactive group to enable electrophilic crosslinking of probes to RNA at their 2′-hydroxyl. The RBRP method used next-generation sequencing and RT-stop detection to identify off-target RNA interactions and map the binding sites of the FDA-approved drugs to their potential RNA targets at near single nucleotide resolution.

In addition to the methodologies highlighted above, small molecule-directed RNA degradation methods such as RiboSNAP [70], proximity-induced nucleic acid degrader (PINAD) [71], and the development of ribonuclease targeting chimeras (RIBOTACS) [72, 73] have also been used to identify small molecule–RNA interactions. These methods incorporate functional groups such as hydroxythiopyridine (HPT) to induce RNA cleavage upon irradiation with an ultraviolet light, an imidazole group which acts as a catalytic chemical degrader of RNA, or by direct degradation of the RNA through the recruitment of RNase-L. RiboSNAP has been limited in its use because only one hydroxy-radical equivalent is produced from each HPT moiety, limiting the RNA cleavage to one event per small molecule [70]. RIBOTACs are still in their infancy, and further development of RNase recruiting ligands and linker optimization is needed to deliver cell-permeable RIBOTACs with good efficacy. Nevertheless, the potential of small molecule directed/induced RNA degradation holds great promise for developing new small-molecule-based RNA therapeutics. For an in-depth overview of the current state of RIBOTACS, we refer the reader to Chapter 9 of this book.

Chem-CLIP, PEARL-seq, and RBRP methods all require the modification of the small molecule of interest with a reactive crosslinking group and an affinity purification handle. Synthesis of these analogs can be challenging, limiting their use in studies with complex small molecules or natural products. In addition, incorporating reactive moieties can result in a loss of binding affinity and selectivity of the small molecule. While these challenges also apply to the analogous techniques used for targeting proteins, there are specific issues that are associated with target engagement studies for RNA. Some of these unique challenges include the complex mechanisms around context-dependent expression and folding, the high rate of RNA turnover, and the highly dynamic structures of RNAs. In addition, detecting RT-stops or pauses can be challenging because many nucleobase modifications can potentially be RT-silent [74]. Furthermore, each new probe generates a different crosslinked lesion that may or may not induce stops, deletions, pauses, or mutagenesis effects during reverse transcription. Taken together, these methods are powerful for mapping RNA–small molecule target engagement; however, they have yet to be widely applied across the field. Thus, the development of robust, reliable, and publicly available methods, datasets, and analysis pipelines is needed to compare the results of experiments done by different laboratories and drive consensus in the field about best practices. The development of reliable *in cellulo* and *in vivo* methods to identify RNA–ligand interactions and enable the mapping of RNA–ligand binding sites to near single nucleotide resolution is needed to streamline the discovery of novel RNA-targeting therapeutics. These methods would ideally be label-free or minimally perturb the small molecule structure and allow for the identification and deconvolution of on-target and off-target interactions of small molecules with both RNA and proteins in cells, although it is unlikely that any one method will fulfill all the desired characteristics.

13.3.3 Unique Challenges Faced in the Development of Functional Assays for Studying Small Molecule–RNA Interactions

The challenge of developing reliable, functional assays is not unique to small molecule–RNA therapeutics. Recently, Lin et al. demonstrated that numerous protein-based clinical drug candidates exhibit cytotoxic effects on cancer cells even when the putative protein target is knocked out with clustered regularly interspaced palindromic repeats (CRISPR)/Cas9 [75]. In additional studies on FDA-approved drugs palbociclib [76], hydroxychloroquine, levofloxacin, and dasatinib [62], potential RNA off-targets for these protein-targeting drugs were identified. These studies highlight the need for improved functional assays that carefully dissect the mechanism of action of small molecule drugs and highlight the importance of genetic validation of drug targets with precise methods such as CRISPR/Cas9 knockouts. Furthermore, methods that extensively map RNA and protein target engagement of small molecules in the context of their function will be indispensable for developing improved functional assays for RNA-targeting small molecules.

The most advanced RNA–small molecule therapeutics, risdiplam and branaplam, were discovered using luciferase reporter assays specifically designed to report on splicing modulation [21, 22, 77]. Similarly, phenotypic screening and resistance profiling led to the discovery and mechanistic characterization of the antimicrobial flavin mononucleotide (FMN) riboswitch binder Ribocil [23]. However, these methods do not apply to all RNA targets. Reliable assays that allow for the readout of functional perturbations invoked by on-target ligand–RNA interactions are currently only readily available for some RNA target classes, and continued development, and careful assay validation is needed. Furthermore, unique challenges are associated with developing accurate functional assays for RNA targets due to the complexity of gene expression regulation in cells. For example, sequence non-conservation between human and non-human species genomes and cell- and tissue-type differences in gene expression and regulation make it difficult to develop broadly applicable models. As exemplified by human and mouse p53, alternative splicing and alternative promoter usage results in 10 mRNA and 13 protein isoforms in humans but only four mRNA and six protein isoforms in mice (Figure 13.3a) [79]. These distinct mRNA isoforms contribute to different disease phenotypes, and accurate incorporation of the desired isoforms in human and mouse-based functional assays is quite challenging.

In addition to the challenges posed by the complexity of gene architecture and alternative splicing, already-developed reporter systems sometimes fail to recapitulate endogenous gene expression accurately. For example, the 3′-UTR in p53 mRNA had been demonstrated to inhibit p53 expression in reporter-based assays [80]. However, work by Mitschka and Mayr demonstrated that deletion of the endogenous 3′-UTR in mouse tissues and human HCT116 cells showed no effect on endogenous p53 mRNA or protein levels, contrary to the previously observed results using luciferase reporter systems [78]. Furthermore, they designed orthogonal green fluorescent protein (GFP-reporter systems and demonstrated that the p53 coding sequences, not the 3′ UTR, have a dominant repressive effect on the reporter gene expression and that the repressive effects of the coding sequence and 3′-UTR are not additive or synergistic (Figure 13.3b). This study highlights the need for careful validation of reporter-based functional assays within the context of endogenous gene regulation. In addition to p53, a recent study by our lab identified small molecules that target a putative G-quadruplex (G4) in the 5′ UTR of the oncogene neuroblastoma RAS viral oncogene homolog (NRAS). A specific ligand identified in a small molecule microarray (SMM) screen stabilized the G4 and repressed translation in a luciferase-based reporter assay; however, it only had moderate effects *in cellulo*. Further investigation of 14 different NRAS-expressing cell lines indicated that the predominantly expressed NRAS variant in these cell lines does not contain the 5′ UTR G4 structure [34]. The above examples exemplify the importance of genetic validation of RNA targets *in cellulo* and highlight a key challenge in developing accurate and reliable functional assays for RNA targeting small molecules.

In addition to the above-highlighted challenges focused on sequence conversation, RNA structure can also be context-dependent. Long-range RNA–RNA and RNA–protein interactions play a vital role in the expression of genes. For example, viral RNA viruses use long-range 3′ UTR-5′ UTR interactions and distal protein–RNA interactions to promote or inhibit viral translation in host cells [81]. These long-range interactions are poorly understood for all RNAs and can dramatically affect gene regulation. Without knowledge of potential long-range interactions, simply including a structured region of RNA in a reporter system can result in functional models that do not accurately recapitulate endogenous gene regulation and expression (Figure 13.3c).

The examples above are just a small subset of the unique challenges encountered when developing functional assays for RNA-targeting small molecules. They exemplify how the field needs to be careful when selecting *in vitro* and *in cellulo* functional assays and ensure thorough genetic validation that these functional models accurately represent *in vivo* endogenous gene expression when determining the

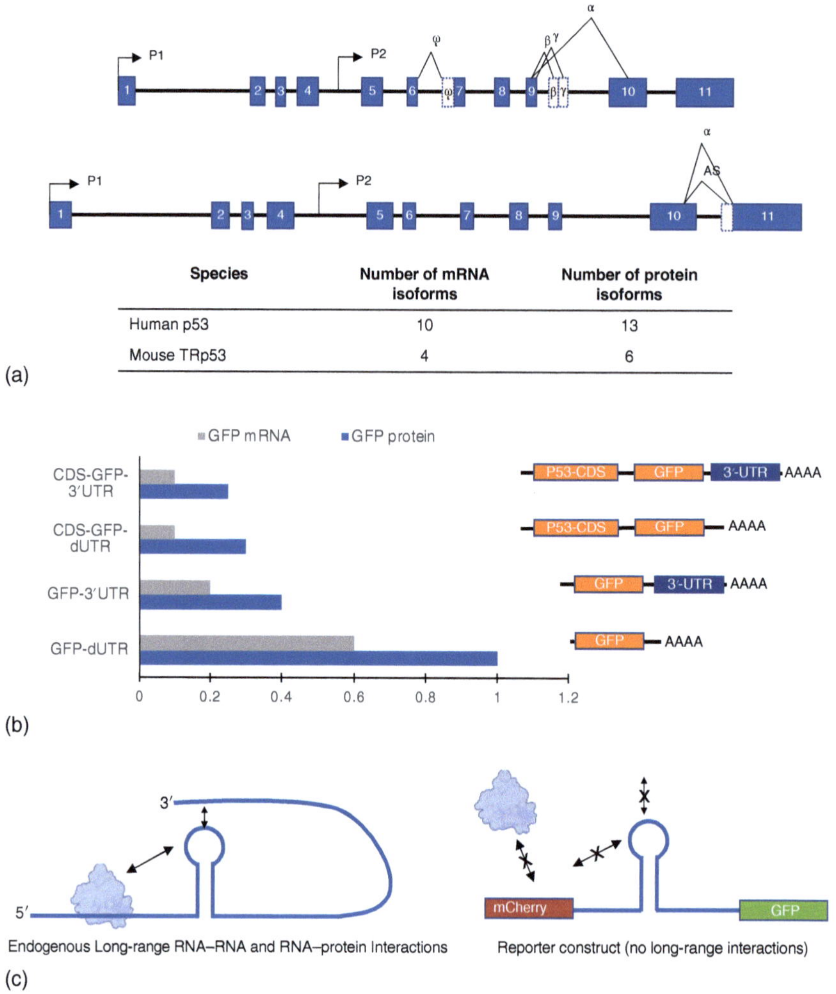

Species	Number of mRNA isoforms	Number of protein isoforms
Human p53	10	13
Mouse TRp53	4	6

Figure 13.3 Complexity of gene architecture and the challenges faced when developing functional models. (a) Comparison of human and mouse p53 gene architecture. The above depiction highlights the transcript and protein isoforms resulting from alternative splicing and promoter usage. Exons are labeled with the exon number and colored blue, and alternative splicing sites are colored orange. The table indicates the number of alternative mRNA transcripts and the resulting number of protein isoforms for human and mouse p53 gene expression. (b) p53-GFP reporter constructs demonstrating the effects of the 3′-UTR and coding sequence on mRNA and protein gene expression. The 3′-UTR has a slight repressive effect on p53 expression in reporter strains. However, this repressive effect is not indicative of endogenous control of p53. The coding sequence has a greater, non-additive repressive effect on p53 expression in p53-GFP reporter systems and more accurately represents endogenous gene expression of p53 in mice and humans. (panel b is an illustrative image [not experimental data] of the results from Mitschka and Mayr Source: Mitschka and Mayr [78]/eLife Sciences Publications Ltd/CC BY 4.0. (c) Endogenous long-range RNA–RNA and RNA–protein interactions (left panel) influence gene expression and are challenging to identify and include in reporter constructs. Reporter constructs without long-range interactions may not accurately recapitulate endogenous gene expression.

mechanism of action and target specificity. Increased development of robust, easily modifiable functional models to probe RNA–ligand interactions and their effect on gene expression at the transcriptional and translational levels will help facilitate the development of novel small molecule–RNA therapeutics. Furthermore, including multiplexed readouts in these models would allow for the identification of potential off-target interactions at both the RNA and protein levels. This would reduce the risk of safety-related clinical attrition of RNA-targeting therapeutics. In summation, further development of robust and widely acceptable biophysical assays, alternative target-engagement methods, and the development of accurate functional assays are needed to streamline the discovery of novel RNA-targeting therapeutics.

13.4 Acquisition of High-Resolution RNA and RNA–Ligand Structures is Needed to Enable the Development and Validation of Computational Tools for RNA–Small Molecule Therapeutic Discovery

Following target engagement and confirmation of the mechanism of action, significant optimization of the hit is typically required to address key parameters such as potency, selectivity, ADME (adsorption, distribution, metabolism, and excretion), and safety. Historically, computational modeling and structure-based design have enabled small molecule optimization in protein-targeting drug discovery [82–84]. These computational tools were developed using data from high-resolution protein structures and protein–ligand complexes available in the protein data bank (PDB) or developed for specific projects. High-resolution structures allow for developing and refining molecular forcefields, docking algorithms, and dynamic simulations of small molecule–biomolecule interactions. However, computational tools for studying RNA-targeting therapeutics have been greatly limited in their development in part due to the paucity of atomic-resolution RNA structures. As of December 2022, there were >195,000 protein structures in the PDB, while only ~6500 structures contained an RNA chain, including over 1200 synthetic RNA constructs with no biological or disease-relevant function. The acquisition of additional atomic resolution structures through X-ray crystallography and cryogenic electron microscopy (cryo-EM) is needed to enable the development and use of computational tools and methods such as molecular modeling, structure-guided design, and RNA structure prediction. Furthermore, with the development of these new tools and the subsequent molecular forcefields, the incorporation of molecular dynamic simulations, machine learning, and artificial intelligence (AI) can aid in the ability to probe RNA dynamics and the effect small molecules can have.

13.4.1 RNA Structure Prediction

Determining which regions of an RNA are structured and ligandable by small molecules is vital for target selection and development of novel RNA–small molecule therapeutics. Previous investigations into the druggability of RNA with small molecules indicated that tertiary RNA structures form ligandable pockets with similar features as protein–ligand pockets [85]. To date, the field has developed tools that predict the secondary structure of regions in the genome, such as Mfold [86–88], RNAfold [89], RNAz [90–92], and ScanFold [93]. Mfold and RNAfold use the minimum free energy (MFE) model based on the Zuker–Stigler algorithm and Turner rules to predict RNA secondary structure [94]. RNAfold also allows for the inclusion of experimental restraints based on chemical probing data from SHAPE-MaP [67, 68, 95, 96] and dimethyl sulfate (DMS) footprinting [97–99] experiments to improve the secondary structure prediction [89]. One of the most widely adopted programs, ScanFold, predicts regions in which base pairing is likely based on scanning window analysis and has been applied to the Zika virus (ZIKV), HIV-1 genomes, and MYC mRNA to successfully identify the structures of known functional motifs and new regions that can form structures in both genomes [93, 100].

Further improvements in the prediction of secondary RNA structure have recently been achieved with the introduction of new computational tools that use multiple sequence analysis, deep-learning, machine-learning-based algorithms, and conditional training methods, such as RNAz [90–92], RNAstructure [101, 102], SPOT-RNA [103], and CONTRAfold [104]. SPOT-RNA is a deep-learning technique comprising an ensemble of two-dimensional deep neural networks and transfer learning, which predicts the secondary structure of RNA based on canonical, noncanonical, and long-range base pairing (i.e. pseudoknots). SPOT-RNA achieved the highest precision compared with twelve other prediction techniques in the independent test of 62 high-resolution X-ray structures [103]. However, these methods are limited and do not provide 3D structural information. The 3D structure of RNA is critical to pocket formation, small molecule binding, and recognition. Furthermore, two RNA molecules can possess similar secondary structures with little sequence identity and exhibit completely different three-dimensional structures and biological functions. This is particularly apparent in the case of chain 9 of the G2099A mutant 5S ribosomal submit of *Haloarcula marismortui* (PDB: 1YJW) and chain B of a signal recognition particle (SRP) molecule (PDB: 1LNG) and highlights the importance tertiary structure has in determining small molecule ligandability [105].

The development of tools to predict the tertiary structure of RNA has been limited compared to secondary structure prediction due to the scarcity of high-quality RNA structural data such as X-ray or cryo-EM data. To date, RNA tertiary structure prediction methods rely on three main computational strategies: Ab initio folding, fragment assembly, and deep-learning-based methods. iFold [106, 107] and SimRNA [108] are *ab initio* folding models that use molecular dynamic simulations or Monte Carlo sampling to predict RNA tertiary structure, respectively. In comparison, FARNA (fragment assembly of RNA) [109], MC-Sym [110], and FARFAR2 (fragment assembly of RNA with full atom refinement) [111] methods predict RNA tertiary structure through the 3D-fragment assembly from a template library of solved 3D RNA motifs. However, these methods are limited in their prediction accuracy due to either the absence of any atomic-level structural information used in the prediction or bias introduced from the limited number of 3D fragments in the template library.

Recently, a deep-learning-based method termed atomic rotationally equivalent scorer (ARES) was reported [112]. ARES is a scoring method that ranks the output of tertiary structure predictions from the FARFAR2 model. ARES ranks the generated tertiary structures based on the 3D coordinates and atom type for each atom in the predicted RNA conformations. The scoring function allows for ranking and identifying the most accurately predicted 3D-RNA conformation. The development of ARES is a significant breakthrough in RNA tertiary structure prediction and the use of artificial intelligence-based models for RNA tertiary structure prediction. As more tertiary RNA structures are solved, new RNA secondary and tertiary structure prediction models can be developed, and current biases and limitations of the existing methods will be significantly reduced [113]. The continued development and inclusion of these methods, especially when AI and machine learning are being applied, has the potential to catalyze and accelerate the field and holds great promise for enabling future discoveries. The reader is referred to Chapters 2 and 3 in this book for in-depth discussions of RNA structure prediction and RNA atomic resolution structures.

13.4.2 Computational Tools for Hit Optimization

In addition to RNA structure prediction, the current absence of high-quality RNA tertiary structures has limited the use and development of computational modeling programs and tools for small molecule docking, virtual ligand screening, and structure-based design. Structure-based design of small molecules has become an industry-standard method for hit optimization. However, the use of structure-based design for RNA–small molecule interactions is almost nonexistent due to the difficulty in obtaining high-quality atomic-resolution RNA–ligand structures. Many commercial modeling and docking programs have modified their molecular forcefields and docking algorithms to accommodate RNA–ligand docking, such as Autodock [114, 115], DOCK [116], Glide [117], and internal coordinate mechanics (ICM) [118]. However, these forcefields still need to be sufficiently refined to represent small molecule–RNA interactions. The development of improved docking methods and forcefields is a very active area of research in the field, and once these methods are further optimized, there is great potential for accelerating hit optimization.

Despite these limitations, Charrette et al. demonstrated how structure-based design could be used to improve the shape complementarity of a 2-aminobenzimidazole viral translation inhibitor that interacts with the IRES of hepatitis C virus (HCV) [119]. In this study, they demonstrated that installing a spiro-cyclopropane off the 2-aminobezimidazole core could fill a small hydrophobic pocket behind the primary binding site of the ligand. The increased shape complementarity of the ligand to the pocket resulted in a five fold improvement in the binding affinity of the ligand. In addition, Connelly et al. used structure-based design to identify three distinct synthetic ligands for the $PreQ_1$ riboswitch, which possessed similar affinities for the RNA aptamer but differed with respect to transcriptional termination activity [36]. This study highlights the importance of understanding the binding mode and interactions of the ligand with the RNA target and how different interactions or binding poses can differentially modulate functional activity.

In addition to structure-based design, commercial software packages have been used for the virtual screening of small molecules against RNA motifs. In one example, researchers from Molsoft used a combination of DOCK and their ICM program to virtually screen the Available Chemicals Directory (ACD) against human immunodeficiency virus trans-acting responsive (HIV TAR) RNA element and found two ligands that inhibit the trans-activator of transcription (Tat)-TAR interaction with a CD_{50} of ~1 μM [120]. Additionally, Stelzer et al. also used ICM to virtually screen a library of small molecules with the dynamic ensemble of HIV-1 TAR element. This study identified six compounds that bind to TAR with high affinity and inhibit its interaction with Tat [121]. ICM has been used by many industrial and academic groups [42], such as Novartis [22], Arrakis [10], and the National Cancer Institute [85], for modeling, docking, and virtual screening of small molecule libraries. However, albeit functional, these programs can result in biased docking scores for RNA–ligand interactions compared to protein–ligand interactions due to the distinct differences between RNA and proteins and the limited structures available for creating accurate RNA-focused forcefields.

Due to the limitations of commercial docking algorithms, new nucleic-acid-based docking algorithms and scoring functions have been developed by academic researchers. RiboDock/rDOCK [122, 123], MORDOR [124], RLDock [125, 126], and NLDock [127] are a few of the many docking programs that are built based on nucleic-acid–ligand interactions and the unique properties of RNA. Feng et al. developed the nucleic acid ligand docking algorithm, NLDock, which generates different binding poses by a distance geometry and matching strategy and then scores each pose with the ITscoreNL function. NLDock was trained on 213 high-resolution nucleic acid–ligand complexes and tested on four diverse test sets and was demonstrated to outperform protein-based programs DOCK, AutoDock, rDOCK, GOLD, and Glide in the docking of small molecules to RNA [127]. However, these methods are still biased and limited in their accuracy due to the limited number of high-quality RNA–ligand complex structures available for developing and optimizing the molecular forcefields and scoring functions used to rank docked small molecules. The source code for many of these programs is publicly available online to enable widespread adoption by computational chemists and encourage their future development and optimization. However, even though programs like NLDock can outperform commercial software like ICM, these computational platforms have not been widely adopted due to the difficulty of installation, limited operating system support, lack of technical support and training, and the absence of user-friendly graphical user interfaces (GUI).

13.4.3 Implementation of Molecular Dynamics Simulations, Machine Learning, and AI Tools to Interrogate RNA–Small Molecule Interactions

In addition to the development of computational tools for small molecule docking, hit optimization, and virtual ligand screening, atomic resolution X-ray, and cryo-EM structures of RNA and RNA–ligand complexes can enable the use of molecular dynamics to probe the perturbations small molecules have on RNA structure and how these perturbations can lead to functional effects. RNA is highly dynamic compared to proteins, and the dynamic structural ensembles are critical for their functions [128]. The use of molecular dynamics simulations can provide vital insights into how small molecules interact with and perturb RNA structure and function. For example, molecular dynamics simulations on the *pfl domain* of the *Thermosinus carboxydivorans* 5-aminoimidazole-4-carboxamide riboside 5′-triphosphate (ZTP) riboswitch provided insights into how the cognate ligand, 5-aminoimidazole-4-carboxamide riboside 5′-monophospahte (ZMP), is essential for the co-transcriptional folding of the aptamer domain and identified important nucleotides that contribute to ZMP recognition and RNA stabilization [129]. In a recent collaborative investigation by our group, structure probing combined with AI-informed molecular dynamics provided insights into the different dissociation pathways of two structurally distinct ligands that bind to the $PreQ_1$ riboswitch. The dynamic simulations and SHAPE-MaP reactivities showed a good correlation between experimentally determined flexibility (i.e. nucleotide reactivity) and C2–C2 distances, indicating the accuracy of the dynamic simulation (Figure 13.4a). Furthermore, this study showed how molecular dynamics simulation of RNA–ligand interactions can illuminate different dissociation trajectories and how these differences contribute to differential stabilization and functional effects (Figure 13.4a) [130]. These examples highlight the potential insights that implementing molecular dynamics simulations can have on our understanding of RNA–small molecule interactions. In addition, one of the first examples of using machine learning to optimize small molecules was recently reported by Grimberg et al. [131]. In this study, they combined deep convolutional networks, Lasso regression, and decision trees to identify chemical features important for phenyl thiazole-containing molecule's affinity to hairpin 91 in the ribosomal peptidyl transferase center (PTC) of *Mycobacterium tuberculosis* (Figure 13.4b, left panel) [131]. Next, based on the features identified in their models and in conjunction with docking, 10 analogs with potentially improved binding affinity to hairpin 91 were identified. Following the synthesis of the predicted analogs, experimental validation of ribosomal activity identified four of the 10 new analogs as potent inhibitors of *M. tuberculosis* ribosomal activity (Figure 13.4b, right panel), highlighting the potential of machine-learning-based models as practical tools for small molecule optimization.

The development of novel computational tools for RNA structure prediction hit optimization and the implementation of molecular dynamics simulations of RNA–ligand complexes will further enable medicinal chemistry efforts for

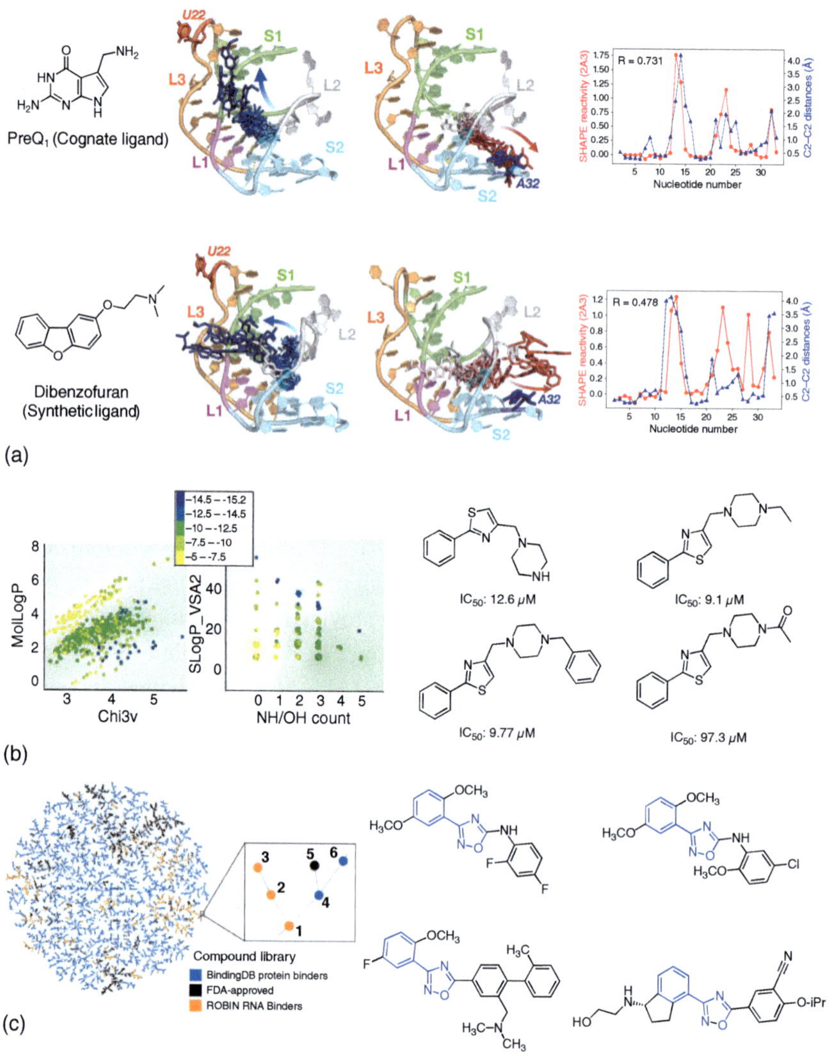
PreQ1 (Cognate ligand)
Dibenzofuran (Synthetic ligand)
U22
S1
L3
L2
L1
S2
A32
R = 0.731
R = 0.478
SHAPE reactivity (2A3)
C2–C2 distances (Å)
Nucleotide number
(a)
MolLogP
Chi3v
SLogP_VSA2
NH/OH count
−14.5 – −15.2
−12.5 – −14.5
−10 – −12.5
−7.5 – −10
−5 – −7.5
IC50: 12.6 μM
IC50: 9.1 μM
IC50: 9.77 μM
IC50: 97.3 μM
(b)
Compound library
BindingDB protein binders
FDA-approved
ROBIN RNA Binders
(c)

Figure 13.4 AI-informed molecular dynamics and machine-learning classification of high-throughput screening (HTS) data informs RNA–ligand interactions and defines RNA-binding chemical space and molecular features contributing to small molecule–RNA binding. (a) AI-augmented molecular dynamics simulation prediction of distinct dissociation pathways for PreQ$_1$ and dibenzofuran ligands from the PreQ$_1$ riboswitch and predicted distal nucleotides (labeled in red and blue) that are important in each ligand's unique dissociation trajectories. Comparison of C2–C2 distances calculated from AI-informed molecular dynamics simulations with experimental structure probing (SHAPE-MaP) reactivities, which indicate specific nucleotide flexibility, showed good correlation, highlighting the accuracy of the AI-augmented molecular dynamics simulations of the RNA–ligand dynamic interactions. Source: Wang et al. [130]/American Chemical Society/CC BY-NC-ND 4.0. (b) Lasso-regression-based classification of chemical features of phenylthiazole analogs correlated with docking scores demonstrated that only two features are sufficient to classify RNA ligand-binding affinity to hairpin 91 in the ribosomal PTC of *M. tuberculosis:* MolLogP vs. Chi3v and SLogP_VSA2 vs. the number of NH/OH showed good correlation with AutoDock docking scores (colored coded: yellow (−5) to blue (−15.2), the more negative, the better the docking score) (left panel). Lasso regression, convolutional neural network (CNN), and decision tree models in combination with AutoDock docking led to the identification of 10 new ligands, four of which were found to induce ribosomal inhibition (right panel). Source: Grimberg et al. [131]/Springer Nature/CC BY 4.0. (c) Visualization of RNA binding small molecules (orange, 2003) within FDA-approved (black, 2350 drugs) and BindingDB (blue, 10,000 ligands) chemical space as a treemap (TMAP). TMAP branches were generated by the classification of ligands with ECFP4 features and highlight areas within known chemical space that contain small molecules that interact with both RNA and proteins and are structurally similar to FDA-approved drugs. One branch from the TMAP containing ligands that are either RNA binding, protein binding, or an FDA-approved drug with the shared core structure (highlighted in blue) is shown. Source: Yazdani et al. [132]/with permission of John Wiley & Sons.

RNA-targeting therapeutics. These tools will enable identification of ligandable RNA structures, prioritization of virtual hits for synthesis, and the interrogation of how small molecules bind and stabilize RNA dynamic ensembles and modulate their function. However, the number of high-quality RNA structures available must increase dramatically for these tools to be developed. The acquisition of more RNA structures will also allow machine-learning models and AI tools to be implemented in the field. For a deeper look at the use of machine learning and other computational tools, we direct the reader to a recent perspective by Bagnolini et al. [133]. These tools could generate a similar impact on the small molecule–RNA drug discovery field that structure-based design has had on protein drug discovery and that AlphaFold2 [134] is predicted to have on protein-targeted drug discovery.

13.5 Deposition of Small Molecule–RNA Interaction Data with Rigorous Experimental Protocols and Controls is Needed

Targeting RNA with small molecules has gained much interest in the past decade. This has resulted in the development of novel screening strategies, biophysical characterization methods, and functional assays. However, with the development of these new technologies comes the responsibility of the researchers to disclose all experimental details and raw data in readily accessible databases. Data deposition enables the generalization, standardization, and adaptation of these new methods throughout the field. Additionally, depositing raw data and experimental conditions allows for increased rigor and reproducibility of reported results and increased efficiency for other researchers. Equally important, data deposition allows for and encourages additional analyses, which can result in new discoveries.

To date, numerous small molecule–RNA interaction datasets have been made available online, including the *R*NA-Targeted *Bi*oactive liga*N*d *D*atabase (R-BIND) [135], nucleic acid ligand database (NALDB) [136], RNAligands [137], SMMRNA [138], and *R*epository *O*f *BI*nders to *N*ucleic acids (ROBIN) [132]. Other databases, such as Inforna [139], are available only to academic users after signing a software use agreement. R-BIND and the recently updated R-BIND 2.0 [140] are a collection of small bioactive molecules reported in the current literature that bind to RNA and have a functional effect. The R-BIND dataset contains extensive and comprehensive information on the small molecule ligand, including RNA target, discovery methods, *in vitro* assays, cell-based assays, and animal model data, if available. Furthermore, NALDB, RNAligands, and SMMRNA are similar to the R-BIND database. They contain curated published data on known nucleic-acid-interacting small molecules from PubMed index research articles and are publicly accessible online. These databases can potentially enable the discovery of new small molecules that interact with RNA and provide insights into what types of chemical matter preferentially interact with RNA.

Despite the benefit of broadly describing successful attempts to target RNA from the literature, these databases are limited by the information publicly disclosed with the original publication. Furthermore, the data published for each ligand is not standardized across the field, restricting the use of these databases. Recently, our laboratory released a new dataset of small molecule–nucleic binders called ROBIN. The ROBIN dataset is the complete data from 36 nucleic acid small molecule microarray screens against a library of ~25,000 small molecules. The ROBIN dataset includes the identity of all hits from the 36 SMM screens, the raw screening data, and *z*-scores for all nucleic acid targets for each compound in the library. This work included several machine-learning models with high predictive value for RNA binding. These models were trained on the small molecule hits from SMM screens to identify RNA-targeting ligands based on distinct chemical features (Figure 13.4b) [132]. Additionally, in this study, a comparative analysis of RNA-binding, FDA-approved drugs, and compounds from the BindingDB database was completed and represented as a tree-map (TMAP) to visualize the shared chemical space of the ligands within these groups (Figure 13.4c). ROBIN is the first collection of compounds published that also includes the raw screening data, which promotes transparency and provides the opportunity for others in the field to use the screening data for novel analyses and the generation of new models to analyze what small molecule features correlate to RNA-binding chemical space.

In addition to screening datasets, the deposition of raw sequencing datasets collected from target engagement studies and functional assays is needed to develop generalized and widely applicable analysis pipelines. One of the significant obstacles to RNA-target engagement studies is the analysis of sequencing data. Each lab has developed its own in-house pipeline, with different cut-offs, data processing steps, and controls. These various analysis pipelines and lack of standardization limit the broad applicability and use of the methods. The RNA sequencing, single-cell RNA sequencing, and proteomics fields benefited greatly from the crowd-sourced development of generalized and standardized analysis pipelines. This same effect can only happen for the RNA-targeting field once researchers publicly release their raw data files with their publications, as exemplified in recent publications by our lab [66] and Fang et al. [62]. Furthermore, the deposition of raw data opens the door to new collaborations, innovation, and the development of standardized protocols and controls across the field and will further enable the advancement of high-quality molecules into clinical development.

13.6 Outlook: The Future of Small Molecule-Based RNA Therapeutics is Bright

Small molecule-based RNA therapeutics is an exciting and rapidly growing area in drug discovery that holds the promise of unlocking new target space. This is exemplified by the foundation of several new biotech start-ups in recent years, along with significant investments from large pharmaceutical companies to study small molecule-based RNA therapeutics. In addition, the recent approval of risdiplam, the granting of orphan drug status for branaplam, and the development of mRNA base vaccines for the COVID-19 pandemic have catalyzed a resurgence of interest in the field. As our understanding of the interplay of RNA structure and dynamics in relation to RNA function grows, the availability of suitable tools and methods to interrogate small molecules will increase. The development of novel biophysical techniques, alternative target engagement methods, and relevant functional assays will help facilitate the identification of small molecule–RNA modulators and their mechanisms of action.

Furthermore, increased acquisition of high-resolution RNA and RNA–ligand structures will enable the development and use of novel computational tools, molecular dynamics simulations, and machine-learning-based models to interrogate ligand–RNA interactions and their functional outcomes. In addition, the continued push from researchers throughout the field to release their raw screening, functional, and sequencing data will enable the generalization of and development of widely applicable techniques to interrogate small molecule–RNA interactions. Equally important, the development of accurate functional models that recapitulate the desired phenotype with standardized protocols is necessary for the continued success of the field. As the knowledge of RNA–small molecule interactions increases and the above-highlighted challenges are addressed, the future of RNA targeting holds the potential to access new target space, identify effective therapeutic intervention points, and develop new medicines for diseases with no cure.

References

1 Warner, K.D., Hajdin, C.E., and Weeks, K.M. (2018). Principles for targeting RNA with drug-like small molecules. *Nat. Rev. Drug Discovery* 17 (8): 547–558.

2 Connelly, C.M., Moon, M.H., and Schneekloth, J.S. Jr., (2016). The emerging role of RNA as a therapeutic target for small molecules. *Cell Chem. Biol.* 23 (9): 1077–1090.

3 Cooper, T.A., Wan, L., and Dreyfuss, G. (2009). RNA and disease. *Cell* 136 (4): 777–793.

4 Meyer, S.M., Williams, C.C., Akahori, Y. et al. (2020). Small molecule recognition of disease-relevant RNA structures. *Chem. Soc. Rev.* 49 (19): 7167–7199.

5 Connelly, C.M., Abulwerdi, F.A., and Schneekloth, J.S. Jr., (2017). Discovery of RNA binding small molecules using small molecule microarrays. *Methods Mol. Biol.* 1518: 157–175.

6 Jordan, D., Yang, M., and Schneekloth, J.S. Jr., (2020). Three-color imaging enables simultaneous screening of multiple RNA targets on small molecule microarrays. *Curr. Protoc. Chem. Biol.* 12 (4): e87.

7 Disney, M.D., Labuda, L.P., Paul, D.J. et al. (2008). Two-dimensional combinatorial screening identifies specific aminoglycoside–RNA internal loop partners. *J. Am. Chem. Soc.* 130 (33): 11185–11194.

8 Rizvi, N.F., Howe, J.A., Nahvi, A. et al. (2018). Discovery of selective RNA-binding small molecules by affinity-selection mass spectrometry. *ACS Chem. Biol.* 13 (3): 820–831.

9 Rizvi, N.F. and Nickbarg, E.B. (2019). RNA-ALIS: methodology for screening soluble RNAs as small molecule targets using ALIS affinity-selection mass spectrometry. *Methods* 167: 28–38.

10 Mukherjee, H., Blain, J.C., Vandivier, L.E. et al. (2020). PEARL-seq: a photoaffinity platform for the analysis of small molecule-RNA interactions. *ACS Chem. Biol.* 15 (9): 2374–2381.

11 Chen, Q., Li, Y., Lin, C. et al. (2022). Expanding the DNA-encoded library toolbox: identifying small molecules targeting RNA. *Nucleic Acids Res.* 50 (12): e67.

12 Benhamou, R.I., Suresh, B.M., Tong, Y. et al. (2022). DNA-encoded library versus RNA-encoded library selection enables design of an oncogenic noncoding RNA inhibitor. *Proc. Natl. Acad. Sci. U.S.A.* 119 (6): e2114971119.

13 Lorenz, D.A. and Garner, A.L. (2017). Approaches for the discovery of small molecule ligands targeting microRNAs. *Top Med. Chem.* 27: 79.

14 Lorenz, D.A., Vander Roest, S., Larsen, M.J., and Garner, A.L. (2018). Development and implementation of an HTS-compatible assay for the discovery of selective small-molecule ligands for pre-microRNAs. *SLAS Discovery* 23 (1): 47–54.

15 Lorenz, D.A., Song, J.M., and Garner, A.L. (2015). High-throughput platform assay technology for the discovery of pre-microRNA-selective small molecule probes. *Bioconjugate Chem.* 26 (1): 19–23.

16 Shortridge, M.D. and Varani, G. (2021). Efficient NMR screening approach to discover small molecule fragments binding structured RNA. *ACS Med. Chem. Lett.* 12 (8): 1253–1260.

17 Tam, B., Sherf, D., Cohen, S. et al. (2019). Discovery of small-molecule inhibitors targeting the ribosomal peptidyl transferase center (PTC) of *M. tuberculosis*. *Chem. Sci.* 10 (38): 8764–8767.

18 Binas, O., de Jesus, V., Landgraf, T. et al. (2021). 19F NMR-based fragment screening for 14 different biologically active RNAs and 10 DNA and protein counter-screens. *ChemBioChem* 22 (2): 423–433.

19 Lee, M.-K., Bottini, A., Kim, M. et al. (2014). A novel small-molecule binds to the influenza A virus RNA promoter and inhibits viral replication. *Chem. Commun.* 50 (3): 368–370.

20 Naryshkin, N.A., Weetall, M., and Dakka, A. (2014). SMN2 splicing modifiers improve motor function and longevity in mice with spinal muscular atrophy. *Science* 345 (null): 688.

21 Ratni, H., Ebeling, M., Baird, J. et al. (2018). Discovery of risdiplam, a selective survival of motor neuron-2 (SMN2) gene splicing modifier for the treatment of spinal muscular atrophy (SMA). *J. Med. Chem.* 61 (15): 6501–6517.

22 Palacino, J., Swalley, S.E., Song, C. et al. (2015). SMN2 splice modulators enhance U1-pre-mRNA association and rescue SMA mice. *Nat. Chem. Biol.* 11 (7): 511–517.

23 Howe, J.A., Wang, H., Fischmann, T.O. et al. (2015). Selective small-molecule inhibition of an RNA structural element. *Nature* 526 (7575): 672–677.

24 Zafferani, M., Muralidharan, D., Montalvan, N.I., and Hargrove, A.E. (2022). RT-qPCR as a screening platform for mutational and small molecule impacts on structural stability of RNA tertiary structures. *RSC Chem. Biol.* 3 (7): 905–915.

25 Childs-Disney, J.L., Yang, X., Gibaut, Q.M.R. et al. (2022). Targeting RNA structures with small molecules. *Nat. Rev. Drug Discovery* 21 (10): 736–762.

26 Morishita, E.C. (2022). Discovery of RNA-targeted small molecules through the merging of experimental and computational technologies. *Expert Opin. Drug Discovery* 1–20.

27 Haga, C.L. and Phinney, D.G. (2022). Strategies for targeting RNA with small molecule drugs. *Expert Opin. Drug Discovery* 1–13.

28 Garner, A.L. (2023). Contemporary progress and opportunities in RNA-targeted drug discovery. *ACS Med. Chem. Lett.* 14 (3): 251–259.

29 Jansson-Löfmark, R., Hjorth, S., and Gabrielsson, J. (2020). Does In Vitro Potency Predict Clinically Efficacious Concentrations? *Clin. Pharmacol. Ther.* 108 (2): 298–305.

30 Abdeldayem, A., Raouf, Y.S., Constantinescu, S.N. et al. (2020). Advances in covalent kinase inhibitors. *Chem. Soc. Rev.* 49 (9): 2617–2687.

31 Owen, D.R., Allerton, C.M.N., Anderson, A.S. et al. (2021). An oral SARS-CoV-2 M^{pro} inhibitor clinical candidate for the treatment of COVID-19. *Science* 374 (6575): 1586–1593.

32 Connelly, C.M., Boer, R.E., Moon, M.H. et al. (2017). Discovery of inhibitors of microRNA-21 processing using small molecule microarrays. *ACS Chem. Biol.* 12 (2): 435–443.

33 Garner, A.L., Lorenz, D.A., Sandoval, J. et al. (2019). Tetracyclines as inhibitors of pre-microRNA maturation: a disconnection between RNA binding and inhibition. *ACS Med. Chem. Lett.* 10 (5): 816–821.

34 Balaratnam, S., Torrey, Z.R., Calabrese, D.R. et al. (2022). Investigating the NRAS 5′ UTR as a target for small molecules. bioRxiv. 2022:2022.01.05.475055.

35 Tran, B., Pichling, P., Tenney, L. et al. (2020). Parallel discovery strategies provide a basis for riboswitch ligand design. *Cell Chem. Biol.* 27 (10): 1241–9 e4.

36 Connelly, C.M., Numata, T., Boer, R.E. et al. (2019). Synthetic ligands for PreQ1 riboswitches provide structural and mechanistic insights into targeting RNA tertiary structure. *Nat. Commun.* 10 (1): 1501.

37 Angelbello, A.J., Benhamou, R.I., Rzuczek, S.G. et al. (2021). A small molecule that binds an RNA repeat expansion stimulates its decay via the exosome complex. *Cell Chem. Biol.* 28 (1): 34–45.e6.

38 Kumar, G.S. and Basu, A. (2016). The use of calorimetry in the biophysical characterization of small molecule alkaloids binding to RNA structures. *Biochim. Biophys. Acta* 1860 (5): 930–944.

39 Vo, T., Paul, A., Kumar, A. et al. (2019). Biosensor-surface plasmon resonance: a strategy to help establish a new generation RNA-specific small molecules. *Methods* 167: 15–27.

40 Arney, J.W. and Weeks, K.M. (2022). RNA–ligand interactions quantified by surface plasmon resonance with reference subtraction. *Biochemistry* 61 (15): 1625–1632.

41 Wicks, S.L. and Hargrove, A.E. (2019). Fluorescent indicator displacement assays to identify and characterize small molecule interactions with RNA. *Methods* 167: 3–14.

42 Zafferani, M., Haddad, C., Luo, L. et al. (2021). Amilorides inhibit SARS-CoV-2 replication in vitro by targeting RNA structures. *Sci. Adv.* 7 (48): eabl6096.

43 Das, B., Murata, A., and Nakatani, K. (2021). A small-molecule fluorescence probe ANP77 for sensing RNA internal loop of C, U and A/CC motifs and their binding molecules. *Nucleic Acids Res.* 49 (15): 8462–8470.

44 Moon, M.H., Hilimire, T.A., Sanders, A.M., and Schneekloth, J.S. Jr., (2018). Measuring RNA–ligand interactions with microscale thermophoresis. *Biochemistry* 57 (31): 4638–4643.

45 Entzian, C. and Schubert, T. (2016). Studying small molecule-aptamer interactions using microscale thermophoresis (MST). *Methods* 97: 27–34.

46 Seidel, S.A.I., Dijkman, P.M., Lea, W.A. et al. (2013). Microscale thermophoresis quantifies biomolecular interactions under previously challenging conditions. *Methods* 59 (3): 301–315.

47 Ofner, C. III, and Schott, H. (1985). Shifts in the apparent ionization constant of the carboxylic acid groups of gelatin. *J. Pharm. Sci.* 74 (12): 1317–1321.

48 Su, Z., Zhang, Y., Gendron, T.F. et al. (2014). Discovery of a biomarker and lead small molecules to target r (GGGGCC)-associated defects in c9FTD/ALS. *Neuron* 83 (5): 1043–1050.

49 Calabrese, D.R., Connelly, C.M., and Schneekloth, J.S. Jr. (2019). Ligand-observed NMR techniques to probe RNA-small molecule interactions. In: *Methods in Enzymology*, vol. 623 (ed. A.E. Hargrove), 131–149. Elsevier.

50 Zhang, Y., Zeng, D., Cao, J. et al. (2017). Interaction of quindoline derivative with telomeric repeat–containing RNA induces telomeric DNA-damage response in cancer cells through inhibition of telomeric repeat factor 2. *Biochim. Biophys. Acta* 1861 (12): 3246–3256.

51 Abulwerdi, F.A., Xu, W., Ageeli, A.A. et al. (2019). Selective small-molecule targeting of a triple helix encoded by the long noncoding RNA, MALAT1. *ACS Chem. Biol.* 14 (2): 223–235.

52 Dremann, D.N. and Chow, C.S. (2019). Chapter 14 - The use of electrospray ionization mass spectrometry to monitor RNA-ligand interactions. In: *Methods in Enzymology*, vol. 623 (ed. A.E. Hargrove), 315–337. Academic Press.

53 Seth, P.P., Miyaji, A., Jefferson, E.A. et al. (2005). SAR by MS: discovery of a new class of RNA-binding small molecules for the hepatitis C virus: internal ribosome entry site IIA subdomain. *J. Med. Chem.* 48 (23): 7099–7102.

54 Aguilar, R., Spencer, K.B., Kesner, B. et al. (2022). Targeting Xist with compounds that disrupt RNA structure and X inactivation. *Nature* 604 (7904): 160–166.

55 Blakeley, B.D., DePorter, S.M., Mohan, U. et al. (2012). Methods for identifying and characterizing interactions involving RNA. *Tetrahedron* 68 (43).

56 Cravatt, B.F., Wright, A.T., and Kozarich, J.W. (2008). Activity-based protein profiling: from enzyme chemistry to proteomic chemistry. *Annu. Rev. Biochem.* 77 (1): 383–414.

57 Backus, K.M., Correia, B.E., Lum, K.M. et al. (2016). Proteome-wide covalent ligand discovery in native biological systems. *Nature* 534 (7608): 570–574.

58 Cisar, J.S. and Cravatt, B.F. (2012). Fully functionalized small-molecule probes for integrated phenotypic screening and target identification. *J. Am. Chem. Soc.* 134 (25): 10385–10388.

59 Sumranjit, J. and Chung, S.J. (2013). Recent advances in target characterization and identification by photoaffinity probes. *Molecules* 18 (9): 10425–10451.

60 Guan, L. and Disney, M.D. (2013). Covalent small-molecule–RNA complex formation enables cellular profiling of small-molecule–RNA interactions. *Angew. Chem. Int. Ed.* 52 (38): 10010–10013.

61 Sexton, A.N., Vandivier, L.E., Petter, J.C. et al. (2022). Determination of RNA-ligand interactions with the photoaffinity platform PEARL-seq. *Methods* 205: 83–88.

62 Fang, L., Velema, W.A., Lee, Y. et al. (2023). Pervasive transcriptome interactions of protein-targeted drugs. *Nat. Chem.* 15 (10): 1374–1383.

63 Yang, W.-Y., Wilson, H.D., Velagapudi, S.P., and Disney, M.D. (2015). Inhibition of non-ATG translational events in cells via covalent small molecules targeting RNA. *J. Am. Chem. Soc.* 137 (16): 5336–5345.

64 Mortison, J.D. (2018). Tetracyclines modify translation by targeting key human rRNA substructures. *Cell Chem. Biol.* 25: 1506.

65 Wang, J., Schultz, P.G., and Johnson, K.A. (2018). Mechanistic studies of a small-molecule modulator of SMN2 splicing. *Proc. Natl. Acad. Sci. U.S.A* 115: E4604.

66 Balaratnam, S., Rhodes, C., Bume, D.D. et al. (2021). A chemical probe based on the PreQ1 metabolite enables transcriptome-wide mapping of binding sites. *Nat. Commun.* 12 (1): 5856.

67 Wilkinson, K.A., Merino, E.J., and Weeks, K.M. (2006). Selective 2′-hydroxyl acylation analyzed by primer extension (SHAPE): quantitative RNA structure analysis at single nucleotide resolution. *Nat. Protoc.* 1 (3): 1610–1616.

68 Smola, M.J., Rice, G.M., Busan, S. et al. (2015). Selective 2’-hydroxyl acylation analyzed by primer extension and mutational profiling (SHAPE-MaP) for direct, versatile and accurate RNA structure analysis. *Nat. Protoc.* 10 (11): 1643–1669.

69 Martin, S., Blankenship, C., Rausch, J.W., and Sztuba-Solinska, J. (2019). Using SHAPE-MaP to probe small molecule-RNA interactions. *Methods* 167: 105.

70 Rzuczek, S.G., Colgan, L.A., Nakai, Y. et al. (2017). Precise small-molecule recognition of a toxic CUG RNA repeat expansion. *Nat. Chem. Biol.* 13 (2): 188–193.

71 Mikutis, S., Rebelo, M., Yankova, E. et al. (2023). *Proximity-Induced Nucleic Acid Degrader (PINAD) Approach to Targeted RNA Degradation Using Small Molecules.* ACS Central Science.

72 Costales, M.G., Suresh, B., Vishnu, K., and Disney, M.D. (2019). Targeted degradation of a hypoxia-associated non-coding RNA enhances the selectivity of a small molecule interacting with RNA. *Cell Chem. Biol.* 26 (8): 1180–6 e5.

73 Costales, M.G., Aikawa, H., Li, Y. et al. (2020). Small-molecule targeted recruitment of a nuclease to cleave an oncogenic RNA in a mouse model of metastatic cancer. *Proc. Natl. Acad. Sci. U.S.A.* 117 (5): 2406–2411.

74 Behm-Ansmant, I., Helm, M., and Motorin, Y. (2011). Use of specific chemical reagents for detection of modified nucleotides in RNA. *J. Nucleic Acids* 2011: 408053.

75 Lin, A., Giuliano, C.J., Palladino, A. et al. (2019). Off-target toxicity is a common mechanism of action of cancer drugs undergoing clinical trials. *Sci. Transl. Med.* 11 (509).

76 Shortridge, M.D., Vidalala, V., and Varani, G. (2022). The kinase inhibitor Palbociclib is a potent and specific RNA-binding molecule. bioRxiv. 2022:2022. 01.20.477126.

77 Cheung, A.K., Hurley, B., Kerrigan, R. et al. (2018). Discovery of small molecule splicing modulators of survival motor neuron-2 (SMN2) for the treatment of spinal muscular atrophy (SMA). *J. Med. Chem.* 61 (24): 11021–11036.

78 Mitschka, S. and Mayr, C. (2021). Endogenous p53 expression in human and mouse is not regulated by its 3′UTR. *eLife* 10: e65700.

79 Kazantseva, M., Mehta, S., Eiholzer, R.A. et al. (2018). A mouse model of the Δ133p53 isoform: roles in cancer progression and inflammation. *Mamm. Genome* 29 (11): 831–842.

80 Haronikova, L., Olivares-Illana, V., Wang, L. et al. (2019). The p53 mRNA: an integral part of the cellular stress response. *Nucleic Acids Res.* 47 (7): 3257–3271.
81 Nicholson, B.L. and White, K.A. (2014). Functional long-range RNA–RNA interactions in positive-strand RNA viruses. *Nat. Rev. Microbiol.* 12 (7): 493–504.
82 Cox, R. and Plemper, R.K. (2016). Structure-guided design of small-molecule therapeutics against RSV disease. *Expert Opin. Drug Discovery* 11 (6): 543–556.
83 Hallenbeck, K., Turner, D., Renslo, A., and Arkin, M.R. (2017). Targeting non-catalytic cysteine residues through structure-guided drug discovery. *Curr. Top. Med. Chem.* 17 (1): 4–15.
84 Ostrem, J.M., Peters, U., Sos, M.L. et al. (2013). K-Ras(G12C) inhibitors allosterically control GTP affinity and effector interactions. *Nature* 503 (7477): 548–551.
85 Hewitt, W.M., Calabrese, D.R., and Schneekloth, J.S. Jr., (2019). Evidence for ligandable sites in structured RNA throughout the protein data bank. *Bioorg. Med. Chem.* 27 (11): 2253–2260.
86 Zuker, M. (2003). Mfold web server for nucleic acid folding and hybridization prediction. *Nucleic Acids Res.* 31 (13): 3406–3415.
87 Zuker, M. (1989). On finding all suboptimal foldings of an RNA molecule. *Science* 244 (4900): 48–52.
88 Zuker, M. and Stiegler, P. (1981). Optimal computer folding of large RNA sequences using thermodynamics and auxiliary information. *Nucleic Acids Res.* 9 (1): 133–148.
89 Hofacker, I.L., Fontana, W., Stadler, P.F. et al. (1994). Fast folding and comparison of RNA secondary structures. *Monatshefte für Chemie /Chemical Monthly* 125 (2): 167–188.
90 Washietl, S., Hofacker, I.L., Lukasser, M. et al. (2005). Mapping of conserved RNA secondary structures predicts thousands of functional noncoding RNAs in the human genome. *Nat. Biotechnol.* 23 (11): 1383–1390.
91 Gruber, A.R., Neuböck, R., Hofacker, I.L., and Washietl, S. (2007). The RNAz web server: prediction of thermodynamically stable and evolutionarily conserved RNA structures. *Nucleic Acids Res.* 35 (suppl_2): W335–W338.
92 Gruber, A.R., Findeiß, S., Washietl, S. et al. (2010). RNAz 2.0: improved noncoding RNA detection. *Biocomputing* 69–79.
93 Andrews, R.J., Roche, J., and Moss, W.N. (2018). ScanFold: an approach for genome-wide discovery of local RNA structural elements-applications to Zika virus and HIV. *PeerJ* 6: e6136.
94 Freier, S.M., Kierzek, R., Jaeger, J.A. et al. (1986). Improved free-energy parameters for predictions of RNA duplex stability. *Proc. Natl. Acad. Sci. U.S.A.* 83 (24): 9373–9377.
95 Siegfried, N.A., Busan, S., Rice, G.M. et al. (2014). RNA motif discovery by SHAPE and mutational profiling (SHAPE-MaP). *Nat. Methods* 11 (9): 959–965.
96 Merino, E.J., Wilkinson, K.A., Coughlan, J.L., and Weeks, K.M. (2005). RNA structure analysis at single nucleotide resolution by selective 2′-hydroxyl acylation and primer extension (SHAPE). *J. Am. Chem. Soc.* 127 (12): 4223–4231.
97 Peattie, D.A. and Gilbert, W. (1980). Chemical probes for higher-order structure in RNA. *Proc. Natl. Acad. Sci. U.S.A.* 77 (8): 4679–4682.

98 Tijerina, P., Mohr, S., and Russell, R. (2007). DMS footprinting of structured RNAs and RNA-protein complexes. *Nat. Protoc.* 2 (10): 2608–2623.

99 Mathews, D.H., Disney, M.D., Childs, J.L. et al. (2004). Incorporating chemical modification constraints into a dynamic programming algorithm for prediction of RNA secondary structure. *Proc. Natl. Acad. Sci. U.S.A.* 101 (19): 7287–7292.

100 O'Leary, C.A., Andrews, R.J., Tompkins, V.S. et al. (2019). RNA structural analysis of the MYC mRNA reveals conserved motifs that affect gene expression. *PLoS One* 14 (6): e0213758.

101 Mathews, D.H. (2004). Using an RNA secondary structure partition function to determine confidence in base pairs predicted by free energy minimization. *RNA* 10 (8): 1178–1190.

102 Reuter, J.S. and Mathews, D.H. (2010). RNAstructure: software for RNA secondary structure prediction and analysis. *BMC Bioinf.* 11: 129.

103 Singh, J., Hanson, J., Paliwal, K., and Zhou, Y. (2019). RNA secondary structure prediction using an ensemble of two-dimensional deep neural networks and transfer learning. *Nat. Commun.* 10 (1): 5407.

104 Do, C.B., Woods, D.A., and Batzoglou, S. (2006). CONTRAfold: RNA secondary structure prediction without physics-based models. *Bioinformatics* 22 (14): e90–e98.

105 Abraham, M., Dror, O., Nussinov, R., and Wolfson, H.J. (2008). Analysis and classification of RNA tertiary structures. *RNA* 14 (11): 2274–2289.

106 Sharma, S., Ding, F., and Dokholyan, N.V. (2008). iFoldRNA: three-dimensional RNA structure prediction and folding. *Bioinformatics* 24 (17): 1951–1952.

107 Krokhotin, A., Houlihan, K., and Dokholyan, N.V. (2015). iFoldRNA v2: folding RNA with constraints. *Bioinformatics* 31 (17): 2891–2893.

108 Boniecki, M.J., Lach, G., Dawson, W.K. et al. (2015). SimRNA: a coarse-grained method for RNA folding simulations and 3D structure prediction. *Nucleic Acids Res.* 44 (7): e63.

109 Das, R. and Baker, D. (2007). Automated *de novo* prediction of native-like RNA tertiary structures. *Proc. Natl. Acad. Sci. U.S.A.* 104 (37): 14664–14669.

110 Parisien, M. and Major, F. (2008). The MC-Fold and MC-Sym pipeline infers RNA structure from sequence data. *Nature* 452 (7183): 51–55.

111 Watkins, A.M., Rangan, R., and Das, R. (2020). FARFAR2: improved de novo Rosetta prediction of complex global RNA folds. *Structure* 28 (8): 963–76.e6.

112 Townshend, R.J., Eismann, S., Watkins, A.M. et al. (2021). Geometric deep learning of RNA structure. *Science* 373 (6558): 1047–1051.

113 Flamm, C., Wielach, J., Wolfinger, M.T. et al. (2022). Caveats to deep learning approaches to RNA secondary structure prediction. *Front. Bioinf.* 2.

114 Morris, G.M., Goodsell, D.S., Halliday, R.S. et al. (1998). Automated docking using a Lamarckian genetic algorithm and an empirical binding free energy function. *J. Comput. Chem.* 19 (14): 1639–1662.

115 Detering, C. and Varani, G. (2004). Validation of automated docking programs for docking and database screening against RNA drug targets. *J. Med. Chem.* 47 (17): 4188–4201.

116 Lang, P.T., Brozell, S.R., Mukherjee, S. et al. (2009). DOCK 6: combining techniques to model RNA–small molecule complexes. *RNA* 15 (6): 1219–1230.

117 Friesner, R.A., Banks, J.L., Murphy, R.B. et al. (2004). Glide: a new approach for rapid, accurate docking and scoring. 1. Method and assessment of docking accuracy. *J. Med. Chem.* 47 (7): 1739–1749.

118 Abagyan, R., Totrov, M., and Kuznetsov, D. (1994). ICM—A new method for protein modeling and design: applications to docking and structure prediction from the distorted native conformation. *J. Comput. Chem.* 15 (5): 488–506.

119 Charrette, B.P., Boerneke, M.A., and Hermann, T. (2016). Ligand optimization by improving shape complementarity at a hepatitis C virus RNA target. *ACS Chem. Biol.* 11 (12): 3263–3267.

120 Filikov, A.V., Mohan, V., Vickers, T.A. et al. (2000). Identification of ligands for RNA targets via structure-based virtual screening: HIV-1 TAR. *J. Comput. Aided Mol. Des.* 14 (6): 593–610.

121 Stelzer, A.C., Frank, A.T., Kratz, J.D. et al. (2011). Discovery of selective bioactive small molecules by targeting an RNA dynamic ensemble. *Nat. Chem. Biol.* 7 (8): 553–559.

122 Afshar, M. and Morley, S.D. (2004). Validation of an empirical RNA-ligand scoring function for fast flexible docking using RiboDock (r). *J. Comput. Aided Mol. Des.*

123 Ruiz-Carmona, S., Alvarez-Garcia, D., Foloppe, N. et al. (2014). rDock: a fast, versatile and open source program for docking ligands to proteins and nucleic acids. *PLoS Comput. Biol.* 10 (4): e1003571.

124 Guilbert, C. and James, T.L. (2008). Docking to RNA via root-mean-square-deviation-driven energy minimization with flexible ligands and flexible targets. *J. Chem. Inf. Model.* 48 (6): 1257–1268.

125 Sun, L.-Z., Jiang, Y., Zhou, Y., and Chen, S.-J. (2020). RLDOCK: a new method for predicting RNA–ligand interactions. *J. Chem. Theory Comput.* 16 (11): 7173–7183.

126 Jiang, Y. and Chen, S.-J. (2022). RLDOCK method for predicting RNA-small molecule binding modes. *Methods* 197: 97–105.

127 Feng, Y., Zhang, K., Wu, Q., and Huang, S.-Y. (2021). NLDock: a fast nucleic acid–ligand docking algorithm for modeling RNA/DNA–ligand complexes. *J. Chem. Inf. Model.* 61 (9): 4771–4782.

128 Dethoff, E.A., Chugh, J., Mustoe, A.M., and Al-Hashimi, H.M. (2012). Functional complexity and regulation through RNA dynamics. *Nature* 482 (7385): 322–330.

129 Yu-nan, H., Kang, W., Yu, S. et al. (2022). Molecular dynamics simulation on the *Thermosinus carboxydivorans* pfl ZTP riboswitch by ligand binding. *Biochem. Biophys. Res. Commun.* 627: 184–190.

130 Wang, Y., Parmar, S., Schneekloth, J.S., and Tiwary, P. (2022). Interrogating RNA–small molecule interactions with structure probing and artificial intelligence-augmented molecular simulations. *ACS Cent. Sci.* 8 (6): 741–748.

131 Grimberg, H., Tiwari, V.S., Tam, B. et al. (2022). Machine learning approaches to optimize small-molecule inhibitors for RNA targeting. *J. Cheminf.* 14 (1): 4.

132 Yazdani, K., Jordan, D., Yang, M. et al. (2022). Machine learning informs RNA-binding chemical space. bioRxiv. 2022:2022.08.01.502065.

133 Bagnolini, G., Luu, T.B., and Hargrove, A.E. (2023). Recognizing the power of machine learning and other computational methods to accelerate progress in small molecule targeting of RNA. *RNA*.

134 Jumper, J., Evans, R., Pritzel, A. et al. (2021). Highly accurate protein structure prediction with AlphaFold. *Nature* 596 (7873): 583–589.

135 Morgan, B.S., Sanaba, B.G., Donlic, A. et al. (2019). R-BIND: an interactive database for exploring and developing RNA-targeted chemical probes. *ACS Chem. Biol.* 14 (12): 2691–2700.

136 Kumar Mishra, S. and Kumar, A. (2016). NALDB: nucleic acid ligand database for small molecules targeting nucleic acid. *Database* 2016.

137 Sun, S., Yang, J., and Zhang, Z. (2022). RNALigands: a database and web server for RNA–ligand interactions. *RNA* 28 (2): 115–122.

138 Mehta, A., Sonam, S., Gouri, I. et al. (2014). SMMRNA: a database of small molecule modulators of RNA. *Nucleic Acids Res.* 42 (Database issue): D132–D141.

139 Disney, M.D., Winkelsas, A.M., Velagapudi, S.P. et al. (2016). Inforna 2.0: a platform for the sequence-based design of small molecules targeting structured RNAs. *ACS Chem. Biol.* 11 (6): 1720–1728.

140 Donlic, A., Swanson, E.G., Chiu, L.-Y. et al. (2022). R-BIND 2.0: an updated database of bioactive RNA-targeting small molecules and associated RNA secondary structures. *ACS Chem. Biol.* 17 (6): 1556–1566.

Index

a

AbsorbArray 57
academic compound libraries 98, 99
acyl imidazoles 10, 12, 363
affinity selection mass spectroscopy (AS-MS) 356
allosteric self-cleaving ribozymes 215
amilorides 100, 102
2-aminobenzimidazole viral translation inhibitor 337
aminoglycosides 2, 22, 36, 53, 54, 58, 68, 72, 94–96, 108, 120, 127, 128, 130, 132, 133, 257, 258, 259, 271, 273
5-aminoimidazole-4-carboxamide riboside 5′-triphosphate 207, 212, 371
2-aminopurine (2-AP) 66, 68
2-aminopyridine-3-carboxylic acid imidazolide (2A3) 10
anti-Shine-Dalgarno sequence 214
antibiotic drug development 210
antibiotics 205–207
antibiotic spectinomycin 22
antisense molecules 2
antisense oligonucleotide (ASO) 2, 41, 72, 74, 78, 93, 119, 127, 151, 183, 227–228, 274
artificial ribonucleases 228
atomic rotationally equivalent scorer (ARES) 337
automated ligand identification system (ALIS) 54, 356
Available Chemicals Directory (ACD) 370

b

base-paring pattern 30
benzimidazoles and purines 100, 101
betacoronaviruses 269, 273
binding site identification and target engagement 72
biolayer interferometry (BLI) 63, 360
biomolecules 31, 34, 51, 70, 71, 97, 130, 297, 367
biosensors 64, 65, 204, 210–211
bleomycin 229–231
bleomycin-based direct degraders *vs.* RiboTACs 242
bleomycin conjugates 142, 230–235, 242, 245
bleomycin degraders 230, 245
  targeting oncogenic precursor microRNA 233–234
  targeting r(CCUG) repeat expansion that causes DM2 233
  targeting the r(CUG) repeat expansion that causes DM1 231–233
branaplam lead generation 79–80
brome mosaic virus tRNA-like structure (BMV TLS) 38

RNA as a Drug Target: The Next Frontier for Medicinal Chemistry, First Edition.
Edited by John Schneekloth and Martin Pettersson.

c

carmofur (1-hexylcarbamoyl-5-fluorouracil) 212, 213
catalytic enzyme-linked click chemistry assay (cat-ELCCA) 297, 356
cell-based RPI detection assays 300, 301
cellular target engagement methods 360–364
cellular thermal shift assays (CETSA) 360
chemical cross-linking and isolation by pull-down (Chem-CLIP, C-Chem-CLIP) 72, 136, 270, 360
chemical probes 10–12, 16, 19, 72, 97, 103, 106, 121
chemical similarity search algorithms 104
chromatin-associated regulatory RNAs (carRNAs) 325
cobalamin (vitamin B12) 2
coding and non-coding RNA 322, 328
cold shock domains (CSD) 290
commercial ligands 108–110
  academic libraries 98–99
  industrial libraries 98
covalent methods 72–74
Covid-19 pandemic 30, 273, 375
cryogenic electron microscopy (cryo-EM) 30, 367
cyanine dyes 68, 69

d

DEAD/DEAH box helicase domains 290
deep learning (DL) 40, 105, 368, 369
designer riboswitches 205, 213–214
Dicer 101, 122, 123, 125, 127, 128, 130, 131, 133, 134, 136, 139, 141, 233, 238, 240–243, 298, 358
dihydropteroate synthase 211
2,5-diketopiperazine (DKP) 261
diphenyl furan (DPF) 100, 103
direct mapping of RNA–RNA interactions 14–17
DNA-encoded libraries (DELs) 56–57, 139–140, 160, 242, 274, 356
double-stranded RNA (dsRNA) 96, 122, 123, 177, 236, 329
double-stranded RNA binding domains (dsRBD) 286–287
Dovitinib-RiboTAC 241, 243
drug discovery
  fragment-based 58–63
  history of 2
Duke RNA-Targeted Library (DRTL) 93
dynamic combinatorial chemistry 101, 103, 258
dystrophia myotonica protein kinase (*DMPK*) gene 229, 294

e

electrospray ionization mass spectrometry (ESI-MS) 51, 360
epitranscriptome 321–336
epitranscriptomics 4, 322, 325, 327, 330, 335
2-ethylquinoline 3-carboxamide moiety 259
eukaryotic expression platforms 214–216

f

first-generation RiboTACs targeting oncogenic miRNAs 236–239
flavin mononucleotide (FMN) 32, 56, 97, 207, 208–209, 364
fluorescence-based assays 66–69, 71, 297
fluorescent indicator displacement (FID) assays 67–69, 127, 359
Fomiversen 227
fragment-based drug design 138, 139
fragment-based drug discovery (FBDD) 58–63
fragment hit optimization 62–63
fragment library design 59
fragment screening method 59
frameshifting activity 254, 269

frameshift-stimulating element (FSE) 255, 256, 264
FSE RNA 256, 258–263, 274
functional assays 4, 49, 75–77, 357, 358, 364–367, 373–375

g
Gag and Gag-pol poly proteins 253, 256
geneticin 271, 273
genome-wide association studies (GWAS) 1, 8
G-quadruplexes (G4) 8, 156, 158, 365
Guanidinoneomycin B 257

h
hereditary transthyretin amyloidosis (hATTR) 227
high resolution structures of RNA
  cryo-EM 37–39
  NMR spectroscopy 34–37
  3D structure prediction and integrative approaches 39–43
  X-ray crystallography 31–34
hit optimization 49, 62–63, 76–78, 369–371
human immunodeficiency virus type 1 (HIV-1) 253, 256
N-hydroxypyridine-2(1*H*)-thione (*N*-HPT) conjugates 229
N-hydroxypyridinethiones 229

i
immucillin-based compounds 212
industrial compound libraries 97, 98
inosine (I) 325, 328–330
internal ribosome entry sites (IRES) 8, 34, 54, 215, 335, 358
in vitro chemiluminescence-based assays 297–300
in vitro fluorescence-based assays 297
iron response elements (IRE) 8
isothermal titration calorimetry (ITC) 70, 358

k
Kennard–Stone algorithm 108
K homology (KH) domains 282, 289–290
knowledge-based *vs.* agnostic screening 49–50

l
lacZ (β-galactosidase) 211
LATS2 130, 132, 133
lead series
  branaplam lead generation 79–80
  hit optimization 77–78
  risdiplam hit-to-lead 78–79
  zotatifin lead generation 80
locked nucleic acids (LNAs) 2, 232
long non-coding RNAs (lncRNAs) 1, 120

m
macrolides 2, 95, 96, 120, 128, 176, 330
mass spectrometry 51–55, 76, 259, 274, 360
merafloxacin 269, 272, 273
messenger RNAs (mRNAs) 7, 75, 80, 120, 121, 203
metastasis associated lung adenocarcinoma transcript 1 (MALAT-1) 33, 103
N^6-methyladenosine (m^6A) 325–330
N-methylation 260, 261
2-methylnicotinic acid imidazolide (NAI) 10
METTL3 325–327, 336
microarray screening 57–58
microRNAs (miRNAs)
  biogenesis 122–123
  cleavage properties 142–144
  degradation and inhibit translation 121
  discovery and identification of 121
  RNA–protein interactions inhibition 140–142
  with small-molecule RNA binders
    pre- and pri-miRNA binders 125–140
    tumor suppressor 124–125

microscale thermophoresis (MST) 70, 359
minimum free energy (MFE) 9, 368
mRNA modifications
  inosine (I) 328–330
  N^6-methyladenosine (m^6A) 325–327
  pseudouridine (Ψ) 327–328
  roles of 322
multivalent ligands 100, 103
muscleblind-like 1 (MBNL1) splicing factor 229

n
nafamostat 272–274
naphthalene diimide (NDI) 101
native riboswitch ligands 95–97
natural ligands 108–110
  aminoglycosides 94–95
  macrolides 96
  native riboswitch ligands 96–97
  tetracyclines 95–96
5-nitroisatoic anhydride (5NIA) 10
non-coding RNAs (ncRNAs) 1, 3, 93, 119, 120, 122, 144, 274, 291, 292, 322, 325, 328, 330, 355
nonmetal-based small molecules 228
nuclear magnetic resonance (NMR)
  for fragment screening 60–61
  spectroscopy 34–37
nucleic acid ligand database (NALDB) 93, 374

o
oncogenes 123, 141, 172, 176, 242, 326, 327, 365
oncogenic pri-microRNAs 231
oxazolidinones 100, 102, 107, 120

p
peptide nucleic acids (PNAs) 2, 140
phage display 63
1,10-phenanthroline-copper complexes 228
phenotypic screens 3, 29, 49, 76, 78, 209, 356, 364
photoaffinity evaluation of the RNA ligation-sequencing (PEARL-seq) 360, 361
Piwi/Argonaute/Zwille (PAZ) domains 290
posttranscriptional modifications of RNA 3, 31, 321, 335
pre- and pri-miRNA binders
  DNA-encoded libraries (DEL) 139–140
  fragment-based drug design 138–139
  intracellular assays 125–127
  specific ligands designs 131–138
  target-based *in vitro* assays 127–131
Programmed Ribosomal Frameshifting (PRF) 253–274
protein-based genetic switches 214
protein data bank (PDB) 29, 106, 367
protein-interacting small molecules 323
proteolysis-targeting chimeras (PROTACs) 162, 235
proximity-induced nucleic acid degrader (PINAD) 363
pseudotyped HIV 261
pseudouridine (Ψ) 321, 325–331
Pumilio (PUF) domains 290

q
quantitative structure–activity relationship (QSAR) 102, 105, 107
quinazoline 100, 101–102, 125
quinoline derivatives 101

r
$r(CCUG)^{exp}$-targeting bleomycin conjugate 230, 233
reactivity-based RNA profiling (RBRP) 328, 331
Resin Bound Dynamic Combinatorial Library (RBDCL) 258, 274
respiratory syncytial virus 253, 254
retroviruses 256

Rev response element (RRE) 8, 70, 95
RGG/RG domains 290
rhodium (II) 9,10-phenanthrenequinone-diimine complexes 228
ribocil-C 32, 97, 209
RiboDock/rDOCK 370
Ribonuclease L (RNase L) 236
ribonuclease targeting chimeras (RiboTACs) 142, 235–244, 271, 363
ribonucleoprotein complexes (RNPs) 2, 31, 281
RiboSNAP 363
ribosomal RNAs (rRNA) 2, 7, 22, 63, 69, 94, 120, 188, 207, 334–335
riboswitches
  antibiotics 205–207
  barriers and future developments 210, 213
  biosensors 210–211
  in drug development 203–205
  of a druggable 208
  fluoride sensor illuminates agonists of fluoride toxicity 211
  landscape of 203
  in proof-of-principle demonstrations 209–210
  SAH sensor reveals an inhibitor of SAH nucleosidase 212–213
  small molecules targeting FMN 208–209
  target 207–208
  ZTP sensor identifies inhibitors of folate biosynthesis 211–212
riboswitches in gene therapy
  barriers and future developments 216–217
  for designer 213–214
  eukaryotic expression platforms 214–216
risdiplam 180–186
  Evrysdi® 183–186
  hit-to-lead 78–79
RNA-binding proteins (RBPs), regulation and dysregulation of 290–296
RNA biopolymer 1, 3
RNA folding problem 9
RNA modifications 66, 321, 322, 327, 328, 335, 336
RNA oligomerization-enabled cryo-EM via installing kissing-loops (ROCK) 38
RNA–protein interactions 2
  cell-based RNA–protein interaction screening 301–302
  cell-based RPI detection assays 300–301
  in vitro chemiluminescence-based assays 297–300
  in vitro fluorescence-based assays 297
  molecular basis
    cold shock domains (CSD) 290
    DEAD/DEAH box helicase domains 290
    double-stranded RNA binding domains (dsRBD) 286–287
    K homology (KH) domains 289–290
    Piwi/Argonaute/Zwille (PAZ) domains 290
    Pumilio (PUF) domains 290
    RGG/RG domains 290
    RNA recognition motifs (RRMs) 282–286
    Sm domains 290
    YT521-B homology domains 290
    zinc finger (ZnF) domains 287–289
  mRNA processing 294
RNA recognition motifs (RRMs) 162, 282–286
RNA sequencing 7, 39, 179, 188, 321, 331, 335, 375
RNA structure
  challenges in studying 8–9
  dealing with heterogeneity 19–22
  direct mapping of RNA–RNA interactions 14–16

RNA structure (*contd.*)
 mapping spatially proximal nucleotides 17
 prediction 355, 357
 querying RNA–small molecule interactions with chemical probing 22
 relevance in disease 8
 structural interrogation of RNA nucleotides via chemical probing 10, 11
RNA target classes 357, 358, 364
RNA-targeted small molecule therapeutics 2
RNA-Targeting BIoactive LigaNd Database (R-BIND) 93
RNA-targeting small molecules 324
 biophysical method 358–360
 cellular target engagement methods 360–364
  functional assays 364–367
 deposition of 373–375
 hit optimization 369–370
 molecular dynamics simulations, machine learning, and AI tools 371–373
 RNA structure prediction 367–369
Rosetta-based FARFAR2 algorithm 39
Rous sarcoma virus (RSV) 253
rRNA modifications 322, 334–335

S
S-adenosylhomocysteine (SAH) 207, 212SARS-Cov-1, 263, 268
SARS-CoV-2 FSE 265, 267, 268, 273
SARS-CoV-2 RNA 36, 41, 270, 271, 274
screening and lead generation techniques, for RNA binders
 binding site identification and target engagement 72
 fluorescence-based assays 66
 functional assays 75
 high-throughput screening (HTS)
  direct MS approaches 52–54
  DNA-encoded libraries (DELs) 56–57
  fragment-based drug discovery (FBDD) 58–63
  indirect MS approaches 54–56
  mass spectrometry 51–52
  microarray screening 57–58
  phage display 63
 isothermal titration calorimetry (ITC) 70–72
 knowledge-based *vs.* agnostic screening 49–50
 microscale thermophoresis (MST) 70
 phenotypic screens 76
 screening funnel for 49, 50
 surface plasmon resonance (SPR) 63
 virtual screening 50–51
Scripps Research Natural Products Discovery Center 94
seed sequence 121
selective 2′-hydroxyl acylation analyzed by primer extension (SHAPE) 10, 17, 266, 363
self-cleaving ribozymes 215, 216
severe acute respiratory syndrome coronavirus 2 (SARS-CoV-2) 102, 253, 357
SHAPE-MaP data 266, 363, 368, 371, 373
site-specific labeling assays (2-AP) 66–68
slippery sequence 254, 256, 263–265, 270
Sm domains 290
small-angle X-ray/neutron scattering (SAXS/SANS) 42, 61
small interfering RNAs (siRNAs)
 drug patisiran 227
 oligonucleotides 119
small-molecule-based RiboTACs 239–242, 244
small-molecule direct degraders 228–235
small-molecule microarray (SMM) 33, 49, 131, 356, 365, 374
Small Molecule Modulators of RNA (SMMRNA) 93, 336, 355

small-molecule RNA targeting
  chemical similarity search algorithms 104
  commercial ligands 97–99, 108–110
  machine-learning tools 105–106
  natural ligands 94–97, 108–110
  principal component analysis 104–105
  QSAR 107
  structure-based ligand design 106
  synthetic ligands 99–100, 103, 108
small molecules targeting FMN riboswitches 208–209
small molecules that degrade RNA
  antisense oligonucleotide degraders 227–228
  ribonuclease targeting chimeras (RiboTACs)
    vs. bleomycin-based direct degraders 242
    discovery of additional small molecule RNase L activators 242–243
    first-generation RiboTACs targeting oncogenic miRNAs 236–239
    Ribonuclease L (RNase L) 236
    small-molecule-based 239–245
  small molecule direct degraders
    bleomycin conjugates 231
    bleomycins 229–231
    N-hydroxypyridine-2(1*H*)-thione (*N*-HPT) Conjugates 229
small non-coding RNAs 120
spinal muscular atrophy (SMA) 2, 3, 74, 120, 151, 180–183
5′ splice site bulge repair 36
stemloops 254
structural interrogation of RNA nucleotides via chemical probing 10–12
structure-based drug design (SBDD) 29, 77
sulfonamides 211, 212
surface plasmon resonance (SPR)
  competition experiments 262
  dealing with nonspecific interactions by 65–66
  for fragment screening 61
  small molecule-RNA interactions 65
survival motor neuron 1 (SMN1) gene 78
synthetic ligands 108–110
  amiloride 102
  benzimidazoles and purines 100–101
  diphenyl furan (DPF) 103
  multivalent ligands 103
  naphthalenes 101–102
  oxazolidinones 102
  quinazoline 101–102
  quinoline derivatives 101–102

t

Targapremir-18a 136
TargapremiR-210 134
target engagement of fragments 62
TAR RNA-binding protein (TRBP) 123, 124
target RNA or regulate RNA function 1
targeting viral enzymes 357
tetracycline repressor (TetR) protein 215
tetracycline-responsive Tet-ON/Tet-OFF systems 214
tetracyclines 95, 96
3D structure prediction and integrative approaches 39–43
transfer RNA (tRNA) 29, 95, 120, 130, 240
  modifications 323, 330–334
tumor suppressor miRNAs 124–125
two-dimensional combinatorial screening (2DCS) 130, 356
tyrosyl-tRNA synthetase (TyrRS) 38

u

untranslated regions (UTRs) 8, 292

v

virtual screening 33, 50–51, 61, 80, 102, 104, 106, 268, 370

w

Watson-Crick base-pairing rules 30, 227

x

X-ray crystallography 3, 30–34, 61, 63, 367

y

YT521-B homology domains 290

z

zinc finger (ZnF) domains 287–289
zotatifin lead generation 80